Focus on Health

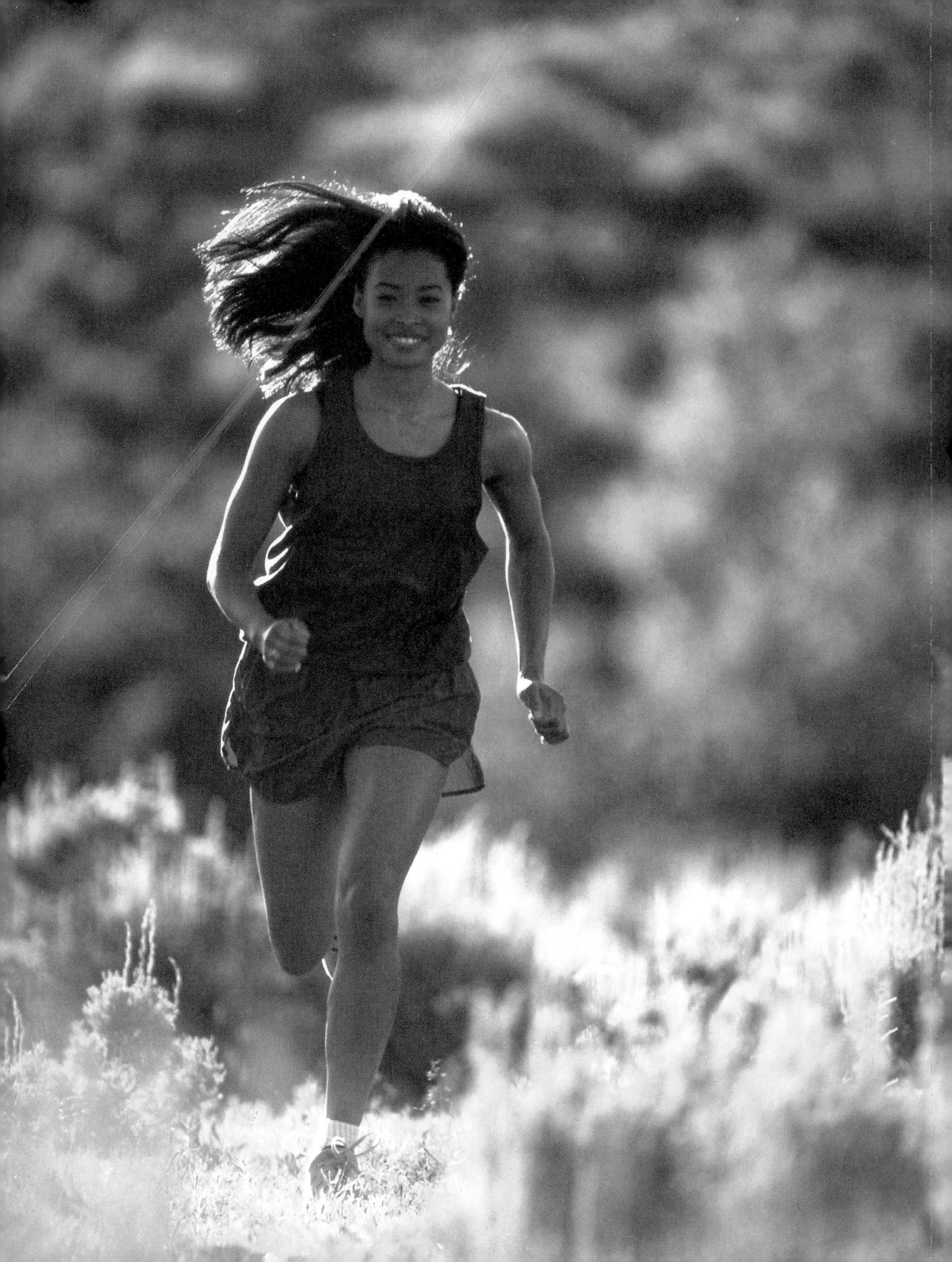

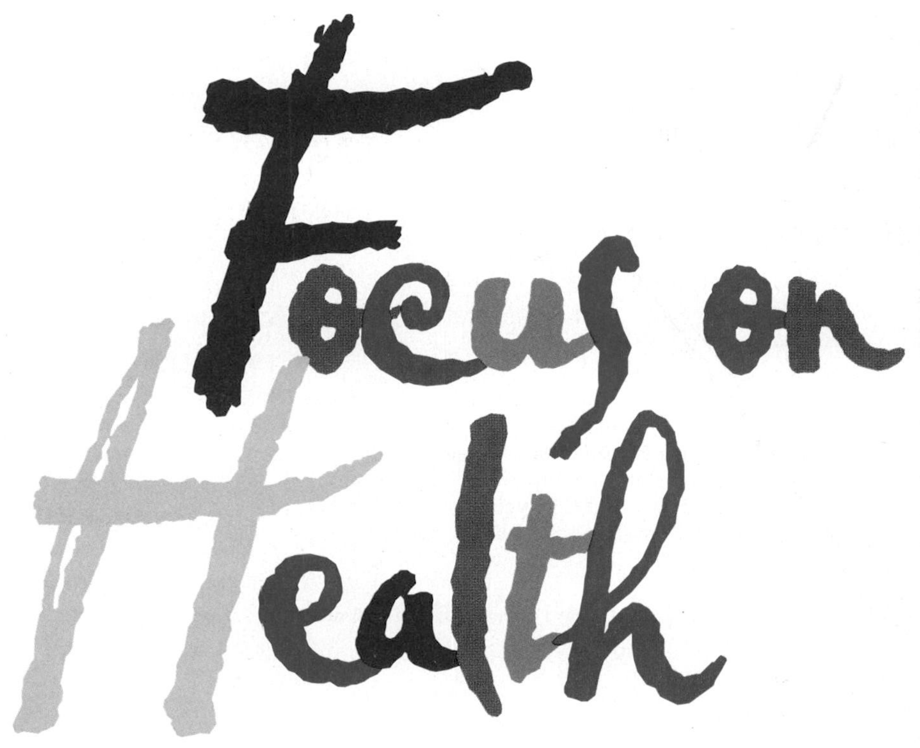

sixth edition

DALE B. HAHN, Ph.D.

WAYNE A. PAYNE, Ed.D.

Both of Ball State University

Muncie, Indiana

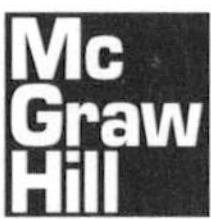

Boston Burr Ridge, IL Dubuque, IA Madison, WI New York San Francisco St. Louis
Bangkok Bogotá Caracas Kuala Lumpur Lisbon London Madrid Mexico City
Milan Montreal New Delhi Santiago Seoul Singapore Sydney Taipei Toronto

To all of our students, with the hope that the decisions they make will be healthy ones.

McGraw-Hill Higher Education

A Division of The **McGraw-Hill** *Companies*

FOCUS ON HEALTH, SIXTH EDITION

Published by McGraw-Hill, a business unit of The McGraw-Hill Companies, Inc., 1221 Avenue of the Americas, New York, NY 10020.

Some ancillaries, including electronic and print components, may not be available to customers outside the United States.

 This book is printed on recycled, acid-free paper containing 10% postconsumer waste.

2 3 4 5 6 7 8 9 0 QPD/QPD 0 9 8 7 6 5 4 3 2

ISBN 0–07–246735–5

Vice president and editor-in-chief: *Thalia Dorwick*
Publisher: *Jane E. Karpacz*
Executive editor: *Vicki Malinee*
Developmental editor: *Carlotta Seely*
Senior marketing manager: *Pamela S. Cooper*
Senior project manager: *Mary E. Powers*
Lead production supervisor: *Sandra Hahn*
Coordinator of freelance design: *Rick D. Noel*
Cover designer: *Rebecca Lloyd Lemna*
Cover photograph: *©International Stock/Tony Demin*
Senior photo research coordinator: *John C. Leland*
Supplement producer: *Sandra M. Schnee*
Media technology producer: *Lance Gerhart*
Compositor: *Shepherd, Inc.*
Typeface: *10.5/12 Minion*
Printer: *Quebecor World Dubuque, IA*

The credits section for this book begins on page 501 and is considered an extension of the copyright page.

www.mhhe.com

Learning to Go: Health

Your online coach for health behavior change

HERE'S HOW IT WORKS

Learning to Go: Health is designed to complement your new McGraw-Hill Personal Health textbook. It uses the Internet and "push technology" to bring lessons that relate to this book directly to your computer. You choose the time of day, and the lessons will automatically appear on your screen. You'll spend 15 minutes a day on one lesson that focuses on a single topic.

This feature is based on the following 4-step system:

1 Core Principle—Focus on one topic per lesson.

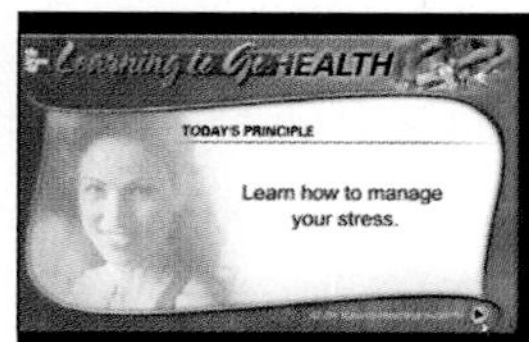

2 Lesson Overview—Review more information about that principle to help yourself learn it.

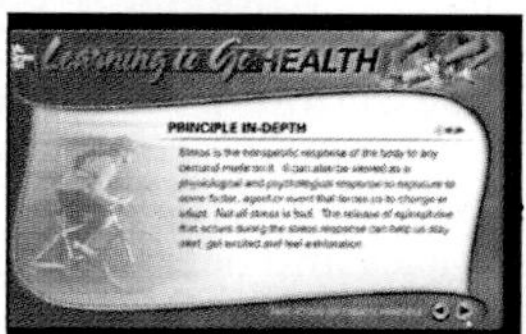

3 Action Steps—Three action steps per lesson help you learn by doing and taking action. Knowledge isn't powerful until you put it into action.

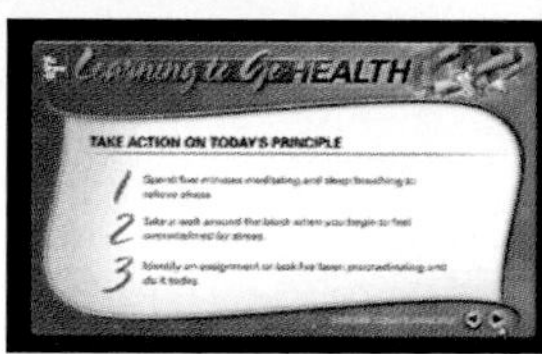

4 Reinforcements—Interact and learn through various means: Quotations, Reality Checks, Health Tips, True or False, Tic-Tac-Toe, and Learn More.

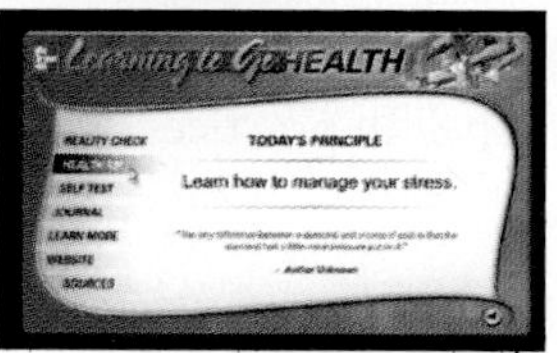

HERE'S HOW TO GET STARTED

- Go to the Online Learning Center for this book at:
  www.mhhe.com/hahn6e
- Click on *Learning to Go: Health.*
- Follow the steps for registration.
- Once you're registered, set your preferences.
- Then you'll be ready for your first lesson!

HealthQuest CD-ROM 4.0

by Robert S. Gold, *University of Maryland–College Park*
and
Nancy L. Atkinson, *University of Maryland–College Park*

In an interactive and personal way, HealthQuest lets you assess your current health and wellness status, determine your health risks, figure your relative life expectancy, explore your health options, and make decisions for positive change!

- How much of a weight difference would an extra candy bar a day make?
- Am I a likely candidate to contract a sexually transmitted disease?
- Are my CPR skills good enough to save someone?

With the help of HealthQuest's consistent organization and easy-to-use interface, all your health and wellness questions are answered.

FEATURES

- New! Updated features to provide the latest information in each unit.
- New! Improved print function allows instructors to make assignments and incorporate the program into the course more easily.
- New! Redesigned to provide graphical interface that appeals to a wide range of students.
- New! Provides web-based user tips and instructor's manual to help students and instructors take full advantage of all the CD's features.
- New! Explorations on CPR and personal drug use that ask you to apply learning to your everyday life.
- New! A variety of new assessments and explorations to provide you with the most current and useful information.
- See how your everyday behavior affects your health risks and life expectancy. Explore HealthQuest's interactive, user-friendly modules. Based on your responses and actions in each module, the "Wellboard" will create for you a database of personal information and generate a population curve plotting your average life expectancy. Assess yourself by answering questions based on your:
  - general demographics
  - family health history
  - personal health history
  - lifestyle
  - preventive health practices

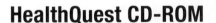

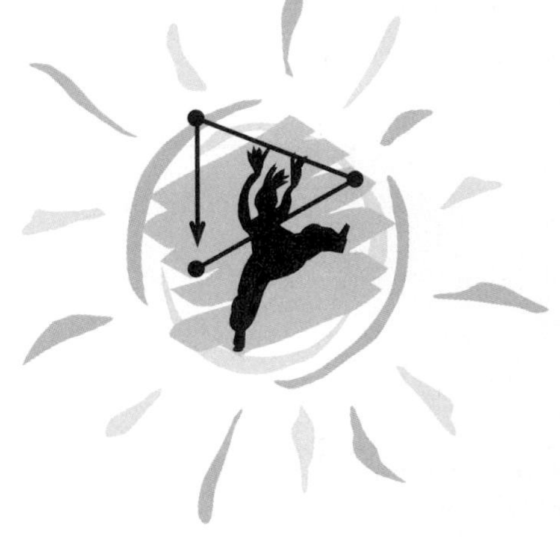

CONTENTS

Wellboard
Alcohol
Cancer
Cardiovascular Health
Communicable Diseases
Fitness
Nutrition and Weight Loss
Other Drugs
Stress Management and Mental Health

Contents *in* Brief

Contents

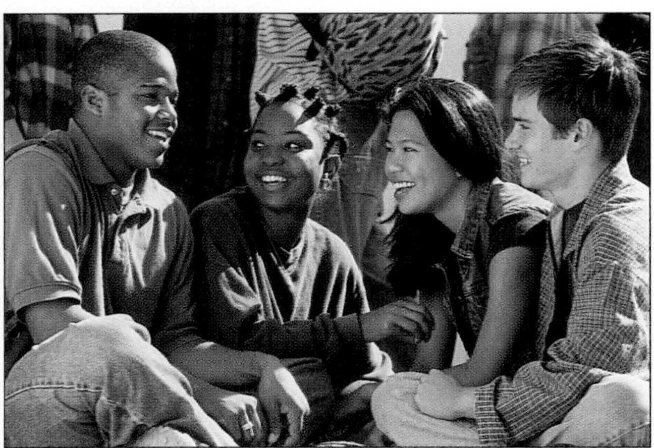

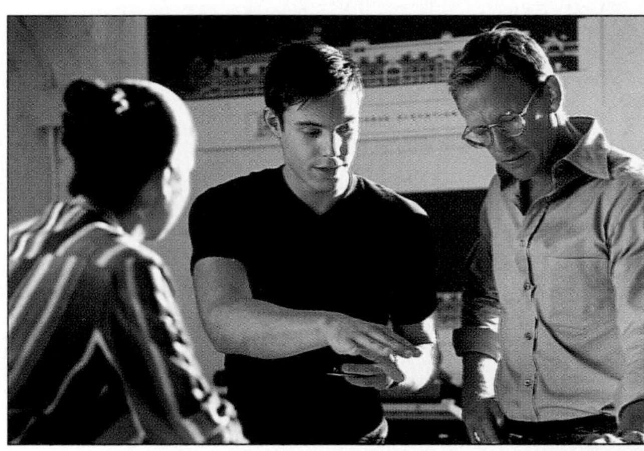

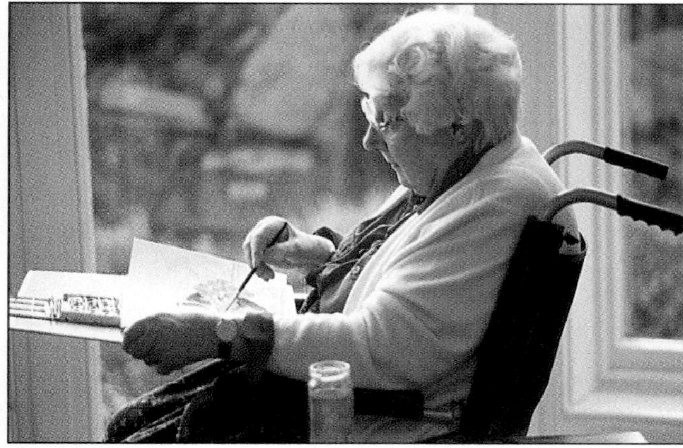

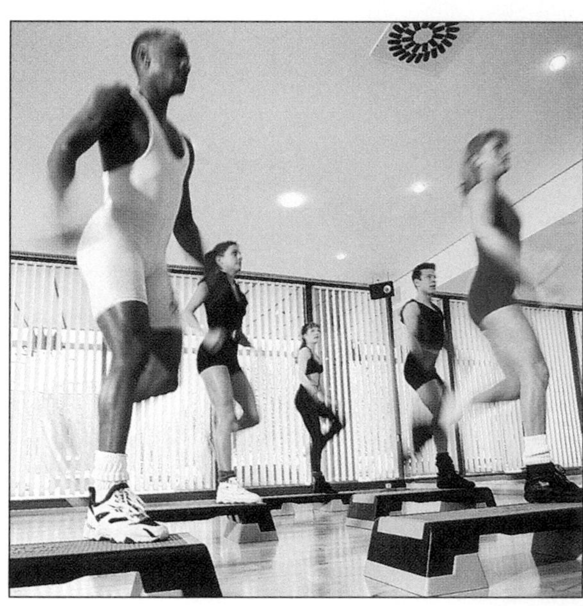

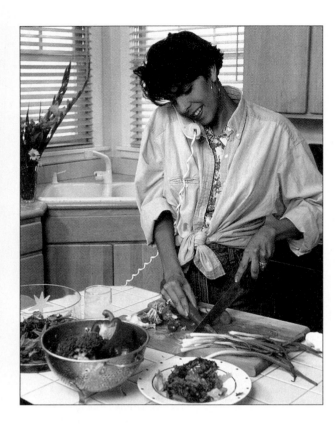

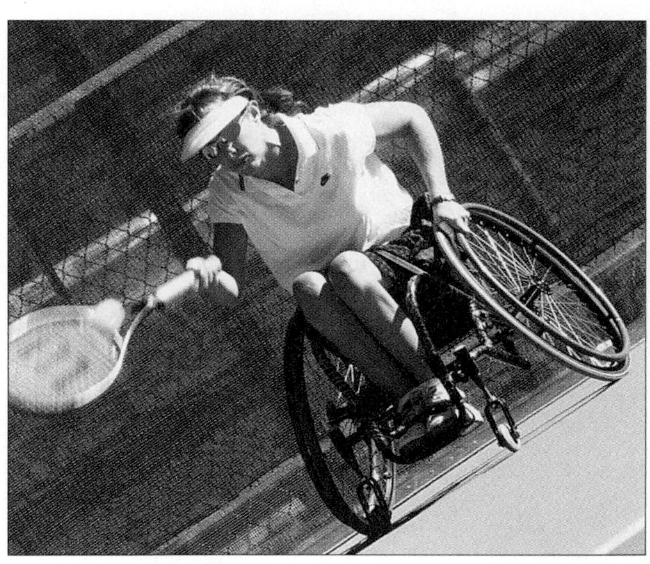

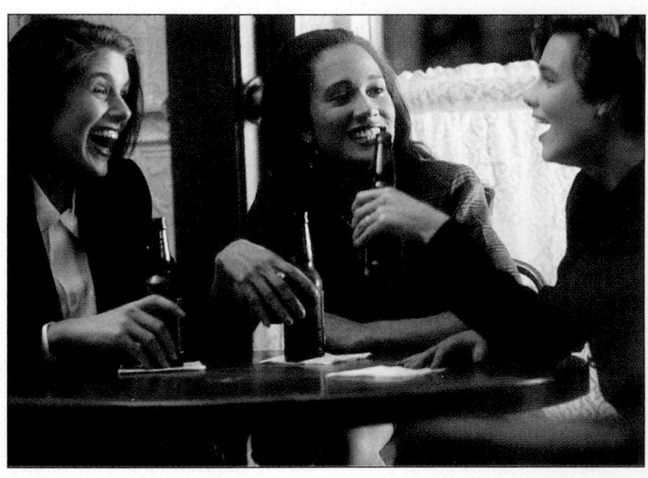

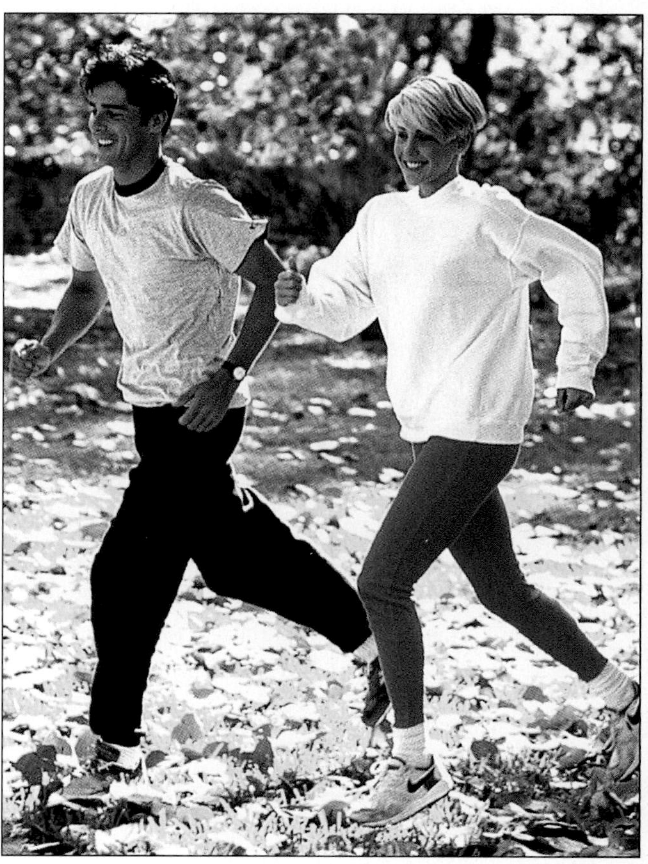

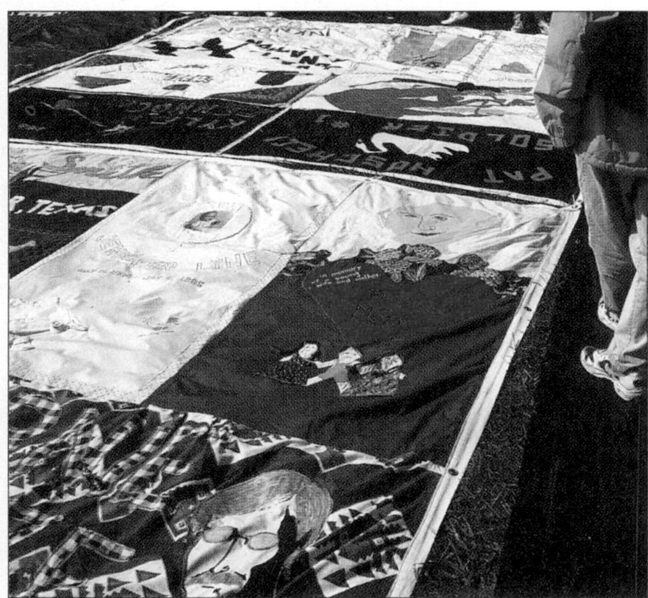

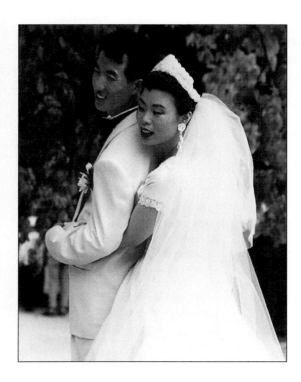

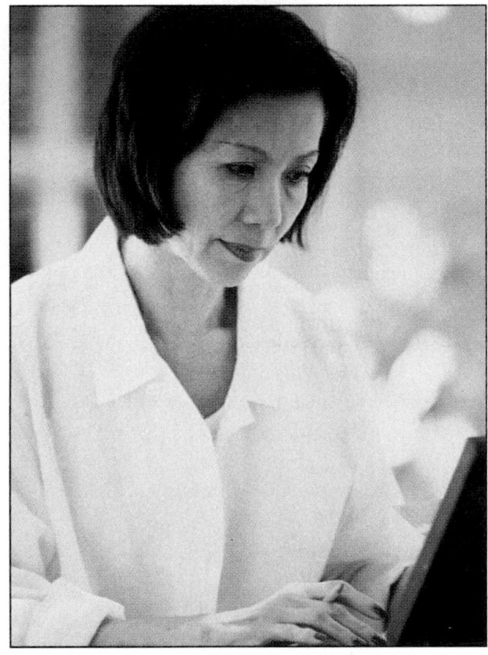

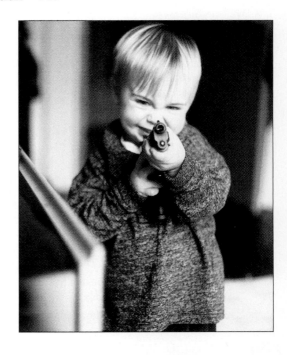

Preface

As a health educator, you know that the personal health course is one of the most exciting courses a college student will take. Today's media-oriented college students are aware of the critical health issues of the new century. They hear about terrorism, substance abuse, sexually transmitted diseases, fitness, and nutrition virtually every day. The value of the personal health course is its potential to expand students' knowledge of these and other health topics. Students will then be able to examine their attitudes toward health issues and modify their behavior to improve their health and perhaps even prevent or delay the onset of certain health conditions.

Focus on Health accomplishes this task with a carefully composed, well-documented manuscript written by two health educators who teach the personal health course to nearly 1000 students each year. They understand the teaching issues you face daily in the classroom and have written this text with your concerns in mind.

This book is written for college students in a wide variety of settings, from community colleges to large four-year universities. The content has been carefully constructed to be meaningful to both traditional- and nontraditional-age students. Special attention has been paid to the increasing numbers of nontraditional students who have decided to pursue a college education. Points in the discussion often address the particular needs of these nontraditional students. *Focus on Health* continues to encourage students of all ages and backgrounds to achieve their goals.

SPECIAL FEATURES

Updated Content

As experienced health educators and authors, we know how important it is to provide students with the most current information available. Throughout each chapter we have included the very latest information and statistics, and the "As we go to Press . . ." feature has allowed us to comment on breaking news right up to press time. In addition, we have introduced many timely topics and issues that are sure to pique students' interest and stimulate class discussion.

HealthQuest Activities

Many chapters contain an activities box to complement the HealthQuest CD-ROM that accompanies the text. These activities allow students to assess their health behavior in each of nine different areas. HealthQuest's exciting graphics and interactive approach will encourage students to learn about topics such as condom use, cancer prevention, and healthy eating behavior as they complete the activities.

OnSITE/InSIGHT

These boxes are designed to spark your students' interest and get them involved. The *Learning to Go: Health* lessons for each chapter challenge students to make positive changes in their health behavior and show them how to get started. The Student Poll features opinion questions and invites students to go online and have their say. Then they have the fun of comparing their responses with those of other college students.

Taking Charge of Your Health

Taking Charge of Your Health behavior change objectives, listed at the beginning of each chapter, help students apply what they learned in the text. These objectives reinforce the concept of self-responsibility and positive behavior change.

Online Learning Center Boxes

Online Learning Center boxes, found on the opening page of each chapter, direct students toward the useful resources available on the Online Learning Center that accompanies this text. These resources include chapter key terms and definitions, learning objectives, additional behavior change objectives, student interactive question-and-answer sites, and self-scoring chapter quizzes. The Online Learning Center boxes also list some of the web links that the student will find on the Online Learning Center.

Eye on the Media

Face it—a student's world revolves around media of all types, especially the web. Students get most of their health information not from instructors and textbooks, but from television, self-help books, popular news magazines, the web, and the radio. To meet students on this familiar ground, we've included Eye on the Media boxes (see the inside front cover for a list of boxes), which take a critical look at these media sources of health information. This feature appears on the first page of each chapter.

Exploring Your Spirituality

Spirituality has become an important focus in health courses. Exploring Your Spirituality boxes (see the inside front cover for a list of boxes) highlight the spiritual dimension of health and its effect on overall wellness. The boxes cover topics such as journal writing, living well with cancer or a chronic infectious disease, making decisions about sex, and having an enjoyable social life without abusing alcohol or other drugs.

Changing for the Better

These unique question-and-answer boxes show students how to put health concepts into practice. Each box begins with a real-life question, followed by helpful tips and practical advice for initiating behavior change and staying motivated to follow a healthy lifestyle.

Integrated Presentation of Aging

Topics of interest to midlife and elderly adults no longer appear in the chapter on death and dying, thus sending a more positive message about aging. Instead, the material has been integrated into appropriate chapters according to subject. For example, Alzheimer's disease is now discussed in Chapter 11, Living with Cancer and Chronic Conditions. This organization allows both traditional- and nontraditional-age students to learn about the physical and emotional changes that take place as we age.

Comprehensive Discussion of Sexuality

The biological and psychosocial origins of sexuality, sexual behavior, and intimate relationships are presented in a single comprehensive chapter. This organization gives the student a better framework for studying these complex topics.

Personal Safety Chapter

With good reason, students are more concerned than ever about issues related to violence and safety both on and off campus. Chapter 16, Protecting Your Safety, delves into critically important current issues such as terrorism; homicide; domestic violence; hate crimes; sexual victimization; and recreational, residential, and motor vehicle safety.

Wellness and Disease Prevention

Throughout this new edition, you will notice that students are continually urged to be proactive in shaping their future health. For example, Chapter 5, Understanding Nutrition and Your Diet, explains the health benefits of following a semivegetarian or other low-fat diet. Chapter 10, Reducing Your Risk of Cardiovascular Disease, opens with a discussion of the "big six" risk factors for heart disease and emphasizes that prevention must begin early. Even the chapter titles themselves invite students to take control of their own health behavior.

"Focus on" Articles

"Focus on" articles examine current issues that students are hearing about in today's news, such as alcohol and violence, volunteering, smokers' rights, and even sex on the Internet. These often controversial health-related topics are a perfect starting point for class or group discussions. Because these essays are set at the end of each chapter, they can be covered or not at the instructor's option.

Attractive Design and Updated Illustration Program

The inviting look, bold colors, and exciting graphics in *Focus on Health* will draw students in with every turn of the page. Photographs are sharp and appealing, drawings are attractive and informative, and anatomical illustrations are accurately rendered and appropriately detailed. In addition, the anatomical illustrations in the cardiovascular disease and sexuality chapters have been reproduced at a large size for greater clarity.

"Exam Prep" Guide

A perforated exam preparation section is included in the back of the book. The multiple-choice questions test students' retention of the material they have read. The critical thinking questions allow them to integrate the concepts introduced in the text with the information presented in class lectures and discussions. This built-in study guide is a good value for students.

Vegetarian Food Pyramid

Many students now follow or are considering a vegetarian diet. To help them understand how such a diet meets nutrient needs, we have printed a vegetarian food pyramid with the USDA Food Guide Pyramid inside the back cover of this textbook. For students who want to significantly reduce but not eliminate meat consumption, a "Focus on" article about the health benefits of following a semivegetarian diet is included in Chapter 5.

New or Expanded Topics

We are committed to making *Focus on Health* the most up-to-date health textbook available. Here is a sampling of topics that are either new to this edition or covered in greater depth than in the previous edition:

Chapter 1 Shaping Your Health

- Top ten causes of death in the United States
- *Healthy People 2010*
- Developing social skills

Chapter 2 Achieving Psychological Wellness

- Depression among college students
- Recent study of St. John's wort for treatment of depression
- Suicide statistics
- Use of pacemakers to treat depression

Chapter 3 Managing Stress

- Variation in response to stressors
- R (risk-taking) personality
- Using journaling to counteract stress
- Terrorism and stress: the anthrax threat

Chapter 4 Becoming Physically Fit

- Osteoporosis in older women
- Level of physical activity required for fitness
- Intensity of training and target heart rate

Chapter 5 Understanding Nutrition and Your Diet

- Balancing fats in your diet
- Cholesterol level and a healthy diet
- Healthy Weight Pyramid and Healthy Eating Pyramid
- Genetically modified foods
- Vegan diet for infants and children
- Food production and international nutritional concerns

Chapter 6 Maintaining a Healthy Weight

- Obesity and overweight
- BOD POD (Body Composition System)
- New weight-loss drugs
- Resources for anorexia and bulimia treatment
- Determining if your food habits are weight-smart

Chapter 7 Making Decisions About Drug Use

- Finding help for drug abuse
- Psychoactive drug categories
- Use/overuse of Ritalin
- New date rape drugs
- OxyContin as drug of abuse

Chapter 8 Taking Control of Alcohol Use

- Negative consequences of alcohol use
- Drinking patterns among college students
- Drinking and driving statistics
- BAC and legal intoxication
- Drugs for treatment of alcoholism

Chapter 9 Rejecting Tobacco Use

- Tobacco use statistics
- States with highest and lowest smoking rates
- Tobacco industry under fire
- Nicotine as an addictive drug
- Cancer statistics
- Smoking cessation

Chapter 10 Reducing Your Risk of Cardiovascular Disease

- Heart disease statistics
- Prevalence of major cardiovascular diseases
- Cardiovascular deaths and heart attacks
- Development of self-contained artificial heart
- Women and heart disease
- Yoga and blood pressure level
- Contributing risk factors
- Congenital heart disease
- Removal of Baycol, a cholesterol-lowering drug, from market

Chapter 11 Living with Cancer and Chronic Conditions

- Cancer incidence and deaths
- Breast cancer updates
- Breast cancer as rare diagnosis in men
- Updated statistics on ovarian, colon and rectal, pancreatic, and skin cancer
- Anti-cancer drugs
- Alzheimer's disease findings

Chapter 12 Preventing Infectious Diseases

- Updated statistics on HIV/AIDS
- Geographic distribution of people living with HIV/AIDS
- Infectious disease and older adults
- West Nile virus update

Chapter 13 Understanding Sexuality

- Patterns of sexual activity among college students
- Updated statistics on cohabitation
- Patterns of single parenthood
- Suicide among gay and lesbian adolescents

Chapter 14 Managing Your Fertility

- Effectiveness rates of birth control methods
- Intrauterine devices
- Condom use
- Injectable contraceptives
- New drugs for medical abortion: mifepristine and methotrexate
- Abortion laws by state
- Contraceptive patch (EVRA)

Chapter 15 Becoming an Informed Health-Care Consumer

- Buying health-care products on the Internet
- New studies of effectiveness of homeopathy
- Changes in use of prescription drugs
- Dietary supplements and health claims
- Medical errors resulting in death

Chapter 16 Protecting Your Safety

- Terrorism and the World Trade Center attacks
- Intentional injury statistics
- Cell phone safety and driving
- Violence against the disabled
- Age factor in fatal motor vehicle crashes
- Terrorism and changes in airline safety requirements

Chapter 17 Accepting Dying and Death

- Advance medical directives
- Living will
- Organ donation

SUCCESSFUL FEATURES

Focus on Health has many unique features that enhance student learning:

Two Central Themes

As mentioned earlier, two central themes—the multiple dimensions of health and the developmental tasks—are presented in Chapter 1. These give students a foundation for understanding their own health and achieving positive behavior change.

Flexibility of Chapter Organization

The sixth edition of *Focus on Health* has 17 chapters. The first stands alone as an introductory chapter that explains the focus of the book. The arrangement of the remaining chapters follows the recommendations of both the users of previous editions of the book and reviewers of this edition. Of course, professors can choose to cover the chapters in any sequence that suits the needs of their courses.

Health Reference Guide

The Health Reference Guide found at the back of the book lists many of the most commonly used health resources. In this edition, we have included many Internet addresses, as well as phone numbers and mailing addresses of various organizations and government agencies. The guide is perforated and laminated, making it durable enough for students to keep for later use.

Pedagogical Aids

In addition to the special pedagogical features listed previously, the teaching aids described here proved to be successful in the earlier editions of this book and have been included in this new edition:

Star Boxes

In each chapter, special material in Star Boxes encourages students to delve into a particular topic or closely examine an important health issue.

Personal Assessment Inventories

Each chapter contains at least one Personal Assessment inventory, beginning with a comprehensive health assessment just before Chapter 1. These self-assessment exercises serve three important functions: they capture students' attention, serve as a basis for introspection and behavior change, and provide suggestions for carrying the applications further.

Definition Boxes

Key terms are set in boldface type and are defined in corresponding boxes. Pronunciation guides are provided where appropriate. Other important terms in the text are set in italics for emphasis. Both approaches facilitate student vocabulary comprehension.

Comprehensive Glossary

At the end of the text, all terms defined in boxes, as well as pertinent italicized terms, are merged into a comprehensive glossary.

Chapter Summaries

Each chapter concludes with a bulleted summary of key concepts and their significance or application. The student can then return to any topic in the chapter for clarification or study.

Review Questions

A set of questions appears at the end of each chapter to aid the student in review and analysis of chapter content.

Think About This . . .

These engaging questions encourage students to apply what they have learned in the chapter by analyzing their own health habits and finding appropriate solutions to the issues raised.

Suggested Readings

Because some students want to know more about a particular topic, a list of annotated readings is given at the end of each chapter. The suggested readings are readily available at bookstores or public libraries.

Mental Disorders Appendix

Categories of mental disorders and therapeutic approaches are outlined in this appendix.

Owner's Manual

Are you looking for health information in the media? Working hard to get in shape? Trying to improve your grade? The great features in *Focus on Health* will help you do all this and more! Let's take a look . . .

ONLINE LEARNING CENTER

Want to get a better grade? This box reminds you about the study aids and other resources available at our free Online Learning Center and describes some of the useful web links you'll find there.

chapter **1**

Shaping Your Health

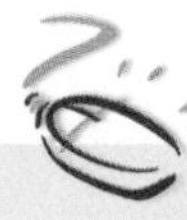

Online Learning Center Resources
www.mhhe.com/hahn6e

Log on to our Online Learning Center (OLC) for access to these additional resources:

- Chapter key terms and definitions
- Learning objectives
- Additional behavior change objectives
- Student interactive question-and-answer sites
- Self-scoring chapter quiz

The OLC also offers web links for study and exploration of health topics. Here are some examples of what you'll find:

- **www.yahoo.com/health** Research hundreds of health-related links and use the Yahoo search engine to zero in on sites of interest.
- **www.healthfinder.gov** Check out this gateway for consumer health and human services information from the U.S. government.
- **www.HealthAtoZ.com** Look here for a searchable database of health information sites that are rated for quality.

Taking Charge of Your Health

- Complete the Comprehensive Health Assessment on p. xxxi. Develop a plan to modify your behavior in the areas in which you need improvement.
- Take part in a new spiritual activity, such as meditating, creating art or music, or appreciating nature.
- To promote the social dimension of your health, try to meet one new person each week during the semester.
- Choose one developmental task you would like to focus on, such as assuming responsibility, and plan the steps you can follow to progress in this area.
- Volunteer to be an assistant in a community service program, such as a literacy project or a preschool program.

Eye on the Media
Where Does Our Health Information Come From?

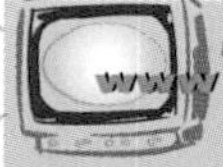

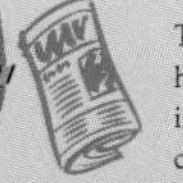

Today our health information comes from a variety of media—some more reliable than others. The following six media groups convey health-related information. Because Eye on the Media will appear in each chapter of this text, this introduction is limited to an overview of these sources. Later chapters will deal with the important issue of which ones are good (in other words, valid and reliable) sources for learning about health.

Radio and Television

When you think of radio, the first thing that may come to mind is your favorite music. But two areas of radio are especially important for news and information: talk radio and National Public Radio (NPR). Talk radio raises the question of validity of information. For example, if you're listening to a talk show about HIV exposure, the perceptions and opinions of the host (which may be strong or even extreme) are an important part of the show. When this point of view is combined with the opinions of callers, whose "facts" may come from unauthoritative sources, what you're hearing is probably not solid information. It's certainly not a good basis for making your health decisions.

EYE ON THE MEDIA

How can you tell whether to trust health information in the media? These boxes take a critical look at coverage of health issues on the web, on television, on the radio, and in print.

EXPLORING YOUR SPIRITUALITY

A healthy body and a healthy mind go hand in hand. This feature will help you tap into your spiritual side to improve your self-esteem, foster good relationships with others, and jump start your physical health.

Social Dimension

Social ability is the third dimension of total health. Whether you identify it as social graces, skills, or insights, you probably have many strengths in this area. Because most of your growth and development has occurred in the presence of others, you can appreciate how this dimension of your health may become even more important in your future development.

The social abilities of many nontraditional-age students may already be firmly established. Entering college may encourage them to develop new social skills that help them socialize with their traditional-age student colleagues. After being on campus for a while, nontraditional-age students often interact comfortably with traditional-age students in such diverse places as the classroom, the student center, and the library. This type of interaction enhances the social dimension of health for both.

Intellectual Dimension

Your ability to process and act on information, clarify values and beliefs, and exercise your decision-making capacity is one of the most important aspects of total health. Coping skills, flexibility, or the knack of saying the right thing at the right time may not serve you as well as the ability to use information or understand a new idea. A refusal to grasp new information or undertake an analysis of your beliefs could hinder the degree of growth and development that your college experience can provide.

Exploring Your Spirituality

Pondering the Meaning of Life

In a survey conducted in May of 1999 by Yankelovich Partners for the Lutheran Brotherhood (an insurance company affiliated with the Lutheran Church), a large, randomly selected sample of American adults was asked a version of the following question: "If you were able to do so, what questions would you ask God or a supreme being?" The most commonly asked question (34%) was: "What is my purpose for being here?" The second (19%) and third (16%) most frequently raised questions were: "Will I have life after death?" and "Why do bad things happen?" The remaining responses reported were: "Is there intelligent life elsewhere?" (7%) and "How long will I live?" (6%). A variety of other questions were asked but not reported on. Twelve percent of the respondents said that they would not (or could not) ask a question, even if given the opportunity.

If it is assumed that these questions are common to the vast majority of Americans (at least on occasion), in the absence of a theology-based belief system, to whom would they be directed? Perhaps to a respected academic, a wise elder, a seasoned veteran of the "school of hard knocks," or a mystic? On the other hand, for those with such a belief system, answers may never be expected. The process of asking in itself may create a sense of inner peace centered on the belief that there is someone (or something) that does have answers to these and other profound questions of life and that eventually those answers will be known.

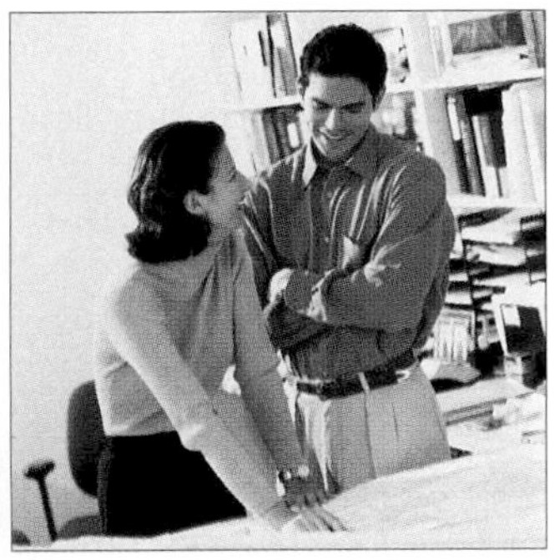

People who feel good about their work often have high self-esteem.

Spiritual Dimension

The fifth dimension of health is spiritual. Although you can include your religious beliefs and practices category, this discussion focuses on your relation other living things, the role of a spiritual direc your life, the nature of human behavior, and yo ingness to serve others.

Many of today's students appear to be search a deeper understanding of the meaning of life. A you may not feel uneasy about the nature of you tual beliefs, many students do feel anxious ab spiritual side of their lives. In fact, one explanat the renewed interest in the spiritual dimension o may stem from its value as a resource for lesseni sonal stress. The spiritual dimension is so signific some health professionals believe it to be the actu of wellness."

Cultivating the spiritual side of your health m you discover how you fit into this universe. You hance your spiritual health in a variety of ways, r which involve opening yourself to new experienc

CHANGING FOR THE BETTER

Learn to put health concepts into practice by following these useful tips. This feature gives you practical advice for making positive changes and staying motivated to follow a healthy lifestyle.

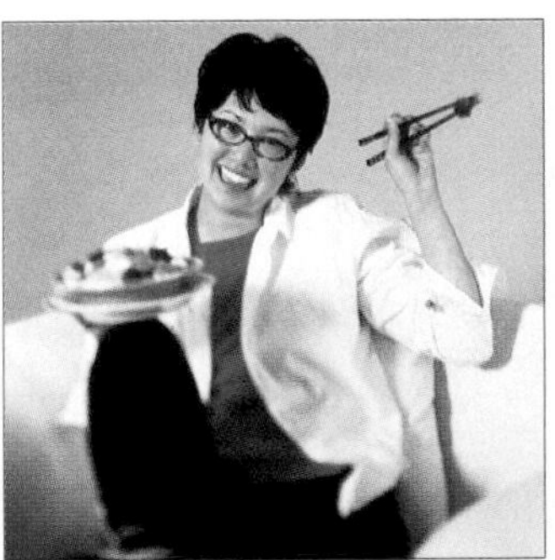

Many students want to change a specific behavior, such as following a more nutritious diet.

help you focus on specific activities for reaching your goals, use the Changing for the Better boxes found in each chapter. For example, see p. 106 Dietary Guidelines for Americans, p. 265 Eat to Lower Your Cancer Risk, and p. 238 Monitoring Your Cholesterol Level. Identify any milestones along the way to your goal. Specify the time, personal resources, and energy you will need to commit to this project.

5. *Devise a plan of action.* As you develop your strategy, adjust your environment to help you replace old cues with new ones. For example, if you are trying to get more sleep, calm yourself before bedtime by reading rather than listening to loud music or watching a TV drama. If you want to improve in your eating behavior, change your walking route so that you avoid passing the campus snack bar.
6. *Chart your progress in your diary or journal.* From day 1, keep a record of how you are doing. Consider making this record visible. For instance, posting an eating record on the refrigerator door is a good motivator for some people.
7. *Encourage your family and friends to help you.* Social support is important in any attempt at behavior change. Your friends may want to join you and change their own behavior. Then you can support each other. But some friends or family members might misunderstand your efforts. They might actually discourage you. If possible, avoid these people—at least while your project is under way.

Changing *for the Better*

Looking Toward the Future: What's Your Game Plan?

After discussing the areas of growth and development from ages 18 to 40 in a personal health class, one student asked: "Just what should I do with all of this growth stuff, anyway?" Some of the responses—from other students and the professor—were as follows:

- Ask others to share their stories with you. Choose people you view as independent, comfortable with their plans, and responsible or established in areas of development where you feel uncertain. Hearing their first-hand accounts can be an excellent way to gain insight into your own future.
- While you are reading, either for recreation or a class assignment, look for aspects of these growth areas in the people being described. Do the same thing with characters depicted in films, plays, or TV programs. For example, think about the character played by Renée Zellweger in *Bridget Jones's Diary* and the college experiences of the main character in the TV program *Felicity*.
- Set aside time to give serious thought to where you are now in each of these developmental areas. Compare your perceived points of progress with what others (friends, professors, family) might see or expect when they think about you and your life experiences. Construct a mental game plan for one or more of the five developmental areas discussed in this chapter.

TALKING POINTS • **What does being an adult mean to you at this point? How would you explain this to your best friend?**

8. *Set up a reward system.* Rewards tend to motivate people. They can be used to reinforce your positive changes. If you achieve success at a particular point in your plan, reward yourself with a special meal, new clothes, or a weekend trip. Pat yourself on the back occasionally for your efforts. Relish your success.
9. *Prepare for obstacles along the way.* No one who achieved anything of importance did it without a few setbacks, so prepare yourself mentally for an occasional obstacle. For example, if you neglect your fitness plan during a long holiday weekend, try to get back on course as soon as possible. Work through your setbacks with a "forgive and forget" attitude.
10. *Revise your plan as necessary.* Try to be flexible in your approach to behavior change. A strategy that works for a while might not work as well after a month or two. So be prepared to reevaluate your goals and try new techniques when necessary.

OnSITE/InSIGHT

Studying personal health can be a fun experience! Use the OnSITE/InSIGHT boxes to guide you to the *Learning to Go: Health* lessons that go with each chapter. Then take the Student Poll and see how your opinions on health issues compare with what other students think.

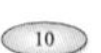

Focus on Health

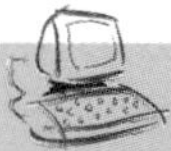

OnSITE/InSIGHT

Learning to Go: Health

Getting tired of your study routine? Click on the Motivator icon for a different slant on studying. Check out these lessons, which make a good match for this chapter:

Lesson 1: Chart a plan for behavior change.
Lesson 2: Strive for multidimensional health.

STUDENT POLL

Thinking about shaping up your health? Go to the Online Learning Center at **www.mhhe.com/hahn6e**. Click on Student Resources to find the Student Poll, where you can answer these questions. Then find out how other students responded.

1. Is improving you health a high priority for you?
2. Do you believe you have control over your own health?
3. Do you take a proactive, preventive approach to your health?
4. Are your eating habits nutritionally sound?
5. Do you consider yourself in good physical shape?
6. Do you search out health information?
7. Is there balance in the different areas of your life?
8. Do you have strong friendships?
9. Do you consider yourself emotionally well balanced?
10. Is being smart important to you?
11. Do you see a spiritual aspect to your everyday life?
12. Is what you're doing today preparing you for your future?
13. Are you career-oriented?
14. Is becoming an adult an important milestone for you?
15. Do you agree that "If you've got your health, you've got everything?

THE COMPOSITION OF HEALTH

Your health is composed of six interacting, dynamic dimensions, each of which provides resources that can be utilized in accomplishing the activities that constitute growth and development within each development area appropriate to young adulthood. Because your health is dynamic, you can modify aspects of its dimensions to help you in your quest for well-being.

Your health is not static. The health you had yesterday no longer exists. The health you aspire to have next week or next year is not guaranteed. However, scientific evidence suggests that what you do today will help determine the quality of your future health. Let's briefly consider each of the six dimensions of health.

hysical Dimension

number of physiological and structural characteristics—cluding your level of susceptibility to disease, body eight, visual ability, strength, coordination, level of enurance, and powers of recuperation—can help you parcipate in the experiences that form the basis of your owth and development. In certain situations the physical mension of your health may be the most important. Perps this is why many authorities have traditionally uated health with the design and operation of the body d the absence of illness or a low level of risk for illness.

motional Dimension

ur emotional makeup can aid in your progress through e various growth areas. The emotional dimension of alth includes the degree to which you are able to cope with stress, remain flexible, and compromise to resolve conflict. This dimension is most closely related to your feelings. How you feel about your family and friends, your life goals and ambitions, and your daily life situations is all tied to the emotional dimension of health.

HealthQuest Activities

- The *How Stressed Are You?* activity in Module 1 lets you look at several areas of your life (including money, school, relationships, and health) and identify stress caused by various events and daily hassles. You can also rate your perceived stress level for each area. Use this feature to find out which area or areas generate the highest levels of stress for you.
- The *CyberStress* activity in the Stress Management and Mental Health Module simulates a stress-filled day. Use it to assess your reactions to daily stressors. Choose the scenario that most closely matches your own. For example, if you work and go to school, you should check both of these choices on the preferences screen. As you are presented with stressful situations, choose the reaction that is closest to how you would react. At the feedback screen, print the screen showing your score. Then evaluate your experience by answering the questions in the *What do you think?* section.

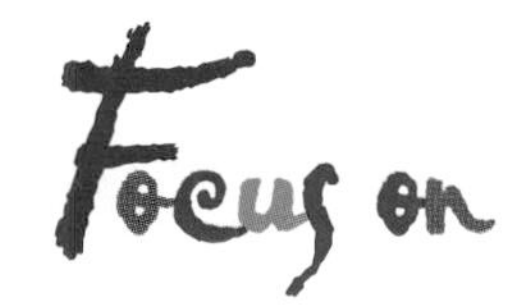

SUPERTWINS: THE BOOM IN MULTIPLE BIRTHS

During World War II their parents gave them patriotic names, such as Franklin, Delano, and Roosevelt, or Franklin D. (for Roosevelt) and Winnie C. (a girl named for Winston Churchill).[1] You may know them as Rachel, Richard, Rebecca, and Ryan or Courtney, Britanny, and Tiffany. They're supertwins—multiple-birth siblings such as triplets, quadruplets, quintuplets, and even sextuplets and more. From 1989 to 1993, an average of 1,057 sets of triplets, 241 sets of quads, and 32 sets of quints were born each year in the United States.[1] More recently, the McCaugheys of Iowa gave birth to septuplets on November 19, 1997. All of their septuplets are home and doing well. Nkem Chukwu and her husband Lyke Louis Udobi of Texas were not as lucky with their octuplets. One of the eight died shortly after delivery in 1998.

Such multiple births are controversial for several reasons, including the increased risk they bring to the mother and the fetuses.

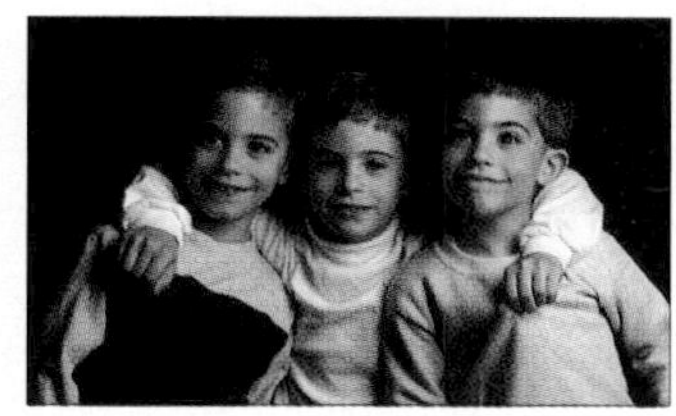

The increased use of fertility drugs and techniques has caused a boom in multiple births. More than 1,000 sets of triplets are born each year in the United States.

The Good, the Bad, and the Unusual

A special type of bonding occurs among multiple-birth siblings that ranges from reading one another's moods to saving another's life, as in the case of twin girls Brielle and Kyrie.[1,2] Kyrie, at 2 pounds 3 ounces, was doing well, but Brielle, the smaller twin, at 2 pounds, had had trouble breathing, an irregular heart rate, and a low blood oxygen level since birth. Then Brielle's condition suddenly became critical. The hospital staff tried every medical procedure they thought might help, to no avail. As a last resort, they put the girls in the same incubator, as some European hospitals do. Amazingly, Brielle's condition immediately improved and within minutes her blood oxygen level was the best it had been since birth. Studies have confirmed that double bedding of multiple-birth babies reduces the length of their hospital stay.[2]

On the darker side, sometimes multiple births, or the prospect of them, are exploited by parents. The Dionne quintuplets, now 60 years old, were the middle 5 of 13 children. When their father sold the rights to exhibit his daughters, the Ontario government made them wards of the state. But the government ended up exploiting them in a bizarre glass playground Quintland-type display, which attracted 10,000 visitors a month. When they were returned to their parents, they were made to feel guilty for their unusual birth and the ensuing familial discord.[3] The surviving quints have written a book about their experiences and have helped teach the world that multiples are not something to be exploited.

Recently, in England, a woman abused fertility drugs by taking them even though she was already fertile and ignoring her physician's instructions while on the drugs. She became pregnant with eight fetuses. She refused to undergo multifetal pregnancy reduction, which would have given the remaining fetuses a better chance of survival, because she had sold her story to a tabloid and would get more money for each baby born. All eight fetuses died at 19 weeks' gestation.[4]

Fertility Drugs and Techniques

Since the birth of the first "test tube baby" (conceived by in vitro fertilization) in 1978, the number of assisted pregnancies and multiple births has escalated. The use of fertility drugs and techniques that stimulate ovulation sometimes causes the release of multiple eggs per cycle.[1,5]

The infertility rate among married couples is 8.5 percent. While this rate has remained relatively constant in recent years, the number of couples seeking help for infertility has tripled.[6] Less than half of the couples who receive fertility treatment ever give birth, but one-fourth of those who *do* achieve a pregnancy give birth to

HEALTHQUEST ACTIVITIES

You received a free HealthQuest CD-ROM with your new copy of *Focus on Health.* This feature provides activities to help you explore HealthQuest and assess your health behavior in areas like cancer prevention, fitness, and nutrition.

"FOCUS ON" ARTICLES

Every day you hear the buzz about hot health topics like vegetarian diets, Internet dating, and fertility drugs that lead to triplets, quadruplets, or more! Read these articles and decide where you stand on these controversial issues.

PERSONAL ASSESSMENTS

Do you eat too much fat? What's the best method of birth control for you if you are sexually active? How compatible are you and your partner? Each chapter in *Focus on Health* includes assessments to help you learn the answers to these questions and many others.

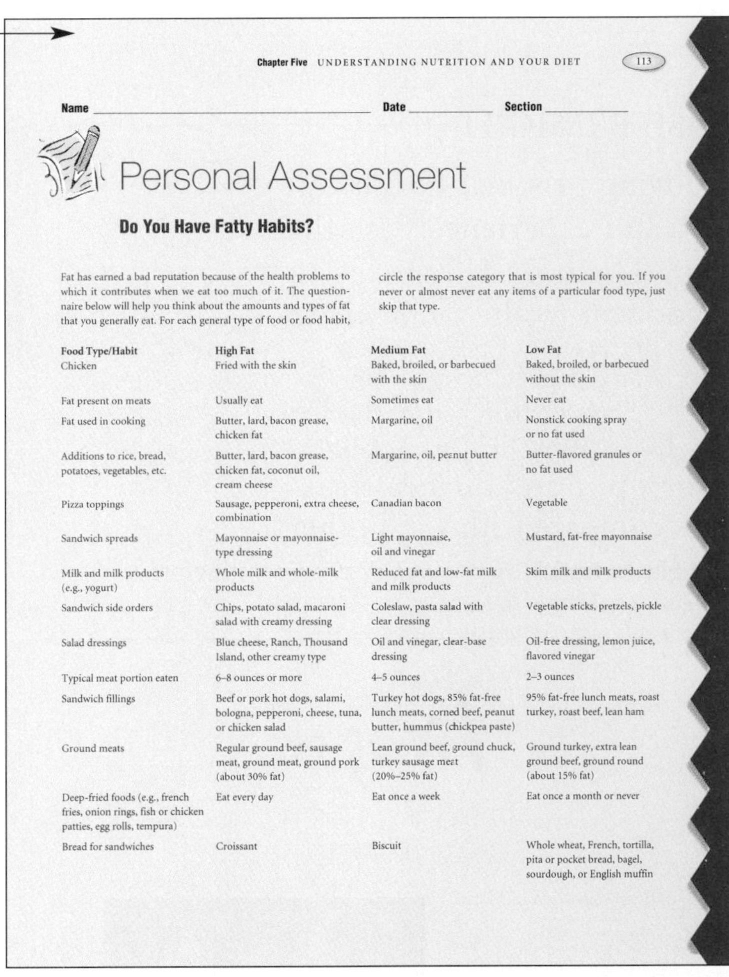

Chapter Five UNDERSTANDING NUTRITION AND YOUR DIET 113

Name ______ Date ______ Section ______

Personal Assessment

Do You Have Fatty Habits?

Fat has earned a bad reputation because of the health problems to which it contributes when we eat too much of it. The questionnaire below will help you think about the amounts and types of fat that you generally eat. For each general type of food or food habit, circle the response category that is most typical for you. If you never or almost never eat any items of a particular food type, just skip that type.

Food Type/Habit	High Fat	Medium Fat	Low Fat
Chicken	Fried with the skin	Baked, broiled, or barbecued with the skin	Baked, broiled, or barbecued without the skin
Fat present on meats	Usually eat	Sometimes eat	Never eat
Fat used in cooking	Butter, lard, bacon grease, chicken fat	Margarine, oil	Nonstick cooking spray or no fat used
Additions to rice, bread, potatoes, vegetables, etc.	Butter, lard, bacon grease, chicken fat, coconut oil, cream cheese	Margarine, oil, peanut butter	Butter-flavored granules or no fat used
Pizza toppings	Sausage, pepperoni, extra cheese, combination	Canadian bacon	Vegetable
Sandwich spreads	Mayonnaise or mayonnaise-type dressing	Light mayonnaise, oil and vinegar	Mustard, fat-free mayonnaise
Milk and milk products (e.g., yogurt)	Whole milk and whole-milk products	Reduced fat and low-fat milk and milk products	Skim milk and milk products
Sandwich side orders	Chips, potato salad, macaroni salad with creamy dressing	Coleslaw, pasta salad with clear dressing	Vegetable sticks, pretzels, pickle
Salad dressings	Blue cheese, Ranch, Thousand Island, other creamy type	Oil and vinegar, clear-base dressing	Oil-free dressing, lemon juice, flavored vinegar
Typical meat portion eaten	6–8 ounces or more	4–5 ounces	2–3 ounces
Sandwich fillings	Beef or pork hot dogs, salami, bologna, pepperoni, cheese, tuna, or chicken salad	Turkey hot dogs, 85% fat-free lunch meats, corned beef, peanut butter, hummus (chickpea paste)	95% fat-free lunch meats, roast turkey, roast beef, lean ham
Ground meats	Regular ground beef, sausage meat, ground meat, ground pork (about 30% fat)	Lean ground beef, ground chuck, turkey sausage meat (20%–25% fat)	Ground turkey, extra lean ground beef, ground round (about 15% fat)
Deep-fried foods (e.g., french fries, onion rings, fish or chicken patties, egg rolls, tempura)	Eat every day	Eat once a week	Eat once a month or never
Bread for sandwiches	Croissant	Biscuit	Whole wheat, French, tortilla, pita or pocket bread, bagel, sourdough, or English muffin

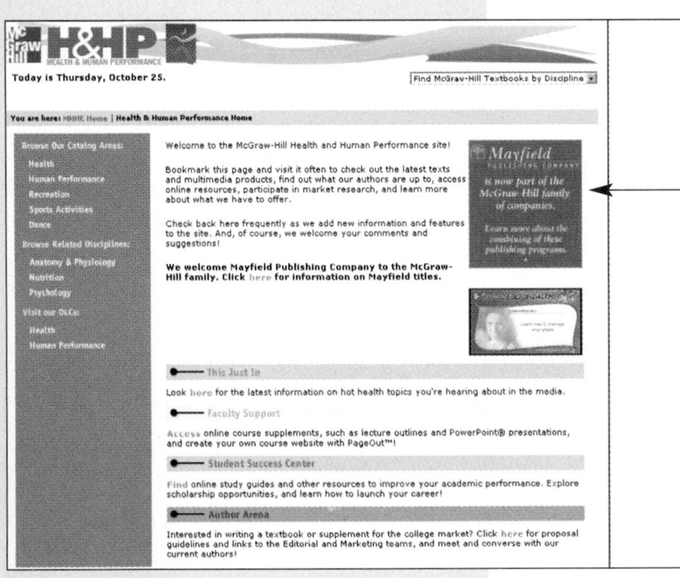

HEALTH & HUMAN PERFORMANCE WEBSITE

www.mhhe.com/hhp

The Personal Health Website is where you'll find a link to the *Focus on Health* website and other resources. Read about the latest "hot" health topics in "This Just In," or link to more self-assessments and updated health information.

ANCILLARIES

Course Integrator Guide

This manual includes all the features of a useful instructor's manual, such as learning objectives, suggested lecture outlines, suggested activities, media resources, and web links. It also integrates the text with all the related resources McGraw-Hill offers, such as the HealthQuest CD-ROM, Online Learning Center, Image Presentation CD-ROM, Healthy Living Video Clips CD-ROM, and Health and Human Performance Website. In addition, the guide includes references to relevant print and broadcast media.

Test Bank

This printed manual includes more than 2,000 questions, including multiple-choice, true-or-false, matching, and critical thinking questions.

Computerized Test Bank CD-ROM

Brownstone's Diploma Computerized Testing is the most flexible, powerful, easy-to-use electronic testing program available in higher education. The Diploma system allows the test maker to create a print version, an online version (to be delivered to a computer lab), or an Internet version of each test. Diploma includes a built-in instructor gradebook, into which student rosters and files can be imported. Diploma is for Windows users, and the CD-ROM includes a separate testing program, Exam IV, for Macintosh users.

Course Management Systems

www.mhhe.com/solutions

Now instructors can combine their McGraw-Hill Online Learning Center with today's most popular course-management systems, such as WebCT, Blackboard, and Top Class. Our Instructor Advantage program offers customers access to a complete online teaching website called the Knowledge Gateway, with prepaid, toll-free phone support and unlimited e-mail support directly from WebCT and Blackboard. Instructors who use 500 or more copies of a McGraw-Hill textbook can enroll in our Instructor Advantage Plus program, which provides on-campus, hands-on training from a certified platform specialist. Consult your McGraw-Hill sales representative to learn what other course management systems are easily used with McGraw-Hill online materials.

HealthQuest 4.0 CD-ROM by Robert S. Gold and Nancy L. Atkinson

The HealthQuest 4.0 CD-ROM helps students explore their wellness behavior using state-of-the-art interactive technology. Students can assess their current health status, determine their risks, and explore options for positive lifestyle change. Tailored feedback gives students a meaningful and individualized learning experience without using valuable classroom time. Modules include the Wellboard (a health self-assessment); Stress Management and Mental Health; Fitness; Nutrition and Weight Control; Communicable Diseases; Cardiovascular Health; Cancer; Tobacco; Alcohol; and Other Drugs. An online instructor's manual presents ideas for incorporating HealthQuest into your course.

Learning to Go: Health by InfoAlly and McGraw-Hill Higher Education

Learning to Go: Health is an Internet-based reinforcement system that periodically delivers interactive lessons directly to users' computers. The lessons help students retain and act on what they learn. This system provides a menu of lessons in personal health, from which instructors can choose content geared to their course. Through *Learning to Go,* students get bite-sized lessons—through overviews, test questions, and other content—that reinforce the main themes taught in class and in the text. Instructors can check students' progress as they move through the course.

Making the Grade Student CD-ROM

Making the Grade is an interactive study tool that enables students to test their mastery of text material with chapter-by-chapter quizzes. Multiple-choice, fill-in-the-blank, and true-or-false questions test students on key facts and concepts. All quizzes are graded instantly, and each includes feedback to explain the correct response. The CD-ROM also offers a Learning Styles Assessment to help students understand how they learn and, based on that assessment, how they can use their study time most effectively. Making the Grade also offers two different guides to the web. The Internet Primer explains the essentials of online research, including how to log on to the web and find information online. For more experienced web researchers, the CD-ROM contains the *McGraw-Hill Guide to Electronic Research,* which shows students how to use web-based information databases and explains how to evaluate the quality of information gathered online.

Online Learning Center

The Online Learning Center to accompany this text offers additional resources for students and instructors.

Resources for the instructor include the following:

- Downloadable PowerPoint presentation
- Lecture outlines
- Interactive web links
- Links to professional resources

Resources for the student include the following:

- Flashcards for learning key terms and their definitions
- Learning objectives and behavior change objectives
- Interactive activities
- Self-scoring chapter quizzes
- Web links for study and exploration of topics in the text
- Student PowerPoint presentation

Image Presentation CD-ROM

The Image Presentation CD-ROM is an electronic library of visual resources. The CD-ROM comprises images from the text displayed in PowerPoint, which allows the user to view, sort, search, use, and print catalog images. It also includes a complete ready-to-use PowerPoint presentation, which allows users to play chapter-specific slideshows.

Transparency Acetates

Seventy-two illustrations and graphics are available as transparency acetates to accompany this text. Attractively printed in full color, these useful tools facilitate learning and classroom discussion. They were chosen specifically to help explain complex concepts, and they serve as helpful aids for educators.

Health and Human Performance Website

www.mhhe.com/hhp

McGraw-Hill's Health and Human Performance website provides a wide variety of information for instructors and students, including monthly articles about current issues, online articles that celebrate diversity, downloadable supplements for instructors, a "how to" technology guide, study tips, and exam-preparation materials. It includes information about professional organizations, conventions, and careers. Additional features include:

- *This Just In*—Offers information on the latest hot topics, the best web resources, and more—all updated monthly.
- *Faculty Support*—Provides downloadable course supplements, such as instructor's manuals and PowerPoint presentations, and allows instructors to create their own course website with PageOut.
- *Student Success Center*—Offers online study guides and other resources to improve students' academic performance. Students can also explore scholarship opportunities and learn how to launch a rewarding career.
- *Author Arena*—Answers instructor's questions about writing a textbook or supplement for the college market. Potential authors can read the McGraw-Hill proposal guidelines, click on links to the Editorial and Marketing teams, and meet our current authors.
- *Self-Assessments*—Provides dozens of self-assessments that help students apply health topics to their own lives.

PageOut: The Course Website Development Center

www.pageout.net

PageOut, free to instructors who use a McGraw-Hill textbook, is an online program that creates custom course websites with the following features:

- A course home page
- An instructor home page
- A syllabus (interactive and customizable, including quizzing, instructor notes, and links to the text's Online Learning Center)
- Web links
- Discussions (multiple discussion areas per class)
- An online gradebook
- Links to student web pages

Contact your McGraw-Hill sales representative to obtain a password.

PowerWeb

www.dushkin.com/online

The PowerWeb website is a reservoir of course-specific articles and current events. Students can visit PowerWeb to take a self-scoring quiz, complete an interactive exercise, click through an interactive glossary, or check the daily news. An expert in each discipline analyzes the day's news to show students how it relates to their field of study.

PowerWeb is packaged with many McGraw-Hill textbooks. Students are also granted full access to Dushkin/McGraw-Hill's Student Site, where they can read study tips, conduct web research, learn about different career paths, and follow fun links on the web.

Primis Online

www.mhhe.com/primis/online

Primis Online is a database-driven publishing system that allows instructors to create content-rich textbooks, lab manuals, or readers for their courses directly from the Primis website. The customized text can be delivered in print or electronic (eBook) form. A Primis eBook is a digital version of the customized text (sold directly to students as a file downloadable to their computer or accessed online by a password).

The AIDS Booklet, sixth edition by Frank D. Cox

www.mhhe.com/catalogs/sem/hhp/student

This booklet provides current facts about HIV/AIDS: what it is, how the virus is transmitted, its prevalence among various population groups, symptoms of HIV infection, and strategies for prevention. It also covers the legal, social, medical, and ethical issues related to HIV/AIDS. Updates are posted to the website.

Annual Editions, edited by Richard Yarian

Annual Editions is an ever-enlarging series of more than seventy volumes, each designed to provide convenient, low-cost access to a wide range of current, carefully selected articles from some of the most important magazines, newspapers, and journals published today. Prominent scholars, researchers, and commentators write the articles, drawn from more than 400 periodical sources. All *Annual Editions* have common organizational features, such as annotated tables of contents, topic guides, unit overviews, and indexes. In addition, a list of annotated websites is included. An Instructor's Resource Guide with testing suggestions for each volume is available to qualified instructors.

Fitness and Nutrition Log

This logbook helps students track their diet and exercise programs. It serves as a diary to help students monitor their behaviors. It can be packaged with any McGraw-Hill textbook for a small additional fee.

FoodWise College Edition

Adapted from the widely tested professional version of FoodWise, this dietary-analysis software has been developed for use in college courses. It offers a variety of functions based on the latest USDA data. A unique tool allows the user to add foods to the database. The program is available for Windows and networks.

Healthy Living Video Clips CD-ROM

The Healthy Living Video Clips CD-ROM contains a collection of digitized video clips from the *Healthy Living: Road to Wellness* telecourse. These clips are brief (2- to 4-minute) segments that can be used to introduce a lecture or to spark classroom discussion. Instructors can incorporate these video clips into their classroom presentations. Links give instructors brief descriptions of each video clip for the corresponding chapter.

Healthy Living Video Library

The McGraw-Hill Video Library contains many quality videotapes, including selected Films for Humanities and all videos from the award-winning series *Healthy Living: Road to Wellness*. Digitized video clips are also available (see Healthy Living Video Clips CD-ROM).

Taking Sides, fifth edition by Eileen L. Daniel and Carol Levine

www.dushkin.com/takingsides

McGraw-Hill/Dushkin's *Taking Sides* series currently comprises twenty-two volumes with an instructor's guide and testing material available for each volume. The *Taking Sides* approach brings together the arguments of leading social and behavioral scientists, educators, and contemporary commentators, forming eighteen to twenty debates, or issues, that present the pros and cons of current controversies in an area of study. An Issue Introduction that precedes the two opposing viewpoints gives students the proper context and historical background for each debate. After reading the debate, students are given other viewpoints to consider in the Issue Postscript, which also offers recommendations for futher reading. *Taking Sides* fosters critical thinking in students and encourages them to develop a concern for serious social dialogue.

Video Library

The McGraw-Hill Video Library contains many quality videotapes, including selected Films for Humanities and all videos from the award-winning series *Healthy Living: Road to Wellness*. Digitized video clips are also available (see Healthy Living Video Clips CD-ROM). The library also features Students on Health Video, a unique video filmed on college campuses across the country, which includes eight brief (8- to 10-minute) segments featuring students involved in discussion and role-play on health issues. Lastly, a new video—McGraw-Hill Health Video—is available. This video features brief clips on a wide range of topics of interest in personal health courses.

ACKNOWLEDGMENTS

The publisher's reviewers made excellent comments and suggestions that were very useful to us in writing and revising this book. Their contributions are present in every chapter. We would like to express our sincere appreciation for both their critical and comparative readings.

For the sixth edition

M. Betsy Bergen
Kansas State University

Sandra Bonneau
Golden West College

Sandra DiNatale
Keene State College

Lisa Everett
Las Positas College

Albert J. Figone
Humboldt State University

Neil E. Gallagher
Towson University

Amy Goff
Scottsdale Community College

Sharrie A. Herbold-Sheley
Lane Community College

Katie Herrington
Jones Junior College

Cathy Kennedy
Colorado State University

Mary Mock
University of South Dakota

Leonid Polyakov
Essex County College

Debra Tavasso
East Carolina University

Jennifer Thomas
Emporia State University

Martin Turnauer
Radford University

Dale Wagoner
Chabot College

Mary A. Wyandt
University of Arkansas

Beverly Zeakes
Radford University

For the fifth edition

John Batacan
Idaho State University

Steve Bordi
West Valley Community College

Judy Drolet
Southern Illinois University–Carbondale

Don Haynes
University of Minnesota–Duluth

Mary Iten
University of Nebraska at Kearney

Emogene Johnson Vaughn
Norfolk State University

Patricia Lawson
Arkansas State University

Rosalie Marinelli
University of Nevada

Marilyn Morton
SUNY-Plattsburgh

Trish Root
North Seattle Community College

Walt Rehm
Cuesta College

Betty Shepherd
Virginia Western Community College

Ladona Tournabene
University of South Dakota

Glenda Warren
Cumberland College

Katie Wiedman
University of St. Francis

For the fourth edition

S. Eugene Barnes
University of Southern Alabama

Anne K. Black
Austin Peay State University

Susan Ceriale
University of California–Santa Barbara

Bridget M. Finn
William Paterson University

Marianne Frauenknecht
Western Michigan University

Edna Gillis
Valdosta State University

Joe Goldfarb
University of Missouri–Columbia

Phil Huntsinger
University of Kansas

Gordon B. James
Weber State University

Sylvia M. Kubsch
University of Wisconsin–Green Bay

Frederick M. Randolph
Western Illinois University

Dell Smith
University of Central Arkansas

B. McKinley Thomas
Augusta State University

Chuck Ulrich
Western Illinois University

For the third edition

Dayna S. Brown
Morehead State University

Diane M. Hamilton
Georgia Southern University

Joe Herzstein
Trenton State College

Rebecca Rutt Leas
Clarion University

Dorinda Maynard
Eastern Kentucky University

Steven Navarro
Cerritos College

Mary Beth Tighe
The Ohio State University

For the second edition

James D. Aguiar
Ithaca College

Carolyn M. Allred
Central Piedmont Community College

Joan Benson
University of Utah

Daniel E. Berney
California State University–Dominguez Hills

Ronnie Carda
Emporia State University

Barbara Funke
Georgia College

William C. Gross
Western Michigan University

Richard Hurley
Brigham Young University

Raeann Koerner Smith
Ventura College

L. Clark McCammon
Western Illinois University

Dan Neal
Southwestern Oregon Community College

David Quadagno
Florida State University

Leslie Rurey
Community Colleges of Spokane

Scott E. Scobell
West Virginia State College

Karen T. Sullivan
Marymount University

Joan Tudor
Chapman University

Stuart L. Whitney
University of Vermont

For the first edition

Sandra L. Bonneau
Golden West College

Richard A. Kaye
Kingsborough Community College

Donald Haynes
University of Minnesota–Duluth

J. Dale Wagoner
Chabot College

SPECIAL ACKNOWLEDGMENTS

The sixth edition of *Focus on Health* is the sixteenth text we have written since the mid-1980s. We could not have accomplished all of this without the help of many people. Among these are our faculty colleagues at Ball State University, who continue to keep us abreast of new information in areas related to personal health. A special thanks goes out to all of you.

Additionally, we want to recognize our administrative colleagues. We are fortunate to have worked with administrators who maintain the vision that (a) textbooks represent important resources for today's college students, and (b) textbooks reflect faculty contributions that shed favorable light on a college community. We very much appreciate the support of Dr. C. Warren Vander Hill, Provost and Vice President for Academic Affairs, and Dr. Ronald L. Johnstone, Dean of the College of Sciences and Humanities at Ball State University.

The list of dedicated people at McGraw-Hill is quite long. Many have played a direct part in influencing the direction of this writing project. Vicki Malinee and Pam Cooper are exceptional people who have championed this project since its inception. They understand clearly the demands authors face as they juggle family, teaching, and writing schedules. They do their best to provide a supportive environment for McGraw-Hill authors.

Another key player is our developmental editor, Carlotta Seely. This edition of *Focus on Health* is the second project we have completed with Carlotta. She has been on top of every detail from the moment we started this revision. We believe that this revised edition of *Focus on Health* is a major reflection of Carlotta's vision and determination. We appreciate her talent, effort, and humor very much.

We also wish to acknowledge the contributions of Virginia Lee Mermel, Joseph Lawler, and Kevin Campbell. Over the years, we have learned the importance of providing professors with a comprehensive, well-written Instructor's Manual and Test Bank. Virginia Lee Mermel and Joseph Lawler have developed an excellent Course Integrator Guide. Kevin Campbell has created an outstanding Test Bank. Both of these ancillaries will benefit experienced instructors as well as new ones.

It is difficult for the authors to know the many people who work on the production end of a textbook project. Our principal connection with this part of McGraw-Hill has been our project manager, Mary Powers. Mary made certain that every manuscript detail was clear and every production deadline met. In addition, the credit for the book's attractiveness goes to the designer, Rebecca Lemna, and the design coordinator, Rick Noel.

Finally, we would like to thank our families for the continued support and love they have given us. Perhaps more than others, our families understand the effort and commitment it takes to write books. We truly appreciate their sacrifices.

Dale B. Hahn
Wayne A. Payne

chapter **1**

Shaping Your Health

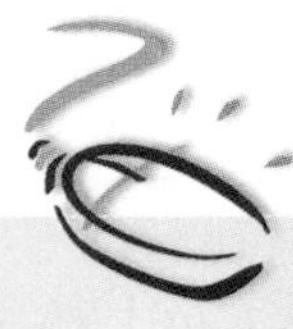

Online Learning Center Resources

www.mhhe.com/hahn6e

Log on to our Online Learning Center (OLC) for access to these additional resources:

- Chapter key terms and definitions
- Learning objectives
- Additional behavior change objectives
- Student interactive question-and-answer sites
- Self-scoring chapter quiz

The OLC also offers web links for study and exploration of health topics. Here are some examples of what you'll find:

- **www.yahoo.com/health** Research hundreds of health-related links and use the Yahoo search engine to zero in on sites of interest.
- **www.healthfinder.gov** Check out this gateway for consumer health and human services information from the U.S. government.
- **www.HealthAtoZ.com** Look here for a searchable database of health information sites that are rated for quality.

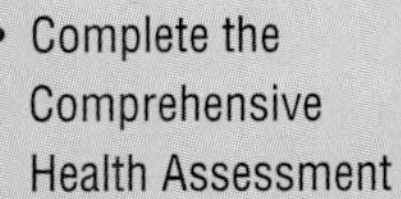

Taking Charge of Your Health

- Complete the Comprehensive Health Assessment on p. xxxi. Develop a plan to modify your behavior in the areas in which you need improvement.
- Take part in a new spiritual activity, such as meditating, creating art or music, or appreciating nature.
- To promote the social dimension of your health, try to meet one new person each week during the semester.
- Choose one developmental task you would like to focus on, such as assuming responsibility, and plan the steps you can follow to progress in this area.
- Volunteer to be an assistant in a community service program, such as a literacy project or a preschool program.

Eye on the Media

Where Does Our Health Information Come From?

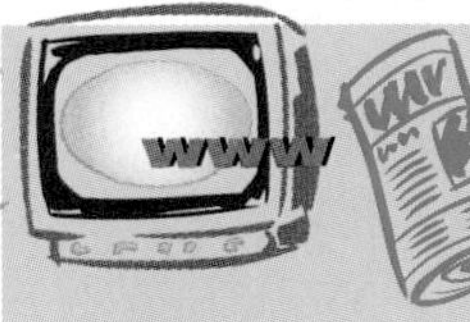

Today our health information comes from a variety of media—some more reliable than others. The following six media groups convey health-related information. Because Eye on the Media will appear in each chapter of this text, this introduction is limited to an overview of these sources. Later chapters will deal with the important issue of which ones are good (in other words, valid and reliable) sources for learning about health.

Radio and Television

When you think of radio, the first thing that may come to mind is your favorite music. But two areas of radio are especially important for news and information: talk radio and National Public Radio (NPR). Talk radio raises the question of validity of information. For example, if you're listening to a talk show about HIV exposure, the perceptions and opinions of the host (which may be strong or even extreme) are an important part of the show. When this point of view is combined with the opinions of callers, whose "facts" may come from unauthoritative sources, what you're hearing is probably not solid information. It's certainly not a good basis for making your health decisions.

Eye on the Media *continued*

NPR, on the other hand, takes a scholarly approach to news, featuring experts who do not always agree on an issue. In general, the news reports on NPR are long enough to present an in-depth, balanced treatment of health-related topics.

Newspapers and Magazines

Let's assume that most people read only one or two newspapers a day—their local paper and perhaps a national newspaper such as *The New York Times* or *USA Today.* If so, the health information they are receiving is typically from wire services like the Associated Press; it is condensed and simplified but accurate within these limitations. When health-related information in newspapers is accompanied by illustrations and original source information (such as a professional journal), it is more helpful to the reader.

Unlike newspapers, magazines are so diverse in terms of ownership, intended audience, and standards of validity that it is difficult to determine the reliability of their health-related content. In general, the national news magazines, such as *Time* and *Newsweek,* are very careful about the accuracy of their reporting, often including primary (original) sources. Their content is considered "state of the art." In contrast, the checkout-lane tabloids, such as *The Globe* and *The National Enquirer,* are known for printing stories with "health" content that few readers take seriously. Between these two extremes is a wide array of general content magazines, such as *The Saturday Evening Post,* and health-oriented magazines, such as *Prevention,* that vary greatly in validity and reliability.

Professional Journals

Your college library probably offers a broad selection of professional journals. Through these publications, the members of an academic discipline share the latest developments and issues in their field with their colleagues and other readers. Because the study of health is so multifaceted, drawing on different disciplines for information, health-related journals are plentiful. The vast majority of articles that appear in publications such as *The New England Journal of Medicine* and *The Journal of the American Dietetic Association* are peer-reviewed. This means that professionals in the particular field review and judge the content of a submitted article to determine whether or not it should be published. Then, if a study being reported was not carefully controlled, or if its underlying theory seems to be flawed, the article is returned to the author(s) for refinement. This process greatly reduces the risk of publishing invalid information. Currently, journals are beginning to appear in fields such as complementary (alternative) health care. When reading such publications, you need to consider whether they are backed by a peer-review process.

Government Documents

Each year various departments of the federal government, particularly the Department of Health and Human Services (DHHS), release the results of research being done under the oversight of its many divisions and agencies. These documents, such as the annual *Surgeon General's Report on Smoking and Health,* become the source of much

CHARTING A PLAN FOR BEHAVIOR CHANGE

As you begin to study health, this is a good time to commit to a health behavior change project. When thinking about making such a change, some students know exactly which behavior they want to alter. Other students are uncertain about which behavior to choose and need to do some self-assessment before they start (Figure 1-1).

Whether or not you think you know how you want to begin, it's a good idea to take the Comprehensive Health Assessment on page xxxi. After you've finished the assessment and calculated your score, you'll know the areas in which you need the most improvement. Knowing that much will at least start to give you a focus. Then browse through this text and take a look at the Personal Assessments in each chapter. For example, if you are thinking about a behavior change in weight management, see the Personal Assessment titled "Is It Time for a Weight-Loss Program?" on p. 145.

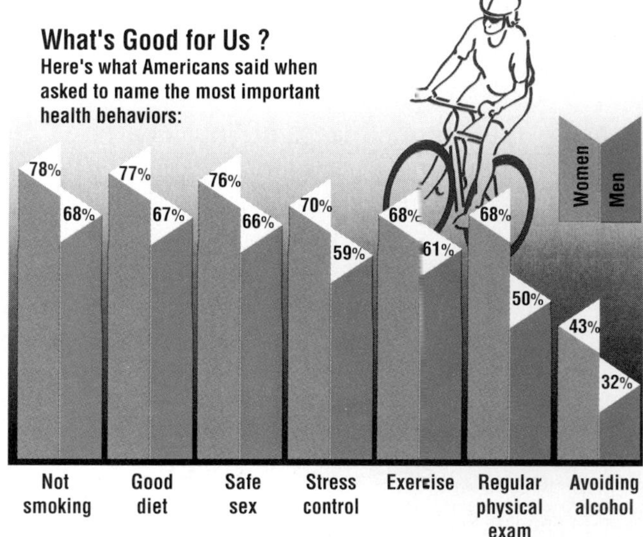

Figure 1-1 People have different ideas about what's good for our health. Which behaviors do you think are most important?

Eye on the Media *continued*

of the health-related news reported by other media sources, including textbooks and professional journals. These publications generally can be purchased through the U.S. Government Printing Office. They are also available through urban public libraries and large university libraries. With few exceptions, the information in these publications is reviewed by the most respected authorities in each field.

Books

Books continue to be a vast source of information on health-related topics. Today's health books, in addition to academic health textbooks such as *Focus on Health,* fall into three categories: reference books, medical encyclopedias, and single-topic trade (retail) books.

Included in the category of reference books are important professional publications such as *The Merck Manual* and the *Physicians' Desk Reference.* These books, intended for professionals in various health fields, contain the most current information on specific aspects of health. Although these books can be purchased by the general public, their content is technical and complex, and their language is often difficult for nonprofessional readers to follow.

More valuable to the typical American household are the various medical (health) encyclopedias, such as *The Johns Hopkins Home Medical Handbook* and *The Mayo Clinic Family Health Book.* Such books usually include a wide array of medical conditions and offer valuable information about health promotion and disease prevention. Their clear writing styles and highly valid information make these books excellent home references.

Single-topic health-related trade books, such as those about diets and health problems, are readily available from retail outlets like bookstores and the Internet. Like magazines, these books are difficult to assess because of their quantity and the varying backgrounds of the authors. Some are very sound in terms of content and philosophy. Others may be misleading and may contain advice that could be dangerous to your health. Included in this group are self-help books, the best-selling health books of all.

The Internet

Today, at least 20% of all U.S. households can access the Internet directly, and more than 50% of all upper-income households can do so. Internet access is also available through libraries, educational institutions, and the workplace. With just a few clicks, you can reach many health-related websites that offer a wide range of health information. Chat rooms provide a forum for individuals to share their personal health experiences. Because the Internet is such an important source of health information for both professionals and the general public, this textbook highlights helpful websites in all chapters. To learn about criteria for assessing the validity and reliability of Internet information, see Chapter 15 (p. 380).

TALKING POINTS • Would you be hesitant to talk to your doctor about health advice you found on the Internet? How would you approach the subject?

Some of the health behaviors students typically want to change are:

- To gain or lose weight
- To stop smoking
- To stop using smokeless tobacco
- To eliminate or reduce caffeine consumption
- To develop better sleeping patterns
- To reduce levels of stress
- To improve physical fitness
- To reduce alcohol consumption
- To eat more nutritiously
- To develop more friendships
- To enhance the spiritual dimension of health

As you plan to change your behavior, using the following 10-step program as a guide can be very helpful:

1. *Establish some baseline data about your behavior.* *Baseline data* is information about your current health and behavior that you can use later for comparison. For example, if you want to lose weight, weigh yourself for three consecutive days early in the morning to pinpoint your starting weight. If you plan to stop smoking, keep track of your smoking patterns for a few days. If you are changing your diet, write down everything you eat for three or four days in a row. It's also a good idea to keep a journal and record your activities and your feelings about the behavior.
2. *Summarize your baseline data.* Identify any patterns you see. Accept this information as an accurate indicator of your current health behavior. Use this textbook to find information about your behavior that can help you plan behavior-change strategies.
3. *Establish some specific goals.* Begin with small steps. For example, if you plan to lose weight, start out with a goal of losing one pound per week for the next three weeks. If you plan to stop smoking, begin by cutting down on your daily intake by five cigarettes. Try to make gradual progress toward your goals.
4. *Make a personal contract to accomplish your goals.* Write down both the starting and ending dates. To

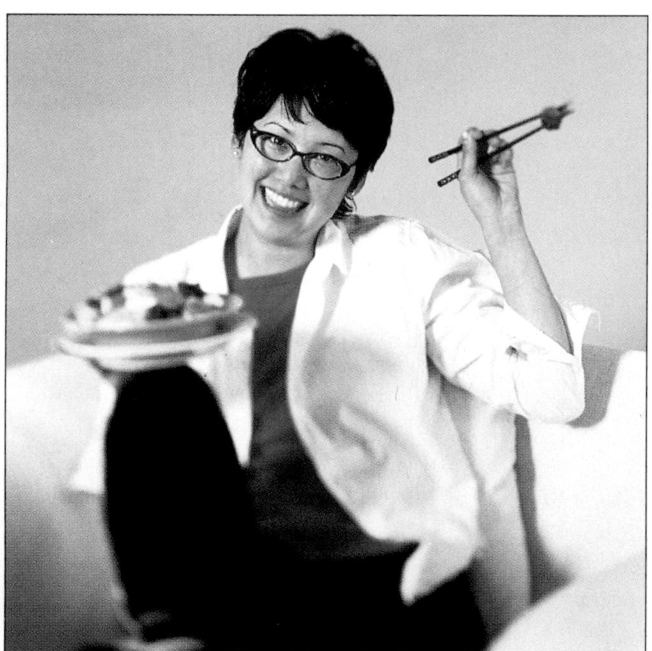

Many students want to change a specific behavior, such as following a more nutritious diet.

help you focus on specific activities for reaching your goals, use the Changing for the Better boxes found in each chapter. For example, see p. 106 Dietary Guidelines for Americans, p. 265 Eat to Lower Your Cancer Risk, and p. 238 Monitoring Your Cholesterol Level. Identify any milestones along the way to your goal. Specify the time, personal resources, and energy you will need to commit to this project.

5. *Devise a plan of action.* As you develop your strategy, adjust your environment to help you replace old cues with new ones. For example, if you are trying to get more sleep, calm yourself before bedtime by reading rather than listening to loud music or watching a TV drama. If you want to improve in your eating behavior, change your walking route so that you avoid passing the campus snack bar.
6. *Chart your progress in your diary or journal.* From day 1, keep a record of how you are doing. Consider making this record visible. For instance, posting an eating record on the refrigerator door is a good motivator for some people.
7. *Encourage your family and friends to help you.* Social support is important in any attempt at behavior change. Your friends may want to join you and change their own behavior. Then you can support each other. But some friends or family members might misunderstand your efforts. They might actually discourage you. If possible, avoid these people—at least while your project is under way.

Changing *for the Better*

Looking Toward the Future: What's Your Game Plan?

After discussing the areas of growth and development from ages 18 to 40 in a personal health class, one student asked: "Just what should I do with all of this growth stuff, anyway?" Some of the responses—from other students and the professor—were as follows:

- Ask others to share their stories with you. Choose people you view as independent, comfortable with their plans, and responsible or established in areas of development where you feel uncertain. Hearing their first-hand accounts can be an excellent way to gain insight into your own future.
- While you are reading, either for recreation or a class assignment, look for aspects of these growth areas in the people being described. Do the same thing with characters depicted in films, plays, or TV programs. For example, think about the character played by Renée Zellweger in *Bridget Jones's Diary* and the college experiences of the main character in the TV program *Felicity*.
- Set aside time to give serious thought to where you are now in each of these developmental areas. Compare your perceived points of progress with what others (friends, professors, family) might see or expect when they think about you and your life experiences. Construct a mental game plan for one or more of the five developmental areas discussed in this chapter.

TALKING POINTS • **What does being an adult mean to you at this point? How would you explain this to your best friend?**

8. *Set up a reward system.* Rewards tend to motivate people. They can be used to reinforce your positive changes. If you achieve success at a particular point in your plan, reward yourself with a special meal, new clothes, or a weekend trip. Pat yourself on the back occasionally for your efforts. Relish your success.
9. *Prepare for obstacles along the way.* No one who achieved anything of importance did it without a few setbacks, so prepare yourself mentally for an occasional obstacle. For example, if you neglect your fitness plan during a long holiday weekend, try to get back on course as soon as possible. Work through your setbacks with a "forgive and forget" attitude.
10. *Revise your plan as necessary.* Try to be flexible in your approach to behavior change. A strategy that works for a while might not work as well after a month or two. So be prepared to reevaluate your goals and try new techniques when necessary.

Now that we've outlined a plan for behavior change, let's look at some of the areas of health that students are concerned about.

HEALTH CONCERNS OF THE NEW DECADE

Throughout this new decade, traditionally defined health problems—heart disease, cancer, accidents, drug use, and mental illness—will continue to be important concerns (Table 1-1).[1] Environmental pollution, violence, health care costs, acquired immunodeficiency syndrome (AIDS), and sexually transmitted diseases will also continue to be significantly important. World hunger, population control, and the threat of terrorism involving nuclear and biological weapons will be great concerns for your generation and those to follow.

The accompanying Star Box lists the top five health issues currently facing college students. Many of these health conditions can be prevented or managed successfully. As you learn more about health, you'll find out how to lower your risk for many of them. Your behavior is within your control, and the choices you make will certainly affect your health. Select a plan of healthful living that incorporates a sound diet, proper exercise, adequate rest, periodic medical checkups, and elimination (or moderation) of drug use (including tobacco and alcohol). This text is designed to provide you with the information and motivation to help you select the lifestyle that will make you a happy and healthy person.

Key Health Issues College Students Face

The American College Health Association, a prominent group of health educators, medical professionals, and college residence hall staff professionals, identified the following as the most critical health issues faced by college students in the 1990s. These concerns continue to be critical in this new decade. They are listed in order of importance:

- *Sexual health concerns,* including topics such as sexually transmitted diseases, relationship issues, unintended pregnancy, and sexual violence
- *Substance abuse,* including a wide range of issues related to the abuse of alcohol, tobacco, and other drugs, and dependency and codependency
- *Mental health concerns,* including stress management, fear of failure, coping skills, complex family relationships, and depression
- *Nutrition issues,* including healthful diets, weight management, chronic disease prevention, and eating disorders
- *Health care services,* including financing and delivering comprehensive, low-cost health services to students and their families

Because these issues will continue to be important, and because of their relevance to you, all are discussed in this text. Many other matters of concern to both traditional-age and nontraditional-age students are also addressed.

DEFINITIONS OF HEALTH

If you asked a room full of people to define health, you'd probably get a variety of responses. Even the experts don't agree on this issue. This section explores the main approaches to this question—both traditional and nontraditional.

Table 1-1 Top 10 Causes of Death (United States, all ages, 1999)*

Cause of Death	Number of Cases
1. Heart disease	724,915
2. Malignant neoplasms	549,787
3. Cerebrovascular diseases	167,340
4. Chronic obstructive pulmonary disease	124,153
5. Unintentional injuries	97,298
6. Diabetes mellitus	68,379
7. Pneumonia and influenza	63,686
8. Alzheimer's disease	44,570
9. Nephritis, nephrotic syndrome, and nephrosis	35,524
10. Septicemia	30,670

*Note: For the first time in many years suicide is not among the 10 leading causes of death. Currently it is in position 11.

Episodic Medicine

When people become ill or are injured, they commonly visit a health care provider for diagnosis and treatment. They are experiencing an "episode" of unhealthfulness. Once this period is over, they feel healthy again. In this context, health can be defined as *the absence of illness, disease, or injury.*

Preventive Medicine

In this approach to health care, patients who are well visit their physicians to identify any potential for illness. By using various tests, the physician attempts to identify and manage early indicators of risk. The goal is to prevent illness from occurring, delay its onset, or lessen its severity. This concept of *risk factor reduction* leads to defining health as *the absence of high-level risk for future illness or disease.*

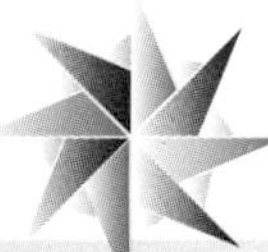

Healthy People 2010

In 1991 a U.S. government document titled *Healthy People 2000: National Health Promotion and Disease Prevention Objectives*[2] outlined a strategic plan for promoting the health of the American public. The plan included 300 health objectives in 22 priority areas. Forty-seven of the 300 objectives were defined as "sentinel" ones—significant goals measuring for the progress of 1990s health promotion objectives.

Progress toward achieving the objectives was assessed near the middle of the decade and reported in a document titled *Healthy People 2000: Midcourse Review and 1995 Revisions*.[3] Although progress was reported in some areas, little or no progress was reported in many. In particular, few gains were made toward achieving the three broadest objectives: (1) increasing the span of healthy life; (2) reducing health differences among Americans; and (3) gaining access to preventive services. A new plan for improving the health of Americans, called *Healthy People 2010*,[4] is currently being reviewed and refined.

Healthy People 2010: Understanding and Improving Health is a health promotion program intended to be implemented at all levels, ranging from individual involvement through multinational cooperative efforts, including *Health for All in the 21st Century*,[5] a World Health Organization health promotion initiative. Although the goals of *Healthy People 2000* and *Healthy People 2010* are similar, the latter focuses on the projected needs of the United States during the first decade of the new century. Newly emerging demographics, such as the increasing number of older adults, and technologies, including new vaccines and HIV antiviral drugs, are better addressed in *Healthy People 2010*.

Central to the design of *Healthy People 2010* are twenty areas in which health promotion activities are critically important, such as mental disability, chronic disease prevention and treatment, increased physical activity, improved nutrition, and more rigorous food and drug safety requirements. Making progress in these areas will allow the nation to reach four "enabling goals": (1) promotion of healthy behavior, (2) protection of health, (3) assurance of access to quality health care, and (4) strengthening of community prevention. When these goals have been achieved, the American public should anticipate two additional benefits: (1) increased years of healthy life, and (2) elimination of health disparities among various segments of the population. The latter two accomplishments were also goals of the earlier programs.

The success of *Healthy People 2010* will not be known for many years. However, if we ultimately reach these goals, Americans can expect an improved quantity and quality of life.

Health Promotion

Similar in theory to preventive medicine, **health promotion** involves an array of health professionals who seek to identify risk for future illness by using noninvasive tests and assessments. Representative of these health promotion specialists are health educators, fitness specialists in exercise science, dietitians, and stress-management specialists. None of these professionals are physicians and as such are limited in the scope of their practices. This approach aims to reduce the likelihood of illness, delay its onset, or lessen its severity. Health is thus defined as existing when risk levels are low or nonexistent.

These three views of health emphasize eliminating sickness or reducing the likelihood of developing illnesses (having a low potential for **morbidity**). They are all directed toward having people live as long as possible (reduction in early **mortality**). These ways of defining health are based on reducing morbidity and mortality.

Wellness

Advocates of this approach suggest that **wellness** has little to do with reducing morbidity and/or mortality. They contend that wellness is achieved by fostering a *wellness lifestyle* that will lead to a sense of well-being, which is subjectively defined. The mechanism for reaching this state is somewhat vague. In fact, many wellness programs seem to be based on the same risk-reduction strategies used in preventive medicine and health promotion. Perhaps "being well" is essentially the same as being healthy.

DEVELOPMENTAL TASKS FOR TODAY'S COLLEGE STUDENTS

Now it's time to consider the various aspects of your life that are made possible by high-level health. This is a multidimensional, or *holistic*, form of health that *empowers* you to grow and develop (Figure 1-2).

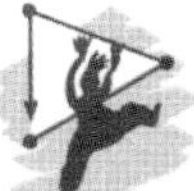

HealthQuest Activities

- Use the Wellboard to report your life score (number of years out of 114) and the score percentages for each of the eight health areas.
- Fill out the Wellboard using data from a fictional college student. On the first assessment screen, change the demographics to show how gender, ethnicity, age, marital status, and community affect average life expectancy.

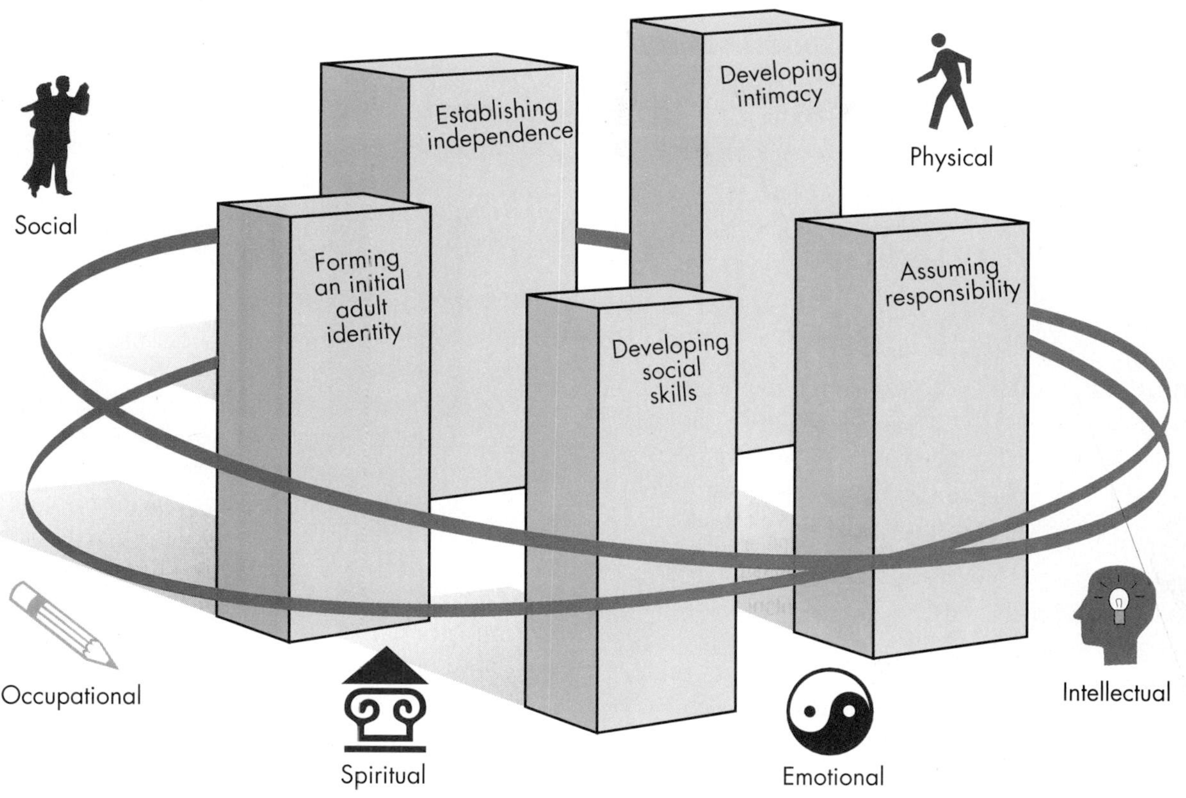

Figure 1-2 Mastery of the developmental tasks through a balanced involvement of the six dimensions of health will lead to your enjoying a more productive and satisfying life.

Whether you are a nontraditional-age or traditional-age student, these are important questions to consider:

1. Compared with your friends, do you see yourself as a fully functioning adult? What new experiences do you need to reach that level and stay there?
2. How independent do you want to be in the future? What decisions do you need to make to reach that point?
3. What is your current level of responsibility—for yourself and for others? What must you do to expand that responsibility to the adult level?
4. Are you developing the social skills necessary to develop comfortable and productive relationships with others in a culturally diverse society?
5. What are your expectations for intimate relationships, such as marriage, long-term friendships, and mentor relationships? Can you handle the responsibilities necessary to sustain them?

Today's college student population is diverse, with ages ranging from 18 to 40 and beyond. In fact, the rapidly growing percentage of **nontraditional-age students** (see the Learning from Our Diversity box on p. 8) is changing the sequence and duration of the traditional

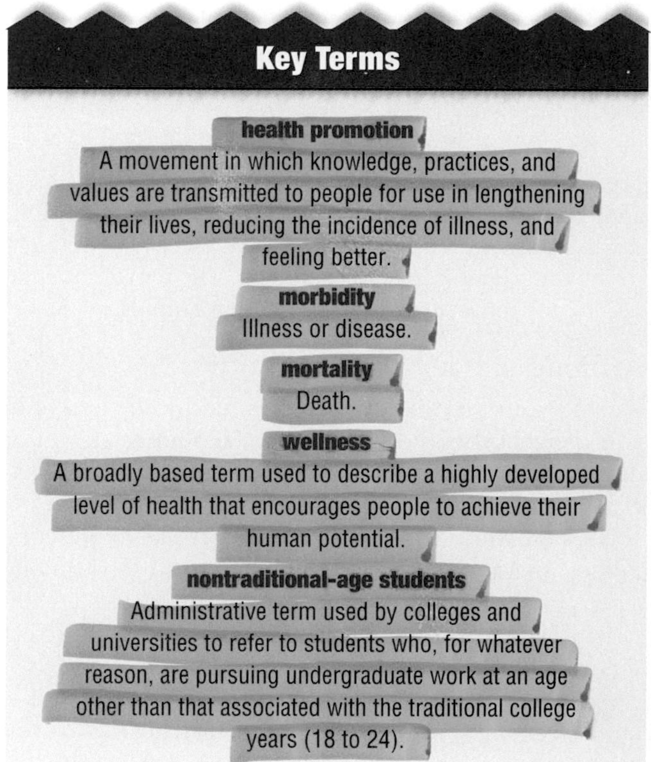

Key Terms

health promotion
A movement in which knowledge, practices, and values are transmitted to people for use in lengthening their lives, reducing the incidence of illness, and feeling better.

morbidity
Illness or disease.

mortality
Death.

wellness
A broadly based term used to describe a highly developed level of health that encourages people to achieve their human potential.

nontraditional-age students
Administrative term used by colleges and universities to refer to students who, for whatever reason, are pursuing undergraduate work at an age other than that associated with the traditional college years (18 to 24).

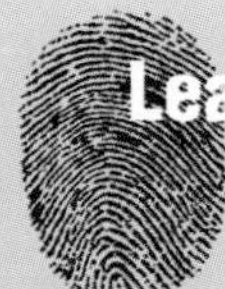

Learning from Our Diversity

Back to the Future: Nontraditional-Age Students Enrich the College Experience

To anyone who's visited an American college campus in the last fifteen years, it's abundantly clear that the once typical college student—white, middle class, between the ages of eighteen and twenty-four—is less of a majority on campus. In most institutions of higher learning, today's student body is a rich tapestry of color, culture, language, ability, and age. Wheelchair-accessible campuses roll out the welcome mat for students with disabilities; the air is filled with the music of a dozen or more languages spoken by students from virtually every part of the world; students in their sixties chat animatedly with classmates young enough to be their grandchildren.

Of all the trends that are changing the face of college enrollment in the United States, perhaps the most significant is the increasing diversity in the age of students now on campus. No longer regarded as oddball exceptions, older students today are both a common and welcome sight in colleges and universities across the country. Many women cut short their undergraduate education—or defer graduate school—to raise children. Divorcees, widows, and women whose children are grown often return to college, or enroll for the first time, to prepare for professional careers. And increasingly, both men and women are finding it desirable, if not essential, to further their education as a means of either keeping their current job or qualifying for a higher position.

Just as children are enriched by the knowledge and experience of their grandparents and other older relatives, so too is today's college classroom a richer place when many of the seats are filled by students of nontraditional age. Without being didactic or preachy, older students can provide valuable guidance and direction to younger classmates who may be uncertain of their career path, or who may be wrestling with decisions about marriage and parenthood. Older students can also serve as role models for young people from unstable homes or disadvantaged backgrounds who may have grown up without consistent adult support. In doing so, nontraditional-age students can gain helpful insights about young people's feelings, attitudes, challenges, and aspirations.

Among the many important benefits of today's increasingly diverse college campus, surely one of the most significant is the enhanced opportunity for intergenerational communication and understanding made possible by the growing numbers of students of nontraditional age.

In your classes, how would you characterize the interactions between traditional-age students and those of nontraditional age? In what ways are they enriching each other's college experience?

TALKING POINTS • You are in charge of a campus event for students of various ages from several cultural groups. How would you go about finding out what would make the event attractive to students with backgrounds different from your own?

areas of growth and development. The lock-step progression toward adulthood that was seen among earlier generations of college students is giving way to a more flexible, nontraditional type of passage.

Of the five developmental tasks discussed here (Figure 1-2), the first four (involving the nurturing of one's adult identity, level of independence, level of responsibility, and social skill development) seem especially pertinent to the traditional-age college student. The remaining task, developing intimate relationships, often unfolds later.

Forming an Initial Adult Identity

During your youth, you were viewed by the adults in your neighborhood or community as someone's son or daughter. That stage is rapidly passing. Both you and society are beginning to look at each other in new ways.

As a maturing adult, you'd probably like to present a unique identity to society. Internally, you're constructing a perception of yourself as the person you wish to be. Externally, you're forming the behavioral patterns to project this identity to others.

The completion of this first developmental task is necessary to have a productive and satisfying life. As you work toward achieving an adult identity, you'll eventually be able to answer the central question of young adulthood: "Who am I?" Many nontraditional-age students are also asking this question as they progress through college.

Establishing Independence

During childhood and adolescence, the primary responsibility for socialization rests with the family. For many years your family was the primary contributor to your knowledge, values, and behavior. By this time, however, you should be demonstrating an interest in moving away from that dependent relationship.

Travel, peer relationships, marriage, military service, and college have been traditional avenues for disengagement from the family. Your ability and willingness to follow one or more of these paths will help you to establish your independence. Your success in these endeavors depends on your willingness to use the resources you have. You will need to draw on various strengths—physical, emotional, social, intellectual, spiritual, and occupational—to undertake the new experiences that will lead you to an increasing level of independence. In a sense, your family laid the foundation for the resources and experiences you will now use to draw yourself away from them.

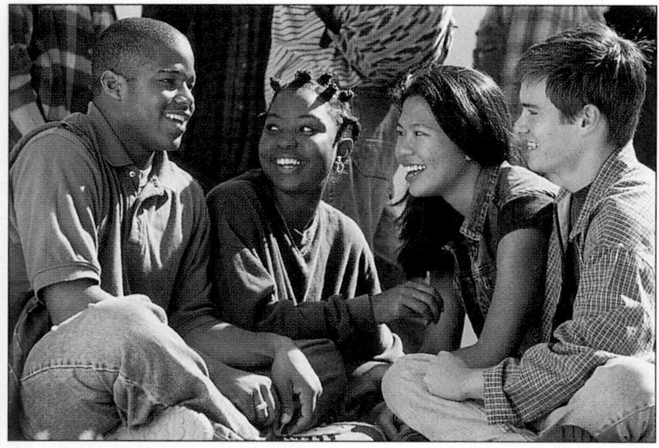

College experiences help students develop important social skills.

Assuming Responsibility

Assuming increasing levels of responsibility is your third developmental task. The opportunity to assume responsibility can come from a variety of sources. You may sometimes accept responsibility voluntarily, such as when you join organizations or establish new friendships. Other responsibilities are placed on you by family members, professors, friends, dating partners, and employers. You may also accept responsibility for doing a particular task for the benefit of someone else, such as when you donate a unit of blood during a campus blood drive.

Developing Social Skills

A fourth developmental task seems especially relevant to traditional-age college students—developing appropriate and dependable social skills. The college experience has traditionally prepared students very well socially, but the interactions involved in friendships, work relationships, or parenting may require that you make an effort to refine a variety of social skills, including communication, listening, and conflict management.

Beyond the social skills required on the college campus are those needed to meet the increasing diversity found in adult life. In the workplace, for example, you will encounter people who differ from you in age, gender, race, ethnicity, marital status, and sexual orientation. You will be expected to interact productively and comfortably in this ever-changing human environment.

Developing Intimate Relationships

After formal studies have been completed, the nearly universal developmental task of establishing one or more intimate relationships becomes important. When defined broadly, intimacy reflects open, deep, caring relationships between you and another in the context of true friendships, marriage or other close relationships, and mentor relationships in the workplace.

People vary in terms of the number of intimate relationships they engage in and the depth of those relationships. Some have several close relationships at the same time, while others seem interested in, or capable of, sustaining only one at a time. What is important is that each person have someone with whom to share close personal thoughts, feelings, and emotions. This connection is helpful throughout life but especially important in the later years, when isolation can become a significant problem.

Once familiar with the five developmental tasks, you will see considerable overlap in their accomplishment. For example, developing and refining your social skills can also enhance your independence from your family. Your willingness to accept increasing responsibility may influence your ability to develop an intimate relationship with someone.

Related Stages

Although not considered developmental tasks, two stages related to them need attention. The first stage, entering or advancing in a career or profession, is generally pursued in the years immediately following the completion of formal studies. College coursework leading to an earned degree, strong recommendations from field-experienced supervisors, and a carefully nurtured network of people already in your field of interest are often required for opening doors into a chosen career path. Professions such as medicine and dentistry also require their own plan for the transition from student to practitioner.

The second stage is making parenting decisions. Regardless of one's ability or desire to reproduce, a wide range of decisions must be made by adults about their role in sustaining the next generation. These decisions may include planning to remain child-free, determining when to begin parenting, deciding on the number and spacing of children, and dealing with infertility. Considerations about adoption, foster care, parenting styles, and child-centered institutions and programs also fall within the scope of this dimension.

In the final analysis, these broad areas of personal growth and development that occur when most people are attending college are intertwined with the overall quality of life. For this reason, the "new" definition of health presented here is based on the contribution health can make to the developmental tasks just discussed.

THE ROLE OF HEALTH

Let's now consider a parallel role for health that complements the more traditional approaches. This role can be summarized in this way: The presence of health supports the activities that constitute your movement into, within, and through the areas of growth and development described. As a result, you feel increasing levels of personal competence, which is the basis for experiencing a meaningful sense of well-being.

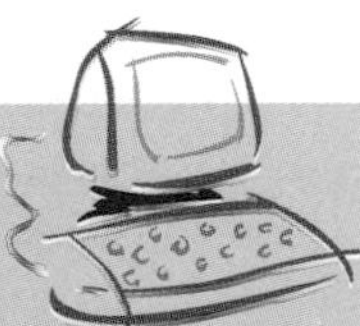

OnSITE/InSIGHT

Learning to Go: Health

Getting tired of your study routine? Click on the Motivator icon for a different slant on studying. Check out these lessons, which make a good match for this chapter:

Lesson 1: Chart a plan for behavior change.
Lesson 2: Strive for multidimensional health.

STUDENT POLL

Thinking about shaping up your health? Go to the Online Learning Center at **www.mhhe.com/hahn6e**. Click on Student Resources to find the Student Poll, where you can answer these questions. Then find out how other students responded.

1. Is improving your health a high priority for you?
2. Do you believe you have control over your own health?
3. Do you take a proactive, preventive approach to your health?
4. Are your eating habits nutritionally sound?
5. Do you consider yourself in good physical shape?
6. Do you search out health information?
7. Is there balance in the different areas of your life?
8. Do you have strong friendships?
9. Do you consider yourself emotionally well balanced?
10. Is being smart important to you?
11. Do you see a spiritual aspect to your everyday life?
12. Is what you're doing today preparing you for your future?
13. Are you career-oriented?
14. Is becoming an adult an important milestone for you?
15. Do you agree that "If you've got your health, you've got everything?

THE COMPOSITION OF HEALTH

Your health is composed of six interacting, dynamic dimensions, each of which provides resources that can be utilized in accomplishing the activities that constitute growth and development within each development area appropriate to young adulthood. Because your health is dynamic, you can modify aspects of its dimensions to help you in your quest for well-being.

Your health is not static. The health you had yesterday no longer exists. The health you aspire to have next week or next year is not guaranteed. However, scientific evidence suggests that what you do today will help determine the quality of your future health. Let's briefly consider each of the six dimensions of health.

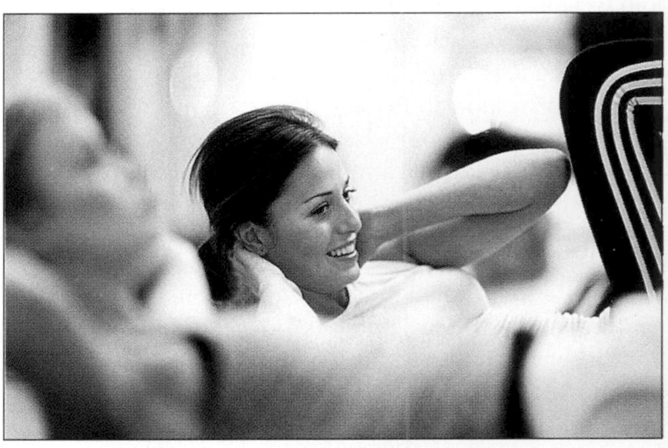

Good physical health helps you develop all the other dimensions of your health.

Physical Dimension

A number of physiological and structural characteristics—including your level of susceptibility to disease, body weight, visual ability, strength, coordination, level of endurance, and powers of recuperation—can help you participate in the experiences that form the basis of your growth and development. In certain situations the physical dimension of your health may be the most important. Perhaps this is why many authorities have traditionally equated health with the design and operation of the body and the absence of illness or a low level of risk for illness.

Emotional Dimension

Your emotional makeup can aid in your progress through the various growth areas. The emotional dimension of health includes the degree to which you are able to cope with stress, remain flexible, and compromise to resolve conflict. This dimension is most closely related to your feelings. How you feel about your family and friends, your life goals and ambitions, and your daily life situations is all tied to the emotional dimension of health.

Your growth and development can be associated with some vulnerability, which may lead to feelings of rejection and failure, reducing your overall productivity and satisfaction. People who consistently try to improve their emotional health appear to lead lives of greater enjoyment than those who let feelings of vulnerability overwhelm them or block their creativity. Specific techniques for improving your emotional health are presented in Chapter 2.

Social Dimension

Social ability is the third dimension of total health. Whether you identify it as social graces, skills, or insights, you probably have many strengths in this area. Because most of your growth and development has occurred in the presence of others, you can appreciate how this dimension of your health may become even more important in your future development.

The social abilities of many nontraditional-age students may already be firmly established. Entering college may encourage them to develop new social skills that help them socialize with their traditional-age student colleagues. After being on campus for a while, nontraditional-age students often interact comfortably with traditional-age students in such diverse places as the classroom, the student center, and the library. This type of interaction enhances the social dimension of health for both.

Intellectual Dimension

Your ability to process and act on information, clarify values and beliefs, and exercise your decision-making capacity is one of the most important aspects of total health. Coping skills, muscular strength, or the knack of saying the right thing at the right time may not serve you as well as the ability to use information or understand a new idea. A refusal to grasp new information or undertake an analysis of your beliefs could hinder the degree of growth and development that your college experience can provide.

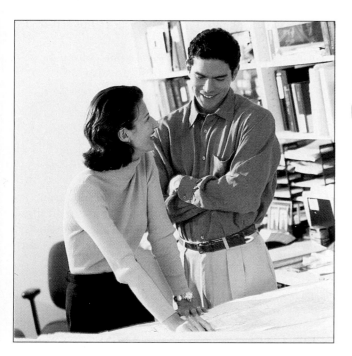

People who feel good about their work often have high self-esteem.

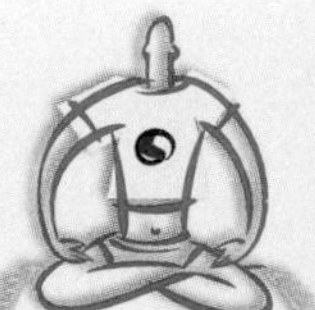

Exploring Your Spirituality

Pondering the Meaning of Life

In a survey conducted in May of 1999 by Yankelovich Partners for the Lutheran Brotherhood (an insurance company affiliated with the Lutheran Church), a large, randomly selected sample of American adults was asked a version of the following question: "If you were able to do so, what questions would you ask God or a supreme being?" The most commonly asked question (34%) was: "What is my purpose for being here?" The second (19%) and third (16%) most frequently raised questions were: "Will I have life after death?" and "Why do bad things happen?" The remaining responses reported were: "Is there intelligent life elsewhere?" (7%) and "How long will I live?" (6%). A variety of other questions were asked but not reported on. Twelve percent of the respondents said that they would not (or could not) ask a question, even if given the opportunity.

If it is assumed that these questions are common to the vast majority of Americans (at least on occasion), in the absence of a theology-based belief system, to whom would they be directed? Perhaps to a respected academic, a wise elder, a seasoned veteran of the "school of hard knocks," or a mystic? On the other hand, for those with such a belief system, answers may never be expected. The process of asking in itself may create a sense of inner peace centered on the belief that there is someone (or something) that does have answers to these and other profound questions of life and that eventually those answers will be known.

Spiritual Dimension

The fifth dimension of health is spiritual. Although you can include your religious beliefs and practices in this category, this discussion focuses on your relationship to other living things, the role of a spiritual direction in your life, the nature of human behavior, and your willingness to serve others.

Many of today's students appear to be searching for a deeper understanding of the meaning of life. Although you may not feel uneasy about the nature of your spiritual beliefs, many students do feel anxious about the spiritual side of their lives. In fact, one explanation for the renewed interest in the spiritual dimension of health may stem from its value as a resource for lessening personal stress. The spiritual dimension is so significant that some health professionals believe it to be the actual "core of wellness."

Cultivating the spiritual side of your health may help you discover how you fit into this universe. You can enhance your spiritual health in a variety of ways, many of which involve opening yourself to new experiences with nature, art, body movement, or music. For many Americans, the spiritual dimension of health is enhanced through an affiliation with a organized religion or belief system. For these people, the existence of a commonly shared doctrine describing the existence of God or an omnipotent Spirit, a familiar set of practices, and a sense of community with others helps provides meaningful answers to life's most profound questions (see the Exploring Your Spirituality box on p. 11). However, such religious affiliation is not essential to enjoying a meaningful spiritual life.

Occupational Dimension

The sixth dimension of health reflects the fact that employment satisfaction is directly related to health. When people feel good about their jobs, they tend to feel good about themselves and are more likely to have a healthier lifestyle. Usually, people have positive feelings about their employment situation if their jobs provide both external rewards (such as adequate salary and benefits) and internal rewards (such as positive social interactions and the opportunity for creative input).

Your future occupation will be linked to your future health status. Many colleges have career counseling offices, where students can talk with professionals about career opportunities. Sometimes during career counseling, students undertake a series of psychological tests to help determine the kinds of jobs that match their personality profiles. Students can also learn about job opportunities in their major areas of study by talking with professors or from volunteer work, student employment or internships, and summer job experiences.

A NEW DEFINITION OF HEALTH

By combining the role of health with the composition of health, this book offers a new and unique definition of health:

> Health is the ability to access and apply resources from the six dimensions of health to the experiences of daily living, thus assuring growth and development and the sense of well-being that it affords.

Remember that this blending of your health resources is a never-ending process. Whether you are a traditional-age or nontraditional-age student, your ability to master the daily demands of living, thus assuring your continued growth and development, hinges on this unique combination of health dimensions.

SUMMARY

- Episodic medicine, preventive medicine, health promotion, and wellness have contributed to our traditional perceptions of health, which are based on morbidity and mortality and their consequences.
- Broadly based programs, such as *Healthy People 2000* and *Healthy People 2010,* seek to improve health by developing risk reduction programs, assuring greater access to health care services, and eliminating disparities that exist between various segments of the population.
- Five important areas of growth and development await people ages 18 to 40, which increasingly characterizes today's college student population.
- A six-dimensional model of health is based on growth and development and complements the traditional health models.
- Health is the ability to apply one's resources from the six dimensions to daily living, assuring growth and development and a sense of well-being.

REVIEW QUESTIONS

1. What is the relationship between the term *episodic medicine* and our most familiar definition of health?
2. How are preventive medicine and health promotion similar? In what important way are they different?
3. What do the terms *morbidity* and *mortality* mean?
4. How does wellness differ from the other definitions of health discussed in this chapter?
5. How does *Healthy People 2010* differ from its predecessor, *Healthy People 2000?*
6. What are the five areas of growth and development discussed in this text? How does each relate to the lives of people between ages 18 and 40?
7. What are the six dimensions of health? How do they relate to the composition of health as discussed in this text?

THINK ABOUT THIS . . .

- There is no perfect version of what an adult should be like. From what you've heard other people say, what type of knowledge, attitudes, and activities characterize a successful, well-adjusted adult? What are your own intentions for adulthood in these areas?
- Few parents want their children to become so independent that all communication, particularly involving advice and various forms of support, would cease. If you are a traditional-age student, how do you think your family perceives your future level of independence? If you are a nontraditional-age student and parent, how have you fostered independence in your children while retaining important ties to them?
- Envision yourself in a conversation with the person who is soon to become your life partner. You are talking about the role of parenting in your partnership. What would you say about the number of children, the spacing between children, and the specific approach to rearing children that would be acceptable to you? If you should decide to be child-free, what would you say to others (including your future partner) if they suggest that your decision is based on selfishness or lack of self-confidence?
- A good college friend shares with you his concerns about the possibility of never marrying (or being in a life partnership). Sensing that these concerns are genuine, and therefore extremely important, what would you tell your friend about the intimacy that can exist in other types of relationships?

REFERENCES

1. Kochanek KD, Smith BL, Anderson RN: Deaths: preliminary data for 1999. *National Vital Statistics Reports,* 49:3, 1–49, 2001.
2. *Healthy people 2000: national health promotion and disease prevention objectives* [Full report, with commentary], Washington, DC, 1991, U.S. Department of Health and Human Services, Public Health Service, DHHS publication no. (PHS) 91-50212.
3. *Healthy people 2000: a midcourse review and 1995 revisions,* Washington, D.C., 1994, U.S. Department of Health and Human Services, Public Health Service, DHHS publication no. (PHS) 94-1232-1.
4. *Developing objectives for healthy people 2010,* Washington, D.C., 1997, U.S. Department of Health and Human Services, Office of Disease Prevention and Health Promotion.
5. *Health for all in the 21st century.* World Health Organization. Geneva, Switzerland, 1979.

SUGGESTED READINGS

Angier N: *Woman: an intimate geography,* Boston, 1999, Houghton-Mifflin.
From unending praise to almost total rejection, this book elicits differing opinions about its blending of information from the biological sciences, cultural anthropology, evolutionary psychology, mythology, history, and other academic fields to explore the subject of being a woman. Even the author's writing style has been praised and criticized. You'll have to read it for yourself and see what you think!

Brown C: *Afterwards, you're a genius: faith, medicine, and the metaphysics of healing.* New York, 1998, Penguin.
In this highly regarded book, the author, who is a journalist, recounts his personal journey into the complex world where rational Western medicine, alternative medicine, and New Age healing interface. You're likely to find the author's uniquely personal and humorous writing style appealing, even if you question some of his conclusions.

Viorst J: *You're officially a grown-up: the graduate's guide to freedom, responsibility, happiness, personal hygiene, and the conquest of fear,* New York, 1999, Simon & Schuster.
This book is from the author of *Alexander and the Terrible, Horrible, No Good, Very Bad Day.* It's an everything-you-need-to-know guide to leaving adolescence and entering the world of adults. This witty book makes a great gift for the college graduate, regardless of age.

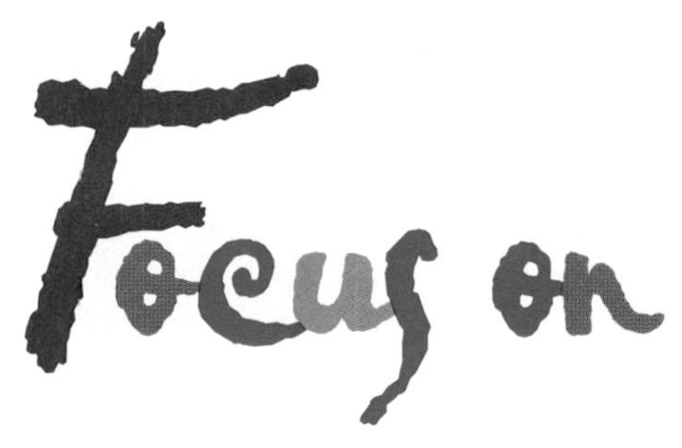

THE DIVERSITY OF TODAY'S COLLEGE STUDENTS

It's the fall of 1970, and you're about to meet Joe College, a student in a freshman health class at State University. Joe is an 18-year-old white man who graduated from City High School last summer in the top half of his class. He lives in State U's dormitory. Because his tuition is being paid by his parents, he can devote himself to his studies and college life on a full-time basis. When Joe looks around his health class, he sees some women and a few minorities and older students, but most of the students are much like himself. Joe College is a typical college student.

Flash forward to today. When you look around your health classroom, what kinds of students do you see? Students like Joe College are probably still there, but they don't make up the overwhelming majority of the student body. The many changes in American society that have taken place over the last 30 years are reflected in today's colleges and universities. Currently, slightly more women than men are graduating from college. As more older people find that they need better skills, more training, or a college degree to keep their present jobs or find new ones, the average age of college students has risen. Also, schools are increasing their efforts in actively recruiting minority students. Finally, recent laws affirming the rights of Americans with disabilities to have access to most public facilities are giving individuals with disabilities the opportunity to attend college.

Causes Behind the Changes

Why are these changes occurring? Several factors seem to be affecting enrollment figures in the United States. Clearly, the changing climate of the economy has influenced enrollment. Corporate trends toward a more streamlined workforce and the gradual shift to a service-oriented marketplace have caused many workers to seek training for new careers or additional training for their current jobs. As a result, people who never thought they would see the inside of a classroom again are drawn back to school.

In response to the economic changes just described, colleges have become more accessible in recent years. The trend toward open admissions, especially at community colleges, has opened the doors of higher education to those who otherwise might be held back by low high school grades or low test scores. Colleges are attempting to meet the needs of these new students with remedial courses and special programs designed to prepare them to meet strong academic standards.

Social changes have also played an important role in the changing demographics on college campuses. The Civil Rights movement of the 1950s and 1960s was instrumental in making a college education available to minorities, and minority enrollment has increased as overall awareness of civil rights becomes more entrenched in society. Students with various physical disabilities are also finding it easier to obtain a college education. The Americans with Disabilities Act, signed into law in 1990, guarantees that people with disabilities will have access to employment, education, and public services. As a result, people with disabilities can pursue careers that were previously inaccessible to them, and many are heading to college to receive training for those careers.

As higher education has become more accessible, an attitude change about going to college has occurred. The feeling that everyone should go to college after high school is now more prevalent. Unfortunately, this emphasis on college has produced a cost to many important skilled trades, such as tool- and dye-making and construction. Students who might have once entered apprentice programs in these areas now feel compelled to seek a college degree. The military services have also experienced a similar effect as more and more high school graduates enter the expanding job market or move on to college campuses.

Practical Implications of Diversity on Campus

With the rise of new populations on campuses, many practical changes have taken place to reflect the needs and interests of those students. For example, most college and universities now offer developmental education programs for students who need skill enhancement in reading, writing, and mathematics. Flexibility in the timing of course offerings is designed to accommodate the employment and parenting demands of nontraditional-age students. Many institutions also provide preschool centers for the children of parents who would otherwise find college attendance more difficult or even impossible.

The college student population is also changing in terms of increased numbers of individuals of different racial backgrounds, ethnic groups, and national origin. In response to these developments, a wider range of courses in areas such as history, literature, fine arts, music, drama, and political science is reflected in course catalogs. Faculty composition is also diversifying; however, in some cases, the pool of qualified applicants is small in relation to demand. Campus libraries have expanded the diversity of their collections to accommodate the changing campus population. Likewise, college bookstores offer a wider range of reading and musical selections. The increasing diversity of today's student bodies has also influenced the number and types of extracurricular offerings. Culturally diverse student associations, student political organizations, honor societies, and interest-based groups such as dance troupes are evident on many college campuses. Greater accessibility to the Internet has brought even the most isolated college campuses into the growing diversity that characterizes the population as a whole.

Changing Campuses and the Study of Health

Why mention the many changes taking place on college campuses in a health text? Because of increasing diversity, students who are studying health (and most other disciplines) need to be aware of issues that affect students of different backgrounds. For example, many people are unaware of the fact that most pharmaceutical research is performed on men and then generalized to apply to women. This is a potentially dangerous practice because women are at greater risk for adverse drug reactions. Another example is the use of complementary (alternative) medical practitioners. Native Americans view health care as a holistic, rather than a symptom-based, process. They are more likely to respond to a healer who looks at both the physical and spiritual person, than to a physician, who focuses only on the body. Similarly, some Mexican Americans will either rely on (or supplement traditional health care with) *curanderismo,* a medical system that combines Western health care practices with folklore, magic, herbalism, and religion. Knowledge of these and other related cultural health care issues will help college students understand all members of our culturally diverse society.

Bringing cultural awareness into the health classroom introduces students to concepts they might not otherwise be exposed to. During your college career, you will encounter students from a variety of backgrounds. They may be young or old, rich or poor, from a rural or urban environment, or from an ethnic group different from yours. Just as your culture has its own unique health concerns, every other culture also has its own set of health concerns, and you need to be aware of them. *Focus on Health* will attempt to address the needs of students from different cultural backgrounds.

TALKING POINTS • When controversial subjects are discussed in class, do you think that your opinions (or how you present them) are affected by the fact that students of different cultural backgrounds are involved in the discussion?

part 1

The Mind

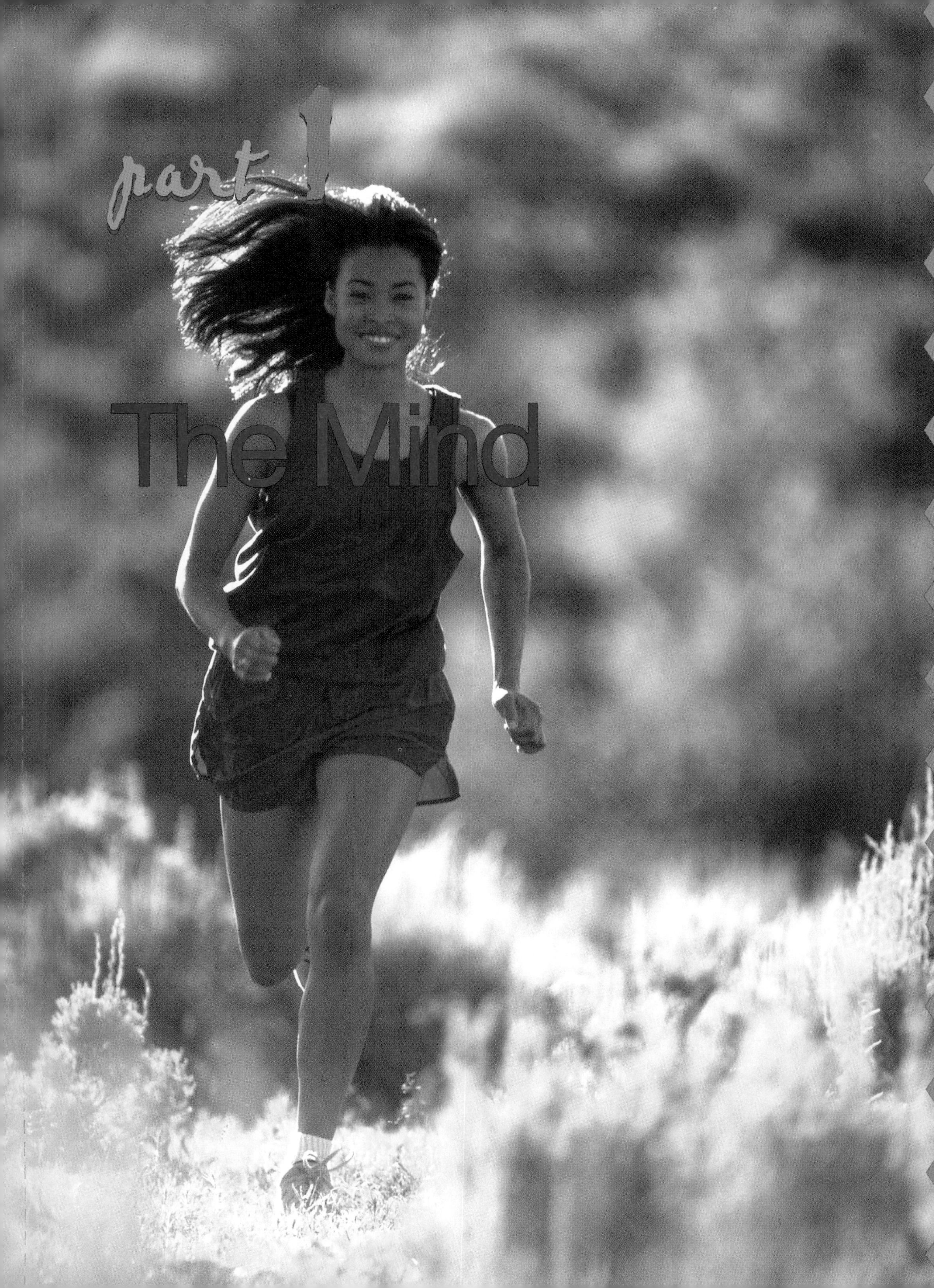

chapter **2**

Achieving Psychological Wellness

Online Learning Center Resources

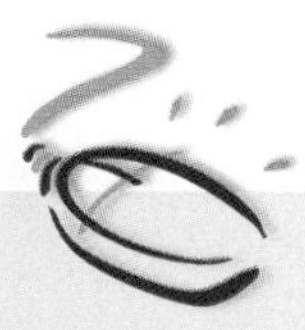

www.mhhe.com/hahn6e

Log on to our Online Learning Center (OLC) for access to these additional resources:

- Chapter key terms and definitions
- Learning objectives
- Additional behavior change objectives
- Student interactive question-and-answer sites
- Self-scoring chapter quiz

The OLC also offers web links for study and exploration of health topics. Here are some examples of what you'll find:

- **www.apa.org** Click here for an encyclopedia of mental health information, including medical diagnostic criteria, descriptions of mental disorders, and common medications used to treat mental disorders.
- **www.shpm.com** Check out this great website by *Self Help and Psychology* magazine for articles on a broad range of emotional health topics.
- **www.metanoia.org/suicide** Don't miss *Suicide: Read This First.*

Taking Charge of Your Health

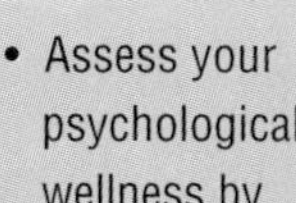

- Assess your psychological wellness by considering the characteristics described on p. 19.
- Think about what your self-concept is like, and list the positive attributes that have shaped it.
- If you are shy, make a special effort to join in a peer group activity that you find interesting.
- Try a new experience to discover new dimensions of your emotional makeup.
- Use dialogue to reach a compromise when you are in a conflict situation.
- Learn to be more proactive in your life by following the four-step process outlined on p. 26.

Eye on the Media

Self-Help Books—Helpful or Hazardous?

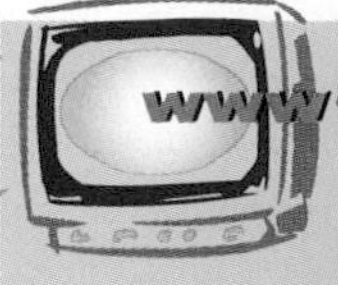

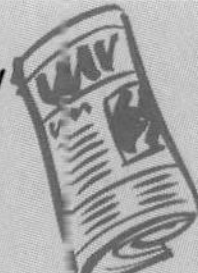

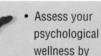

Americans purchase thousands of self-help books each day. These books give them access to information that was once limited to a much smaller segment of the population, mainly professionals. Hundreds of titles focus on improving your psychological well-being. They offer advice on intimate relationships, coping with stress, gender-related issues, and building self-esteem. Many of these books have accompanying audiotapes, computer programs, and workbooks to complement the books' content. Workbooks that let readers chart their progress in changing their behavior (by following the book's advice) are especially popular.

It's difficult to know how effective self-help books are in helping people maintain or regain their psychological well-being. There are almost no scientific studies on the subject. One thing that's certain, though, is that the publishers are skilled at marketing their product. They know that the book titles need to be appealing; for example, *Awaken the Giant Within: How to Take Immediate Control of Your Mental, Emotional, and*

Eye on the Media *continued*

Financial Destiny (by Anthony Robbins); *Alter: A Simple Path to Emotional Wellness* (by Judy Curley); and *Emotional Blackmail: When the People in Your Life Use Fear, Obligation, and Guilt to Manipulate You* (by Susan Forward). They carefully design the dust jackets to catch the eye of consumers. Also, they feature glowing summaries, such as this one for *Emotional Blackmail: When the People in Your Life Use Fear, Obligation, and Guilt to Manipulate You:*

> Susan Forward knows what pushes our hot buttons. Just as John Gray illuminates the communications gap between the sexes in *Men Are From Mars, Women Are From Venus,* and Harriet Lerner describes an intricate dynamic in *The Dance of Anger,* so Susan Forward presents the anatomy of a relationship damaged by manipulation, and gives readers an arsenal of tools to fight back.

Publishers also highlight reviews by people who have read the book and tried its strategies. Here's one "reader's review" for the same book:

> An absolute MUST READ for everyone! Susan's book is fantastic. The information is priceless. I was trapped in a fog for many years, and after reading this book, my eyes opened WIDE. Now, I not only see how others manipulate with emotions, but also how I've manipulated myself! This should be a part of the infamous "Manual" we should get when we're born.

With this type of strong marketing and no objective way to measure how effective self-help books are, how can we judge their usefulness? The American Psychological Association (APA) says the answer is clear—we can't. After reviewing the limited research done on the subject, the APA presented these conclusions:

- Some self-help books on psychological wellness do appear to be helpful, based on anecdotal reports (reports based on personal experience, such as the one you just read), but why this should be so is unclear.
- There appears to be little relationship between the academic credentials of the authors and the effectiveness of their books, again based on anecdotal reports of helpfulness.
- There appears to be little relationship between successful clinically based approaches to enhancing psychological well-being and books designed to depict how to use these approaches in a nonclinical setting, such as the home or with friends or coworkers.

What all this means to you, the reader, is that you're truly on your own when you're browsing through self-help books at your favorite bookstore or checking out titles on the Internet. Does the author have good credentials and experience in his/her field? Is he/she affiliated with a respected university or organization? Of course, that's not everything—and certainly not a guarantee. But it's a good way to start.

People who are emotionally healthy have a high level of self-esteem. For them, social interaction is comfortable and rewarding. Adequate self-esteem is so important that it is sometimes equated with psychological wellness. But don't expect to feel personally fulfilled by everything. There will always be situations in which you must act against your own best interests for the sake of others. And if you should be faced with a serious health problem, your strong self-esteem will help you, but it won't completely offset this challenge.

CHARACTERISTICS OF A PSYCHOLOGICALLY WELL PERSON

A psychologically well person is one who is capable of using resources from each of the six dimensions of health (see Chapter 1) to feel good about life and other people. A more specific yardstick for measuring emotional health comes from the National Mental Health Association. This group describes emotionally well people as having three fundamental characteristics:[1]

- They feel comfortable about themselves. They are not overwhelmed by their own feelings, and they can accept many of life's disappointments in stride. They experience the full range of human emotions (for example, fear, anger, love, jealousy, guilt, and joy) but are not overcome by them.
- They interact well with other people. They are comfortable with others and are able to give and receive love. They are concerned about others' well-being and have relationships that are satisfying and lasting.
- They are able to meet the demands of life. Emotionally healthy people respond appropriately to their problems, accept responsibility, plan ahead without fearing the future, and are able to establish reachable goals.

It's important to realize that emotionally well people are not perfect. At times, they experience stress, frustration, self-doubt, failure, and rejection. What distinguishes the emotionally well person is resilience—the ability to recapture a sense of psychological wellness within a reasonable time after encountering a difficult situation.

EMOTIONAL AND PSYCHOLOGICAL WELLNESS

Is there a difference between emotional and psychological wellness? Many people don't think so. They believe that both reflect the absence of emotional illness and psychopathological conditions. However, other people think that emotional health refers specifically to the feelings people have in response to changes in their environment. These feelings, such as anger, jealousy, joy, disappointment, compassion, and sympathy, are familiar, healthy emotions. Responses to change vary from one person to the next and reflect each person's values. Emotionally healthy people feel good about their responses. Those who are less emotionally well feel negative about their responses.

In contrast to emotional health, some people think that psychological health refers more broadly to the development and functioning of a wide array of mental abilities, such as language, memory, perception, and awareness. For example, a person who believes he is being followed by government agents has faulty perception, so he would be considered not psychologically healthy. People who are psychologically healthy deal rationally with the world, have a fully functional personality, and resolve conflicts constructively. Finally, the psychophysical (mind-body) interface of the psychologically healthy person is sound.

Specific forms of psychological disfunction, including schizophrenic disorders, and forms of psychotherapy, are discussed in the Appendix.

Normal Range of Emotions

Do you know people who seem to be "up" all the time? These people appear to be confident, happy, and full of good feelings 24 hours a day. Although some people are like that, they are truly the exceptions. For most people, emotions are more like a roller coaster ride. Sometimes they feel good about themselves and others, but other times nothing seems to go right. This is normal and healthy. Life has its ups and downs, and the concept of the "normal range of emotions" reflects these changes.

Self-Esteem

The key to overall psychological wellness is self-esteem. When people have positive self-esteem, they feel comfortable in social situations and with their own thoughts and feelings. They get along with others, cope in stressful situations, and make contributions when they work with others. Strong self-esteem may offset self-defeating or self-destructive behavior problems. For example, a young woman who is slightly overweight but has high self-esteem would be unlikely to go on an unhealthy crash diet to conform to the currently fashionable thin body image. As you will see when you complete the Personal Assessment on p. 33, people with high levels of self-esteem find a comfortable balance between their idealized self and where they actually are.

The foundation of positive self-esteem can be traced to childhood.[2] Interactions that young children experience can create powerful messages about their self-

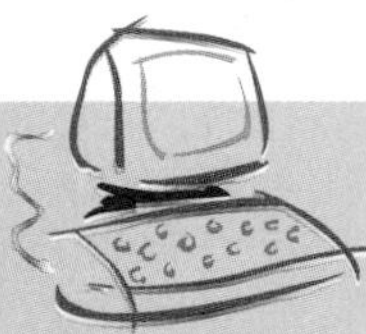

OnSITE/InSIGHT

Learning to Go: Health

Did you know that emotional health is just as important as physical health? Click on the Motivator icon to explore these lessons, which are ideal for this chapter:

Lesson 3: Boost your emotional health.
Lesson 4: Expand your communication skills.
Lesson 5: Approach your life proactively.
Lesson 6: Get a handle on mood disorders.
Lesson 7: Battle against depression.
Lesson 8: Seek both emotional and psychological wellness.

STUDENT POLL

What do you think about your own psychological wellness? Go to the Online Learning Center at **www.mhhe.com/hahn6e**. Click on Student Resources to find the Student Poll. There you can answer these questions and then compare your responses to those of other students.

1. Do you consider your range of emotions to be normal?
2. Are you able to maintain good self-esteem?
3. Do you like to try new things?
4. Is relaxing difficult for you?
5. Do you practice positive self-talk?
6. Do you interact well with others?
7. Do you have a good relationship with your family?
8. Have you ever suffered from depression?
9. Do you avoid confrontation?
10. Does voicing your opinion come easily to you?
11. Do you often feel lonely?
12. Is it important to you to be proactive?

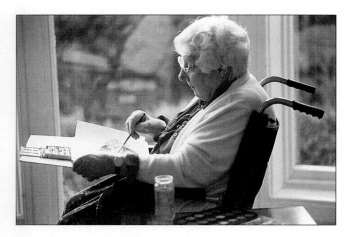

Expressing creativity helps people improve their self-esteem.

worth. Warm and supportive physical and emotional contact, communication that emphasizes talking "with" rather than "to" the child, and gradual loosening of control so that more and more decisions are made by the child tell children that they are competent and valued. Children's emerging self-esteem, then, is strongly influenced by their parents' behavior. Children from less supportive or overly protective home environments will eventually seek positive feedback from other sources.

As important as parents and others (including peers) are to the development of self-esteem in children, people eventually become responsible for enhancing their own self-esteem. The extent to which people wish to nurture their self-esteem varies. However, many want to take an active role in developing a more solid sense of self-worth.

Hardiness

Hardiness and self-esteem work together to ensure psychological wellness.[3] Hardiness exists when a person consistently shows three important traits. First, hardy people possess a high level of *commitment* to something or someone; this commitment is the basis for their value orientation and sense of purpose in life. Maintaining this sense of commitment provides structure and direction, even in the face of a wide variety of stressors (see Chapter 3). Second, a sense of *control* characterizes hardy people. By possessing the ability to orchestrate the events in their lives, hardy people reduce their chance of feeling helpless and vulnerable when change is imposed from outside. Third, hardy people welcome *challenge*. They have the ability to take control of change and shape it to enhance their personal growth and fulfillment.

Hardiness may be more common among some types of people than others. Nevertheless, a high level of hardiness can be developed by focusing on signals from the body, assessing and responding to previous stressors, and engaging in activities that strengthen commitment, control, and challenge.

CHALLENGES TO PSYCHOLOGICAL WELLNESS

In spite of their best efforts to be hardy and resilient, many people have a less than optimal level of psychological wellness. Depression is the most common and one of the most treatable of these dysfunctional emotional states. Loneliness, shyness, and thoughts of suicide are also challenges to high-level psychological wellness. Although this chapter focuses on psychological well-being rather than emotional illness, it's important to examine these conditions. At some time during our lives, most of us will either have emotional problems ourselves or know someone who is experiencing them.

Depression

Depression is an emotional state characterized by feelings of sadness, melancholy, dejection, worthlessness, emptiness, and hopelessness that are inappropriate and out of proportion to reality.[4] The common symptoms of depression are listed in the Star Box below. One key indicator of depression is the long-term presence of some of these symptoms. Everyone feels down or blue at times, but depression is characterized by a chronic state of feeling low (see the Changing for the Better box on p. 22 and 27).

In the United States, approximately 30% to 40% of all college students self-report symptoms of depression, and 5% of health center prescriptions are for antidepressants. Students with depression commonly have a number of compounding problems, including family problems and difficulty with social relationships. Depression is a common factor related to most suicides.

Types of depression

According to mental health experts, there are two main types of depression. When depression develops after a

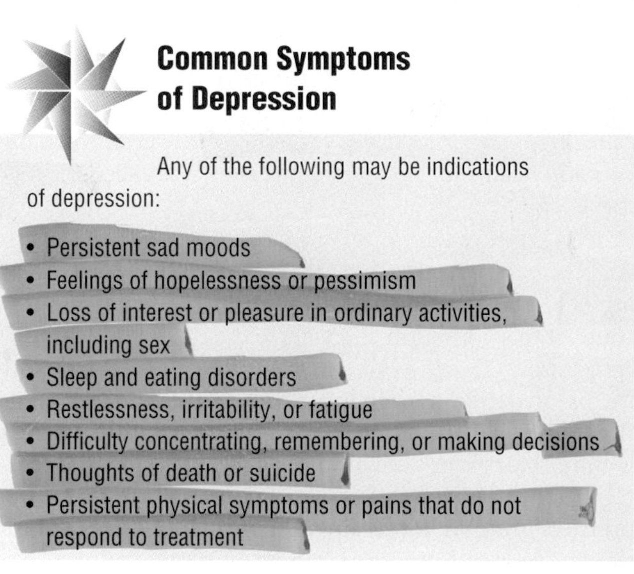

Common Symptoms of Depression

Any of the following may be indications of depression:

- Persistent sad moods
- Feelings of hopelessness or pessimism
- Loss of interest or pleasure in ordinary activities, including sex
- Sleep and eating disorders
- Restlessness, irritability, or fatigue
- Difficulty concentrating, remembering, or making decisions
- Thoughts of death or suicide
- Persistent physical symptoms or pains that do not respond to treatment

Changing *for the Better*

Taking the First Step in Fighting Depression

Making the transition to college has been very tough for me. I feel down a lot, and I'm starting to think I'll never get rid of this feeling. Where do I go for help?

- Seek help from your university health center, personal physician, or community health center.
- Try your university mental health counseling and treatment programs.
- Family and social service agencies can identify mental health specialists.
- Check the telephone book for private psychologists or psychiatric clinics.
- Talk with a trusted professor.
- Contact one of the organizations listed below.

The Depression/Awareness, Recognition and Treatment Program (operated by the National Institute of Mental Health)
5600 Fishers Lane
Room 15-C-05
Rockville, MD 20857
(301) 460-3062

The National Foundation for Depressive Illness
P.O. Box 2257
New York, NY 10016-2257
(800) 248-4344
www.depression.org

The National Mental Health Association
1021 Prince Street
Alexandria, VA 22314
(703) 684-7722
www.nmha.org

Changing *for the Better*

Fostering Your Emotional Growth

As a 32-year-old college student, I feel as though I'm being pulled in too many different directions. Sometimes I think I'm losing my sense of self or wonder if I ever had one. What can I do to help myself grow emotionally?

Emotional growth requires two things from you—knowledge about yourself and willingness to undertake new activities and experiences and learn from them. People who actively promote their psychological wellness take steps toward this end. For example, many keep journals to record the events of the day. More important, they note how they felt about these events and how they managed any associated stress. Others join support groups, which allow them to interact empathetically (sharing their feelings and experiences) with others. Such groups create a sense of community that enriches the psychological well-being of all involved.

Many people find that counseling helps them maintain or reestablish a sense of psychological well-being. Growth-enhancing skills can be developed in individual or group counseling sessions, with a variety of effective counseling strategies used. As a college student, you have access to counseling services that are both dependable and affordable. Contacting the campus health center or psychological services center for referral may be the first step in improving your psychological well-being.

period of difficulty, such as a divorce or loss of a job, it is called *secondary* or *reactive depression.* However, when depression begins for no apparent reason, it is called *primary depression* and is caused by changes in brain chemistry. When taken in combination, these two forms of depression are incapacitating enough to be classified as *major depression*. The duration and depth of major depression is in contrast to a condition characterized by chronic periods of "blueness" that is clinically labeled as *dysthymia.* Both forms of major depression can be successfully treated through a combination of approaches, and recovery within 2 years is not uncommon, although never assured.

Today, the most effective treatments for major depression are psychotherapy and antidepressant medications. The psychotherapy model of choice is usually a form of cognitive-based therapy (CBT), in which the depressed person learns how to recognize and deal with life situations in a constructive fashion. Drug therapy typically involves one or more of four classes of antidepressive medications: monoamine oxidase (MAO) inhibitors, tricyclic antidepressants, selective serotonin reuptake inhibitors (SSRIs) such as Prozac, and the new serotonin/norepinephrine reuptake inhibitors such as Serzone and Effexor.[5] Recent research indicates that both psychotherapy and antidepressants can be effective when used alone or in combination.[6] This contrasts with the heavy reliance on antidepressive medication alone favored during the past decade.

Only a small percentage (about 33%) of depressed people ever seek help. This is unfortunate in light of the high rate of successful treatment. The Changing for the Better box above lists several resources for people with depression.

Some people try to treat their depression by taking over-the-counter substances such as St. John's wort. This popular form of self-treatment should be viewed with caution and should be used only after consultation with your physician (see Star Box on p. 23).

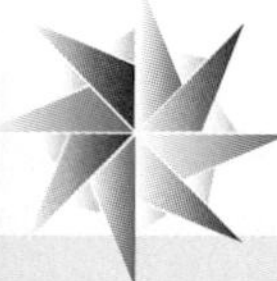

St. John's Wort for the Treatment of Depression

In a 1998 study conducted for Celestial Seasonings, it was reported that 97% of adults between ages 18 and 54 use (or have used) an herbal dietary supplement as an aid to better health. One of the most commonly used substances (17%) was St. John's wort, a dietary supplement reported to be effective in treating mild to moderate depression. Since 17 million Americans are classified as clinically depressed and an additional 10 million experience dysthymia, a less severe but chronic form of depression, the market potential for St. John's wort is sizable.

St. John's wort was introduced in the United States via Germany, where it had been researched (23 studies) and used effectively by physicians in the treatment of depression for many years. Even today in Germany, St. John's wort is a prescribed medication that is closely monitored by physicians and manufactured under governmental supervision to ensure potency. In contrast, the St. John's wort marketed in the United States is an over-the-counter dietary supplement that is not regulated by the Food and Drug Administration (FDA). It is manufactured in a variety of formulations by companies ranging from large pharmaceutical houses with international name recognition to small regional laboratories and is sold under many brand names. This lack of supervision in formulation and manufacturing was clearly evident in a recent study commissioned by the *Los Angeles Times,* in which it was found that the amount of active ingredient, hypericum, in seven of the ten largest-selling brands of St. John's wort ranged from 65% below to 135% above the labeled amount.

In 1997, a meta-analysis of twenty-three studies conducted in Europe was undertaken by the National Center for Complementary and Alternative Medicine. Results of this assessment suggested that St. John's wort was effective in treating mild to moderate depression when compared to antidepressants.[7] However, the design of many of these studies was questioned.

In a more recent and carefully controlled study involving 200 patients at Vanderbilt University Hospital, St. John's wort was found to be no more effective than a placebo in treating clinical depression. Experts believe that this finding is more reliable than that reported in 1997 and that, once accepted by the general public, it will result in less time being lost through self-treating of depression with an ineffective dietary supplement.[7] Additionally, in spite of the popularity of St. John's wort, an extensive review of the pharmacological and toxicological literature conducted in 2001 indicates that little is known about its potential adverse reactions with either prescription or OTC medications,[8] although concern has been noted regarding adverse interactions with surgical anesthetics.

Loneliness

Many depressed people display signs of loneliness, but loneliness is not always associated with depression. People are said to be lonely if they want close personal relationships but cannot establish them. It's possible to feel isolated and friendless even when you are around many people every day. In fact, loneliness is common among college students.

The difference between "being alone" and "feeling lonely" is important. Many people enjoy being alone occasionally to relax, exercise, read, enjoy music, or just think. These people can appreciate being alone, but they can also interact comfortably with others when they wish. However, when being alone or isolated is not enjoyable and seeking close relationships is very difficult, loneliness can produce serious feelings of rejection.

One unfortunate aspect of loneliness is that it tends to continue in people year after year unless they actively try to change it. Chronically lonely people frequently cope with their loneliness by becoming consumed by their occupations or by adopting habit-forming behaviors that increase their sense of loneliness (such as drinking alcohol).

Fortunately, there are successful techniques to help most lonely people. Counseling can help them change how they think about themselves when they interact with others. Another technique involves teaching people important social skills, such as starting a conversation, taking social risks, and introducing themselves. Through social skills training, people can also learn how to talk comfortably on the telephone, give and receive compliments, and enhance their appearance. If you need help in this area, contact your campus counseling center or health center.

Shyness

Is loneliness the result of an inability to interact comfortably with others, something brought about by shyness? If so, why are some people so shy? Some argue that shyness is a genetic part of a person's temperament. They believe that shy people do not want to be shy, have not been conditioned to avoid contact with others, and have not had unpleasant experiences with others. Instead, they are genetically predisposed to feel uncomfortable with other people. So shy people cope by avoiding such situations. Even if shyness is a genetic trait, social skills counseling and training can help those who are shy. Today, clinicians label shyness as *social anxiety.* When identified as a component of "type D" personality, shyness may play a role in the progression of some forms of cardiovascular disease and cancer.[9]

TALKING POINTS • You've noticed that one of your friends always seems to avoid doing anything new. What would you say to this person about the importance of new experiences?

Suicide

One of the tragedies of our times is the high incidence of suicide. In 1999 the last year for which statistics are available, 30,575 people in the United States killed themselves, including 3,885 between the ages of 15 and 25 years.[10] Among young people (including college students), suicides are the third leading cause of death (accidents and homicides being first and second).

What separates the potentially suicidal person from the nonsuicidal person is the degree of despair and depression the person feels and the person's ability to cope with it. Suicidal people tend to become overwhelmed by a range of destructive emotions, including anxiety, anger, loneliness, loss of self-esteem, and hopelessness. They may believe that death is the only solution to all of their problems.

Some college students have committed suicide in a mistaken attempt to resolve academic failure, relationship difficulties, or problems of unemployment. This "solution" is tragic for them and for their families and friends.

Suicide prevention

Many communities currently recognize the need to provide or expand suicide prevention services. Most suicide prevention centers operate 24-hour hotlines and are staffed through volunteer agencies, mental health centers, public health departments, or hospitals. Staff members have extensive training in the counseling skills required to deal with suicidal people. Phone numbers for these services can be found in the telephone directory.

It is critically important to be alert for signs suggesting suicidal tendencies in the people you know. A family member, friend, or residence hall neighbor should be guided toward professional intervention if signs of suicidal intentions begin to cluster in a short time. Any combination of changes in appetite, sleep patterns, concentration, and routine activities should be noted. In addition, increases in agitation, social withdrawal, feelings of hopelessness and self-reproach, and guilt are also cause for concern. A person who is openly talking about or planning a suicide, giving away prized possessions, suggesting that he or she is no longer loved and supported by others, or experiencing extreme humiliation should be called to the attention of intervention experts immediately.

TALKING POINTS • How would you approach a friend who is displaying suicidal tendencies to discuss his or her need for professional intervention?

ENHANCING PSYCHOLOGICAL WELLNESS

Most people have the opportunity to function at an enhanced level of psychological well-being. This state is often achieved by improving certain skills and abilities, including improving verbal and nonverbal communication, learning to use humor effectively, developing better conflict resolution skills, and taking a proactive approach to life. This section explores each of these facets of psychological well-being enhancement.

Improving Communication

Communication can be viewed in terms of your role as sender or receiver. In sending messages, you can enhance the effectiveness of your *verbal* communication in several ways. First, take time before speaking to understand what needs to be said. For example, does the audience/listener need information, encouragement, humor, or something else? Try to focus on the most important thoughts and ideas. Talk *with,* rather than at, listeners to encourage productive exchanges. Begin all verbal exchanges on a positive note, and maintain a positive environment. Use "minimal encouragers," such as short questions, to gain feedback. Avoid using slanted language, which can be destructive to communication. Recognize when other forms of communication, such as e-mail messages or handwritten notes, would be better for transmitting information or ideas.

You also need to be a skilled listener. First, listen attentively in order to hear everything that is being said. Then listen selectively, filtering out information that is repetitious or unrelated to the main point. In a polite way, stop the speaker at certain points and ask him or her to repeat or rephrase the information. This technique helps you to understand what the speaker really means rather than focusing on your own responses.

Communication skills are also very important in your personal life, especially in your intimate relationships. An approach to improving your skills in this area is outlined in the Changing for the Better box on p. 25.

Strengthening your *nonverbal* communication skills may also enhance your psychological well-being. One way to do this is by using facial expressions. For example, a smile usually opens lines of communication. Eye contact is also important, although staring is undesirable. Practice using effective eye contact by studying your facial expressions in the mirror. Keeping a comfortable distance from the people you are speaking to, wearing appropriate clothing, and maintaining good posture all contribute to effective communication.

Changing *for the Better*

Communication Counts in a Close Relationship

My partner and I have been living together for 2 years. We get along well most of the time, but when we try to talk about problems, we just can't connect. How do we learn to communicate better?

- Schedule the conversation so that you and the other person will be prepared for it.
- Choose a neutral setting to lessen the possibility of hostility.
- Set aside any preoccupations before starting the discussion.
- State your position clearly and nonaggressively.
- Keep your tone, manner of speaking, and body language respectful.
- Focus on the topic at hand.
- Be specific when you praise or criticize.
- Listen to what the other person is saying—not just the words but the feelings behind them.
- Avoid using trigger words that might turn a discussion into an argument.
- Suggest and ask for ideas about a course of action that will help resolve the problem.

If you follow these suggestions, you'll be taking into account the psychological well-being of the other person and yourself. This creates a sense of equality within the intimate relationship. Since both of you will be aware of this fact, you'll begin on a positive note.

Using Humor Effectively

Having a sense of humor is an important component of high-level psychological wellness. It means recognizing that life is not meant to be one long, boring exercise. Part of the reason for living is to have fun. So it's a good idea not take yourself or your life situations too seriously.

Recognizing the humor in everyday situations and being able to laugh at yourself will make you feel better about yourself. People who build humor into their daily lives generally feel positive, and others enjoy being around them. Some researchers have suggested that recovery from an injury or illness is enhanced when patients maintain a sense of humor.[11] In the medical field, *therapeutic humor* can be used effectively with other forms of therapy, as demonstrated in the film *Patch Adams.*

Improving Conflict Management Skills

In spite of our best efforts to avoid it, conflict regularly occurs when people interact. In fact, it is the presence of conflict, and the change that arises from its resolution, that leads to growth. The ability to meet and resolve conflict reflects a mature state of psychological wellness. However, some forms of conflict resolution are more effective than others. The following discussion describes different approaches to conflict resolution.

Many people believe that a *hostile aggressive* approach to conflict resolution, in which the parties involved use force to win, is the least emotionally mature way of resolving differences. For example, attacking others for simply disagreeing shows both hostility and aggression. Whether the weapon used is a loud voice or a physical blow, this approach usually leads to more and deeper conflict.

Submission is another unacceptable technique for resolving conflict. When one person involved in the conflict gives in, the disagreement may appear to have been resolved. Yet the accommodating party generally remains angry. The conflict is merely driven temporarily out of sight and is likely to reappear later in a more intense form. Ask yourself, for example, "How long would I be willing to do only what others want, rather than what I would enjoy doing, before I became angry and resentful?"

Another emotionally immature approach to conflict resolution is *withdrawal.* Simply walking out of a room to avoid further disagreement is an example of this method. This approach may calm the atmosphere, but it rarely leads to a true and constructive resolution of the conflict. Withdrawal can be constructive if it provides time for one or both people to rethink the conflict situation and return to it later, using a more constructive approach.

One positive conflict resolution approach is *persuasion.* In this method, one or both parties use words to explain their reasons for the position they are taking. Pointing out the advantages of pursuing one course of action versus another is an example of persuasion. The idea is to make a convincing presentation, so that the other party involved will be motivated to resolve the conflict—by accepting the position being advanced. If all parties involved are given an opportunity to have the floor, this approach to conflict resolution can be constructive.

Perhaps the most mature conflict resolution technique is *dialogue.* In this approach, a verbal exchange of facts, opinions, and perceptions takes place so that the pros and cons of each of the positions being advanced can be weighed. The goal is to reach an acceptable compromise that all parties involved have helped to formulate. An example of this approach is the lengthy negotiation process that comes before the signing of peace accords between nations. When dialogue is used, often there are no losers in the traditional sense. Instead, the compromise position allows all parties to contribute to a healthier relationship.

Taking a Proactive Approach to Life

In addition to the approaches already discussed, the plan that follows is intended to give you even greater control in enhancing your self-esteem. A key to psychological wellness is the ability to control the outcomes of your experiences and thus learn about your own emotional resources. Figure 2-1 shows a four-step process that continues throughout life: constructing perceptions of yourself, accepting these perceptions, undertaking new experiences, and reframing your perceptions based on new information. With some thought and practice, this process can be undertaken regularly by most people.

Constructing mental pictures

Actively taking charge of your emotional growth begins with constructing a mental picture of what you're like. Use the most recent and accurate information you have about yourself—what is important to you, your values, and your competencies.

To construct this mental picture, set aside a period of uninterrupted quiet time for reflection. Even in the midst of a busy schedule, most people can find several moments to complete a task that is important.

Before proceeding to the second step, you also need to construct mental pictures about yourself in relation to *other people and material objects,* including your residence and college or work environment, to clarify these relationships.

For example, after graduating from college with a degree in fine arts, Allison moved to a large city to become a jewelry designer. Two years later, her small business was thriving and she was living in a spacious loft apartment with room for her studio. Still, Allison felt that something was missing. She constructed a mental picture in which she saw herself as a resourceful, creative, independent person who was comfortable in her new surroundings. However, Allison realized that she wanted a partner to share her success and her life.

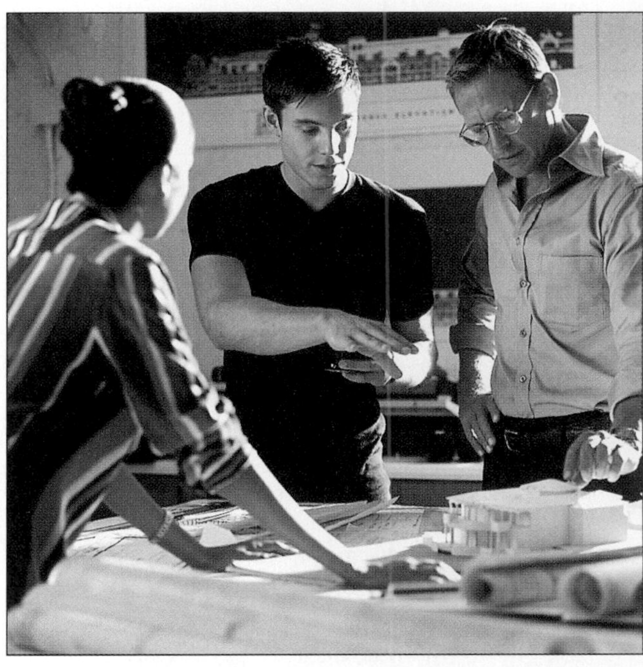

Participating in an internship in a career field that interests you could be a challenging new experience.

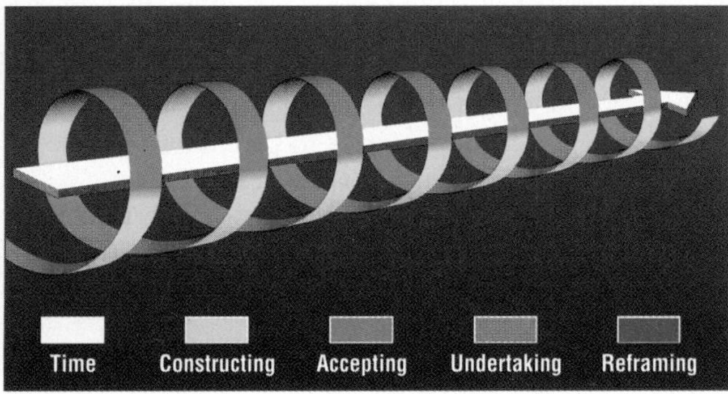

Figure 2-1 If you visualize the growth of the emotional dimension of health as a four-step process, you will see that continued emotional growth occurs in cycles throughout your life.

Accepting mental pictures

The second step of the plan involves an *acceptance* of these perceptions. This implies a willingness to honor the truthfulness of the perceptions you have formed about yourself and other people. For example, Allison should acknowledge her professional success and her artistic ability, but she must also accept the fact that she has been unable to establish the long-term romantic relationship she wants.

Like the first step, the second one requires time and commitment. Controlling emotional development is rarely a passive process. You must be willing to be *introspective* (inwardly reflective) about yourself and the world around you.

Undertaking new experiences

To mature emotionally, you must progress beyond the first two steps of the plan and test your newly formed perceptions. This *testing* is accomplished by *undertaking a new experience* or by reexperiencing something in a different way.

Learning from Our Diversity

Students Find Their Differences Rewarding

On most college campuses today, students encounter classmates with different backgrounds—race, ethnicity, sexual orientation, and age. In addition, since the Americans with Disabilities Act was passed in 1990, students with disabilities are increasingly represented on many campuses. This changing student population makes the college campus the perfect place to prepare yourself for the growing diversity in the larger community and throughout the world.

Although some college students strongly resist diversity, most find that interacting with people who are different from themselves can be rewarding. Still, there's a tendency for students from diverse backgrounds or with special needs to form their own organizations and sign up for certain programs. That creates a situation in which both inclusion and isolation exist. Isolation becomes a challenge for the entire college community—to nurture respect for the diversity that's so important in today's society.

Every student is unique. Some students are willing to step outside their individual comfort zones and celebrate the diversity that surrounds them. For them, the college years can be a time of accelerated personal growth that prepares them to interact socially and work effectively with others throughout life.

New experiences do not necessarily require high levels of risk, foreign travel, or money (see Learning from Our Diversity, above). They may be no more "new" than deciding to move from the dorm into an apartment, to change from one shift at work to another, or to pursue new friendships. The experience itself is not the goal; rather, it's a means of collecting information about yourself, others, and the objects that form your material world.

For instance, Allison volunteered to teach art therapy classes to chronically ill patients at a local hospital. This work was enjoyable and fulfilling for her, and she formed friendships with a few of the other hospital volunteers. Allison also met and began dating Mark, a staff physical therapist.

Reframing mental pictures

When you have completed the first three steps in the plan, the new information about yourself, others, and objects becomes the most current source of information. Regardless of the type of new experience you have undertaken and its outcome, you are now in a position to modify the initial perceptions constructed during the first step. Then you will have new insights, knowledge, and perspectives.

Allison reframed her mental pictures in light of the changes that had taken place in her life. Her volunteer work gave her a renewed appreciation for art. Also, she now saw herself as part of a circle of friends and as a partner in a long-term relationship with Mark. With her proactive approach to life, Allison had created challenges for herself that allowed her to change and grow.

If you are a parent, you also need to consider the challenge of fostering the emotional growth of your child (see Changing for the Better box on p. 28).

Changing *for the Better*

Reaching Out to Someone Who's Depressed

I have a close friend who's been under a lot of stress lately. Her parents are expecting her to make the dean's list, and she's trying very hard. Whenever she's not studying, she's sleeping. She seems depressed and never wants to go out. How can I help?

- Help your friend manage her time effectively.
- Try to be present when she wants to discuss her problems.
- Help her find a balance between any remaining interest in work and play.
- Encourage her to set daily goals, starting with small ones.
- Work with your friend to plan a calendar for both routine and special activities.
- If she asks you, suggest ways that she can cope more effectively.
- Find or organize a support group for depressed people in which your friend can participate.
- Try to offset any tendency she may have toward being critical of herself and others.
- Help her find ways to complete tasks.
- If necessary, help her schedule hours for sleep and other low-level activities.
- Arrange to share pleasant and nutritious meals with your friend.
- Give her permission not to do everything perfectly.
- Help plan her daily activities so that the important activities are done first.
- Be patient, personable, and forgiving.

TALKING POINTS • **How would you tell a friend that you think she should seek professional help for depression?**

Changing *for the Better*

Children's School Success and Self-Confidence Work Together

My daughter, who's in third grade, has been struggling with math. Lately, her other grades, even in subjects she likes, seem to be falling. What can I do to help her get back on track?

- Encourage your daughter and your other children to learn, and emphasize the positive aspects of school.
- Read to young children, and have them read to you.
- Keep a variety of age-appropriate books on hand for your children.
- Set specific times and locations for homework to be done. If your daughter's homework is finished ahead of time, let her use the extra time to read something of her choice.
- Talk to your children about their school day, and listen to them. Encourage them to tell you specific things that happened, not just say "yes" or "no" to your questions.
- Get to know your children's teachers, and take part in the classroom activities when invited to do so.
- Become an active member of an organization that promotes the teaching-learning environment, such as the Parent-Teacher Association (PTA).
- Provide nutritious food, safe play areas, and opportunities for contact with other children when school is not in session.
- Set limits regarding appropriate behavior and enforce them.
- Praise your children's successes, and encourage them during their struggles.

For many years, professionals in education and mental health have recognized the relationship between school success and children's self-esteem. For some children, the school experience has a negative effect on their self-concept and sense of self-worth. Parental involvement and support, guided by respect for the child, can do much to make the total school experience better.

REFLECTIONS OF PSYCHOLOGICAL WELLNESS

What characterizes people who have developed their psychological wellness most fully? The following discussion suggests three areas in which psychological wellness is evident. These include (1) movement toward fulfilling the highest level of need (as defined by Maslow), (2) development of a mature level of faith, and (3) expression of creativity in the context of a world that often restricts creative expression.

Maslow's Hierarchy of Needs

One of the most familiar ideas in developmental psychology is Abraham Maslow's model of need fulfillment. Maslow views emotional growth in terms of inner needs and motivation. He lists motivational requirements in the following order: physiological needs, safety needs, belonging and love needs, esteem needs, and **self-actualization** needs (Figure 2-2).[12] Maslow distinguishes between the lower *deficiency needs* and the higher *being needs.* People do not seek the higher needs until the lower demands have been reasonably satisfied. Accordingly, people who are hungry, feel unsafe, or have few friends will be highly unlikely to have high self-esteem until their lower needs have been met.

The people who are emotionally healthiest and most effective are those whose lives embody *being values,* such as truth, beauty, goodness, faith, wholeness, and love. Maslow labels these as "Theory Z" people, or **transcenders.** Self-actualization, the highest level of self-development, is clearly evident in the personality of transcenders, who are described as follows:[12]

- Transcenders have more peak or creative experiences and naturally speak the language of being values.
- Transcenders are more responsive to beauty, are more holistic in their perceptions of humanity and the cosmos, adjust well to conflict situations, and work more wholeheartedly toward goals and purposes.
- Transcenders are innovators who are attracted to mystery and the unknown and see themselves as people who live according to transcendent values, such as unconditional acceptance, love, honesty, and forgiveness.
- Transcenders tend to fuse work and play. They are less attracted by the rewards of money and objects and more motivated by the satisfaction of being and service values.
- Transcenders are more likely to accept others with an unconditional positive regard, and they tend to be more oriented toward spiritual reality.

From these descriptions, it's clear that there is a strong connection between self-esteem, transcendence, and self-actualization.

Spiritual or Faith Development

A fully developed sense of self-esteem may involve accepting yourself as a person of **faith.** Many older adults say that they believe in something (such as the universal truths of beauty, honesty, and love) or someone greater than themselves and that this belief brings them great comfort and a sense of support. Many report that because of their personal level of faith, they do not fear death; they know that their lives have had meaning within the context of their deeply held beliefs. Such

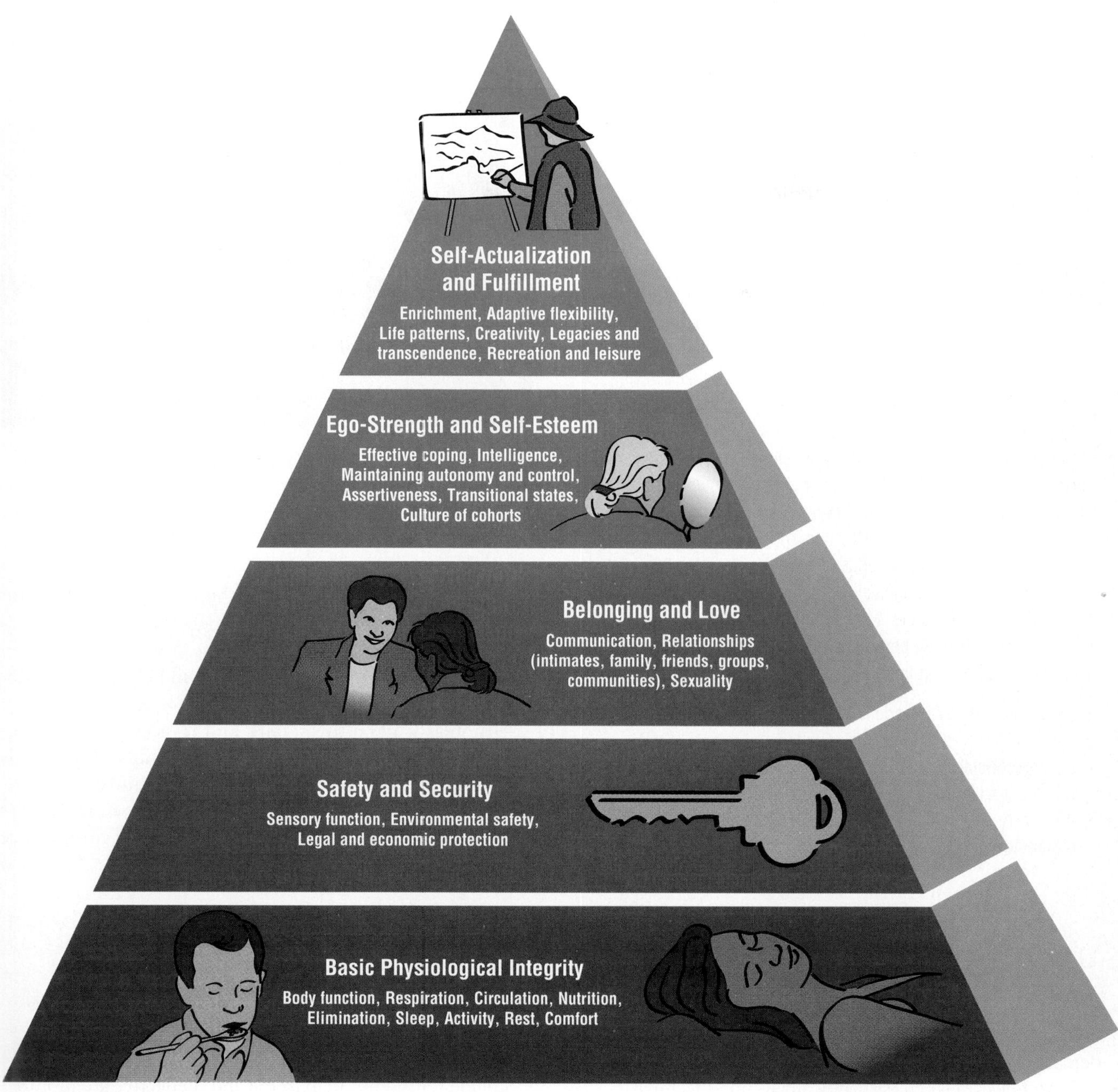

Figure 2-2 Maslow's hierarchy of needs.

people would urge younger people to search for the strength and the direction that faith provides.

As a resource for the spiritual dimension of health, faith provides a basis on which a belief system can mature and an expanding awareness of life's meaning can be fostered. Faith also gives meaning (or additional meaning) to your vocation (your life's work) and helps you better understand the consequences of your vocational efforts. For example, a college student might choose to major in education instead of marketing because he or she would find greater spiritual fulfillment in teaching than in business. In addition, faith in something (or

Key Terms

self-actualization
The highest level of personality development; self-actualized people recognize their roles in life and use personal strengths to reach their fullest potential.

transcenders
Self-actualized people who have achieved a quality of being ordinarily associated with higher levels of spiritual growth.

faith
The purposes and meaning that underlie an individual's hopes and dreams.

Exploring Your Spirituality

How Does Your Faith Affect Your Life?

James Fowler describes faith as a fundamental universal, but infinitely varied, value response in the human experience.[13] Faith can include religious practice, but it can also be quite distinct from it. Faith is the most fundamental stage in the human quest for the meaning of life. It's a developing focus of the total person that gives purpose and meaning to life.

By the time people reach college age, their faith may have already placed them in uncomfortable situations. Taking seriously their responsibility for their own commitments, lifestyles, beliefs, and attitudes, they've had to make some difficult personal decisions. This demands objectivity and a certain amount of independence. It requires finding a balance between personal aspirations and a developing sense of service to others. Finally, the symbols and doctrines of faith must be translated into personalized spiritual concepts that become part of everyday living.

- Have you had any experiences that show you're growing in your faith?
- Do you consider yourself more spiritual or less spiritual than your friends or family members?
- What school-related experiences have affected the spiritual dimension of your health most powerfully?

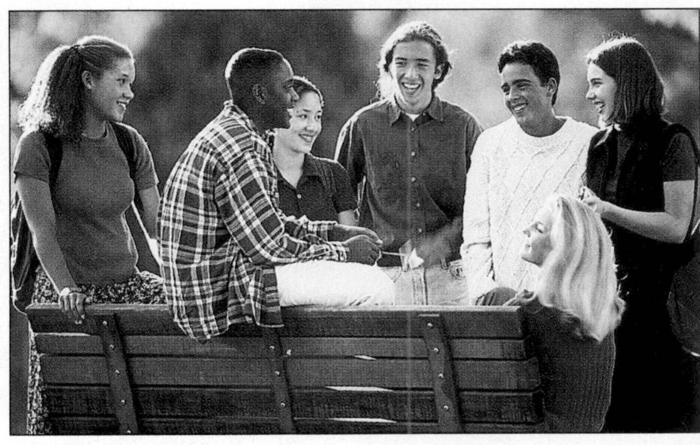

Spending leisure time with others helps you become self-actualized.

someone) influences many of the experiences that you will seek throughout life and tempers your emotional response to these experiences.[13] The questions posed in Exploring Your Spirituality (p. 30) will help you consider how your faith affects your own life.

In nearly all cultures, faith and its accompanying belief system provide individuals and groups with rituals and practices that foster a sense of community—"a community of faith." In turn, the community nurtures the emotional stability, confidence, and sense of competence needed for living life fully.

SUMMARY

- Emotionally well people feel comfortable about themselves and other people and are able to meet the demands of life.
- *Emotional wellness* refers specifically to one's feelings in response to change, whereas *psychological wellness* refers more broadly to the adequate development and proper functioning of mental abilities.
- Emotions are not always constant; people experience a normal range of emotions.
- A sense of self-esteem may be the essence of emotional maturity.
- Hardiness reflects the existence of confidence and commitment and an ability to build on challenge.
- Depression can be recognized by the presence of characteristic symptoms.
- Loneliness results from the absence of adequate human contact.
- Shyness may be a basic component of temperament, yet social skills counseling can help shy people learn to interact more comfortably with others.
- Suicide represents an extreme and ineffective attempt to cope with life's problems.
- Effective verbal and nonverbal communication skills can be learned and used to enhance psychological well-being.
- Humor can contribute to psychological wellness and well-being.
- Conflict management skills include a variety of approaches, some of which are more effective than others.
- A four-step plan can be used to foster greater emotional growth and enhanced psychological wellness.
- According to Maslow, the ability to meet basic human needs establishes a basis for pursuing higher emotional needs.
- People who possess a mature faith recognize the existence of guiding values in their lives.

REVIEW QUESTIONS

1. What are the characteristics of an emotionally healthy person?
2. How is psychological health related to but different from emotional health?
3. What is meant by the "normal range of emotions"?
4. Define *self-esteem*. List strategies that can be used to improve self-esteem.
5. What are three characteristics of hardy people?
6. What is depression, and what are the behavioral patterns of depressed people? How do major depression and dysthymia differ? How do the terms *primary* and *secondary* relate to major depression?
7. What is the important component missing in the lives of lonely people? What skills can such people learn to ease their sense of loneliness?
8. On the basis of current understanding, what is the most likely origin of shyness? What personality type includes shyness as one of its recognizable components?
9. What behavioral characteristics indicate a suicidal tendency? How should someone who observes these traits in another person respond?
10. What are several characteristics of effective verbal communication?
11. What nonverbal cues encourage positive communication? What nonverbal cues detract from positive interpersonal communication?
12. What message is given to others by those who allow humor to be a part of their social interaction?
13. Which techniques are the more effective approaches to conflict management? Which are less effective?
14. Identify and explain the four components of the cyclic process that will help you enhance your emotional growth.
15. In what order are human needs encountered as one moves toward self-actualization?
16. What aspects of life are brought into focus as the spiritual dimension of health matures?

THINK ABOUT THIS . . .

- How close do you come to meeting the characteristics of an emotionally healthy person?
- Are you ready to undertake a new experience? What kind of experience will it be?
- Do you take yourself too seriously at times?
- How proactive are you in enhancing the emotional dimension of your health?

REFERENCES

1. *Mental health and you,* 2000, National Mental Health Association.
2. Berne P, Savary L: *Building self-esteem in children,* 1996, Crossroad Herder & Herder.
3. Pengilly JW, Dowd ET: Hardiness and social support as moderators of stress, *J. Clin Psychol,* 2000, 56(6):813–820.
4. *Diagnostic and statistical manual of mental disorders: DSM-IV-TR,* American Psychiatric Association, 2000.
5. *Physicians' desk reference* (5th ed), 2001, Medical Economics Company.
6. DeRubeis R et al: Medications versus cognitive behavior therapy for severely depressed outpatients: meta-analysis of four randomized comparisons, *Am J Psychiatry* 156(7):1007–1013, 1999.
7. *St John's wort,* National Institutes of Health, National Center for Complementary and Alternative Medicine, NCCAM Clearinghouse, 2001.
8. Greeson JM, Sanford B, Monti DA: St. John's wort (Hypercum perforatum): a review of the current pharmacological, toxicological, and clinical literature, *Psychopharmacology (Berl),* 153(4):402–414, 2001.
9. Denollet J: Personality and risk of cancer in men with coronary heart disease. *Psychol Med,* 28(4):991–995, 1998.
10. Kochanek KD, Smith BL, Anderson RN: Deaths: preliminary data for 1999, *National Vital Statistics Report,* 49(3):1–27, 2001.
11. Berk LS et al: Modulation of neuroimmune parameters during the eustress of humor-associated mirthful laughter, *Altern Ther Health Med,* 7(2):67–72, 2001.
12. Maslow A: *The farthest reaches of human nature,* 1983, Peter Smith.
13. Fowler J: *Faith development and pastoral care,* 1987, Fortress Press.

SUGGESTED READINGS

Forward S: *Emotional blackmail: when the people in your life use fear, obligation, and guilt to manipulate you,* 1998, HarperCollins.

Is it possible for you to allow others, even those you love, to take control of your life? Susan Forward believes that this happens frequently. She claims that it is often done in a way that erodes your psychological well-being and deteriorates your health in all its dimensions. This book explores the techniques and consequences of being emotionally blackmailed by someone very close to you.

Gersten D, Dossey L: *Are you getting enlightened or losing your mind: how to master everyday and extraordinary spiritual experiences,* 1998, Three Rivers Publishing.

Where is the fine line between profound psychological disorders, such as schizophrenia, and the equally unfamiliar and uncomfortable spiritual experiences that some report? Are near-death experiences, out-of-body experiences, visitation by angels, and cases of spontaneous healing the products of spiritual connectedness, or are they illnesses to be diagnosed and treated? Dennis Gersten, MD, a practicing psychiatrist, helps the reader distinguish between dysfunction and spiritual transformation.

Gurley J: *Alter: a simple path to emotional wellness,* 1998, Footprint Press.

The author of this book believes that just as a computer can access incredible stores of information, you can tap into vast stores of self-knowledge through your unconscious mind. The idea is to use a "rub plate" to free the mind from the disturbing chatter, stress, anxiety, and emotional blinders that block access to our own store of personal information.

As we go to Press...

The use of surgically implanted electronic stimulators (pacemakers) for regulation of heart conductivity and stomach smooth muscle activity is well established. Currently, a new use for this technology is nearing approval by the FDA. Vagus nerve stimulation (VNS) is being assessed as a method of treating severe depression.

VNS involves the implantation of a stopwatch-size electrical device in the chest (immediately under the skin and below the collar bone) with an electrical wire leading to the vagus nerve. This nerve carries both motor and sensory fibers from the brain to a variety of structures within the chest area, including the heart. In VNS once every 30 seconds an electrical current is sent into the sensory fibers of the nerve for transmission. When the electrical impulses reach the mood areas in the brain, they alter neurotransmitter activity to produce an elevated mood, thus reducing the symptoms of depression. Used in Europe for some time, VNS appears to be both effective and safe in the management of depression.

Name ______________________ Date __________ Section __________

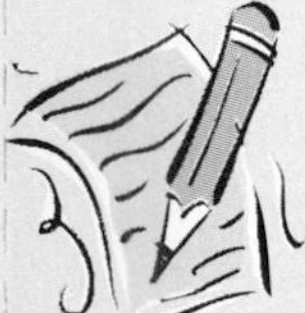

Personal Assessment

How Does My Self-Concept Compare with My Idealized Self?

Below is a list of fifteen personal attributes, each portrayed on a 9-point continuum. Mark with an X where you think you rank on each attribute. Try to be candid and accurate; these marks will collectively describe a portion of your sense of self-concept. When you are finished with the task, go back and circle where you *wish* you could be on each dimension. These marks describe your idealized self. Finally, in the spaces on the right, indicate the difference between your self-concept and your idealized self for each attribute.

Decisive					Indecisive				____
9	8	7	6	5	4	3	2	1	
Anxious					Relaxed				____
9	8	7	6	5	4	3	2	1	
Easily influenced					Independent thinker				____
9	8	7	6	5	4	3	2	1	
Very intelligent					Less intelligent				____
9	8	7	6	5	4	3	2	1	
In good physical shape					In poor physical shape				____
9	8	7	6	5	4	3	2	1	
Undependable					Dependable				____
9	8	7	6	5	4	3	2	1	
Deceitful					Honest				____
9	8	7	6	5	4	3	2	1	
A leader					A follower				____
9	8	7	6	5	4	3	2	1	
Unambitious					Ambitious				____
9	8	7	6	5	4	3	2	1	
Self-confident					Insecure				____
9	8	7	6	5	4	3	2	1	
Conservative					Adventurous				____
9	8	7	6	5	4	3	2	1	
Extroverted					Introverted				____
9	8	7	6	5	4	3	2	1	
Physically attractive					Physically unattractive				____
9	8	7	6	5	4	3	2	1	
Lazy					Hardworking				____
9	8	7	6	5	4	3	2	1	
Funny					Little sense of humor				____
9	8	7	6	5	4	3	2	1	

To Carry This Further . . .

1. Overall, how would you describe the discrepancy between your self-concept and your self-ideal (large, moderate, small, large on a few dimensions)?
2. How do sizable gaps for any of your attributes affect your sense of self-esteem?
3. Do you think that any of the gaps exist because you have had others' ideals imposed on you or because you have thoughtlessly accepted others' ideals?
4. Identify several attributes that you realistically believe can be changed to narrow the gap between your self-concept and your self-ideal and, thus, foster a well-developed sense of self-esteem.

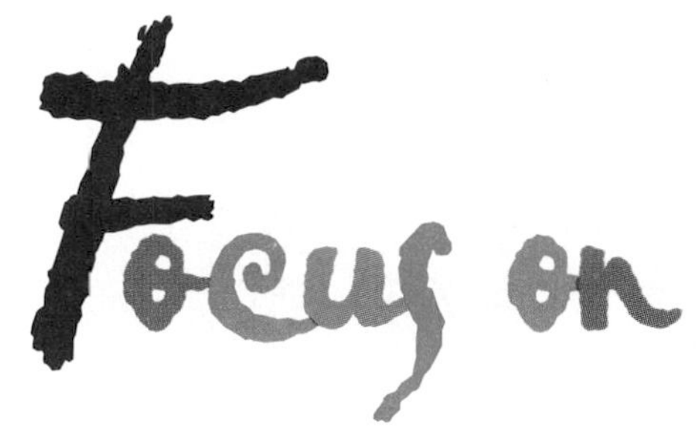

LENDING A HELPING HAND: BECOMING A VOLUNTEER

From now on in America, any definition of a successful life must include serving others.
—Former President George H. W. Bush

For nearly 40 years, two federally funded voluntary agencies, Peace Corps and VISTA (Volunteers in Service to America), have provided American adults of all ages an opportunity to put their idealism into action by using their skills in service to others. More recently, a third avenue for extending services to others, AmeriCorps, was established. This agency is a paid service initiative that lowers the cost of college for participants. Today, thousands of programs at the local, state, national, and international levels provide a similar opportunity.

Americans traditionally have expended their time, talents, and energy in support of others more freely than have the citizens of many other highly industrialized nations. Recent examples of this admirable American response were the clean-up efforts following devastating tornadoes in Oklahoma, assistance to those affected by the massive earthquake damage in Turkey, and victims of flooding in North Carolina following Hurricane Floyd. Less visible are the thousands of American volunteers who serve on committees, babysit, coach, and lead scout troops. Various international programs also provide opportunities for Americans to volunteer in other countries. Two such programs are Amigos de las Americas (a program for teens to live and volunteer in Latin America) and World Teach (a program for college graduates to teach English in a foreign country). The monetary value of this free (or nearly free) service given by Americans is difficult to determine accurately, but most recently it was estimated to be worth at least $200 billion per year.[1]

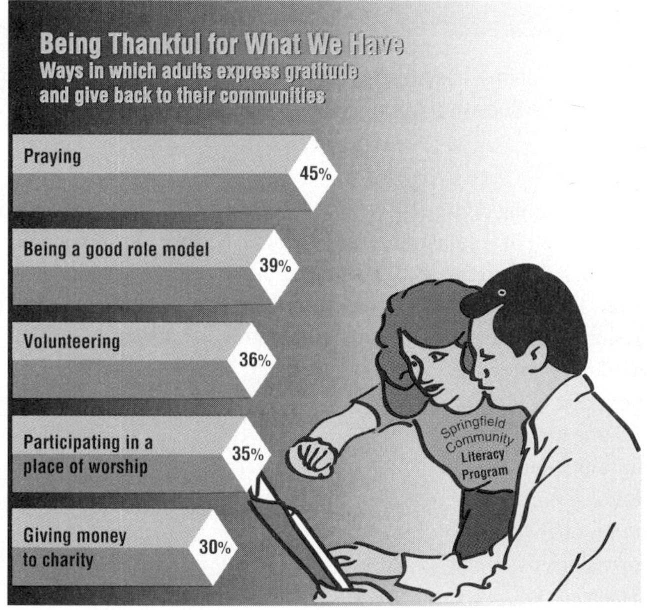

Many of us have been fortunate enough not to experience poverty, serious illness, or lack of education. Do you think it's important to express gratitude by giving something back to your community?

Helping Others and Improving Yourself

Although volunteer service benefits those in need, volunteering is also good for the volunteer. It provides companionship, friendship, and fellowship in working toward a common goal. Volunteer service allows us to use skills and talents that we normally don't use at our daily jobs. It encourages us to branch out, learn new things, and become more well-rounded. The decision to become a volunteer fosters decision making and expands the scope of the volunteer's self-directed behavior. Most important, volunteering brings people of diverse backgrounds together, makes those being served feel a greater sense of self-worth, and raises the aspirations of all involved.

Today, the importance of volunteering, referred to as *service learning,* is reflected in the fact that many colleges and high schools are requiring its inclusion in their curricula.[2,3] Students who have participated in volunteering programs appear to profit in terms of their academic performance, perhaps because of the time management skills and discipline involved. They also report an increased sense of concern for the well-being of others and a greater ability to respond empathetically, as well as sympathetically, to people in need.

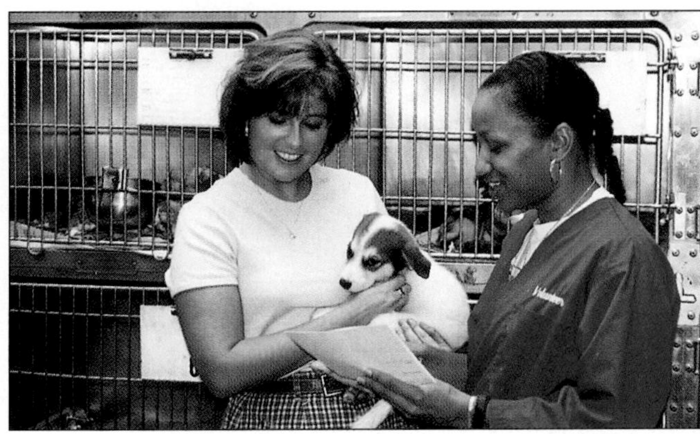

Jaquette Johnson helps animals and their new owners by volunteering as an adoption counselor at the Humane Society of Missouri.

Employers are beginning to notice—and value—the inclusion of volunteering on the transcripts of recent graduates. It is important to note, however, that volunteering is not necessarily highly regarded by employers unless it leads to skill development that is relevant to the organization.[4] Some members of the academic community question the appropriateness of *requiring* students to volunteer. Perhaps offering opportunities for students to volunteer (for credit) and to develop job-related skills is a good reason to include it in the curricula. Volunteering broadens the volunteer's world and sharpens his or her focus, combining to enhance both occupational performance and psychological well-being.

Diversity Among Volunteers

Volunteers are a very diverse group. Examples of recent American Institute of Public Service Jefferson Award recipients include a 14-year-old who teaches English to Latino immigrant children and a 106-year-old woman who has logged more than 128,000 volunteer hours (equal to 64 years of 40-hour work weeks) with the Red Cross. The many volunteers who do not receive official recognition for their efforts are just as important. Millions of Americans volunteer their expertise, time, and energy in various ways. Many "silent" volunteers are lobbying for the preservation of free speech and privacy on the Internet, participating in Habitat for Humanity, working on behalf of abused or neglected animals, and participating in countless other types of service.

Ways to Volunteer

No matter what your interests, abilities, or time commitments, there is much that you, as a college student, can do. Just a few of the volunteer opportunities you might consider include the following:

AIDS
Arts/cultural enrichment
Business assistance
Citizenship
Civic affairs
Consumer services/legal rights
Day care/Head Start
Disaster response/emergency preparedness
Drug abuse/alcoholism
Education
Employment
Health issues
Law enforcement/crime prevention
Literacy
Mental health
Nutrition
Physical environment
Psychosocial support services
Recreation and sports
Teen pregnancy prevention
Parenting
Transportation and safety
Animal welfare
Women's crisis centers

You can make a difference alone, with a few friends, or as part of an established organization. The Student Environmental Action Coalition (with chapters at 2,300 high schools and colleges), VISTA, Peace Corps, United Way, the Salvation Army, and the American Red Cross are just a few of the national organizations that need volunteers. To volunteer, contact one of these agencies or your local church, hospital, nursing home, city recreation department, or scout council directly.

For Discussion . . .

Do you currently volunteer? Why or why not? If you decided to become a volunteer, what areas of work would interest you most? Can you think of a volunteer who has touched your life? How do you feel about compulsory service as a component in college and high school curricula? Should time spent volunteering be counted as a contribution for income tax purposes (as is a monetary contribution to a nonprofit agency would)?

References

1. Wofford H, Waldlman S, Bandow D: AmeriCorps the beautiful? *Policy Review* 79:28–36, 1996.
2. Sax L, Justin A: The benefits of service: evidence from undergraduates, *EducationalRecord,* Summer/Fall:25–33, 1997.
3. Calderon J: Making a difference: service-learning as an activism catalyst and community builder, *American Association for Higher Education Bulletin* 52(1):7–9, 1999.
4. Larry Beck: Personal interview with Larry Beck, Associate Director, Career Services, Ball State University, September 27, 1999.

chapter **3**

Managing Stress

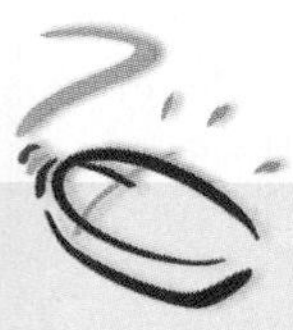

Online Learning Center Resources

www.mhhe.com/hahn6e

Log on to our Online Learning Center (OLC) for access to these additional resources:

- Chapter key terms and definitions
- Learning objectives
- Additional behavior change objectives
- Student interactive question-and-answer sites
- Self-scoring chapter quiz

The OLC also offers web links for study and exploration of health topics. Here are some examples of what you'll find:

- **www.teachhealth.com** Get information on recognizing stress, take a self-test for determining your stress level, and learn stress-management techniques.
- **www.stressrelease.com/strssbus.html** Read the facts about workplace stress and what you can do about it.
- **www.cyberpsych.com/stress.html** Don't miss *Reality Check: 20 Questions to Screw Your Head on Straight.*

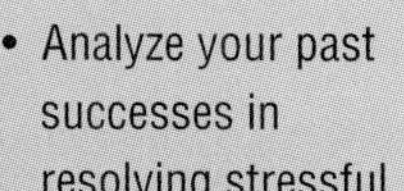

Taking Charge of Your Health

- Analyze your past successes in resolving stressful situations, noting the resources that were helpful to you.
- Prioritize your daily goals in a list that you can accomplish, allowing time for recreational activities.
- Counteract a tendency to procrastinate by setting up imaginary (early) deadlines for assignments and rewarding yourself when you meet those dates.
- Add a new physical activity, such as an intramural team sport, to your daily schedule.
- Replace a damaging coping technique that you currently use, such as smoking, with an effective alternative, such as diaphragmatic breathing or yoga.
- List the positive aspects of your life, and make them the focus of your everyday thoughts.
- Explore the stress-reduction services that are available in your community, both on and off campus.

Eye on the Media

New Technology, New Stresses

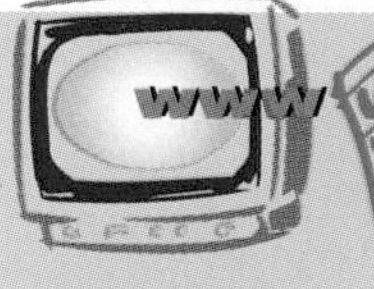

Over the past thirty years, the technology explosion has created a massive volume of information and a faster pace of life—in the workplace, in the classroom, and at home. Advances in technology offer many advantages, including saving time and increasing convenience. Would you want to go back to a world without e-mail, answering machines, the Internet, and cell phones? Probably not. Yet these technologies also produce stressors.

E-Mail: Correspondence of all types is increasingly being sent via computer. People who rarely exchanged written correspondence are now dropping lines via e-mail. At the office, a worker may arrive in the morning and find a long list of electronic correspondence that needs to be answered. Forwarded memos and messages, sent for informational purposes, may not require a reply, but they still need to be read and sometimes require action.

Voice Mail and Answering Machines: Sometimes it's hard to ignore the blinking light on the office phone. It's a constant reminder that you've missed a call and need to respond to it. To make that light stop blinking, you've got to listen to the message.

Eye on the Media *continued*

Automated Voice Message System: Many phone calls that we now make—to companies, community agencies, and even some homes—produce a familiar menu of choices. After listening to several choices, such as "For your current balance, press 3," you might like to wait for the final choice, "To speak to a company representative, please remain on the line." These automated services generate feelings ranging from annoyance to anger. For the caller who wants to talk to a knowledgeable person about an important question or concern, listening to the entire menu and waiting to talk to a "real" person can be stressful.

Junk Mail: Much of today's mail is unsolicited and unwanted, such as, an application for a credit card, a request for financial support, or a clothing catalog. A pile of junk mail may be the first stressor you encounter at the end of a stress-filled day at school or work. It's something that needs to be dealt with, if only sorted through and thrown away.

Fax Machines: Faxing is fast, convenient, and inexpensive. It can also be stressful, such as, when the fax number is unknown and can't be located or the line is constantly busy. Poor print quality, especially for graphics, can also produce frustration. Also, the "urgent" message on a fax suggests that an immediate reply is expected.

Call Waiting: Some people find call waiting to be irritating. First, their phone conversation is interrupted so that the person they are speaking to can check to see who the other caller is. The first caller needs to wait until the conversation can be resumed or is told that he or she will be called back later. This juggling of call priorities creates stress for both parties—the called party may feel the need to talk to both callers, and the original caller may be annoyed if his or her call becomes a lower priority than the new call.

Palm Pilots: For many busy people, it's convenient to carry a small electronic appointment book that interfaces with their personal computer. But when a person's schedule is recorded in a device that can be easily damaged or incapacitated (e.g., when power supplies run low), this information can be lost in an instant.

Pagers and Cell Phones: With electronic pagers and cell phones becoming so common, many people—employees, clients, and children—find themselves on call virtually all the time. The increasing pressure to keep in touch makes it more difficult to get away from it all. Even the enjoyment of watching a movie in a theater or dining in a quiet restaurant is often interrupted by the beeping of pagers and ringing of cell phones. Some people consider these interruptions necessary; others think they are simply annoying and intrusive.

Listservs: As valuable and informative as listservs can be, the amount of sharing on a single topic can become overwhelming as membership grows. Even the process of disaffiliating from the service can be complicated and stressful.

Internet: The Internet literally puts a world of information at your fingertips. But this can be somewhat daunting. Suddenly, you realize just how much information is out there. How can you get the right information? How is it that your computer searches through 25,000 sites without capturing the particular information you need? Why must you wait so long for pages to be loaded? Why does your on-line service always seem to be overloaded when you want to log on?

Clearly, these new technologies offer many advantages. But, like the technologies that preceded them, they create new stresses. Accepting that fact and developing a technology-friendly attitude will keep your stress level down as you make the new technology work for you.

TALKING POINTS • If you're at the library studying for an exam and someone nearby is having a long conversation on his cell phone, how would you tell that person that he is disturbing you?

Change is a part of daily living. Each person, institution, and situation in your environment holds the potential for change, which sometimes seems threatening. Taking control of this change or adjusting to it can be challenging, stimulating, and rewarding—contributing to your sense of well-being. But if you handle change poorly, stress can result, producing unpleasant experiences and the potential for harm to your health.

STRESS AND STRESSORS

On your college campus, you probably hear people talking about how much **stress** they feel. Certainly, for both traditional-age and nontraditional-age college students, the demands of school, work, marriage, and parenting can produce feelings of distress that detract from wellness. Students with disabilities face these and additional stressors (see Learning from Our Diversity box on p. 39).

Although you've experienced stress, you may not understand what it is and how it works. Hans Selye, the originator of stress theory, described stress as "the nonspecific response of the body to any demand made on it."[1] Stress can be viewed as a physical and emotional response that occurs when people are exposed to change. The events that produce stress are called **stressors.** Stressors are the cause, and stress is the effect.

Variation in Response to Stressors

Because individuals are unique, what is a stressor for one person might not be a stressor for another. For example,

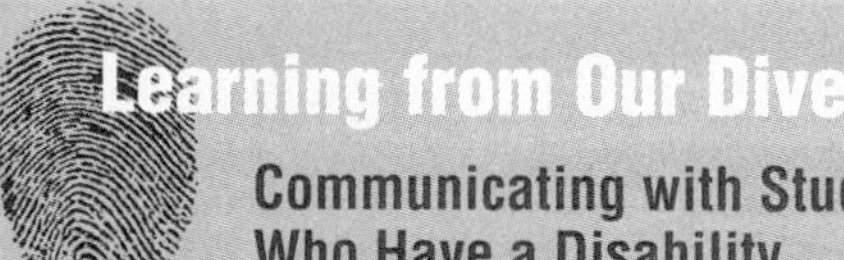

Communicating with Students Who Have a Disability

For many college students, interacting with classmates who have a disability is uncomfortable and stressful. The students with the disability feel this discomfort, and it is a source of stress for them. They are also dealing with the demands of college in the context of their unique disability.

What approach could be taken to minimize the discomfort for all parties involved? The following list contains some suggestions:

- Remember that everyone is a *person first*. In addition, that person may have a disability. Think in terms of a student with a learning disability, not a learning-disabled student.
- Always make *eye contact* with the person. This simple courtesy is very important in assuring the individual with a disability that he or she is a part of your college experience.
- *Talk with* the person with the disability rather than with the accompanying attendant or assistant.
- Keep in mind that the person in the attendant/assistant role may know only certain aspects of the individual with a disability.
- Don't "*fake it*" or "*smile it off.*" If you can't understand the person with a disability, simply say: "I'm sorry. Give that to me one more time."
- If verbal communication is very difficult or simply ineffective, *do what it takes* to interact with the person with a disability. For example, sit down at the computer and write a note.
- If you think that the person with a disability needs assistance, just ask: "*May I assist you?*" The worst that can happen is that the person might say no. If the person says yes, he or she might even tell you how you can help.
- *Don't generalize* from a single negative and stressful experience about interacting with someone with a disability. Expect no more or no less from that person than you would from your able-bodied classmates.

if the bookstore is out of a textbook that you need for an upcoming assignment, you'll be affected by this situation; however, someone who already has the book will not. In other words, events themselves are neutral. They only become stressors when individuals interpret them as such. And, of course, not everyone sees the same event in the same way. Therefore some people could be more *stressed* than others. This variation results from the unique information that each person applies in making decisions about certain situations. When people refer to "stress," they commonly mean the *distress* associated with fear, anger, anxiety, and uncertainty regarding changing events.

Stress can usually be categorized as *acute* (associated with a single isolated event), *episodic* (related to a particular series of events, such as taking examinations), or *chronic* (such as being a parent of active young children).

Positive or negative stressors

Stressors produce the same generalized physical response whether an individual views the stressor as good or bad. Poor academic performance, loss of a friend, or being the only minority student on the dorm floor can cause stress, just as giving birth, receiving a promotion, or starting a new romance can be stressors. In each case, the effect on the body's physical systems is similar.

Selye coined the word **eustress** to mean positive stress. Stressors that produce eustress can enhance longevity, productivity, and life satisfaction. An example might be the mild stress that helps you stay alert during a midterm examination or the anticipation you feel on the first day of a new job. Some suggest that a personality type, type R (risk taking) or type T (thrill-seeking), may "require" the regular occurrence of high-risk activities as positive stressors. Recent research suggests that this behavior may be caused by a genetic predisposition.[2]

Selye calls harmful, unpleasant stress **distress.** If distress is not controlled, it can result in physical and emotional disruption, illness, and even death.

TALKING POINTS • How would you go about telling a professor that your grades are slipping because of family problems?

Key Terms

stress
The physiological and psychological state of disruption caused by the presence of an unanticipated, disruptive, or stimulating event.

stressors
Factors or events, real or imagined, that elicit a state of stress.

eustress
Stress that enhances the quality of life.

distress
Stress that diminishes the quality of life; commonly associated with disease, illness, and maladaptation.

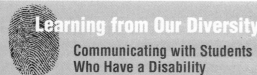

Stress and Disease

If the effects of a stressor are not minimized or resolved, the human body becomes exhausted, and an emotional and physical breakdown results. Depending on the strength of the stressor and the resistance of the person, this breakdown may occur quickly or may extend over many years, leading to stress-related diseases and disorders. Among the major diseases that have some origin in unresolved stress are hypertension, stroke, heart disease,[3] depression, alcoholism, and gastrointestinal disorders. Other stress-related disorders are migraine headaches, allergies, asthma, anxiety, insomnia, impotence, and menstrual irregularities. Cigarette smoking, overeating or undereating, and underactivity are partly related to unresolved stress. Even the immune system, which protects the body from infection and disease, may be weakened by stress.

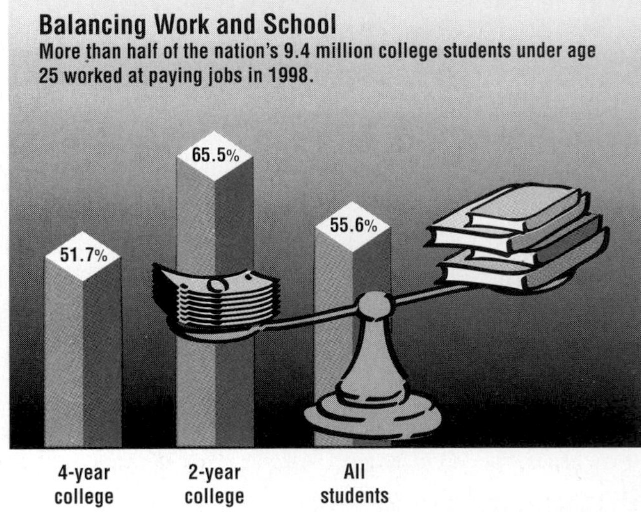

Figure 3-1 Percentages of college students who also work at paying jobs. (Statistics cited are the most recent available.)

COLLEGE STRESSORS

For some people who have not attempted college work, the idea that college life is stressful may seem strange. After all, isn't college the good life? Yet college students know that their experience is serious because it is preparing them for life and their career. For the part-time nontraditional-age student who comes to campus at night and returns to work, family, and community responsibilities during the day, college classes can be especially stressful (Figure 3-1). (To find out how stressed you are, see the Personal Assessment on p. 53.)

TALKING POINTS • As a part-time student with a full-time job, how would you explain to a classmate why you keep saying no when you're asked to go out for coffee with a group of students?

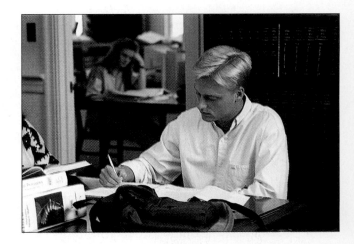

College life presents many stressors, such as studying for exams.

In college and university settings, stressors can arise from a variety of areas, including the following:

- Financial needs that can only be met by scholarships, loans, or employment during the academic year.
- School policies that seem to make going to school too complicated, such as the inconvenient scheduling of classes and the restrictions on parking
- Expectations of faculty regarding various course requirements, such as attendance, out-of-class participation, and the type of examinations given by a particular instructor
- Personal goals that become unachievable, such as making an athletic team, earning a desired grade point average, or graduating with honors
- Uncertainties about previously held beliefs, including those related to religion, sexual abstinence, and politics
- Interpersonal relationships and decisions about dating, roommates, or being older than other students
- Availability of a job, acceptance into graduate or professional school, and the approach of real-world responsibilities
- Family expectations about whether school is being taken seriously enough or money is being used wisely
- Time management, particularly as it relates to excessive and unproductive computer use.[4]

Education is not a passive process. It demands your active participation and effort. At times, the college experience may demand more than you believe you can give. Not surprisingly, it frequently becomes the source of many stressors.

Employment also presents stressors that must be confronted and resolved. Although different from stressors associated with college, work-centered stressors hold the same potential for causing physical and emotional illness and challenges to an individual's well-being.[5] For advice on coping with stress in the workplace, read the Focus on box on p. 57.

GENERALIZED PHYSIOLOGICAL RESPONSE TO STRESSORS

Once you're under the influence of a stressor, your body responds in certain predictable ways. For example, if you're asked to stand in front of a group and talk, your heart rate increases, your throat becomes dry, your palms sweat, and you may feel dizzy or light-headed. You would have similar feelings if you were told that you had lost your job or when the roller coaster begins its ascent up the first hill. These different stressors all elicit certain common physical reactions.

Selye described the typical physical response to a stressor in his **general adaptation syndrome** model. He stated that the human body moves through three stages when confronted by stressors: alarm reaction, resistance, and exhaustion.

Alarm Reaction Stage

Once exposed to any event that is seen as threatening, the body immediately prepares for difficulty with an alarm reaction. The involuntary changes described in Figure 3-2 are controlled by hormonal and nervous system functions and quickly prepare the body for the **fight-or-flight response.**[1]

Resistance Stage

The resistance stage reflects the body's attempt to reestablish its internal balance, or *homeostasis.* The high level of energy seen in the initial alarm stage cannot be maintained very long. So the body attempts to reduce the intensity of the initial response to a more manageable level. This is accomplished by reducing the production of adrenocorticotropic hormone (ACTH) (see p. 42), allowing *specificity of adaptation* to occur. Specific organ systems, such as the cardiovascular and digestive systems, become the focus of the body's response.[1]

The alarm stage gives way to the less damaging resistance stage, because of effective coping or because the status of the stressor changes. As control over the stressful situation is gained, homeostasis becomes reestablished in movement toward full recovery. When the *recovery stage* is complete, the body has returned to its prestressed state and there is minimal evidence of the stressor's existence.[1]

If the resistance stage is prolonged, the body may show clinical signs of the demands made on it by the continuing presence of stressors. At such times the person may begin to display the **psychogenic** and **psychosomatic** disorders associated with chronic stress. (See the Changing for the Better box on p. 43, which lists different types of headaches, some of which are worsened by stress.)

Exhaustion Stage

Body adjustments resulting from long-term exposure to a stressor often lead to overload. Specific organs and body systems that were called on during the resistance stage may not be able to resist a stressor indefinitely. Exhaustion results, and the stress-producing hormone levels again rise. In extreme or chronic cases of stress, exhaustion can become so pronounced that death may occur.

THE STRESS RESPONSE

Why could something as familiar as a telephone ringing late at night cause a person to feel fear and near-panic? Why is it that your hands sweat, your muscles tense, and your appetite leaves as you wait in the hallway outside the classroom where your final examination is to be held? Is the "cotton-mouth" feeling described by athletes a valuable aid to performance? The answers are simple and based on the body's primitive interpretation of reality. The body is looking for energy because it believes that all change is threatening and can be confronted by running, fighting, scaring the "adversary" away, or engaging it in sexual activity (the flight, fight, fright, or folly response). For these responses, the body simply needs energy for physical activity.[6]

Key Terms

general adaptation syndrome
A sequenced physiological response to the presence of a stressor; the alarm, resistance, recovery, and exhaustion stages of the stress response.

fight-or-flight response
The reaction to a stressor by confrontation or avoidance (sometimes called the flight, fight, fright, or folly [or 4F] response).

psychogenic
Pertaining to mind-induced (emotional) changes in physical function, without evidence of structural change to body tissues.

psychosomatic
Pertaining to mind-induced (emotional) changes in both physical function and the normal structure of body tissues.

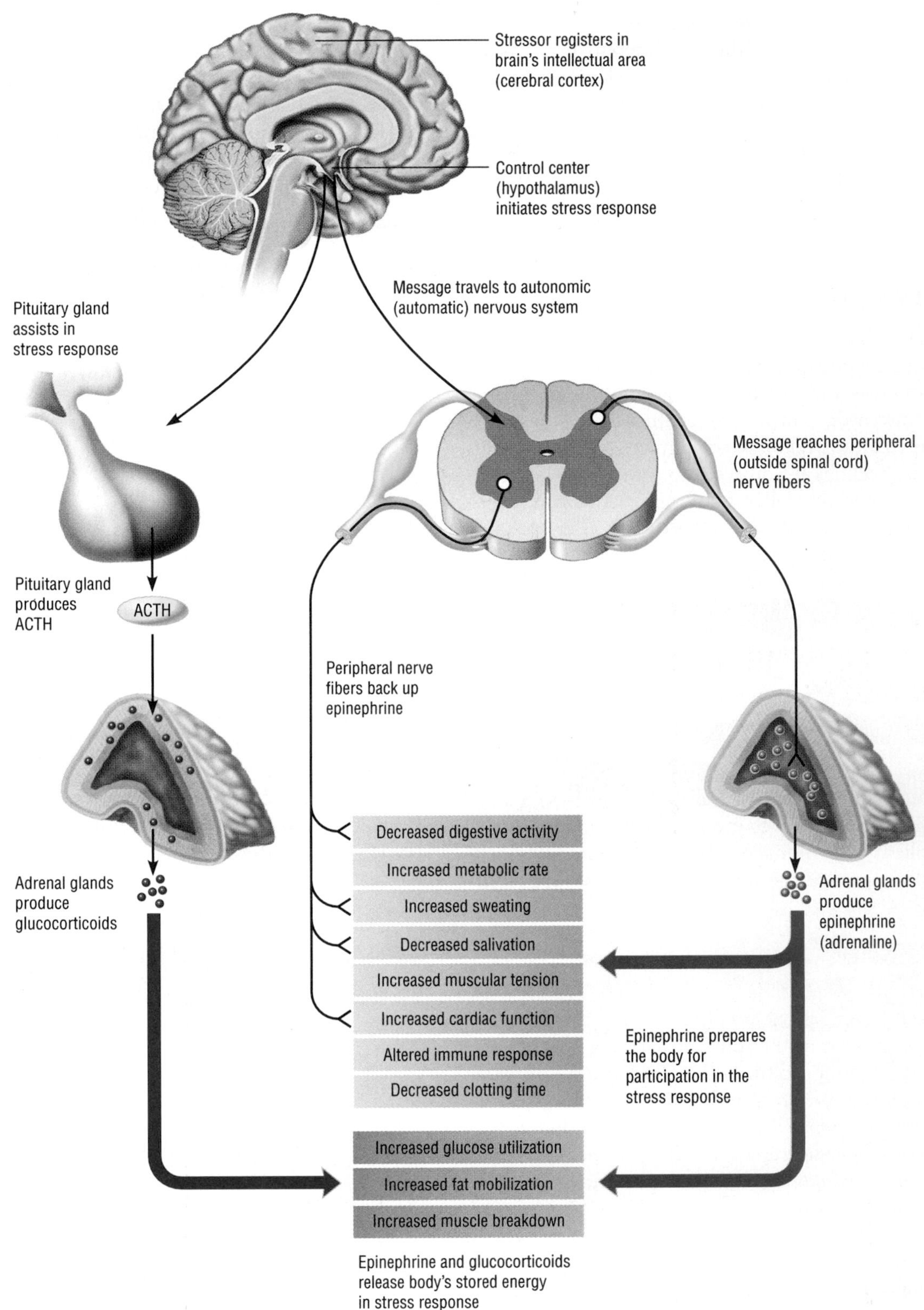
Stressor registers in brain's intellectual area (cerebral cortex)
Control center (hypothalamus) initiates stress response
Message travels to autonomic (automatic) nervous system
Pituitary gland assists in stress response
Message reaches peripheral (outside spinal cord) nerve fibers
Pituitary gland produces ACTH
ACTH
Peripheral nerve fibers back up epinephrine
Decreased digestive activity
Increased metabolic rate
Increased sweating
Decreased salivation
Increased muscular tension
Increased cardiac function
Altered immune response
Decreased clotting time
Adrenal glands produce glucocorticoids
Adrenal glands produce epinephrine (adrenaline)
Epinephrine prepares the body for participation in the stress response
Increased glucose utilization
Increased fat mobilization
Increased muscle breakdown
Epinephrine and glucocorticoids release body's stored energy in stress response

Figure 3-2 The stress response: physiological reactions to a stressor.

Changing *for the Better*

When Do Headaches Need Attention?

I never used to get headaches, but now I seem to have them a lot, especially around midterm and exam weeks. Is this something to be concerned about?

An estimated 45 million Americans have frequent, bothersome headaches. If you have chronic headache symptoms or symptoms that are especially painful, you should seek medical help. Headaches can have many causes, including stress. The three most common categories are described here

Tension

Description
A dull, constricting pain centered in the hatband region. Pain may be on both sides of the head and extend down the neck to the shoulders. Produced by stress, eye strain, muscle tension, sinus congestion, temporomandibular joint dysfunction, nasal congestion, or caffeine withdrawal.

Treatment
Nonnarcotic pain relievers, muscle relaxants, relaxation exercises, massage.

Prevention
Preventive relaxation exercises, certain antidepressant medications.

Migraine

Description
Throbbing pain on one side of the head, usually preceded by visual disturbances. Sensitivity to lights and sounds; nausea and dizziness. More common in women. A genetic predisposition may exist.[7] Can last from a few hours to 2 days.

Treatment
Three oral prescription medications (Imitrex, Maxalt, and Zomig) are now available. Imitrex is available as a nasal spray. An over-the-counter medication, Excedrin Extra Strength, is effective for many.

Prevention
Avoidance of certain foods, including red wines, other alcoholic beverages, ripened cheeses, chocolate, cured meats, and monosodium glutamate (MSG). In some cases, prescription medications are recommended.

Cluster

Description
Focused, intense pain near one eye, often producing a red and teary eye and a runny nose. Headaches occur daily for weeks or months. They mainly affect men and last up to 2 hours.

Treatment
Oxygen and/or ergot compounds during the headache.

Prevention
Avoidance of alcohol and nitrite-containing foods. Various prescription medications, including antidepressants, steroids, ergotlike compounds, or heart-regulating drugs.

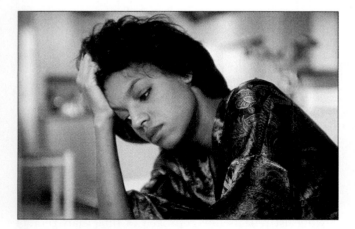

Financial concerns, work and school deadlines, and family responsibilities can all trigger the stress response.

Stressors

For a state of stress to exist, a person must first be confronted by change, real or imagined. Any change holds the potential for becoming a stressor and stimulating the stress response (Figure 3-2).

PSYCHONEUROIMMUNOLOGY

Clinical observation and laboratory studies show that the emotional component of stress (e.g., anxiety and depression) and the disruption of social support systems contribute to the weakening of the immune response and the development of some illnesses. For example, high levels of stress can predispose individuals to the development of colds; when immunizations are given during periods of stress, they may be less effective than if given when stress is not a factor. What is not known, however, is which mechanisms stressors use in altering immune system function. Are the emotional, nervous system, and endocrine components of the stress response all influenced by a single stressor?

Or is a combination of stressors necessary for seeing clinical evidence of immune system depression? In addition, it is not clear whether studies done with immune cells removed from the body reflect what actually occurs in the body and whether studies done with animals can be applied to humans.

Despite these limitations, theoretical explanations for a strong relationship between stress and immune system function exist. Experts in the field of **psychoneuroimmunology** are aggressively pursuing clinical studies to clarify which pathways are involved and which forms of management, including social support, can be used to support the immune system during periods of stress.[8]

Personality Traits

Can personality play a role in making people more or less prone to stress? If so, what outlook on life is considered to be the most stress-producing? The answer to the latter question has changed over the past three decades.

The initial, and still widely recognized, theory describing personality's role in fostering stress was that of type A and type B personalities. In this model, time-dependence (hurry sickness) was related to high levels of stress and, eventually, to heart disease.

Today, the type A/B concept of time-dependence as the most influential personality trait associated with high levels of stress has given way to concern over high levels of *anger* and *cynicism.* Anger is the intense feeling of rage and fury that accompanies an event or a change. Some people always seem to be angry, and the resulting stress on the body is detrimental to both their physical and emotional health. In fact, an association between stress-induced behavioral patterns and cardiovascular disease and insulin resistance syndrome (associated with diabetes mellitus type II), is well established.[9]

Closely related to anger is cynicism, the second personality trait that fosters high levels of stress. This trait is associated with deeply held dislike and distrust of others and their ideas. Cynics have nothing good to say about others. They are, perhaps, profoundly angry about their relationships with others and can express this feeling only by being very critical. Like anger, cynicism places the body under chronic stress and erodes the physical and emotional well-being of the person. As mentioned on page 39, R (risking-taking) and T (thrill-seeking) personality types are also related closely to stress. In persons with these genetically predisposed personality types, a form of neurotransmitter-influenced dependency may exist.

TALKING POINTS: • How would you speak honestly with a friend who seems chronically angry and cynical to help that person recognize that these feelings can be dangerous?

Time Management

For many college students, the most significant problem about being a student is everything that interferes with academics, including campus activities, athletics, employment, marriage, parenting, and relaxation time. Ultimately, the problem becomes an issue of priorities and time management so that academic demands can be met. Without question, *effective time management* is at the heart of balancing the demands of the college experience. The Personal Assessment on p. 55 will assist you in determining how you are currently using your time.

Procrastination is the purposeful, though sometimes unrecognized, putting off of important tasks, often at the time they *should* be done. It expresses itself in a variety of ways. For example, some college students put off working on important course assignments until the very last minute, leaving little time to meet the deadline (or do a good job). Others establish time tables for several projects but don't leave enough time for doing quality work. Some students place the responsibility for their work on others, for example, by not starting to write a paper until they can bounce their ideas off others (whose expertise they believe is needed).

A final example of procrastination occurs when students blame others for interfering with their ability to stay on task. This approach is seen when students blame their school, their residence hall friends, and their employers for depriving them of time needed for academic requirements. The motivations to procrastinate are subtle. They include anxiety or fear that the required work will not be done well (regardless of time) and a general sense of apathy.

Procrastination is sometimes fostered by the tendency to spend too much valuable time engaged in *maintenance tasks,* such as organizing materials on your desk, taking a nap, or going to lunch or dinner. The rationalization is that these things are a necessary part of getting ready for the work to be done. In contrast, *progress tasks* move you into your academic work, such as reviewing notes prior to the next class meeting, running database searches, and visiting professors for clarification of assignments. Although time-consuming, progress tasks are valuable in terms of efficient use of time and quality of work.

Specific techniques can be used to structure your time in ways that enhance academic progress. The following list reflects one approach to time management taken by many successful college students:

1. *Investigate Time Use:* Make a time/activity log for 1 week. Include descriptive entries for each half-hour period of the day to see where and how you are using time. Then analyze the log to identify how you misuse time (e.g., procrastination, overuse of maintenance tasks).

2. *Organize Activities:* Next, divide the day into blocks so that related activities can be scheduled together. Clearly identify the blocks for your major areas of responsibility, such as academics, employment, recreation, family activities, and socializing.
3. *Establish a Time Schedule:* For each block of activities, determine the amount of time you can assign to each block. Then, within that block, fill in the amount of time to be allotted to each specific activity. For example, on a particular day 3 hours may be assigned to review and refine class notes, with 1 hour given to a particular course and 40 minutes each to three other courses.
4. *Privatize Time:* State your intentions about doing serious and time-consuming schoolwork. Post a "Do Not Disturb" sign on your door. Leave the social atmosphere of your home, residence hall room, or apartment to work in a public area such as libraries, empty classrooms, and some coffee shops.

Review and modify this process to fit your requirements. Time management is not impossible for most college students. In fact, it is an effective approach used by the more successful (and busier) students on the typical college campus.

Test Anxiety

As examination time approaches, *test anxiety* may appear. For some students, the days and hours before major examinations are filled with real, but generalized, feelings of discomfort because they think that they will not perform well. Often, this situation is the result of poor time management. Those students who know that they will experience test anxiety may be prompted to use time-management strategies to reduce this problem. If this approach doesn't work for you, and you still feel test anxiety, contact your college's psychological services center. Most schools offer group sessions that explore methods of preparing for and taking examinations at no expense to students.

TALKING POINTS • How would you explain to a classmate that he is spending too much time on maintenance tasks before an important test and not enough time on progress tasks?

COPING: REACTING TO STRESSORS

It is no longer socially acceptable to escape stressors through negative dependency behavior, withdrawal, or aggressiveness. Negative dependency behaviors are still too frequently used by many people (Figure 3-3). Currently, the emphasis is on lifestyle management techniques that are not only effective but also supportive of overall health.

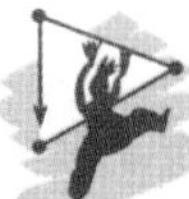

HealthQuest Activities

- The *How Stressed Are You?* activity in Module 1 lets you look at several areas of your life (including money, school, relationships, and health) and identify stress caused by various events and daily hassles. You can also rate your perceived stress level for each area. Use this feature to find out which area or areas generate the highest levels of stress for you.
- The *CyberStress* activity in the Stress Management and Mental Health Module simulates a stress-filled day. Use it to assess your reactions to daily stressors. Choose the scenario that most closely matches your own. For example, if you work and go to school, you should check both of these choices on the preferences screen. As you are presented with stressful situations, choose the reaction that is closest to how you would react. At the feedback screen, print the screen showing your score. Then evaluate your experience by answering the questions in the *What do you think?* section.

Stress-Management Techniques

Experts in stress management have proposed several effective techniques for coping with stress. Each of these techniques is described in the material that follows, with specific instructions provided for some. You will not know whether a particular coping approach is effective for you until you study the technique and use it for an adequate time.

Self-hypnosis

Techniques designed to increase awareness, induce mental relaxation, and enhance self-directedness are taught by trained professionals to people who can be hypnotized. These techniques, which can be learned in one lesson, are self-administered in daily sessions lasting from 10 to 20 minutes. Beware of unqualified practitioners, who frequently sell their services through newspaper advertisements. Contact professional organizations, such as psychological or psychiatric associations, for a list of qualified therapists.

Key Term

psychoneuroimmunology
A newly emerging field of human biology and clinical medicine that studies the functional interfaces among the mind, nervous system, and immune system.

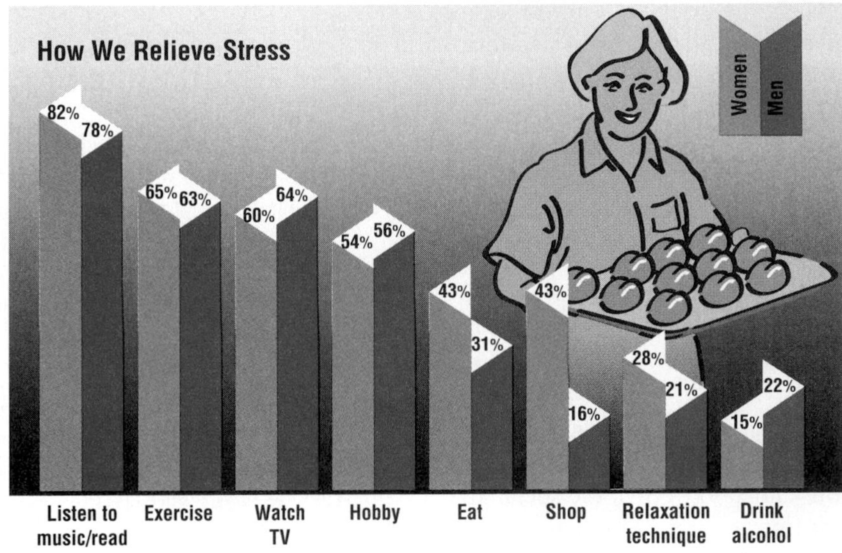

Figure 3-3 People have different ways of relaxing and relieving stress, such as cooking, reading a mystery novel, or swimming. How do you cope with stress?

The relaxation response

The "relaxation response," a technique developed by Herbert Benson, M.D., is a method of learning to quiet the body and the mind. The relaxation technique centers on exhalation and allowing the body to relax while sitting in a comfortable position. It can be learned in a single session but requires a commitment to practice. Effective for many people, the technique is described in Dr. Benson's book *The Relaxation Response.*[10]

Progressive muscle relaxation

Pioneered by the work of Edmund Johnson (author of *You Must Relax*),[11] progressive muscle relaxation (PMR) is a procedure in which each of several muscle groups is systematically contracted and relaxed. The theory is that by learning to recognize the difference between contracted and relaxed muscles, you can purposely place certain muscles into a controlled state of stress-reducing relaxation.

PMR is based on the appropriate use of positioning, breathing, and concentration. The position of choice is lying on the floor, with the hands at the sides and the palms facing upward. Once a comfortable position has been assumed, alternating periods of inhalation and exhalation are begun. During inhalation, the muscles are contracted. During exhalation, the muscle groups are relaxed. Concentration is focused on the "feelings" of relaxation that accompany the release of tension during each exhalation. Once mastered, the basics can be done in almost any setting, including a moving car, at a desk, and in a college classroom. Depending on a person's level of expertise, contractions last from a maximum of 100 seconds to a minimum of 5 seconds. The face, jaw, neck, shoulders, upper chest, hands and forearms, abdomen, lower back, buttocks, thighs, calves, and feet are tightened and then relaxed progressively. To the extent possible, each muscle group within the area is included.

Quieting

Quieting involves using a set of specific responses, such as striving for a positive mental state, an "inner smile," and a deep exhalation, with the tongue and shoulders relaxed, as soon as the onset of stress is noted. This technique can be practiced at any time and is easily learned. Its main advantage is that it produces an immediate feeling of "being on top of" the stress. The technique can be learned by reading *QR: The Quieting Reflex,* by Charles Stroebel, M.D., Ph.D.[12]

Yoga

An ancient exercise program for the mind and body, yoga can be learned from a qualified instructor in 1 to 13 months. It is practiced daily in a quiet setting in sessions lasting 15 to 45 minutes. Yoga can alter specific physiological functions, enhance flexibility, and free the mind from worry. Many good yoga books, classes, and videotapes are available.

Diaphragmatic breathing

A coping technique that combines elements of relaxation and quieting is diaphragmatic breathing. Aspects of this practice are seen in the Lamaze approach to childbirth, yoga, and tai chi. Although no single explanation for its effectiveness can be given, when practiced regularly, diaphragmatic breathing produces relaxation that buffers the powerful stress response. A three-component approach to the practice of diaphragmatic breathing is described below:

1. **Assume a comfortable position.** Lie on the floor with arms by your sides, eyes closed, back straight. Begin breathing from the diaphragm, rather than by lifting the chest.
2. **Concentrate.** The ability to concentrate is important. It is most easily mastered by following the pathway of air as it enters the body and flows deeply into the lower levels of the lungs, followed by the flattening of the stomach as the air leaves the lungs. Each ventilation can be fragmented into four distinct steps: (1) take air into your lungs through the nose and mouth, (2) pause slightly before exhaling, (3) release the air to flow out via the path from which it entered, and (4) pause slightly after exhalation before repeating step 1.
3. **Visualize.** Diaphragmatic breathing promotes relaxation most fully when it is practiced in conjunction with visualization. What is visualized varies from person to person, but many feel that envisioning the air (or clouds) entering the body with each breath, traveling down the path taken by the air, and leaving through the nostrils is very effective. Extending the image of the air flowing throughout the entire body (energy breathing), rather than only into the lungs, is even more effective.

Once mastered, diaphragmatic breathing quiets the body. Experienced users of this technique can temporarily lower their breathing from a typical rate of 14 to 18 breaths per minute to as few as 4 breaths per minute. With this technique, the entire nervous system is slowed, in direct opposition to its role in the stress response.

Transcendental meditation

Transcendental meditation (TM) allows the mind to transcend thought effortlessly when the person recites a mantra, or a personal word, twice daily for 20 minutes. It is a seven-step program taught by trained professionals. TM centers are listed in the telephone directory under Transcendental Meditation.

Biofeedback

Biofeedback is a system for monitoring and controlling specific physiological functions, such as heart rate, respiratory rate, and body temperature. Training with an experienced instructor and appropriate monitoring instruments requires weekly sessions that last 1 hour or longer over 12 or more weeks. When used with other tension-reduction techniques, biofeedback provides reinforcement of stress-reduction goals. For more information, contact the Biofeedback Society of America, 4301 Owens Street, Wheat Ridge, CO 80033.

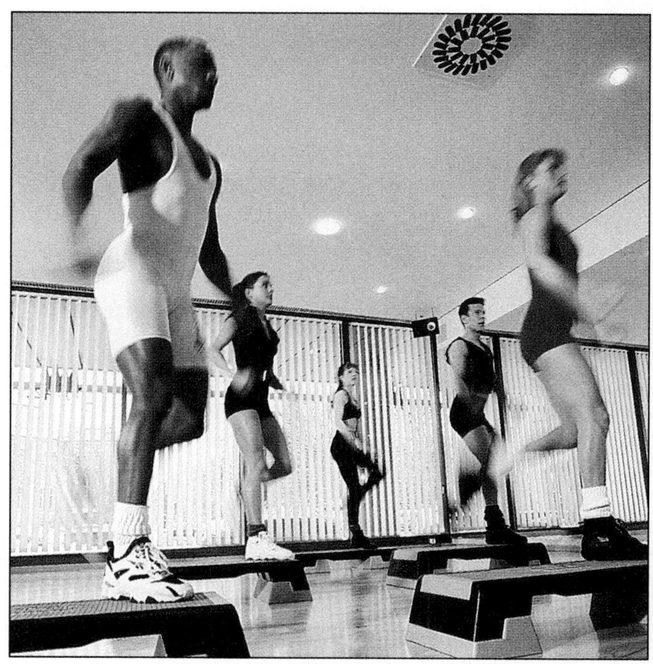

Regular physical activity reduces stress and promotes relaxation.

Exercise

Various movement activities are intended to reduce stress, expend energy, promote relaxation, provide enjoyment through social contact, and produce biological opiates. Running, jogging, lap swimming, walking, rope skipping, cycling, stair climbing, and aerobic dancing are all excellent ways to burn the energy produced by the stress response. Equipment needs, facilities, and required skills vary. Three to four sessions per week lasting a half-hour per session are sufficient for most people. Health and fitness clubs also offer exercise programs.

Art, dance, and poetry therapy

As an aid to emotional, physical, and spiritual health, the arts can be used to enhance an individual's sense of well-being. Qualified professional therapists in these fields work one-on-one or in group sessions. Although the methods used may vary, the idea is to foster a sense of peace through the art form and a focus for the troubled person's thoughts and energy during times of illness or stress.

A Realistic Perspective on Stress and Life

It's important to approach life with a tough-minded optimism based on hope and anticipation and understand that life will never be free of stress. To develop this type of realistic approach to today's fast-paced, demanding lifestyle, use the following guidelines:[13]

- **Don't be surprised by trouble.** Anticipate problems, and see yourself as a problem solver.

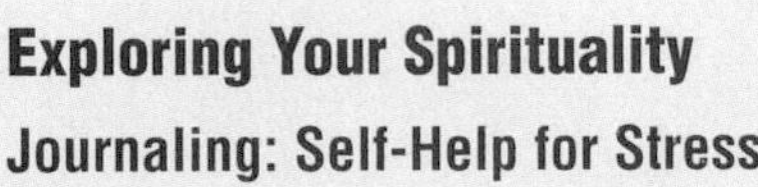

Exploring Your Spirituality

Journaling: Self-Help for Stress

Feeling anxious about your college experience? Trying to put past events in perspective? Want to record your experiences? Focused, regular writing—journaling—is growing in popularity as a way to approach these issues.

Writing in a journal each day slows down your pace. You sit and reflect. You connect with an experience by recalling details you may have forgotten, then write them down. For 15 to 30 minutes a day, you pause to make sense of your life.

Journaling generally gets easier the more you do it, so start by writing about nonthreatening topics. Try this: Each day, ask yourself a simple question, and then write the answer in your journal. As you gain experience, you may want to tackle more difficult issues.

Here are some journaling tips. Use an easy-to-carry spiral-bound notebook with a thick cover, so you can write anywhere. Or you may want to set aside a regular time and place so you won't be disturbed. Once you start writing, keep your pen moving continuously. Don't go back to correct spelling or punctuation. That will only slow you down and distract you from your thoughts, which are more important than perfect writing. Don't share your journal with others. This will inhibit your writing, making it less "you."

One powerful form of journaling is therapeutic, or healing, journaling, in which the individual writes about a traumatic event for 15 to 30 minutes a day, on three or four consecutive days. Studies by James W. Pennebaker, M.D., and colleagues noted lowered blood pressure and heart rates in healthy people who wrote about their deepest feelings for 20 minutes on three consecutive days.

Therapeutic writing can be very difficult and should be approached with caution. In particular, if you have been under medical treatment, check with your health-care professional before you begin a therapeutic journaling program. If you write about private events, you can shred or burn your pages. Whether you keep them or not has no bearing on the therapeutic impact.

Want to know more about journaling? *Personal Journaling Magazine* (www.journalingmagazine.com) is a good place to start. You'll find that journaling takes many forms, including memoirs, dream journals, chronicles of daily life, and "blogging" on the Internet.

In college, most of the things you write, such as papers and reports, are assigned and judged by an instructor. But when you write in a journal, it's for yourself—no judgments, no grades.

Tired of being stressed out all the time? Want to clear out the cobwebs in your head? Take out paper and pen and embark on one of the most exciting trips you'll ever take—the journey into yourself.

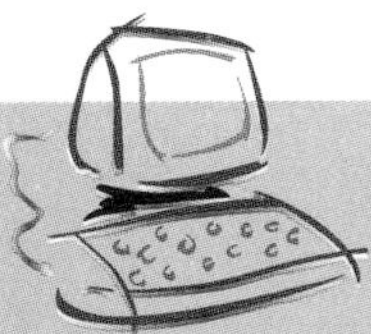

OnSITE/InSIGHT

Learning to Go: Health

Want to reduce your stress load? Click on the Motivator icon, and check out this lesson for some interesting suggestions:

Lesson 9: Learn how to manage your stress.

STUDENT POLL

Feeling as if your life is out of control? Go to the Online Learning Center at **www.mhhe.com/hahn6e**. Click on Student Resources to find the Student Poll. There you can answer these questions and see how other students responded.

1. Do you seek help or talk to someone when you're faced with stress?
2. Do you practice stress-management techniques?
3. Has your stress level increased since you started college?
4. Are you working while going to school?
5. Have you ever participated in yoga or other relaxation classes?
6. Do you keep a journal?
7. Do you take time for quieting or breathing exercises?
8. Is it important to you to take a break or reassess your schedule when projects pile up?
9. Do you suffer from physical symptoms, such as headaches or sleep problems, when you're stressed?
10. Do you seek out positive-thinking people?
11. Are you an overachiever?
12. Do you arrange free time for yourself?
13. Are there constant changes in your life?
14. Are you able to say "no" to requests when you're already overextended?
15. Do you find it acceptable to make mistakes or fail?

- **Search for solutions.** Act on a partial solution, even when a complete solution seems distant.
- **Take control of your own future.** Set out to accomplish all of your goals. Don't view yourself as a victim of circumstances.
- **Move away from negative thought patterns.** Don't extend or generalize difficulties from one area into another.
- **Rehearse success.** Don't disregard the possibility of failure. Instead, focus on the things that are necessary and possible to ensure success.
- **Accept the unchangeable.** The direction your life takes is only partly the result of your own doing. Cope as effectively as possible with the events over which you have no direct control.
- **Live each day well.** Combine activity, contemplation, and a sense of cheerfulness with the many things that must be done each day. Celebrate special occasions.
- **Act on your capacity for growth.** Undertake new experiences, and extract from them new information about your interests and abilities.
- **Allow for renewal.** Make time for yourself. Take advantage of opportunities to pursue new and fulfilling relationships. Foster growth of your spiritual nature.
- **Tolerate mistakes.** Both you and others will make mistakes. Recognize that these can cause anger or frustration, and learn to avoid feelings of hostility.

With a realistic and positive outlook on life, you'll need less coping time to live a satisfying and productive life. Change in all aspects of life is inevitable. With good health, change should be anticipated, nurtured, and incorporated into your maturing sense of well-being.

SUMMARY

- Stress is the physiological and emotional response to the presence of a stressor. Stressors are events that generate the stress response.
- Distress and eustress reflect similar physiological responses but different emotional interpretations.
- Uncontrolled stress can lead to a variety of illnesses. Since the effects of stress are cumulative, stress-related health problems can develop slowly.
- The college experience can generate stressors from several different areas, including finances, classroom requirements, and personal expectations.
- In today's world, even the media, which deliver information to us, can cause as much or more stress than the messages they deliver.
- The general adaptation syndrome consists of three distinct stages: alarm, resistance, and exhaustion. Ideally, exhaustion from excessive stress will not occur and recovery will follow.
- An intricate interplay involving the brain, the nervous system, and the endocrine system results in a series of physiological changes that prepare the body to respond to stressors.
- The stress response mobilizes energy for the fight-or-flight response.
- Stress that is chronic in nature can generate both psychogenic and psychosomatic conditions.
- Experts in psychoneuroimmunology are gaining insight into the mechanisms through which the mind influences the nervous system and the effectiveness of the immune system.
- Chronic feelings of anger and cynicism can be central to the development of stress.
- Ineffective time management may be the single most powerful stressor influencing college students. To overcome this problem, effective time management techniques can be learned.
- A variety of coping techniques can be easily learned and used to reduce stress.
- Therapeutic techniques such as art, dance, and poetry therapy may aid in stress reduction by enhancing the spiritual dimension of health.
- An optimistic outlook on life may protect some people from the potentially damaging effects of stressors. A less stressful life also enhances health and fosters a greater sense of well-being.

REVIEW QUESTIONS

1. What is the difference between stress and stressors?
2. How do distress and eustress differ? In what way are they similar?
3. Which familiar health conditions are often attributed to chronic unresolved stress? To what extent are the effects of stress cumulative?
4. How does the college experience contribute to the stress level of students?
5. In what predictable manner does the stress response unfold? What is the role of the endocrine system? What are the principal energy stores used during the stress response? What is the role of epinephrine and the

glucocorticoids in relationship to the energy needs associated with the stress response?
6. What is psychoneuroimmunology? To date, what has research found in regard to immune function and the occurrence of stress?
7. How do anger and cynicism contribute to stress? How do type R people use the stress response?
8. What coping techniques have proved helpful when used on a regular basis? How do various modern technologies contribute to the high levels of stress reported by many Americans?
9. What are some techniques for improving time management? What is the difference between a maintenance task and a progress task?
10. What traits characterize the optimistic lifestyle?

THINK ABOUT THIS . . .

- Can you remember a stressful experience you had recently in which your body responses clearly followed the pattern of Selye's general adaptation syndrome? How long did you remain in each of the specific stages?
- If the body's response to stressors is similar for distress and eustress, how do we learn to distinguish between the two?
- Do you have a realistic perception about the potentially stressful nature of life?
- Which dimension of your health (physical, emotional, social, intellectual, spiritual, and occupational) do you most frequently rely on when confronted with a stressful situation?
- If you believe that the enhancement of your stress-management skills will be important to you in the future, which of the suggested coping strategies could you most comfortably develop? When can you start to develop these skills?

REFERENCES

1. Selye H: *Stress without distress,* 1975, New American Library.
2. Suhara T et al: Dopamine D2 receptors in the insular cortex and the personality trait of novelty seeking. *Neuroimage,* 13(5):891–985, 2001.
3. Williams RB et al: Central nervous system serotonin function and cardiovascular responses to stress, *Psychosom Med,* 63(2):300–305.
4. Kubey RW, Lavin MJ, Barrows JR: Internet use and collegiate academic performance decrements: early findings, *J Commun,* 51(2):366–382, 2001.
5. Probst TM, Brubaker TL: The effects of job insecurity on employee safety outcomes: cross-sectional and longitudinal explorations, *J Occup Health Psychol,* 139–159, 2001.
6. Saladin K: *Anatomy and physiology: the unity of form and function,* ed 2, 2000, McGraw-Hill.
7. Ulrich V et al: The inheritance of migraine with aura estimated by means of structural equation modeling, *J Med Genet,* 36(3):225–227, 1999.
8. Elenkov I et al: Stress, corticotropin-releasing hormone, glucocorticoids, and the immune/inflammation response: acute and chronic effects, *Ann NY Acad Sci,* 866:1–11, discussion 11–13, 1999.
9. Keltikangas-Jarvinen L, Ravaja, Viikari J: Indentifying Cloninger's temperament profiles as related to the early development of the metabolic cardiovascular syndrome in young men, *Arterioscler Thromb Vasc Biol,* 19(8):1998–2006, 1999.
10. Benson H (with MZ Klipper): *The relaxation response,* 2000, Wholecare.
11. Jacobson E: *You must relax,* 1991, National Foundation for Progressive Relaxation.
12. Stroebel C: *QR: the quieting reflex,* 1983, Berkley.
13. McGinnis L: *The power of optimism,* 1990, Harper & Row.

SUGGESTED READINGS

Burke L: *Seven steps to stress-free teaching: a stress prevention planning guide for teachers,* 1999, Educators' Lighthouse.
In this book, an experienced teacher shares her step-by-step approach to reducing the stress of classroom teaching. Included are specific techniques to use for classroom management, time management, and parental pressure. The author also addresses aspects of the personal life of teachers and how they can be structured to avoid conflict with professional responsibilities. If you're an education major, you'll find this book helpful in planning your career as a classroom teacher.

Jevne R, Williams D: *When dreams don't work: professional caregivers and burnout,* 1998, Baywood Publishing.
In this book, the term *caregivers* is broadened to include a wide array of social service fields, such as teaching, social work, law enforcement, and other public service–centered occupations. Special attention is given to the motivations of people who enter these fields and to the emotional, social, and spiritual forces that precipitate the burnout often experienced by those who work in these fields. If you're considering a career in one of the helping professions, you may find this book a valuable source of information.

Mayer J: *Time management for dummies,* ed 2, 1999, IDG Books Worldwide.
The author, a recognized authority in the field of time management, focuses on areas such as organizing work space, establishing a daily planning process, efficient use of the telephone and other electronic equipment, setting goals, and making time for family activities.

1,001 perfectly legal ways to get exactly what you want, when you want it, every time, 1999, FC&A Publishing.
Sometimes the lack of a detail or certain obscure information makes daily life more stressful than it needs to be. This book supplies such information on topics ranging from financial management and child rearing to pet care. It promises readers that they will have more money in their pockets, more time and fun in their lives, and less stress after reading this book.

As we go to Press...

Shortly after the September 11, 2001, terrorist attacks on the World Trade Center in New York City and the Pentagon in Washington, letters and packages containing a mysterious white powder began appearing in several areas of the country. The substance, later identified as anthrax, was found in Boca Raton, Florida; New York City; Washington, DC; and Reno, Nevada. The offices of Dan Rather at CBS in New York and Senator Tom Daschle in Washington were two high-profile targets.

As news of these events was broadcast on TV, Americans saw technicians wearing respirators and protective clothing as they tested sites for anthrax spores, gloved postal employees handling mail, and congressional staff members waiting for anthrax testing.

Signs of panic soon began appearing throughout the country. Doctors were flooded with requests for anthrax testing. Pharmacists noted a run on Cipro, used for treatment of inhalation anthrax, with sales doubling and tripling the normal level in some instances. In response, the maker of Cipro, Bayer A.G., planned to triple its normal production of the drug. One airline stopped serving sweetener and creamer to passengers because these substances could be mistaken for anthrax powder. Meanwhile, government officials were trying to reassure the public that there was no need for alarm, but their sometimes conflicting reports and advice only seemed to add to the anxiety of many.

At the time of this writing, three people in the United States have died from the dangerous form of anthrax (inhalation), and several people have been infected with the highly treatable cutaneous (skin) type. Although no definite link has yet been established between the September 11 attacks and these apparent acts of bioterrorism, many people have no doubt that there is a connection and are feeling the stress every day as they do something as simple as open their mail or touch their computer keyboard.

Name ______________________ **Date** ____________ **Section** ____________

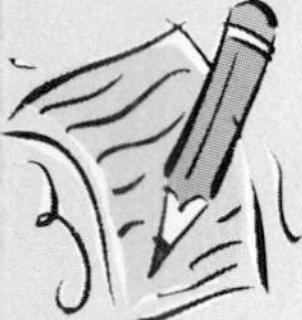

Personal Assessment

How Stressed Are You?

You must know how much stress you are under and what events are triggering your feelings of stress before you can begin to cope effectively. In the following stress test, developed by researchers at Carnegie Mellon University, you can obtain a rough measure of the level of stress you are under. The questions reflect some of the most familiar perceptions of people who are experiencing distress.

The higher your total score on this test, the higher your level of stress. In the general population, the average score for men was 12 and for women was 14.

Other stress assessments indicate that difficult or unexpected life events, such as the death of a family member, arrest and incarceration, the demands of school or work, a pregnancy (yours or your partner's), a serious illness or injury, and even marriage, are among the greatest sources of stress for most adults. How familiar are you with these events?

In the last month, how often have you felt:	Never	Almost never	Sometimes	Fairly often	Very often
Upset because of something that happened unexpectedly?	0	1	2	3	4
Unable to control the important things in your life?	0	1	2	3	4
Nervous and "stressed"?	0	1	2	3	4
Unable to cope with all the things you had to do?	0	1	2	3	4
Angered because of things that were beyond your control?	0	1	2	3	4
That difficulties were piling up so high that you could not overcome them?	0	1	2	3	4
Confident about your abilities to handle your personal problems?	4	3	2	1	0
That things were going your way?	4	3	2	1	0
Able to control irritations in your life?	4	3	2	1	0
That you were on top of things?	4	3	2	1	0

TOTAL SCORE: ____________

Name ______________________ **Date** __________ **Section** __________

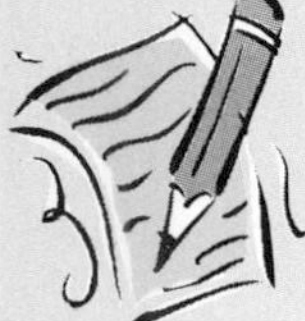

Personal Assessment

Do You Manage Your Time Effectively?

This assessment is designed to help you determine how you are spending your nonsleeping hours. With this information, you will be able to assess the effectiveness of your time management. In particular, you will be able to judge whether you are scheduling enough time for your academic responsibilities.

In 1 week, there are 168 hours available for different uses. You need 6 to 8 hours of sleep per day. If 6 hours is used as a realistic figure for daily sleep, that makes 42 hours a week for sleep. So the remaining (nonsleeping) time for 1 week is 126 hours.

Directions: Calculate the number of hours per day that you spend in each of the activity categories listed on the right. Then multiple each figure by 7 to determine the number of hours spent weekly for each activity. Add all these figures together. Then subtract this total from 126. The result is the number of hours remaining for your classes and classwork.

1. Hours spent getting ready to begin the day _____ × 7 = _____
2. Hours spent "on the road" (going to and from class, work, and other locations) _____ × 7 = _____
3. Hours spent doing planned exercise _____ × 7 = _____
4. Hours spent eating (meals and snacks) _____ × 7 = _____
5. Hours spent watching television and videos _____ × 7 = _____
6. Hours spent on the Internet, excluding school-related assignments and research _____ × 7 = _____
7. Hours spent in extracurricular activities or employment _____ × 7 = _____
8. Hours spent "hanging out" with friends _____ × 7 = _____

TOTAL _____

After subtracting the total hours from 126, you will see how many hours are available for class attendance, research, writing, and test preparation. Are you showing signs of poor time management?

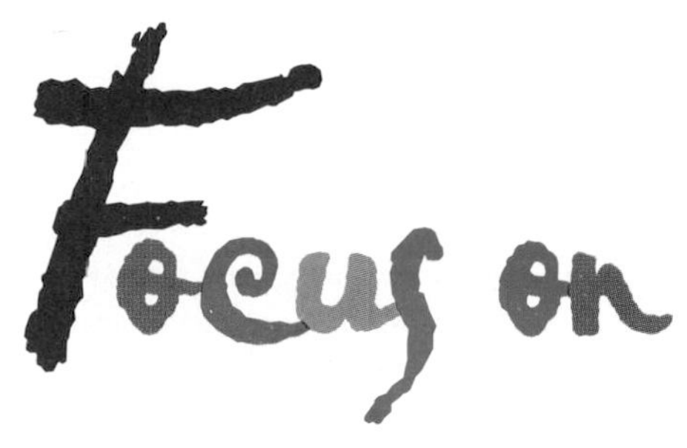

MANAGING WORK-RELATED STRESS

When someone is introduced to you, the first thing you learn is the person's name. Next, you usually find out something about that person's occupation. Since Americans identify people with the jobs they perform, our self-identity is linked to our occupations. As a result, anything that threatens our job or job performance can be a threat to our sense of personal worth.

Job stress is becoming a part of everyday life. In a 1999 study for *The Wirthin Report,* 67 percent of the respondents reported that their work was very stressful or moderately stressful. Only 10 percent said that their work was not stressful. If left unchecked, employment-related stress can have negative effects on our feelings of well-being and the structure and function of our bodies. The cardiovascular and immune systems are particularly vulnerable to work-related stress.[1,2]

Sources of Job Stress

Since work-related stress can be a significant problem, it is important to identify what specific things can cause stress in the workplace, such as the following:

- Conflicts with colleagues, supervisors, or workers under your supervision
- Changes in work routine
- Deadlines
- Too much (or too little) responsibility
- Lack of control over work methods and planning
- Long working hours
- Repetitive tasks
- Excessive or rhythmic noise
- Poor time management or organization
- Working with hazardous equipment or substances
- Threat of pay reduction or unemployment
- Lack of necessary resources

Nearly everyone has to deal with these issues at one time or another in the workplace. Although these stressors may vary from job to job, and individuals may react to them in different ways, they still produce an effect.

Job Stress Among Older Workers

In general, older workers are hit hardest by job stress. Technological advances tend to cause more stress for them, especially workers who have been performing a similar routine for a long time and are suddenly forced to assimilate new technology into their daily work. Older workers are also prime targets for layoffs.[3] As a result, some are leaving the workforce at an earlier age than expected. This situation may produce both financial and psychological stress.

Stress in the Modern Workplace

Throughout the last twenty-five years, corporate mergers and buyouts have eliminated entire companies and thousands of jobs, new technology has caused a drastic increase in the pace of work, and heightened competition has forced individual employees to take on much heavier workloads. All of this adds up to increased stress.

Technology

Today's workers must deal with stressors that are unique to our time. The most obvious is the drastic increase in workplace technology. Workers must be more knowledgeable about the new machines they use, and so reeducation becomes necessary. Personal computers and computer networks, which are constantly increasing workplace efficiency and speed, also contribute to job stress. Getting more work done in a specified time means more profit for a company, but it also leads to the expectation that more work will continue to be accomplished in less time. Therefore the person working at the computer may be asked to perform more and more tasks in a workday. The increased productivity resulting from computer use can lead to the elimination of many jobs, since one worker may now be able to do the work that was once done by two or more people.

The computer may also contribute to physical problems. Constant work on a keyboard places excess stress on the fingers, hands, and wrists. This, in turn, may contribute to arthritic conditions or *carpal tunnel syndrome.* The simple act of sitting at the computer for extended periods with the body in a fixed position puts stress on the muscles and bones of the back, neck, and limbs.[4]

Problems caused by repetitive motions, unusual body postures, or holding static joint positions over extended periods are referred to as *repetitive strain injuries* (RSIs).[5] The risk of developing RSIs is increased during periods of emotional stress or deadline pressure. RSIs can also develop because of improper placement of equipment (e.g., a keyboard). Company production goals based on quotas, such as counting workers' keystrokes, may influence employees to work through needed break periods to meet the expected work output.

Downsizing

The corporate practice of eliminating jobs to cut costs—downsizing—can contribute greatly to job stress.[3] This practice affects both rank-and-file workers and management; everyone is vulnerable. Often, cuts are made with little or no regard to an employee's years of service or experience (or senior employees are "let go" as a way of saving money). This lack of job security has been an important contributor to job stress over the last decade.

The fear of being unemployed and the difficult transition following unemployment causes workers and their families to develop a variety of stress-induced conditions, including anxiety and depression. These families also often display higher than normal rates of divorce and drug and alcohol abuse.

One extreme expression of the impact of work-related stress is death resulting from cardiovascular disease, particularly heart attack. As long ago as 1982, this trend was reported in the Swedish workforce.[6] Autopsies on these heart attack victims, some of whom were as young as 29, showed that no significant risk factors were present except for high levels of chemicals (e.g., epinephrine) that are released in response to stress. Other industrialized nations, including the United States, are observing signs of this trend in their workforces.

Downsizing has been a stated goal of many U.S. corporations and agencies, including IBM, Boeing, Apple Computer, and NASA. Recently, AT&T announced a "reduction in force" anticipated to be as high as 40,000 employees.

Competition

Although there are more than enough jobs being created to offset those lost through downsizing, many new jobs offer lower pay, fewer benefits, and less desirable working conditions. As a result, competition for good jobs is growing keener. A college education is no longer enough, More than 20 percent of adults hold at least a bachelor's degree, and over 40 percent of adults have some college experience. The most current statistics available (1994–1995 academic year) indicate that over 14 million students are currently enrolled at institutions of higher education.[7] Workers whose jobs are cut are facing competition from new college graduates, who will often work for less money, and from others who have been laid off. New graduates are competing with displaced workers, who usually have a wealth of work experience.

This uncertainty in the workplace has led many people to broaden their knowledge to become more competitive within their chosen field or to change careers altogether. This has resulted in a booming business for colleges and universities. According to the most current data available, over 26 percent of all college students enrolled in the United States are over the age of 24.[7] Many of these nontraditional-age students (and a great many traditional-age students) face the challenge of succeeding at school while trying to raise a family or hold down a job. It is becoming increasingly common for students to attend classes either before or after working a full shift at a regular job. Job stress is thus compounded with classroom stress.

Reducing Work-Related Stress

Since work-related stress appears to be increasing in most professions, it is important to recognize the physical signs of stress and reduce job stress when possible. Here are a few things you can do to reduce the effects of work-related stress:

- *Recognize when stress is getting to you.* Be able to identify early warning signs that you may be under heavy stress. Emotional signs may include anxiety, lack of interest, and irritability. Mental fatigue, physical exhaustion, and frequent illness may be physical manifestations of stress. Know yourself well enough to recognize when stressors are affecting you.
- *Control your environment when you can.* Not every work situation can be controlled, but managing some situations can help reduce stress. Try not to schedule stressful work activities in succession. Break larger jobs down into smaller parts. Rearrange your work area to keep things fresh.
- *Know the things you cannot control and deal with them.* Becoming angry or obsessed over a situation you can't do anything about only increases your stress level. Developing a flexible attitude toward situations on the job that are not flexible is a healthy approach.
- *Take a break.* Schedule some down time to keep yourself refreshed. If your breaks are scheduled for you, don't use them to get extra work done. When performing repetitive tasks, step away from the task whenever you can. If you work at a computer terminal, get up occasionally and move around.
- *Get some exercise.* Physical activity can be healthy for the mind and the body. Exercise can actually increase energy levels and strengthen physical resistance to stress.
- *Make your workplace safe.* Take safety precautions when possible. If safety equipment is available, use it. Staying safe on the job can prevent stressful situations that may occur because of an injury, such as missed work, decreased productivity, and physical pain.

If you notice that stress on the job is affecting you physically or mentally, see your family doctor or a qualified mental health professional as soon as possible. Work-related stress does not have to become an overwhelming factor in your life. Managing stress is an important skill that all employees must learn to master. Set aside time to assess your problems and devise strategies to deal with your stressful situations.

REFERENCES

1. McCann BS, Benjamin CA, et al: Plasma lipid concentrations during episodic occupational stress, *Ann Behav Med,* 21(2):103–110, 1999.
2. DeGucht V, Fischler B, Demanet C: Immune dysfunction associated with chronic professional stress in nurses, *Psychiatry Res,* 85(1):105–111, 1999.
3. Reissman DB, Orris P, et al: Downsizing role demands, and job stress, *J Occup Environ Med,* 41(4):289–293, 1999.
4. Tittiranonda P, Burastero S, Rempel D: Risk factors for musculoskeletal disorders among computer users, *Occup Med,* 14(1):17–38, 1999.
5. Nainzadeh N, Malantic-Lin A, et al: Repetitive strain injury (cumulative trauma disorder): causes and treatment, *Mt Sinai J Med,* 66(3):192–196, 1999.
6. Alfredsson L, Karasek R, Theorell T: Myocardial infarction risk and psychosocial work environment: an analysis of the male Swedish working force, *Soc Sci Med,* 16(4):463–467, 1982.
7. U.S. Bureau of the Census: *Statistical abstract of the United States: 1999* (119th ed), 1999, Washington, D.C.

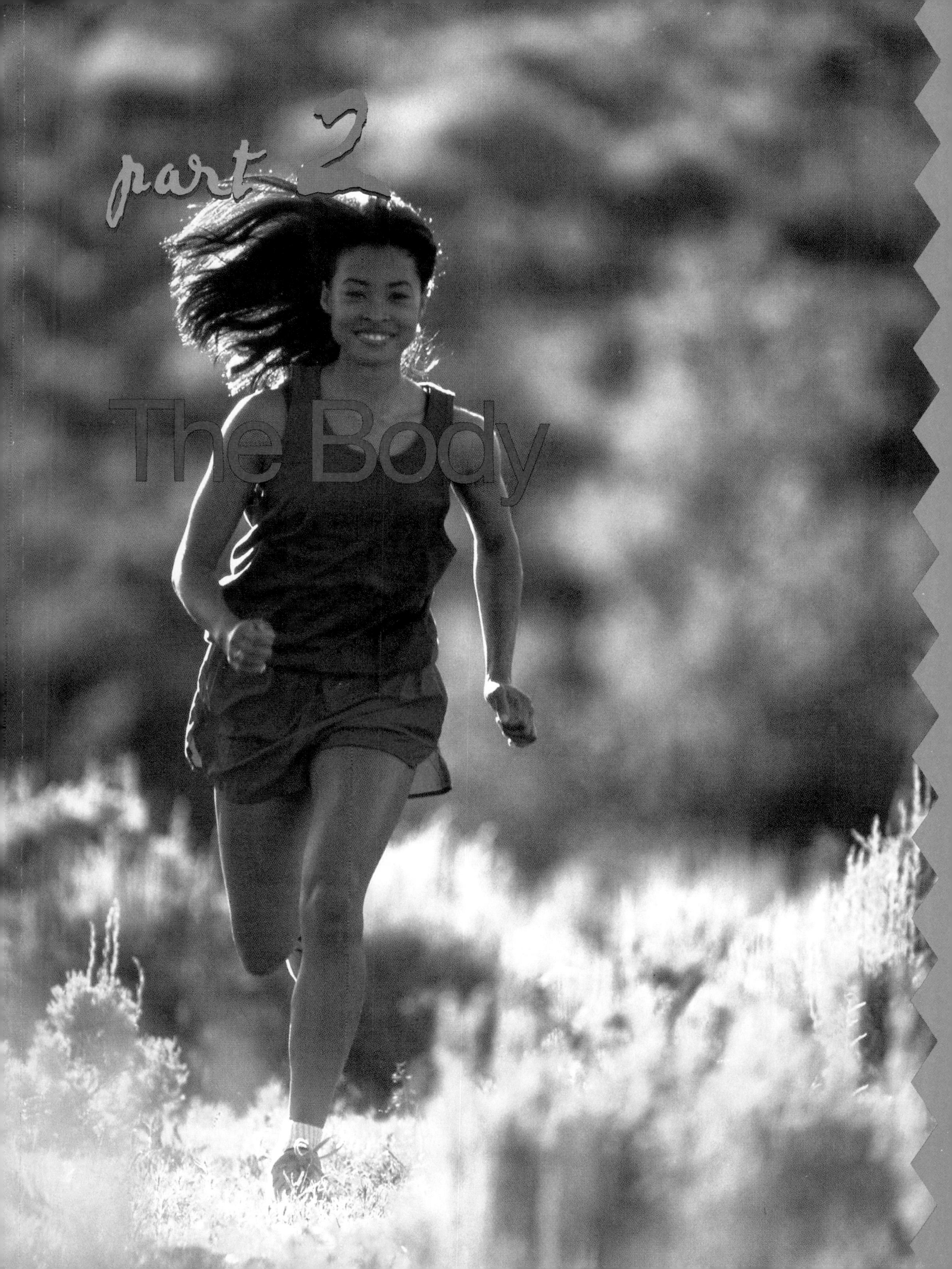
part 2
The Body

chapter **4**

Becoming Physically Fit

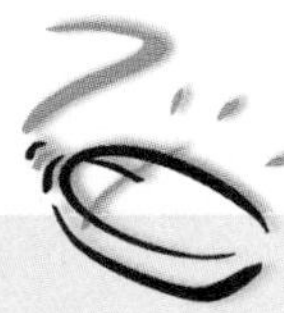

Online Learning Center Resources

www.mhhe.com/hahn6e

Log on to our Online Learning Center (OLC) for access to these additional resources:

- Chapter key terms and definitions
- Learning objectives
- Additional behavior change objectives
- Student interactive question-and-answer sites
- Self-scoring chapter quiz

The OLC also offers web links for study and exploration of health topics. Here are some examples of what you'll find:

- **www.primusweb.com/fitnesspartner** Use this jumpsite to find fitness information on topics ranging from nutrition to equipment.
- **www.netsweat.com** Click on this site for a fitness message board where you can post a question for discussion.
- **www.hoptechno.com/book11.htm** Find guidelines for a personal exercise program from the President's Council on Physical Fitness and Sports.

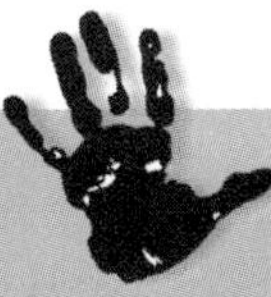

Taking Charge of Your Health

- Assess your level of fitness by completing the National Fitness Test on p. 83.
- Start a daily stretching program based on the guidelines in this chapter.
- Implement or maintain a cardiorespiratory fitness program that uses the most recent American College of Sports Medicine recommendations.
- Examine your athletic shoes to determine their appropriateness for the fitness activities you do (see Choosing an Athletic Shoe on p. 74).
- Monitor your physical activities for potential danger signs indicating that you should consult an athletic trainer, physical therapist, or physician.
- For 2 weeks, keep track of the amount of sleep you are getting. Determine whether this is enough sleep, and make adjustments accordingly.

Eye on the Media

Magazines Feature Readers' Choice—Health News

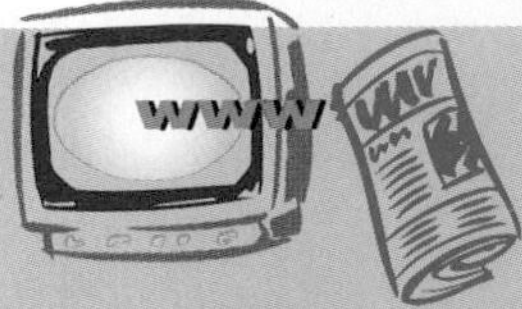

In the past decade, popular magazines have initiated or greatly expanded their coverage of health issues. This is especially true for the magazines that cover national and international news. In fact, it is difficult to pick up a major news magazine (such as *Time, Newsweek,* or *U.S. News & World Report*) and *not* find one or two articles about health issues. Occasionally, these magazines have cover stories on topics such as fitness, obesity, smoking, prescription drugs, the environment, herbal supplements, growth and development, and sexuality.

This inclusion of health issues did not come about without careful consideration by the media moguls. Readers have been routinely surveyed by publishers about their preferences for topics. Since readers have reported that they want more coverage of health issues, magazine publishers have complied.

Fortunately, the health editors and writers for these major publications generally do an excellent job of preparing their news reports. Most try to consult (and then quote) health researchers who are experts in

Eye on the Media *continued*

their fields. Many reports in the popular news magazines present the results of health-related research that has been published in scientific journals or presented at professional meetings.

You, the consumer (reader), should be aware, however, that magazine articles may not give the most complete coverage of a health issue or may exaggerate the threat posed by certain diseases. Most health issues that are hot news items can be viewed from more than one perspective. Be inquisitive about finding out if there are conflicting views about stories that interest you. Find and read the original sources identified in the magazine article. Many of these original sources are available in your college library or on the Internet. If you have additional questions, ask professors, nutritionists, physical therapists, or physicians. Used in this way, magazine articles can provide an excellent first step in your quest to discover new information concerning your health.

TALKING POINTS • If you had a strong reaction to a news magazine's treatment of a certain health issue, would you consider writing a letter to the editor expressing your opinion?

When your day begins early in the morning, then you go to class or work or immerse yourself in family activities, and your day does not end until after midnight, you must be physically fit to keep up the pace. Even a highly motivated college student must have a conditioned, rested body to maintain such a schedule.

OK, let's simplify things a bit. The paragraph above reflects how college health professors might view the value of fitness—it helps people function well enough to cope with their hectic lifestyles. But what motivates students to value fitness? Quite simply, students say that overall body fitness helps them look and feel better.

Many college students want to look in the mirror and see the kind of body they see in the media: one with well-toned muscles, a trim waistline, and no flabby tissue, especially on the arms and legs. Students become motivated to start fitness programs because they hope that they can build a better body for themselves. Through their efforts to do so, students usually start to feel better, both physically and mentally. They realize that change is possible, since they see it happening to their bodies with each passing week. "Go for it" and "Just do it" then become more than just sports marketing phrases; they become reminders that the activities that lead to fitness are a meaningful part of their lives. Fitness actually becomes fun (Figure 4-1).

Fortunately, you don't have to be a top-notch athlete to enjoy the health benefits of physical activity. In fact, even a modest increase in your daily activity level can be rewarding. The health benefits of fitness can come from regular participation in moderate exercise, such as brisk walking or dancing[1] (see HealthQuest Activities).

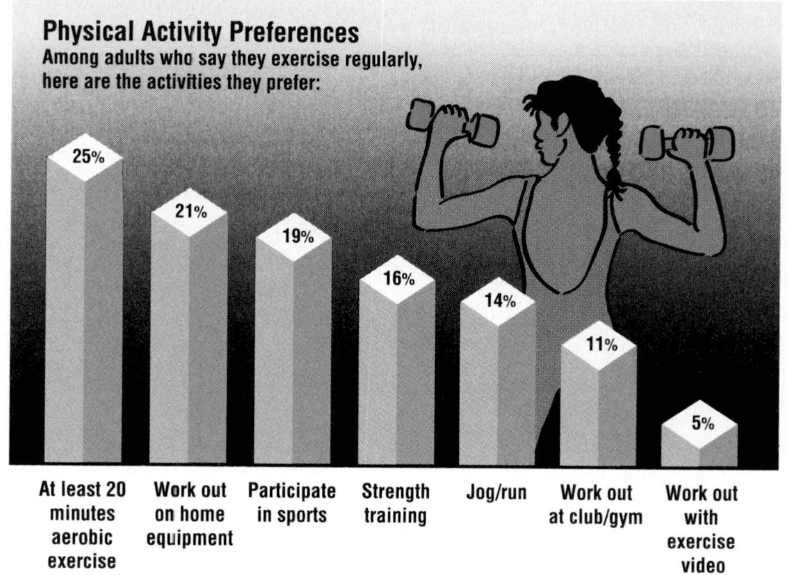

Figure 4-1 Running or working out in a gym is not for everyone. Which physical activities fit your preferences and lifestyle?

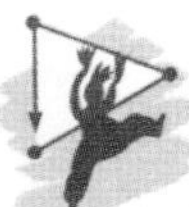

HealthQuest Activities

- The *How Fit Are You?* exercise in the Fitness module will help you determine your current level of fitness in four major areas: body composition, cardiorespiratory capacity, muscular strength, and flexibility. Complete the series of questions about how much you exercise, what types of training you do, how intensely you exercise, and your body size. After you complete the questions, *HealthQuest* will give you feedback in each of the four areas mentioned above. Then develop an individual plan for improving or maintaining your current fitness level.
- The *Exercise Interest Inventory* in the Fitness module allows you to rate your feelings about certain aspects of exercise. *HealthQuest* provides feedback about the activities and exercises you would most enjoy, based on your individual needs and preferences. First, write down the five fitness activities that you like best or those you participate in most often. After each one, indicate your motivation for engaging in that particular activity. For example, you could list "enjoyment," "habit," or "convenience." When you have completed the *Exercise Interest Inventory,* compare the two lists. Any surprises? What factors had you not considered to be influential in your choice of exercise?

COMPONENTS OF PHYSICAL FITNESS

Physical fitness is achieved when "the various systems of the body are healthy and function efficiently so as to enable the fit person to engage in activities of daily living, as well as in recreational pursuits and leisure activities, without unreasonable fatigue."[2] The following sections focus on cardiorespiratory endurance, muscular strength, muscular endurance, flexibility, and body composition.

Cardiorespiratory Endurance

If you were limited to improving only one area of your physical fitness, which would you choose—muscular strength, muscular endurance, or flexibility? Which would a dancer choose? Which would a marathon runner select? Which would an expert recommend?

The experts, exercise physiologists, would probably say that another fitness dimension is even more important than those listed above. They regard improvement of your heart, lung, and blood vessel function as the key focal point of a physical fitness program. **Cardiorespiratory endurance** forms the foundation for whole-body fitness.

Cardiorespiratory endurance increases your capacity to sustain a given level of energy production for a prolonged period. It helps your body to work longer and at greater levels of intensity.

Your body cannot always produce the energy it needs for long-term activity. Certain activities require performance at a level of intensity that will outstrip your cardiorespiratory system's ability to transport oxygen efficiently to contracting muscle fibers. When the oxygen demands of the muscles cannot be met, **oxygen debt** occurs. Any activity that continues beyond the point at which oxygen debt begins requires a form of energy production that does not depend on oxygen.

This oxygen-deprived form of energy production is called **anaerobic** (without oxygen) **energy production,** the type that fuels many intense, short-duration activities. For example, rope climbing, weight lifting for strength, and sprinting are short-duration activities that quickly cause muscle fatigue; they are generally considered anaerobic activities.

Activities not generally associated with anaerobic energy production (walking, distance jogging, and bicycle touring) become anaerobic activities when they are increased in intensity or continued for an extended period.

If you usually work or play at low intensity but for a long duration, you have developed an ability to maintain **aerobic** (with oxygen) **energy production.** As long as your body can meet its energy demands in this oxygen-rich mode, it will not convert to anaerobic energy production. Thus fatigue will not be an important factor in determining whether you can continue to participate. Marathon runners, serious joggers, distance swimmers, cyclists, and aerobic dancers can perform because of their highly developed aerobic fitness. The cardiorespiratory systems of these aerobically fit people take in, transport, and use oxygen in the most efficient manner possible.

Besides allowing you to participate in activities such as those mentioned, aerobic conditioning (cardiorespiratory endurance conditioning) may also provide certain structural and functional benefits that affect other dimensions of your life (see Exploring Your Spirituality on p. 65). These recognized benefits (see the Star Box on p. 66) have received considerable documented support. Some data, for example, strongly suggest that aerobic fitness can increase life expectancy[3] and reduce the risk of developing cancer of the colon, heart, uterus, cervix, and ovaries.[4]

Muscular Strength

Muscular strength is essential for your body to accomplish work. Your ability to maintain posture, walk, lift, push, and pull are familiar examples of the constant demands you make on your muscles to maintain or in-

Exploring Your Spirituality

Harnessing the Spirit: The Saga of Lance Armstrong

In July 2001, American cyclist Lance Armstrong won his third straight Tour de France, the most grueling cycling event in the world. As amazing as this feat may seem, an even bigger victory for Lance Armstrong was his conquest of cancer. In October 1996, Armstrong was diagnosed with advanced testicular cancer and given less than a 50% chance of survival. At the time of diagnosis, the cancer had already spread to his abdomen, lungs, and brain.

However, before starting aggressive cancer therapy, Armstrong declared himself "a cancer survivor, not a cancer victim." He convinced himself, his family, and his medical support team that he could beat the long odds facing him. He even established the Lance Armstrong Foundation (**www.laf.org**) before he had surgery and chemotherapy. He battled through his therapy without giving up hope that the cancer would be defeated.

Along the way, many doubted whether Armstrong would ever compete again at the world-class level. Armstrong proved his doubters wrong by winning not only the 1999 race, but also the 2000 and 2001 Tour de France races. He became a world celebrity and chronicled his battle with testicular cancer in his best-selling book *It's Not about the Bike: My Journey Back to Life* (Putnam) and followed this with a cycling training book called *The Lance Armstrong Performance Program: Seven Weeks to the Perfect Ride* (Rodale Press).

Clearly, Armstrong's powers of the mind and spirit worked to help him overcome his physical barriers. His success story has undoubtedly inspired others to take charge of their lives by doing their best to rise above mental and physical barriers to pursue the dreams that sometimes seem impossible.

crease their level of contraction. The stronger you are, the greater your ability to contract muscles and maintain a level of contraction sufficient to complete tasks.

Muscular strength can be improved best by training activities that use the **overload principle.** By overloading, or gradually increasing the resistance (load, object, or weight) your muscles must move, you can increase your muscular strength. The following three types of training exercises are based on the overload principle.

In **isometric** (meaning "same measure") **exercises,** the resistance is so great that your contracting muscles cannot move the resistant object at all. So your muscles contract against immovable objects, usually with increasingly greater efforts. Because of the difficulty of precisely evaluating the training effects, isometric exercises are not usually used as a primary means of developing muscular strength. These exercises can be dangerous for people with hypertension.

Progressive resistance exercises, also called *isotonic* or *same-tension* exercises, are currently the most popular type of strength-building exercises. Progressive resistance exercises include the use of traditional free weights (dumbbells and barbells), as well as Universal, Body Master, and Nautilus machines. People who perform progressive resistance exercises use various muscle groups to move (or lift) specific fixed resistances or weights. Although during a given repetitive exercise the weight resistance remains the same, the muscular contraction effort required varies according to the joint angles in the range of motion. The greatest effort is required at the start and finish of the movement.

Key Terms

cardiorespiratory endurance
The ability of the heart, lungs, and blood vessels to process and transport oxygen required by muscle cells so that they can contract over a period of time.

oxygen debt
The physical state that occurs when the body can no longer process and transport sufficient amounts of oxygen for continued muscle contraction.

anaerobic energy production
The body's means of energy production when the necessary amount of oxygen is not available.

aerobic energy production
The body's means of energy production when the respiratory and circulatory systems are able to process and transport a sufficient amount of oxygen to muscle cells.

muscular strength
The ability to contract skeletal muscles to engage in work; the force that a muscle can exert.

overload principle
The principle whereby a person gradually increases the resistance load that must be moved or lifted; this principle also applies to other types of fitness training.

isometric exercises
Muscular strength training exercises in which the resistance is so great that the object cannot be moved.

progressive resistance exercises
Muscular strength training exercises in which traditional barbells and dumbbells with fixed resistances are used.

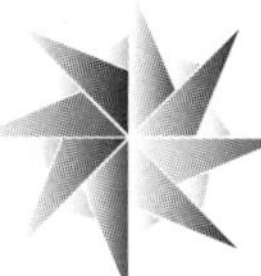

Structural and Functional Benefits of Cardiorespiratory (Aerobic) Fitness

Aerobic fitness can help you do the following:

- Complete and enjoy your daily activities.
- Strengthen and increase the efficiency of your heart muscle.
- Increase the proportion of high-density lipoproteins in your blood.
- Increase the capillary network in your body.
- Improve **collateral circulation.**
- Control your weight.
- Stimulate bone growth.
- Cope with stressors.
- Ward off infections.
- Improve the efficiency of your other body systems.
- Bolster your self-esteem.
- Achieve self-directed fitness goals.
- Reduce negative dependence behavior.
- Sleep better.
- Recover more quickly from common illnesses.
- Meet people with similar interests.
- Receive reduced insurance premiums.

Isokinetic (meaning "same motion") **exercises** use mechanical devices that provide resistances that consistently overload muscles throughout the entire range of motion. The resistance will move only at a preset speed, regardless of the force applied to it. For the exercise to be effective, a user must apply maximal force.[2] Isokinetic training requires elaborate, expensive equipment.

Thus the use of isokinetic equipment may be limited to certain athletic teams, diagnostic centers, or rehabilitation clinics. The most common isokinetic machines are Cybex, Orthotron, Biodex, Mini-Gym, and Exergenie.

Which type of strength-building exercise (machines or free weights) is most effective? Take your choice, since all will help develop muscular strength. Some people prefer machines because they are simple to use, do not require stacking the weights, and are already balanced and less likely to drop and cause injury.

Other people prefer free weights because they encourage the user to work harder to maintain balance during the lift. In addition, free weights can be used in a greater variety of exercises than weight machines.

Muscular Endurance

Muscular endurance is a component of physical fitness associated with strength. When muscles contract and their individual muscle fibers shorten, energy is needed. Energy production requires that oxygen and nutrients be delivered by the circulatory system to the muscles. After these products are transformed into energy by individual muscle cells, the body must remove the potentially toxic waste by-products.

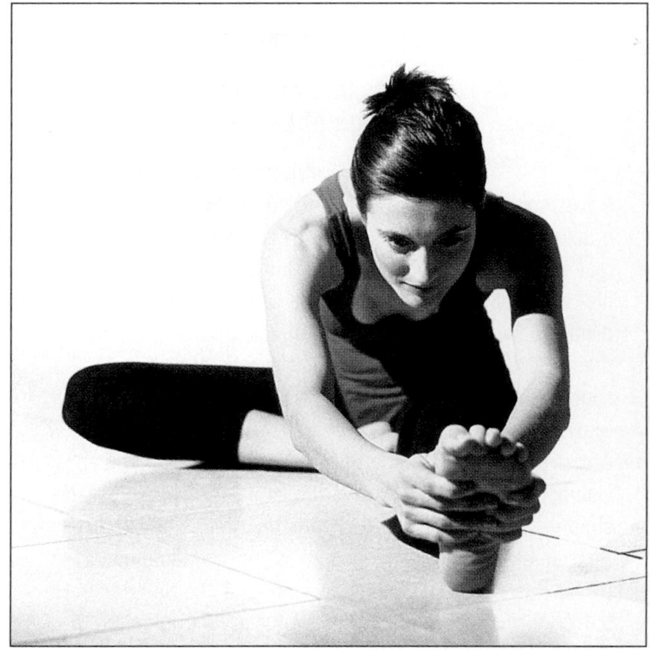

Static stretching can help you develop and maintain flexibility.

Amateur and professional athletes often wish to increase the endurance of specific muscle groups associated with their sports activities. This can be achieved by using exercises that gradually increase the number of repetitions of a given movement. However, muscular endurance is not the physiological equivalent of cardiorespiratory endurance. For example, a world-ranked distance runner with highly developed cardiorespiratory endurance and extensive muscular endurance of the legs may not have a corresponding level of muscular endurance of the abdominal muscles.

Flexibility

The ability of your joints to move through their natural range of motion is a measure of your **flexibility.** This fitness trait, like so many other aspects of structure and function, differs from point to point within your body and among different people. Not every joint in your body is equally flexible (by design), and over the course of time, use or disuse will alter the flexibility of a given joint. Certainly, gender, age, genetically determined body build, and current level of physical fitness will affect your flexibility.

Inability to move easily during physical activity can be a constant reminder that aging and inactivity are the foes of flexibility. Failure to use joints regularly will quickly result in a loss of elasticity in the connective tissue

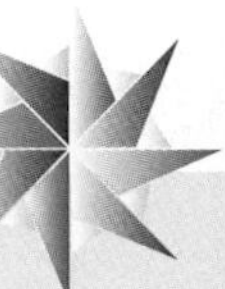

Guidelines for Static Stretching

Take the following precautions to reduce the possibility of injury during stretching:

- Warm up using a slow jog or fast walk before stretching.
- Stretch only to the point at which you feel tightness or resistance to your stretching. Stretching should not be painful.
- Be sure to continue normal breathing during a stretch. Do *not* hold your breath.
- Use caution when stretching muscles that surround painful joints. Pain is an indication that something is wrong—it should not be ignored.

and shortening of muscles associated with the joints. Benefits of flexibility include improved balance, posture, and athletic performance and reduced risk of low back pain.

As seen in young gymnasts, flexibility can be highly developed and maintained with a program of activity that includes regular stretching. Stretching also helps reduce the risk of injury. Athletic trainers generally prefer **static stretching** to **ballistic stretching** for people who wish to improve their range of motion. Guidelines for stretching are given in the Star Box above.

Body Composition

Body composition is the makeup of the body in terms of muscle, bone, fat, and other elements.[2] Of particular interest to fitness experts are percentages of body fat and fat-free weight. Health experts are especially concerned about the large number of people in our society who are overweight and obese. Increasingly, cardiorespiratory fitness trainers are recognizing the importance of body composition and are including strength-training exercises to help reduce body fat. (See Chapter 6 for further information about body composition, health effects of obesity, and weight management.)

AGING PHYSICALLY

The period between 45 and 64 years of age brings with it a variety of subtle changes in the body's structure and function. When life is busy and the mind is active, these changes are generally not evident. Even when they become evident, they are not usually the source of profound concern. Your parents, older students in your class, and people with whom you will be working are, nevertheless, experiencing these changes.

- Decrease in bone mass and density
- Increase in vertebral compression
- Degenerative changes in joint cartilage
- Increase in adipose tissue—loss of lean body mass
- Decrease in capacity to engage in physical work
- Decrease in visual acuity
- Decrease in basal energy requirements
- Decrease in fertility
- Decrease in sexual function

For some midlife adults these health concerns can be quite threatening, especially for those who view aging with apprehension and fear. Some middle-aged people reject these physical changes and convince themselves they are sick. Indeed, *hypochondriasis* is much more common among midlife people than among young people.

Two medical conditions influenced by physical activity, osteoporosis and osteoarthritis, deserve careful examination and are discussed in the following sections.

Osteoporosis

Osteoporosis is a condition often seen in late middle-aged women. However, it is not fully understood why menopausal women are so susceptible to the increase in calcium loss that leads to fracture of the hip, wrist, and vertebral column. Half of all women over the age of 50 will likely suffer an osteoporosis-realted fracture.

Key Terms

collateral circulation
The ability of nearby blood vessels to enlarge and carry additional blood around a blocked blood vessel.

isokinetic exercises
Muscular strength training exercises in which machines are used to provide variable resistances throughout the full range of motion.

muscular endurance
The ability of a muscle or muscle group to function over time; supported by the respiratory and circulatory systems.

flexibility
The ability of joints to function through an intended range of motion.

static stretching
The slow lengthening of a muscle group to an extended stretch; followed by holding the extended position for a recommended period.

ballistic stretching
A "bouncing" form of stretching in which a muscle group is lengthened repetitively to produce multiple quick, forceful stretches.

osteoporosis
Loss of calcium from the bone, seen primarily in postmenopausal women.

The endocrine system plays a large role in the development of osteoporosis. At the time of menopause, a woman's ovaries begin a rapid decrease in the production of *estrogen,* one of two main hormones associated with the menstrual cycle. This lower level of estrogen may decrease the conversion of the precursors of vitamin D into the active form of vitamin D, the form necessary for absorbing calcium from the digestive tract. As a result, calcium may be drawn from the bones for use elsewhere in the body.

Premenopausal women have the opportunity to build and maintain a healthy skeleton through an appropriate intake of calcium. Current recommendations are for an intake of 1200 mg of calcium per day. Three to four daily servings of low-fat dairy products should provide sufficient calcium. Adequate vitamin D must also be in the diet because it aids in the absorption of calcium.

Many women do not take in an adequate amount of calcium. Calcium supplements, again in combination with vitamin D, can be used to achieve recommended calcium levels. It is now known that calcium carbonate, a highly advertised form of calcium, is no more easily absorbed by the body than are other forms of calcium salts.

In premenopausal women, calcium deposition in bone is facilitated by exercise, particularly exercise that involves movement of the extremities. Today, women are encouraged to consume at least the recommended servings from the milk group and engage in regular physical activity that involves the weight-bearing muscles of the legs, such as aerobics, jogging, or walking.

Postmenstrual women who are not elderly can markedly slow the resorption of calcium from their bones through the use of hormone replacement therapy (HRT). When combined with a daily intake of 1500 mg of calcium, vitamin D, and regular exercise, HRT almost eliminates calcium loss. Women will need to work closely with their physicians in monitoring the use of HRT because of continuing concern over the role of HRT and the development of breast cancer.

Osteoarthritis

Arthritis is an umbrella term for more than 100 forms of joint inflammation. The most common form is **osteoarthritis.** It is likely that as we age, all of us will develop osteoarthritis to some degree. Often called "wear and tear" arthritis, osteoarthritis occurs primarily in the weight-bearing joints of the knee, hip, and spine. In this form of arthritis, joint damage can occur to bone ends, cartilaginous cushions, and related structures as the years of constant friction and stress accumulate.

The object of current management of osteoarthritis (and other forms) is not to cure the disease but rather to reduce discomfort, limit joint destruction, and maximize joint mobility. Aspirin and nonsteroidal anti-inflammatory agents are the drugs most frequently used to treat osteoarthritis.

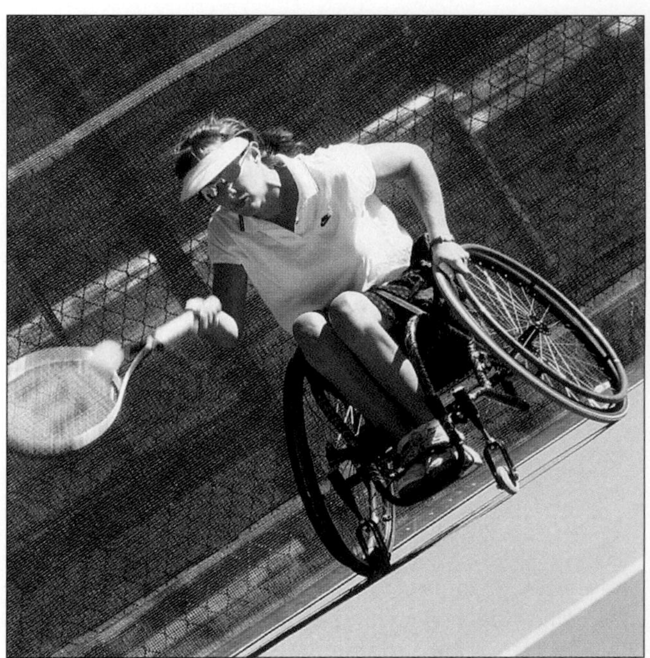

Cardiorespiratory fitness is essential for optimal heart, lung, and blood vessel function.

It is now believed that osteoarthritis develops most commonly in people with a genetic predisposition for excessive damage to the weight-bearing joints. Thus the condition seems to "run in families." Further, studies comparing the occurrence of osteoarthritis in those who exercise and those who do not demonstrate that regular movement activity may decrease the likelihood of developing this form of arthritis.

DEVELOPING A CARDIORESPIRATORY FITNESS PROGRAM

For people of all ages, cardiorespiratory conditioning can be achieved through many activities. As long as the activity you choose places sufficient demand on the heart and lungs, improved fitness is possible. In addition to the familiar activities of swimming, running, cycling, and aerobic dance, many people today are participating in brisk walking, rollerblading, cross-country skiing, swimnastics, skating, rowing, and even weight training (often combined with some form of aerobic activity) (see Learning from Our Diversity, p. 69). Regardless of age or physical limitations, you can select from a variety of enjoyable activities that will condition the cardiorespiratory system. Complete the Personal Assessment at the end of this chapter to determine your level of fitness.

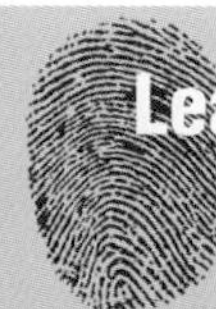

Learning from Our Diversity

A Different Kind of Fitness: Developmentally Disabled Athletes Are Always Winners in the Special Olympics

In America, as in many other countries around the world, physical fitness and athletic prowess carry a high degree of prestige, whereas lack of conditioning and poor sports performance often draw scorn and rejection. As anyone knows who's ever been picked last when sides were being chosen for a schoolyard game, few things are more damaging to youthful self-esteem than being the player nobody wants.

Some of these children blossom into accomplished athletes as they gain coordination or are inspired and guided by caring coaches. Others, lacking strong interest in sports, turn to less physical arenas in which they can excel—drama, debating, music, computers, science.

But what about people who want to be athletes at almost any cost, but who have no realistic hope of attaining the standards of athletic accomplishment set for those in top physical condition? The Joseph P. Kennedy Foundation created an arena in which these athletes could compete when it established the Special Olympics in 1968. Joseph Kennedy was the father of President John F. Kennedy, whose older sister Rosemary was virtually shut away from the world when her family discovered she was mentally disabled. Many people at that time shared the Kennedy's view that the kindest way to treat family members who were developmentally disabled was to "protect" them from stares and whispers by keeping them at home or placing them in institutions or residential facilities. Spearheaded by President Kennedy's sister Eunice Kennedy Shriver, the Special Olympics was intended to change the old attitudes toward developmentally disabled people by giving them an opportunity to compete at their own level and to celebrate their victories publicly.

Now, nearly thirty years later, the Special Olympics holds both winter and summer games and boasts participation of more than 1 million developmentally disabled athletes in 140 countries around the world. The contests are open to athletes between the ages of eight and sixty-three, some of whom have proved wrong the specialists who claimed they would never walk, let alone compete internationally. "Mainstream" Olympic champions like figure-skating silver medalist Brian Orser and a host of well-known entertainers have attended opening-day ceremonies to cheer and inspire the special athletes.

But medals aren't what the Special Olympics is all about. No matter where a Special Olympian finishes in a contest, he or she is applauded and celebrated for the accomplishment of playing the game and seeing it through. The oath taken by each participant in the Special Olympics aptly states the credo of this remarkable group of athletes: "Let me win. But if I cannot win, let me be brave in the attempt."

In what ways other than physical conditioning do you think a developmentally disabled person might benefit from participating in the Special Olympics? What can the rest of us learn from these athletes' courage and perseverance?

Many people think that any kind of physical activity will produce cardiorespiratory fitness. Golf, bowling, hunting, fishing, and archery are considered to be forms of exercise. However, these activities would generally fail to produce positive changes in your cardiorespiratory and overall muscular fitness; they may enhance your health, be enjoyable, and produce some fatigue after lengthy participation, but they do not meet the fitness standards recently established by the American College of Sports Medicine (ACSM), the nation's premier professional organization of exercise physiologists and sport physicians.[1]

The ACSM's most recent recommendations for achieving cardiorespiratory fitness were approved in 1998 and include six major areas: (1) mode of activity, (2) frequency of training, (3) intensity of training, (4) duration of training, (5) resistance training, and (6) flexibility training. These recommendations are summarized in the following sections. You may wish to compare your existing fitness program with these standards.

Mode of Activity

The ACSM recommends that the mode of activity be any continuous physical activity that uses large muscle groups and can be rhythmic and aerobic in nature. Among the activities that generally meet this requirement are continuous swimming, cycling, aerobics, basketball, cross-country skiing, rollerblading, step training (bench aerobics), hiking, walking, rowing, stair climbing, dancing, and running. Recently, water exercise (water or aqua aerobics) has become a popular fitness mode, since it is especially effective for pregnant women and elderly, injured, or disabled people. (The Focus On Box at the end of this chapter provides more information about exercise during pregnancy.)

Key Term

osteoarthritis
Arthritis that develops with age; largely caused by weight bearing and deterioration of the joints.

Endurance games and activities, such as tennis, racquetball, and handball, are fine as long as you and your partner are skilled enough to keep the ball in play; walking after the ball will do very little for you. Riding a bicycle is a good activity if you keep pedaling. Coasting will do little to improve fitness. Softball and football are generally less than sufficient continuous activities—especially the way they are played by weekend athletes.

Regardless of which continuous activity you select, it should also be enjoyable. Running, for example, is not for everyone—despite what some accomplished runners say! Find an activity you enjoy. If you need others around you to have a good time, get a group of friends to join you. Vary your activities to keep from becoming bored. You might cycle in the summer, run in the fall, swim in the winter, and play racquetball in the spring. To help you maintain your fitness program, see the suggestions in the accompanying Changing for the Better box.

Changing *for the Better*

How to Stick to Your Exercise Program

I know that working out is important, but with a full load of classes and my activities, I either don't have the time or the energy. I just can't seem to stick with any routine I start. How can I make exercise part of my life?

- Fit your program into your daily lifestyle.
- Exercise with your friends.
- Incorporate music into your activity.
- Vary your activities frequently; crosstrain.
- Reward yourself when you reach a fitness goal.
- Avoid a complicated exercise program; keep it simple.
- Measure your improvement by keeping a log or diary.
- Take some time off to rest and recuperate.
- Keep in mind how important physical activity is to your life and health.

Frequency of Training

Frequency of training refers to the number of times per week a person should exercise. The ACSM recommends three to five times per week. For most people, participation in fitness activities more than five times each week does not significantly improve their level of conditioning. Likewise, an average of only two workouts each week does not seem to produce a measurable improvement in cardiorespiratory conditioning. Thus, although you may have a lot of fun cycling twice each week, do not expect to see a significant improvement in your cardiorespiratory fitness level from doing so.

Intensity of Training

How much effort should you put into an activity? Should you run quickly, jog slowly, or swim at a comfortable pace? Must a person sweat profusely to become fit? These questions all refer to **intensity** of effort.

The ACSM recommends that healthy adults exercise at an intensity level of between 65% and 90% of their maximum heart rate (calculated by subtracting your age from 220). This level of intensity is called the **target heart rate (THR).** This rate refers to the minimum number of times your heart needs to contract (beat) each minute to have a positive effect on your heart, lungs, and blood vessels. This improvement is called the *training effect.* Intensity of activity below the THR will be insufficient to make a significant improvement in your fitness level.

Although intensity below the THR will still help you expend calories and thus lose weight, it will probably do little to make you more aerobically fit. On the other hand, intensity that is significantly above your THR will probably cause you to become so fatigued that you will be forced to stop the activity before the training effect can be achieved. For persons who are quite unfit, the 1998 ACSM recommendations permit intensity levels as low as 55%.

Choosing a particular THR between 65% and 90% of your maximum heart rate depends on your initial level of fitness. If you are already in relatively good physical shape, you might want to start exercising at 75% of your maximum heart rate. A well-conditioned person might select a higher THR for his or her intensity level, whereas a person with a low fitness level will still be able to achieve a training effect at a lower THR of 65% of maximum.

In the accompanying Star Box, the younger person would need to participate in a continuous activity for an extended period while working at a THR of 160 beats per minute. The older person would need to function at a THR of 117 beats per minute to achieve a positive training effect.

Determining your heart rate is not a complicated procedure. Find a location on your body where an artery passes near the surface of the skin. Pulse rates are difficult to determine by touching veins, which are more superficial than arteries. Two easily accessible sites for determining heart rate are the *carotid artery* (one on either side of the windpipe at the front of your neck) and the *radial artery* (on the inside of your wrist, just above the base of the thumb).

You should practice placing the front surface of your index and middle fingertips at either of these locations and feeling for a pulse. Once you have found a regular pulse, look at the second hand of a watch. Count the number of beats you feel in a 10-second period. Multiply this number by 6. This number is your heart rate. With a little practice, you can become very proficient at determining your heart rate.

What's Your Target Heart Rate?

The target heart rate (THR) is the recommended rate for increasing cardiorespiratory endurance. To maintain a training effect, you must sustain activity at your THR. To calculate your THR, subtract your age from 220 (the maximum heart rate) and multiply by .65 to .90. Here are two examples:

For a 20-year-old person who wants a THR of 80% of maximum
Maximum heart rate: $220 - 20 = 200$
$200 \times .80 = 160$
THR = 160 beats per minute

For a 40-year-old person who wants a THR of 65% of maximum
Maximum heart rate: $220 - 40 = 180$
$180 \times .65 = 117$
THR = 117 beats per minute

Duration of Training

The ACSM recommends that the **duration** of training be between 20 and 60 minutes of continuous or intermittent aerobic activity. Intermittent activity can be accumulated in 10-minute segments throughout the day. This is especially helpful for persons who cannot take a single large chunk of time during the day to devote to an exercise program.

However, for most healthy adults the ACSM recommends moderate-intensity activity levels with longer duration times, perhaps 30 minutes to an hour. For healthy adults who train at higher intensity levels, the duration of training will likely be shorter, perhaps 20 minutes or more.[1] Adults who are unfit or have an existing medical condition should check with their fitness instructor or physician to determine an appropriate duration of training.

Resistance Training

Recognizing the important fact that overall body fitness includes muscular fitness, the ACSM recommends resistance training in its current standards. The ACSM suggests participation in strength training of moderate intensity two or three times a week. This training should help develop and maintain a healthy body composition—one with an emphasis on lean body mass. The goal of resistance training is not to improve cardiorespiratory endurance but to improve overall muscle strength and endurance. For the average person, resistance training with heavy weights is not recommended because it can induce a sudden and dangerous increase in blood pressure. See the Changing for the Better box on p. 72 for safety precautions to observe during strength training.

The resistance training recommended by the ACSM includes one set of 8 to 12 repetitions of 8 to 10 different exercises. These exercises should be geared to the body's major muscle groups (legs, arms, shoulders, trunk, and back) and should not focus on just one or two body areas. Isotonic (progressive resistance) or isokinetic exercises are recommended (see p. 65). For the average person, resistance training activities should be done at a moderate-to-slow speed, use the full range of motion, and not impair normal breathing. With just one set recommended for each exercise, resistance training is not very time-consuming. The ACSM, however, indicates that multiple sets could provide greater benefits, if time is available.

Flexibility Training

To develop and maintain a healthy range of motion for the body's joints, the ACSM suggests that flexibility exercises be included in one's overall fitness program. These exercises should stretch the major muscle groups of the body and be undertaken a minimum of two to three times per week. Stretching should be done according to safe and appropriate techniques. (See the Guidelines for Static Stretching on p. 67.)

Warm-up, Workout, Cooldown

Each training session consists of three basic parts: the warm-up, the workout, and the cooldown.[2] The warm-up should last 10 to 15 minutes. During this period, you should begin slow, gradual, comfortable movements related to the upcoming activity, such as walking or slow jogging. All body segments and muscle groups should be exercised as you gradually increase your heart rate. Near the end of the warm-up period, the major muscle groups should be stretched. This preparation helps protect you from muscle strains and joint sprains.

Key Terms

frequency
The number of times per week one should exercise to achieve a training effect.

intensity
The level of effort put into an activity.

target heart rate (THR)
The number of times per minute the heart must contract to produce a training effect.

duration
The length of time one needs to exercise at the THR to produce a training effect.

Changing *for the Better*

Considering Strength Training? Think Safety . . .

I'm a 22-year-old college student thinking about starting a strength-training program. What kinds of safety precautions should I take?

- Warm up appropriately.
- Use proper lifting techniques.
- Always have a spotter if you are using free weights.
- Do not hold your breath during a lift.
- Avoid single lifts of very heavy weights.
- Before using a machine (such as Nautilus, Universal, or Cybex), be certain you know how to use it correctly.
- Seek advice for training programs from properly licensed or certified experts.
- Work within your limitations; avoid showing off.

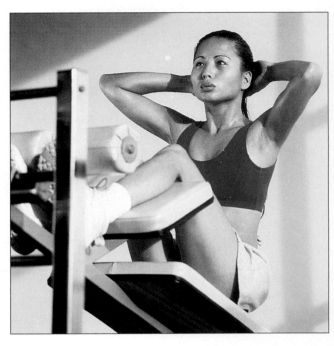

Strength training helps you develop and maintain a healthy body composition.

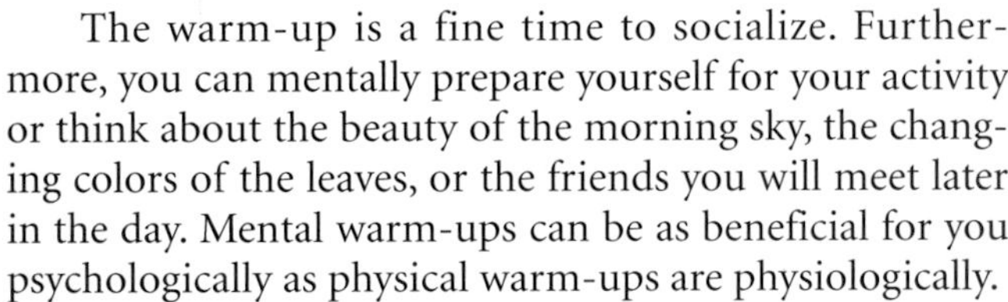

The warm-up is a fine time to socialize. Furthermore, you can mentally prepare yourself for your activity or think about the beauty of the morning sky, the changing colors of the leaves, or the friends you will meet later in the day. Mental warm-ups can be as beneficial for you psychologically as physical warm-ups are physiologically.

The second part of the training session is the workout, the part of the session that involves improving muscular strength and endurance, cardiorespiratory endurance, and flexibility. Workouts can be tailor-made, but they should follow the ACSM guidelines discussed earlier in this chapter.

The third important part of each fitness session, the cooldown, consists of a 5- to 10-minute session of relaxing exercises, such as slow jogging, walking, and stretching. This activity allows your body to cool and return to a resting state. A cooldown period helps reduce muscle soreness.

Exercise for Older Adults

An exercise program designed for younger adults may be inappropriate for older people, particularly those over age fifty. Special attention must be paid to matching the program to the interests and abilities of the participants. The goals of the program should include both social interaction and physical conditioning.

Older adults, especially those with a personal or family history of heart problems, should have a physical examination before starting a fitness program. This examination should include a stress cardiogram, a blood pressure check, and an evaluation of joint functioning. Participants should learn how to monitor their own cardiorespiratory status during exercise.

Well-designed fitness programs for older adults will include activities that begin slowly, are monitored frequently, and are geared to the enjoyment of the participants.[5] The professional staff coordinating the program should be familiar with the signs of distress (excessively elevated heart rate, nausea, breathing difficulty, pallor, and pain) and must be able to perform CPR. Warm-up and cooldown periods should be included. Activities to increase flexibility are beneficial in the beginning and ending segments of the program. Participants should wear comfortable clothing and appropriate shoes and should be mentally prepared to enjoy the activities.

A program designed for older adults will largely conform to the ACSM criteria specified in this chapter. However, except for certain very fit older adults (such as runners and triathletes), the THR should not exceed 120 beats per minute. Also, because of possible joint, muscular, or skeletal problems, certain activities may have to be done in a sitting position. Pain or discomfort should be reported immediately to the fitness instructor.

Fortunately, properly screened older adults will rarely have health emergencies during a well-monitored fitness program. Of course, for some older adults, individual fitness activities may be more enjoyable than supervised group activities. Either choice offers important benefits.

Low Back Pain

A common occurrence among adults is the sudden onset of low back pain. Each year, 10 million adults develop

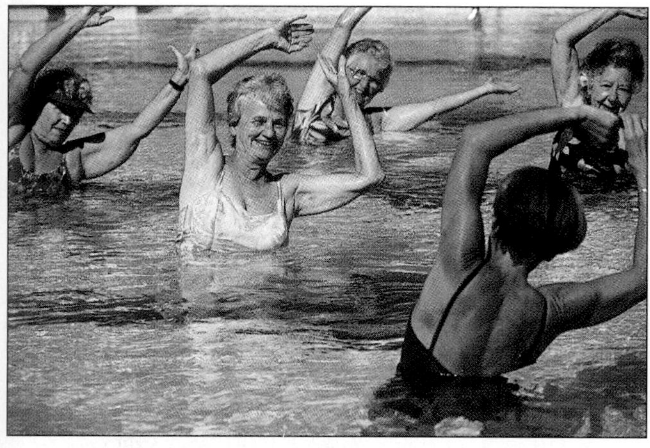

Well-designed fitness programs are beneficial to older adults.

this condition, which can be so uncomfortable that they miss work, lose sleep, and generally feel incapable of engaging in daily activities. Eighty percent of all adults who have this condition will experience these effects two to three times per year.

Although low back pain can reflect serious health problems, most low back pain is caused by mechanical (postural) problems. As unpleasant as low back pain is, the problem usually corrects itself within a week or two. The services of a physician, physical therapist, or chiropractor are not generally required after an initial visit.

By engaging in regular exercise, such as swimming, walking, and bicycling, and by paying attention to your back during bending, lifting, and sitting, you can minimize the occurrence of this uncomfortable and incapacitating condition. Commercial fitness centers and campus recreational programs are starting to offer specific exercise classes geared to muscular improvement in the lower back and abdominal areas.

FITNESS QUESTIONS AND ANSWERS

Along with the six necessary elements to include in your fitness program, you should consider many additional issues when you start a fitness program.

Should I See My Doctor Before I Get Started?

This issue has probably kept thousands of people from ever beginning a fitness program. The hassle and expense of getting a comprehensive physical examination is an excellent excuse for people who are not completely sold on the idea of exercise. A complete examination, including *blood analysis, stress test, cardiogram, serum lipid analysis,* and *body fat analysis,* is a valuable tool for developing some baseline physical data for your medical record.

Is this examination really necessary? Most exercise physiologists do not think so. The value of these measurements as safety predictors is questioned by many professionals.

A good rule of thumb to follow is to undergo a physical examination if (1) you have an existing medical condition (for example, diabetes, obesity, hypertension, heart abnormalities, or arthritis), (2) you are a man over age 40 or a woman over age 50,[6] or (3) you smoke.

TALKING POINTS • If your screening tests indicate that you cannot start a vigorous fitness program, are you prepared to ask your doctor about alternative activities?

How Beneficial Is Aerobic Exercise?

One of the most popular fitness approaches is aerobic exercise, including aerobic dancing. Many organizations sponsor classes in this form of continuous dancing and movement. The rise in popularity of televised and videotaped aerobic exercise programs reflects the enthusiasm for this form of exercise. Because extravagant claims are often made about the value of these programs, the wise consumer should observe at least one session of the activity before enrolling. Discover for yourself whether the program meets the criteria outlined earlier in this chapter: mode of activity, frequency, intensity, duration, resistance training, and flexibility training.

Street dancing, swing dancing, and Latino dancing are fast becoming some of the most popular aerobic excercises. Popularized by rap music, hip-hop music, and the growth of vigorous dancing in music videos, these forms of dancing provide an excellent way of having fun and developing cardiorespiratory fitness. Have you experienced the exhilaration that results from an hour or two of dancing?

What Are Low-Impact Aerobic Activities?

Because long-term participation in some aerobic activities (for example, jogging, running, aerobic dancing, and rope skipping) may damage the hip, knee, and ankle joints, many fitness experts promote low-impact aerobic activities. Low-impact aerobic dancing, water aerobics, bench aerobics, and brisk walking are examples of this kind of fitness activity. Participants still conform to the principal components of a cardiorespiratory fitness program. THR levels are the same as in high-impact aerobic activities.

The main difference between low-impact and high-impact aerobic activities is the use of the legs. Low-impact aerobics do not require having both feet off the ground at the same time. Thus weight transfer does not occur with the forcefulness seen in traditional high-impact aerobic

Choosing an Athletic Shoe

Aerobic Shoes

When selecting shoes for aerobic dancing, J. Lynn Reese, president of J. Lynn & Co. Endurance Sports, Washington, DC, advises the following:

- Check the width of the shoe at the widest part of your foot. The bottom of the shoe should be as wide as the bottom of your foot; the uppers shouldn't go over the sides.
- Look for leather or nylon uppers. Leather is durable and gives good support, but it can stretch. Nylon won't stretch and gives support, but it's not as durable. Canvas generally doesn't offer much support.
- Look for rubber rather than polyurethane or black carbon rubber soles. Treads should be fairly flat in the forefoot. If you dance on carpet, you can go with less tread; if you dance on gym floors, you may need more grab.

Basketball Shoes

What's most important when choosing a basketball shoe? John Burleson, of the Sports Authority, offers this advice:

- Cushioning. Cushioning is especially important in the forefoot area. Each shoe manufacturer has its own cushioning "system." For example, Nike has "Air," and Reebok promotes its "Hexalite" material, composed of hexagonal air chambers.
- Side support. Side support, also called lateral and medial support, is important for making quick directional changes.
- Fit of heel cup. Try on the shoe, and then put your little finger in behind the heel. It should fit snugly.
- Traction. Keep in mind the surface on which you play most often. More traction is needed on asphalt than on hardwood.
- Socks should be breathable and pull moisture away from the foot.
- "Rope" laces are more convenient than the more traditional flat laces because pulling on the ends will tighten up the laces on the whole shoe at once.

Running Shoes

Need new running shoes? Here's advice from Jeff Galloway, former Olympic runner and founder and president of Phidippides International aerobic sports stores, headquartered in Atlanta.

- Take time to shop, and find a knowledgeable salesperson. Good advice is crucial.
- Check the wear pattern on your old shoes to see whether you have floppy or rigid feet. Floppy-footed runners wear out their soles on the outside and inside edges; rigid-footed runners wear out soles predominantly on the outside edges. Floppy-footed runners can sacrifice cushioning for support; rigid-footed runners can sacrifice support for cushioning.
- Know whether your feet are curved or straight and whether you have high arches or are flatfooted. The shoe should fit the shape of your foot.

Walking Shoes

Have you joined the millions of people who walk for fitness? If so, and if you are ready for a pair of athletic walking shoes, shoe manufacturer Nike has the following advice for you:

- Note where most of your weight falls on your foot when you walk. Are you landing mostly on the heel or on the forefoot? This is where you will want cushioning.
- As with all other types of athletic shoes, take the time to find a knowledgeable salesperson who will provide good advice.
- Go for comfort. Stride in the different types of shoes at your typical walking pace and identify the shoes that are most comfortable.
- Choose shoes that are comfortable in the forefoot area, which will be carrying much of your weight.
- All-leather uppers are satisfactory for most walkers. If you are a serious walker, consider shoes with breathable uppers made of material such as mesh.

Crosstraining Shoes

Crosstraining shoes are a hybrid, an all-purpose shoe for those who participate in a variety of fitness activities, such as basketball, weight lifting, or light trail hiking. If you tend to specialize in one type of activity (such as basketball), consider buying shoes designed specifically for that activity (for example, high-top basketball shoes for ankle support). To shop for an all-purpose crosstraining shoe, Nike recommends that you keep the following points in mind: (*continued*)

activities. In addition, low-impact activities may include exaggerated arm movements and the use of hand or wrist weights. All of these variations are designed to increase the heart rate to the THR without damaging the joints of the lower extremities. Low-impact aerobics are excellent for people of all ages, and they may be especially beneficial to older adults.

In-line skating (rollerblading) is one of the fastest-growing participant fitness activities. This low-impact activity has cardiorespiratory and muscular benefits similar to those of running without the pounding effect that running can produce. Rollerblading requires important safety equipment: sturdy skates, knee and elbow pads, wrist supports, and a helmet.

- Once again, comfort is paramount. Try to simulate the activity when you try on the shoe, such as rolling from side to side for court sports, fast movement for walking or running, or walking an incline for light hiking.
- If you tend toward one activity (such as running), look for crosstraining shoes that support that activity (for example, heel and forefoot cushioning for running).
- If you intend to use the shoes for activities with lots of lateral movement, such as court sports or aerobic classes, look for good lateral support.

Aerobic Shoes (*below*)
Flexibility: More at ball of foot than running shoes; less flexible than court shoes or running shoes; sole is firmer than running shoes. Uppers: Most are leather or leather-reinforced nylon. Heel: Little or no flare. Soles: Rubber if you dance on wood floors; polyurethane for other surfaces. Cushioning: More than court shoes; less than running shoes. Tread: Should be fairly flat, especially on forefoot; may also have "dot" on the ball of the foot for pivoting.

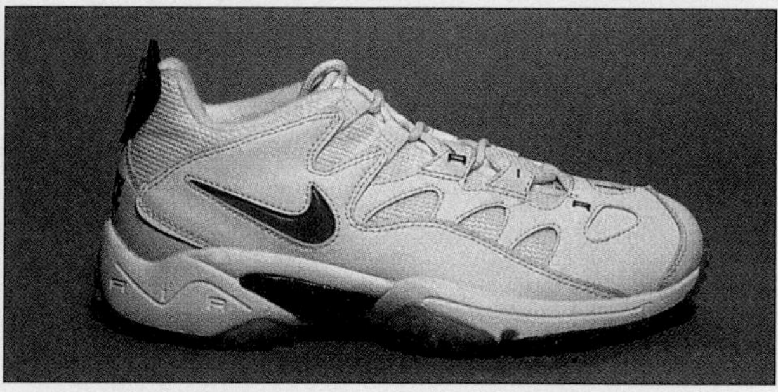

Basketball Shoes (*above right*)
Soles: Can be made from rubber for durability, EVA for lightweight cushioning, or polyurethane, which is both lightweight and durable. Flexibility: Should be most flexible in the forefoot, for making jump shots. Cushioning: Should absorb shock in the ball of the foot, for landing from jump shots. Heel: A snug-fitting heel cup is essential to keep the ankle in place; the shoe can be high-, mid-, or low-cut, depending on the amount of ankle support desired. Tread: For playing outdoors, the sole should be harder and the tread deeper; a smoother tread works well for playing on a court. Uppers: Can be made of leather for durability or nylon or other synthetics for breathability.

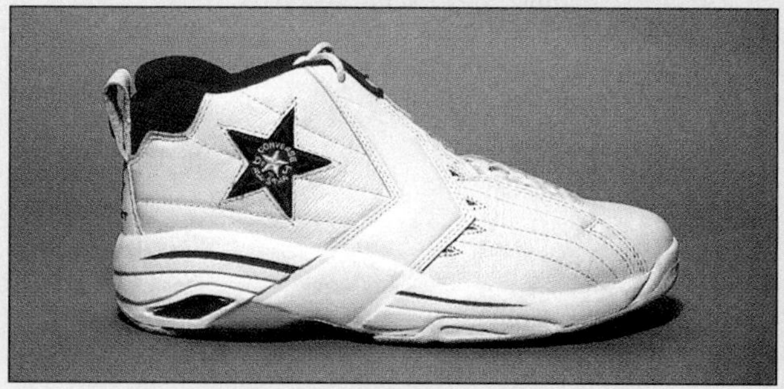

Running Shoes (*below*)
Heel: Flare gives foot broader, more stable base. Soles: Usually carbon-based for longer wear. Cushioning: More than court shoes, especially at heel. Tread: "Waffle" or other deep-cut tread for grip on many surfaces.

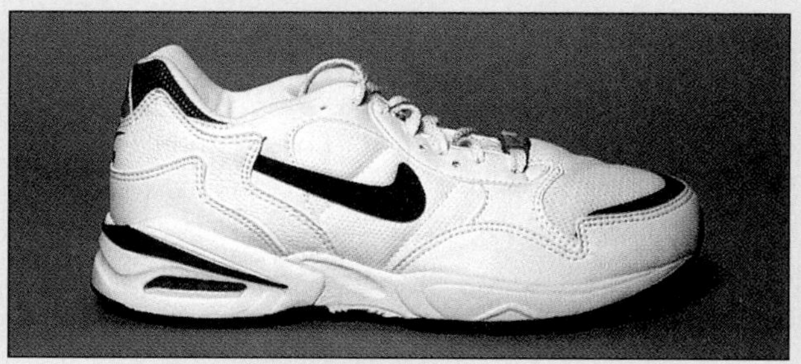

Walking Shoes
Cushioning: Can be forefoot and heel, or primarily forefoot or heel. Heel: May have some flare, similar to running shoes. Soles: Typically polyurethane for durability. Tread: Some tread for traction, but slightly flatter than running shoes.

Crosstraining Shoes
Cushioning: Can be forefoot and heel, or primarily forefoot or heel. Tread: Can be moderate to aggressive.

What Is the Most Effective Means of Fluid Replacement During Exercise?

Despite all the advertising hype associated with commercial fluid replacement products, for an average person involved in typical fitness activities, water is still the best fluid replacement. The availability and cost are unbeatable. However, when activity is prolonged and intense, commercial sports drinks may be preferable to water because they contain electrolytes (which replace lost sodium and potassium) and carbohydrates (which replace depleted energy stores). However, the carbohydrates in sports drinks are actually simple forms of sugar. Thus sports drinks tend to be high in calories, just like regular soft drinks. Regardless of the drink you choose, exercise physiologists recommend that you drink fluids before and at frequent intervals throughout the activity.

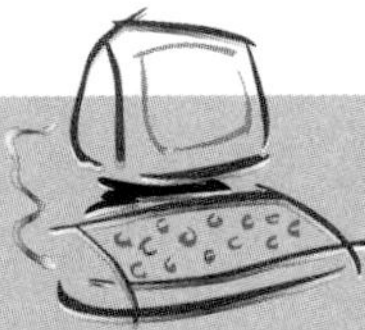

OnSITE/InSIGHT

Learning to Go: Health

Looking for a workout routine that's right for you? Click on the Motivator icon to find these lessons, which offer valuable information and suggestions:

Lesson 10: Discover the benefits of physical fitness.
Lesson 11: Uncover the components of physical fitness.
Lesson 12: Create a fitness program that works for you.
Lesson 13: Choose the right athletic shoe.
Lesson 14: Promote sound sleep for fitness.

STUDENT POLL

Is physical fitness a part of your life or still on your "to do" list? Go to the Online Learning Center at **www.mhhe.com/hahn6e**. Click on the Student Resources. Then go to the Student Poll, where you can answer these questions and find out how other students responded to them.

1. Do you exercise on a regular basis?
2. Is exercise something you enjoy?
3. Do you use exercise videos?
4. Do you feel better when you exercise than when you don't?
5. Can you determine your heart rate?
6. Do you exercise while watching TV?
7. Do you average about 7 hours of sleep a night?
8. Do you find it difficult to stick with an exercise or fitness plan?
9. Do you work out or exercise with friends?
10. Do you practice flexibility exercises?
11. Is warm-up/cooldown a part of your fitness routine?

What Effect Does Alcohol Have on Sport Performance?

It probably comes as no surprise that alcohol use is generally detrimental to sport performance. Alcohol consumption, especially excessive intake the evening before a performance, consistently decreases the level of performance. Many research studies have documented the negative effects of alcohol on activities involving speed, strength, power, and endurance.[7] Lowered performance appears to be related to a variety of factors, including impaired judgment, reduced coordination, depressed heart function, liver interference, and dehydration.

What Level of Physical Activity Is Necessary to Produce Fitness?

According to the surgeon general's report on physical activity and health,[6] moderate amounts of physical activity can produce significant health benefits, including lowering the risk of premature death, coronary heart disease, hypertension, colon cancer, and diabetes. Even a variety of simple activities, such as gardening, walking, raking leaves, or dancing, that consistently increase a person's daily activity levels can be as helpful for the majority of Americans as are activities such as jogging, swimming, and cycling.

What Are the Risks and Benefits of Androstenedione?

Androstenedione ("andro") and creatine have recently received much attention for their use as possible **ergogenic aids.** Ergogenic aids are supplements taken to improve athletic performance.[8] Andro is a steroid-like precursor to the male hormone testosterone. When taken into the body, andro stimulates the body to produce more of its natural testosterone. Increased levels of testosterone help a person build lean muscle mass and recover from injury more quickly.

Andro's primary use as an ergogenic aid is to build muscle tissue, improve overall body strengh, and boost performance, especially in anaerobic sports. Andro is banned by the National Football League (NFL), the National Collegiate Athletic Association (NCAA), and the IOC. The health concerns that most physicians attribute to andro are similar to those of anabolic steroids (see p. 77).

St. Louis Cardinal baseball player Mark McGwire's admitted use of andro put this supplement in the national spotlight in the summer of 1998. That was the season when McGwire rocked the baseball world by surpassing Roger Maris's home run record by hitting seventy home runs. It is interesting, though, that during the 1999 baseball season McGwire opted to stop using andro but still managed to hit nearly seventy home runs.

What Are the Risks and Benefits of Creatine?

Creatine is an amino acid found in meat, poultry, and fish. In a person's body, creatine is produced naturally in the liver, pancreas, and kidneys. Typically, people get one to two grams of creatine each day from their food intake.[8] As an ergogenic aid, creatine performs its work in the muscles, where it helps restore the compound adenosine triphosphate (ATP). ATP provides quick energy for muscle contractions. It also helps to reduce the lactic acid buildup that occurs during physical exertion. This buildup causes a burning sensation that limits the amount of intense activity one can perform.

Early studies suggest that creatine can help athletes in anaerobic sports, which require short, explosive bursts of energy. However, the increase in performance has been small, the long-term health impacts are unknown, studies have been restricted to highly trained subjects (not recreational athletes), and damage to kidneys is possible with high dosages. Users are cautioned to consume ample amounts of water to prevent cramping and dehydration.

All in all, creatine is unlikely to prove as potentially dangerous as androstenedione. If additional studies should indicate that creatine can consistently improve performance, this substance might be banned by many sports federations. At the time of this writing, the safest, most prudent recommendation is for athletes to spend their time and energy improving their training programs rather than looking for a solution in a bottle.

How Worthwhile Are Commercial Health and Fitness Clubs?

The health and fitness club business is booming. Fitness clubs offer activities ranging from free weights to weight machines to step walking to general aerobics. Some clubs have saunas and whirlpools and lots of frills. Others have course offerings that include wellness, smoking cessation, stress management, time management, dance, and yoga. The atmosphere is friendly, and people are encouraged to have a good time while working out.

If your purpose in joining a fitness club is to improve your cardiorespiratory fitness, measure the program offered by the club against the ACSM standards. If your primary purpose is to meet people and have fun, request a trial membership for a month or so to see whether you like the environment.

Before signing a contract at a health club or spa, do some careful questioning. Find out when the business was established, ask about the qualifications of the employees, contact some members for their observations, and request a thorough tour of the facilities. You might even consult your local Better Business Bureau for additional information. Finally, make certain that you read and understand every word of the contract.

What Is Crosstraining?

Crosstraining is the use of more than one aerobic activity to achieve cardiorespiratory fitness. For example, runners may use swimming, cycling, or rowing periodically to replace running in their training routines. Crosstraining allows certain muscle groups to rest and injuries to heal. Also, crosstraining provides a refreshing change of pace for the participant. You will probably enjoy your fitness program more if you vary the activities.

What Are Steroids and Why Do Some Athletes Use Them?

Steroids are drugs that can be legally prescribed by physicians for a variety of health conditions, including certain forms of anemia, inadequate growth patterns, and chronic debilitating diseases. Steroids can also be prescribed to aid recovery from surgery or burns. **Anabolic steroids** are drugs that function like the male sex hormone testosterone. They can be taken orally or by injection.

Anabolic steroids are used by athletes who hope to gain weight, muscular size and strength, power, endurance, and aggressiveness. Over the last few decades, many bodybuilders, weightlifters, track athletes, and football players have chosen to ignore the serious health risks posed by illegal steroid use.

The use of steroids is highly dangerous because of serious, life-threatening side effects and adverse reactions. These effects include heart problems, certain forms of cancer, liver complications, and even psychological disturbances. The side effects on female steroid users are as dangerous as those on men. Figure 4-2 shows the adverse effects of steroid use.

Steroid users have developed a terminology of their own. Anabolic steroids are called "roids" or "juice." "Roid rage" is an aggressive, psychotic response to chronic steroid use. "Stacking" is a term that describes the use of multiple steroids at the same time.

Most organizations that control athletic competition (for example, the NCAA, The Athletics Congress, the NFL, and the IOC) have banned steroids and are testing athletes for illegal use. Many athletes finally seem to be getting the message and are steering clear of steroids.

TALKING POINTS • If you suspected a young person you know was using steroids, what strategies would you use to encourage the person to change his or her behavior?

Are Today's Children Physically Fit?

Major research studies published during the last 10 years have indicated that U.S. children and teenagers lead very sedentary lives. Children ages 6 to 17 score extremely poorly in the areas of strength, flexibility, and cardiorespiratory endurance. In many cases, parents are in better shape than their children.

This information presents a challenge to educators and parents to emphasize the need for strenuous play activity. Television watching and parental inactivity were implicated as major reasons in these studies. For students

Key Terms

ergogenic aids
Supplements that are taken to improve athletic performance.

anabolic steroids
Drugs that function like testosterone to produce increases in weight, strength, endurance, and aggressiveness.

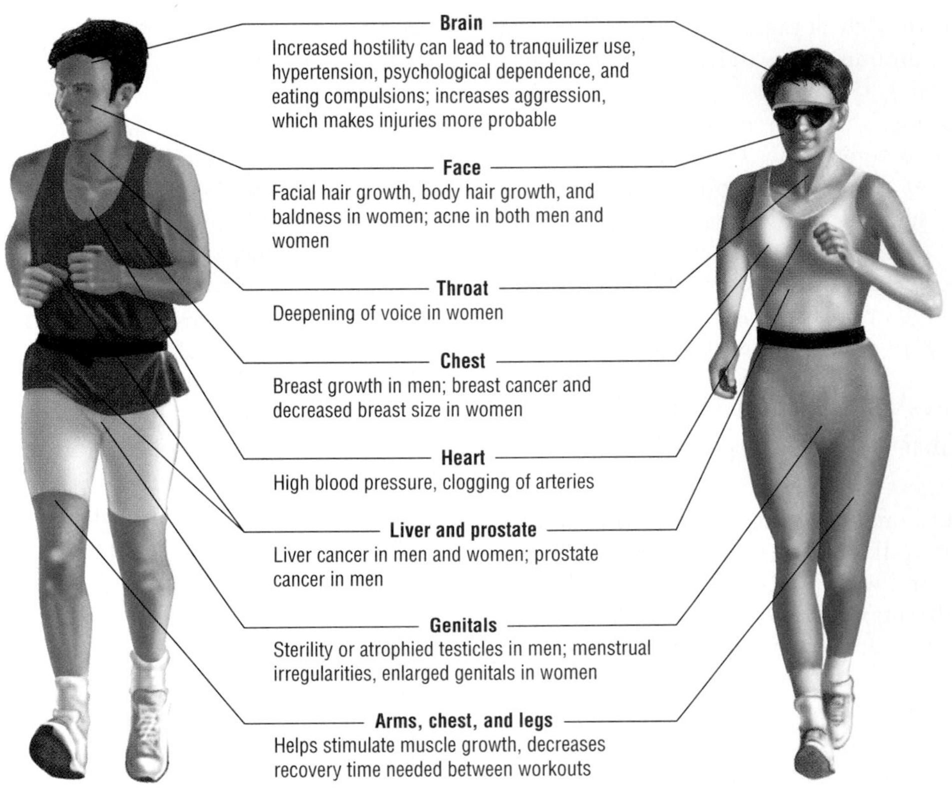
Brain
Increased hostility can lead to tranquilizer use, hypertension, psychological dependence, and eating compulsions; increases aggression, which makes injuries more probable
Face
Facial hair growth, body hair growth, and baldness in women; acne in both men and women
Throat
Deepening of voice in women
Chest
Breast growth in men; breast cancer and decreased breast size in women
Heart
High blood pressure, clogging of arteries
Liver and prostate
Liver cancer in men and women; prostate cancer in men
Genitals
Sterility or atrophied testicles in men; menstrual irregularities, enlarged genitals in women
Arms, chest, and legs
Helps stimulate muscle growth, decreases recovery time needed between workouts

Figure 4-2 Adverse effects of steroids on various parts of the body.

reading this text who are parents or grandparents of young children, what can you do to encourage more physical activity and less sedentary activity?

TALKING POINTS • What can you do to encourage children to become more active participants in physical activities?

How Does Sleep Contribute to Overall Fitness?

Although sleep may seem to be the opposite of exercise, it is an important adjunct to a well-planned exercise program. Sleep is so vital to health that people who are unable to sleep sufficiently (those with insomnia) or who are deprived of sleep experience deterioration in every dimension of their health. Fortunately, exercise is frequently associated with improvement in sleeping.

The value of sleep is apparent in a variety of positive changes in the body. Dreaming is thought to play an important role in supporting the emotional dimension of health. Problem-solving scenarios that occur during dreams seem to afford some carryover value in actual coping experiences. A variety of changes in physiological functioning, particularly a deceleration of the cardiovascular system, occur while you sleep. The feeling of being well rested is an expression of the mental and physiological rejuvenation you feel after a good night's sleep.

The amount of sleep needed varies among people. In fact, for any person, sleep needs vary according to activity level and overall state of health. As we age, the need for sleep appears to decrease from the six to eight hours young adults require. Elderly people routinely sleep less than they did when they were younger. This decrease may be offset by the short naps older people often take during the day. For all people, however, periods of relaxation, daydreaming, and even an occasional afternoon nap promote electrical activity patterns that help regenerate the mind and body.

How Do I Handle Common Injuries That May Be Caused by My Fitness Activities?

For the most part, emergency care for injuries that pertain to the bones or muscles should follow the RICE acronym.[9] Depending on the type and severity of the injury, the importance of rest (R), ice (I) or cold application, compression (C), and elevation (E) cannot be overstated. Each type of injury identified in Table 4-1 has a particular RICE protocol to follow. Any significant injury should be reported to your college student health center,

Table 4-1 Common Injuries Associated with Physical Activity

Injury	Condition
Achilles tendinitis	A chronic tendinitis of the "heel cord," or muscle tendon, located on the back of the lower leg just above the heel. It may result from any activity that involves forcefully pushing off with the foot and ankle, such as in running and jumping. This inflammation involves swelling, warmth, tenderness to touch, and pain during walking and especially running.
Ankle sprains	Stretching or tearing of one or several ligaments that provide stability to the ankle joint. Ligaments on the outside or lateral side of the ankle are more commonly injured by rolling the sole of the foot downward and toward the inside. Pain is intense immediately after injury, followed by considerable swelling, tenderness, loss of joint motion, and some discoloration over a 24- to 48-hour period.
Groin pull	A muscle strain that occurs in the muscles located on the inside of the upper thigh just below the pubic area and that results from either an overstretch of the muscle or from a contraction of the muscle that meets excessive resistance. Pain will be produced by flexing the hip and leg across the body or by stretching the muscles in a groin-stretch position.
Hamstring pull	A strain of the muscles on the back of the upper thigh that most often occurs while sprinting. In most cases, severe pain is caused simply by walking or in any movement that involves knee flexion or stretch of the hamstring muscle. Some swelling, tenderness to touch, and possibly some discoloration extending down the back of the leg may occur in severe strains.
Patellofemoral knee pain	Nonspecific pain occurring around the knee, particularly the front part of the knee, or in the kneecap (patella). Pain can result from many causes, including improper movement of the kneecap in knee flexion and extension; tendinitis of the tendon just below the kneecap, which is caused by repetitive jumping; bursitis (swelling) either above or below the kneecap; and osteoarthritis (joint surface degeneration) between the kneecap and thigh bone. It may involve inflammation with swelling, tenderness, warmth, and pain associated with movement.
Quadriceps contusion "charley horse"	A deep bruise of the muscles in the front part of the thigh caused by a forceful impact or by some object that results in severe pain, swelling, discoloration, and difficulty flexing the knee or extending the hip. Without adequate rest and protection from additional trauma, small calcium deposits may develop in the muscle.
Shin splints	A catch-all term used to refer to any pain that occurs in the front part of the lower leg or shin, most often caused by excessive running on hard surfaces. Pain is usually caused by strain of the muscles that move the ankle and foot at their attachment points in the shin. It is usually worse during activity. In more severe cases it may be caused by stress fractures of the long bones in the lower leg, with the pain being worse after activity is stopped.
Shoulder impingement	Chronic irritation and inflammation of muscle tendons and a bursa underneath the tip of the shoulder, which results from repeated forceful overhead motions of the shoulder, such as in swimming, throwing, spiking a volleyball, or serving a tennis ball. Pain is felt when the arm is extended across the body above shoulder level.
Tennis elbow	Chronic irritation and inflammation of the lateral or outside surface of the arm just above the elbow at the attachment of the muscles that extend the wrist and fingers. It results from any activity that requires forceful extension of the wrist. Typically occurs in tennis players who are using faulty techniques hitting backhand ground strokes. Pain is felt above the elbow after forcefully extending the wrist against resistance or applying pressure over the muscle attachment above the elbow.

an athletic trainer, a physical therapist, or a physician. See the Star Box on p. 80 for exercise danger signs you should be aware of.

What Is the Female Athlete Triad?

In the early 1990s, the American College of Sports Medicine identified a three-part syndrome of disordered eating, **amenorrhea** (lack of menstruation), and osteoporosis as

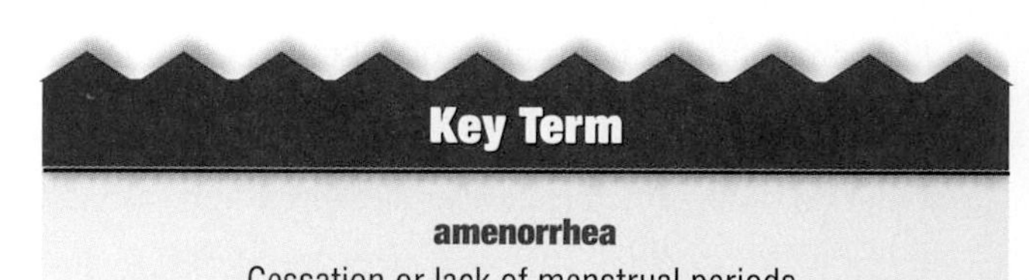

amenorrhea
Cessation or lack of menstrual periods.

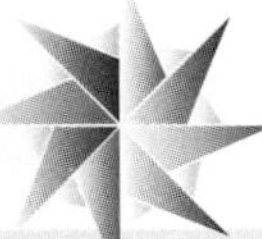

What Are the Common Exercise Danger Signs?

- A delay of over one hour in your body's return to a fully relaxed, comfortable state after exercise.
- A change in sleep patterns.
- Any noticeable breathing difficulties or chest pains. Exercising at your THR should not initiate these problems. If these effects occur, consult a physician.
- Persistent joint or muscle pain. Any lingering joint or muscle pain might signal a problem. Seek the help of an athletic trainer, a physical therapist, or your physician.
- Unusual changes in urine composition or output. Marked color change in your urine could signal possible kidney or bladder difficulties. Drink plenty of water before, during, and after you participate in your activity.
- Anything unusual that you notice after starting your fitness program. Examples are headaches, nosebleeds, fainting, numbness in an extremity, and hemorrhoids.

the female athlete triad.[10] The conditions of this syndrome appear independently in many women, but among female athletes they appear together. The female athlete triad is most likely to be found in athletes whose sport activities emphasize appearance (for example, diving, ice skating, or gymnastics).

Parents, coaches, athletic trainers, and teammates should be watchful for signs of the female athlete triad. This syndrome has associated medical risks, including inadequate fuel supply for activities, inadequate iron intake, reduced cognitive function, altered hormone levels, reduced mental health, early onset of menopause, increased likelihood of skeletal trauma, altered blood fat profiles, and increased vulnerability to heart disease.[10] Vitally important is an early referral to a physician who is knowledgeable about the female athlete triad. The physician will likely coordinate efforts with a psychologist, a nutritionist, or an athletic trainer to improve the health of the athlete and prevent recurrences.

SUMMARY

- Physical fitness allows one to engage in life's activities without unreasonable fatigue.
- The health benefits of exercise can be achieved through regular moderate exercise.
- Fitness is composed of five components: cardiorespiratory endurance, muscular strength, muscular endurance, flexibility, and body composition.
- The American College of Sports Medicine's program for cardiorespiratory fitness has six components: mode of activity, frequency of training, intensity of training, duration of training, resistance training, and flexibility training.
- The target heart rate refers to the number of times per minute the heart must contract to produce a training effect.
- Training sessions should take place in three phases: warm-up, workout, and cooldown.
- Fitness experts are concerned about the lack of fitness in today's youth.
- Dancing, step aerobics, and rollerblading are currently popular aerobic activities.
- College students who are interested in fitness should understand the important topics of steroid use, crosstraining, fluid replacement, the female athlete triad, and proper sleep.

REVIEW QUESTIONS

1. Identify the five components of fitness described in this chapter. How does each component relate to physical fitness?
2. What is the difference between anaerobic and aerobic energy production? What types of activities are associated with anaerobic energy production? With aerobic energy production?
3. List some of the benefits of aerobic fitness.
4. Describe the various methods used to promote muscular strength. How do "andro" and creatine differ?
5. What does the principle of overload mean in regard to fitness training programs?
6. Identify the ACSM's six components of an effective cardiorespiratory fitness program. Explain the important aspects of each component.
7. Under what circumstances should you see a physician before starting a physical fitness program?
8. Identify and describe the three parts of a training session.
9. Describe some of the negative consequences of anabolic steroid use.
10. How does adequate sleep help improve ones fitness?

THINK ABOUT THIS . . .

- What are your attitudes toward physical fitness? Do you participate in a regular physical fitness program? Why or why not?
- Does your present level of fitness allow you to carry out the activities your schedule demands effectively? Are there things that you would like to do but cannot because of your current level of fitness?
- Describe your level of fitness, taking into consideration cardiorespiratory endurance, strength, and flexibility.
- After determining your own target heart rate, calculate the THR for a parent or older friend. Talk to these people about starting their own fitness programs. Be ready to help with encouragement and accurate information. They may look to you as a role model for their own health.
- Design a physical fitness plan for yourself, taking into consideration all of the dimensions of body structure and function and the five components of an effective fitness program described in this chapter. What are the chances that you will continue this program after college?

REFERENCES

1. American College of Sports Medicine: Position stand on the recommended quantity and quality of exercise for developing and maintaining cardiorespiratory and muscular fitness and flexibility in healthy adults, *Med Sci Sports Exerc* 30(6):975–991, 1998.
2. Prentice WE: *Fitness for college and life,* 1999, McGraw-Hill.
3. Fit, fitter, fittest, *Harvard Medical School Health Letter* 15(4):2, 1990.
4. Simon HB: Can you run away from cancer? *Harvard Medical School Health Letter* 17(5):5–7, 1992.
5. An exercise prescription for older people, *Harvard Heart Letter* 8(10):1–4, 1998.
6. U.S. Department of Health and Human Services: *Physical activity and health: a report of the surgeon general,* 1996, Centers for Disease Control and Prevention, National Center for Chronic Disease Prevention and Health Promotion.
7. Williams MH: Alcohol and sport performance, *Sports Science Exchange* 4(40):1–4, 1992.
8. The creatine craze, *UC Berkeley Wellness Letter* 14(3):6, 1998.
9. Arnheim DD, Prentice WE: *Essentials of athletic training,* 1999, McGraw-Hill.
10. Stevens WC, Brey RA, Harris JE, Fowlkes-Godek S: The dangerous trio: a case study approach to the female athletic triad, *Athletic Therapy Today,* 2(2):30–36, 1997.

SUGGESTED READINGS

Cooper KH: *Antioxidant revolution,* 1997, Thomas Nelson Inc.

This book, written by Dr. Kenneth H. Cooper (the "father of aerobics"), examines the benefits of antioxidant supplementation combined with aerobic exercise. Cooper contends that vitamin C, vitamin E, beta-carotene, and other antioxidants strengthen the body's tissues by counteracting the effects of unstable oxygen molecules.

Fitness Magazine (editor) with K Andes: *The complete book of fitness: mind, body, spirit,* 1999, Three Rivers Press.

Written in an easy-to-read style, this book is a primer on fitness. It's an encyclopedia-like reference organized into four major sections: strength training, cardiovascular training, diet and nutrition, and wellness. You can use this book to customize a fitness program for your lifestyle, present fitness level, and body type.

Fitness Magazine (editor) with G Graves: *Pregnancy fitness,* 1999, Three Rivers Press.

This book provides the fitness information every expectant mother needs as she progresses through her pregnancy. It is based on the premise that exercise will help a woman have a healthier pregnancy, an easier delivery, and a faster postpartum recovery. *Pregnancy Fitness* is effectively illustrated and designed for women of every fitness level.

Kaehler K (with CK Olson): *Real-world fitness,* 1999, Golden Books Publishing Co.

Kathy Kaehler is a well-recognized fitness instructor. She works with many celebrities, appears regularly on the *Today* show, and has made several fitness videos. The author describes ways to become fit with exercises that can be done in the home or dorm room. Kaehler is a good motivator and a firm believer in the cumulative effect of short sessions of exercise.

Prentice WE: *Fitness and wellness for life,* 1999, McGraw-Hill.

This highly recommended, comprehensive textbook covers all aspects of fitness and wellness. It provides particularly well-written coverage of strength training and stretching activities. The author's unique background as a scholar, athletic trainer, and physical therapist strengthens the credibility of the book.

Name ______________________ **Date** __________ **Section** __________

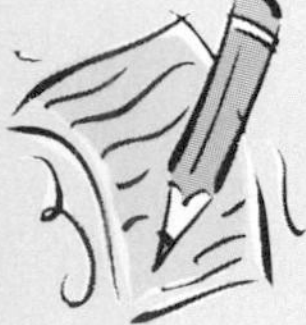

Personal Assessment

What Is Your Level of Fitness?

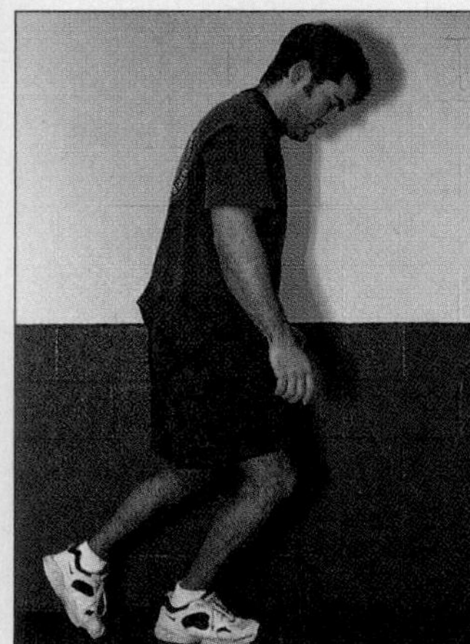

You can determine your level of fitness in thirty minutes or less by completing this short group of tests based on the National Fitness Test developed by the President's Council on Physical Fitness and Sports. If you are over 40 years old or have chronic medical disorders such as diabetes or obesity, check with your physician before taking this or any other fitness test. You will need another person to monitor your test and keep time.

Three-Minute Step Test

Aerobic capacity. Equipment: 12-inch bench, crate, block, or stepladder; stopwatch. Procedure: face bench. Complete 24 full steps (both feet on the bench, both feet on the ground) per minute for 3 minutes. After finishing, sit down, have your partner find your pulse within 5 seconds, and take your pulse for 1 minute. Your score is your pulse rate for 1 full minute.

Scoring standards (heart rate for 1 minute)

Age	18–29		30–39		40–49		50–59		60+	
Gender	F	M	F	M	F	M	F	M	F	M
Excellent	<80	<75	<84	<78	<88	<80	<92	<85	<95	<90
Good	80–110	75–100	84–115	78–109	88–118	80–112	92–123	85–115	95–127	90–118
Average	>110	>100	>115	>109	>118	>112	>123	>115	>127	>118

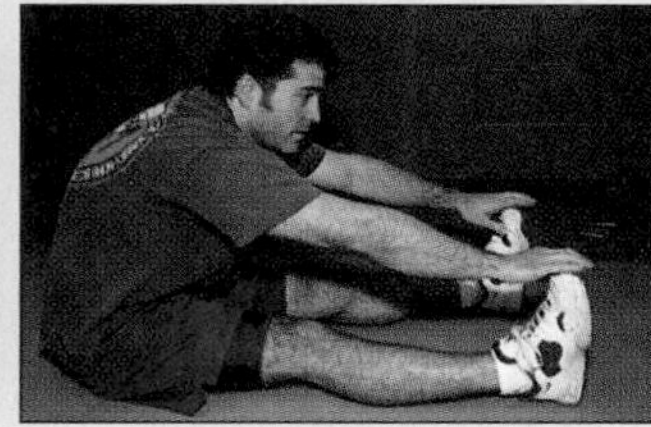

Sit and Reach

Hamstring flexibility. Equipment: yardstick; tape. Between your legs, tape the yardstick to the floor. Sit with legs straight and heels about 5 inches apart, heels even with the 15-inch mark on the yardstick. While in a sitting position, slowly stretch forward as far as possible. Your score is the number of inches reached.

Scoring standards (inches)

Age	18–29		30–39		40–49		50–59		60+	
Gender	F	M	F	M	F	M	F	M	F	M
Excellent	>22	>21	>22	>21	>21	>20	>20	>19	>20	>19
Good	17–22	13–21	17–22	13–21	15–21	13–20	14–20	12–19	14–20	12–19
Average	<17	<13	<17	<13	<15	<13	<14	<12	<14	<12

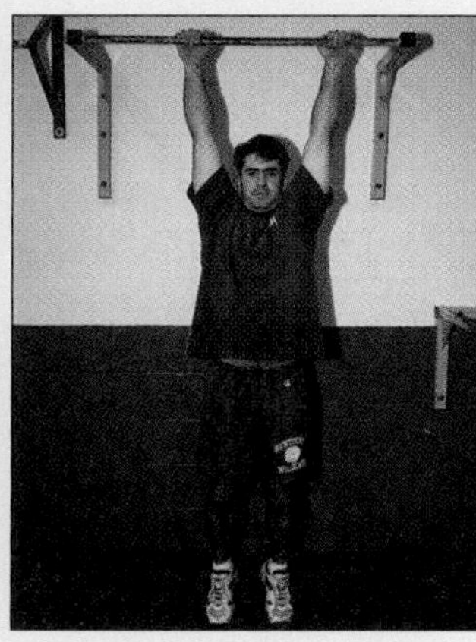

Arm Hang

Upper body strength. Equipment: horizontal bar (high enough to prevent your feet from touching the floor); stopwatch. Procedure: hang with straight arms, palms facing forward. Start watch when subject is in position. Stop when subject lets go. Your score is the number of minutes and seconds spent hanging.

Scoring standards (heart rate for 1 minute)

Age	18–29		30–39		40–49		50–59		60+	
Gender	F	M	F	M	F	M	F	M	F	M
Excellent	>1:30	>2:00	>1:20	>1:50	>1:10	>1:35	>1:00	>1:20	>:50	>1:10
Good	:46–1:30	1:00–2:00	:40–1:20	:50–1:50	:30–1:10	:45–1:35	:30–1:00	:35–1:20	:21–:50	:30–1:10
Average	<:46	<1:00	<:40	<:50	<:30	<:45	<:30	<:35	<:21	<:30

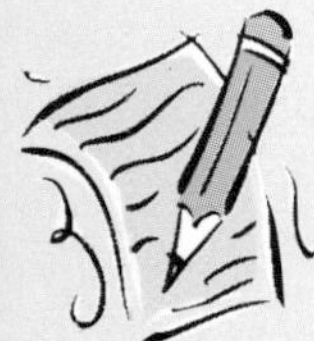

Personal Assessment *continued*

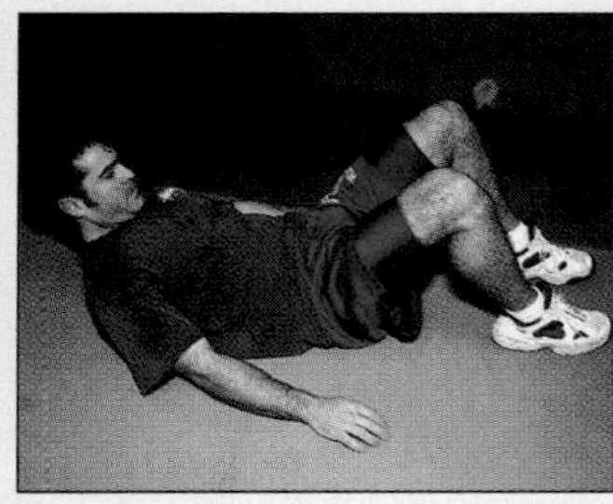

Curl-Ups

Abdominal and low back strength. Equipment: stopwatch. Procedure: Lie flat on upper back, knees bent, shoulders touching the floor, arms extended above your thighs or by your sides, palms down. Bend knees so that the feet are flat and 12 inches from the buttocks. Curl up by lifting head and shoulders off the floor, sliding hands forward above your thighs or the floor. Curl down and repeat. Your score is the number of curl-ups in 1 minute, without breaking a beat.

Scoring standards (number in 1 minute)

Age	18–29		30–39		40–49		50–59		60+	
Gender	F	M	F	M	F	M	F	M	F	M
Excellent	>45	>50	>40	>45	>35	>40	>30	>35	>25	>30
Good	25–45	30–50	20–40	22–45	16–35	21–40	12–30	18–35	11–25	15–30
Average	<25	<30	<20	<22	<16	<21	<12	<18	<11	<15

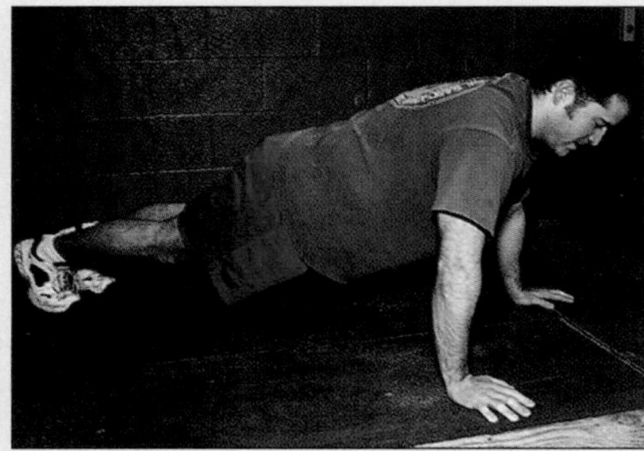

Push-Ups (Men)

Upper body strength. Equipment: stopwatch. Assume a front-leaning position. Lower your body until chest touches the floor. Raise and repeat for 1 minute. Your score is the number of push-ups completed in 1 minute, without breaking a beat.

Scoring standards (number in 1 minute)

Age	18–29	30–39	40–49	50–59	60+
Excellent	>50	>45	>40	>35	>30
Good	25–50	22–45	19–40	15–35	10–30
Average	<25	<22	<19	<15	<10

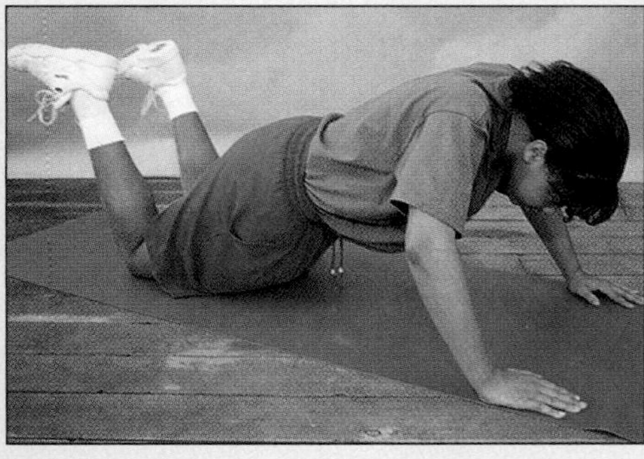

Modified Push-Ups (Women)

Upper body strength. Equipment: stopwatch. Assume a front-leaning position with knees bent up, hands under shoulders. Lower your chest to the floor, raise, and repeat. Your score is the number of push-ups completed in 1 minute, without breaking a beat.

Scoring standards (number in 1 minute)

Age	18–29	30–39	40–49	50–59	60+
Excellent	>45	>40	>35	>30	>25
Good	17–45	12–40	8–35	6–30	5–25
Average	<17	<12	<8	<6	<5

To Carry This Further . . .

Note your areas of strengths and weaknesses. To improve your fitness, become involved in a fitness program that reflects the concepts discussed in this chapter. Talking with fitness experts on your campus might be a good first step.

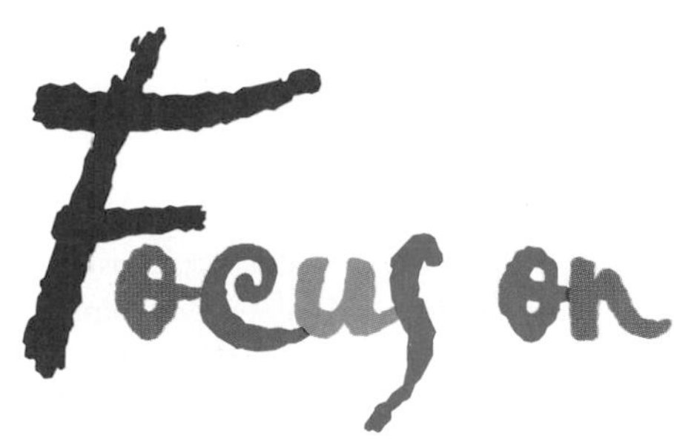

STAYING FIT DURING PREGNANCY

Like many other attitudes, our thinking on fitness during pregnancy has changed in recent years.[1] No longer is a pregnant woman treated as fragile. A woman needs to be quite careful when carrying a baby, but these days a doctor is more likely to advise against a sedentary lifestyle for a healthy pregnant woman. Exercise during pregnancy can increase a woman's muscle strength, making delivery of the baby easier and faster. Exercise can also help control her weight, making it easier to get back to normal weight after delivery. The baby may benefit from the mother's exercise program as well.

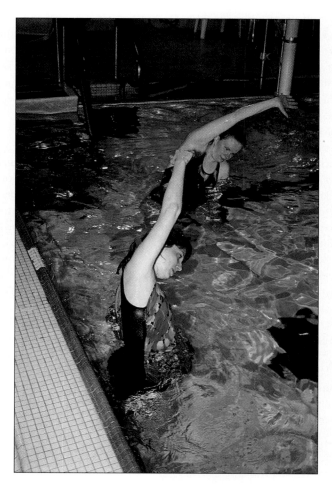

Water exercise is especially beneficial to pregnant women.

Importance of Exercise for Pregnant Women

Exercise in general is beneficial to the human body, and it is even more important for pregnant women to exercise regularly.[2] During pregnancy a woman's entire body undergoes many physical changes. Muscles are stretched, joints are loosened, and tissues are subjected to stress. If a woman is in good physiological condition, she is more likely to handle these changes with few complications.[3] The baby may also benefit: studies have shown that women who exercise during pregnancy tend to give birth to healthier babies.[2]

Types of Exercise

The types of exercises a woman should perform during pregnancy will vary with the individual and with the stage of pregnancy. General exercises that increase overall fitness and stamina should be practiced, as well as exercises that strengthen specific muscle groups. Muscles of the pelvic floor, for example, should be exercised regularly, since these muscles will be supporting most of the extra weight of the baby. The pelvic floor muscles are involved with control of the bladder and rectum and with controlling increases in pressure within the abdominal cavity resulting from pushing during labor.[3] General exercises for the pelvic floor muscles include Kegel exercises. These exercises involve the contraction of pelvic floor muscles, and they can be performed by squeezing and then relaxing the anal sphincter.[3] These exercises work on the sphincters (rings of muscle) that control the openings of the urethra and anus.

The abdominal muscles are responsible for supporting the load of the growing fetus in the front of the mother's body. They are also used for pushing during delivery. These muscles must be kept in good shape so they can adequately support the increased weight.[3] Muscles involved in maintaining good posture, such as the back and leg muscles, should also be exercised. Efficient breathing should be practiced as well.

A variety of exercises is available, including walking, swimming, stretching, and strengthening exercises.[2] Yoga and tai chi are also good forms of exercise for pregnant women. The muscles of the pelvic floor, abdomen, and back are especially subject to stress and strain during pregnancy and delivery, so certain exercises can also be performed to strengthen these muscles. Exercises can also be performed to speed up recovery after delivery.[4] Such postpartum exercises can be started in some cases within 24 hours after delivery. Exercises can even be started before conception if a pregnancy is anticipated.

Hydrotherapy is becoming a popular option for expectant mothers. Exercising in the water helps reduce stress on joints. Water also provides more resistance than air, so muscles get a better workout. No special equipment is needed, but various props such as weights or fans can be used to increase resistance. Immersion in water has also been shown to decrease blood pressure, reduce heart rate, and reduce tissue swelling in pregnant women.[5] Exercising in water may also reduce the risk for pregnant women of getting overheated or tired. The water must not be too warm, however, since water that is too hot (around 97.8 F or above) may damage the nervous system and brain of the fetus.[2]

Risks to the Fetus

Although exercise during pregnancy has definite advantages, there are some drawbacks that must be considered as well. Studies suggest that exercise can be harmful to the fetus in some cases. Women who undergo exercise for long periods may experience a prolonged increase in core body temperature (a condition called *hyperthermia*), which may in turn increase the body temperature of the fetus. It is thought that such increases in fetal temperature may in turn put the baby at risk for congenital malformations. It has been shown that fever-induced hyperthermia is related to congenital malformation in many mammals, and recent studies suggest that this may be true for humans as well.[5] If fever from illness can increase the expectant mother's core temperature enough to produce malformations in the fetus, then it is possible that an increase in the mother's core temperature resulting from prolonged exercise may have similar effects. Fortunately, exercise over short periods (15 minutes or less) is not likely to raise the mother's core temperature enough to cause problems.[5]

Exercising Safely

If the expectant mother exercised regularly before becoming pregnant, she may have to alter her exercise routine. Intense, high-impact workouts should be avoided in favor of moderate exercise, since very intense workouts may reduce blood flow to the fetus and deprive it of nutrients. Sports that involve sudden stops, such as basketball or tennis, should be avoided, and certain strenuous sports may eventually result in birth complications.[2] Exercises that involve lying on the back should not be performed after the first trimester of pregnancy, since they may reduce blood flow to the mother's heart and the heart of the fetus. Deep knee bends, sit-ups and toe touches should be avoided, as well as downhill skiing, rock climbing, and horseback riding.[6] Exercises should be chosen that minimize the risk of injury to the fetus and the mother. Because of the changes in the mother's weight distribution during the course of pregnancy, she should be especially aware of balance during workouts. Exercises that may put her at risk of losing her balance and falling should be avoided, especially during the last trimester.[2]

Once safety factors have been accounted for, the healthy pregnant woman still has an array of options to choose from for her exercise routine. As with any workout program, she should consult her physician before beginning. Her obstetrician can tell her which exercises will be most beneficial and can also give tips to reduce potential injury to her and her baby. The obstetrician can give the expectant mother guidelines concerning safe levels of exertion and duration times of exercise as well.

For Discussion . . .

Do you think exercise during pregnancy is a good idea or not? Do the benefits outweigh the risks?

References

1. Kaehler K, Tivers C: *Primetime pregnancy: the proven program for staying in shape before and after your baby is born,* 1997, Contemporary Books.
2. Marti J, Hine A: *The alternative health and medicine encyclopedia,* 1995, Gale.
3. Noble E: *Essential exercises for the childbearing year,* 1982, Houghton Mifflin.
4. Parr R, Rudnitsky DA: *Rob Parr's post-pregnancy workout,* 1997, Berkeley Publishing Group.
5. Cefalo RC, Moos M-K: *Preconceptional health care: a practical guide,* 1995, Mosby.
6. Williams, RD: Healthy pregnancy, healthy baby, *FDA Consumer* 33(2):18–23, 1999.

chapter **5**

Understanding Nutrition and Your Diet

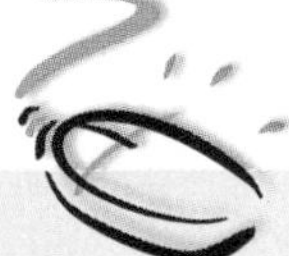

Online Learning Center Resources

www.mhhe.com/hahn6e

Log on to our Online Learning Center (OLC) for access to these additional resources:

- Chapter key terms and definitions
- Learning objectives
- Additional behavior change objectives
- Student interactive question-and-answer sites
- Self-scoring chapter quiz

The OLC also offers web links for study and exploration of health topics. Here are some examples:

- **www.nalusda.gov/fnic** Check out this site to find United States Department of Agriculture information on food safety, dietary guidelines, and more.
- **www.healthtouch.com** Look at this site for information on vitamins and supplements and health resources.
- **www.olen.com/food** Learn how much fat is in that Big Mac or Pizza Hut pepperoni pizza (answer: 31g/29g), and find nutritional information from nearly twenty national restaurants.

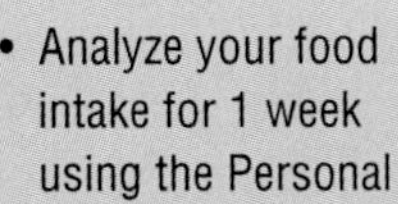

Taking Charge of Your Health

- Analyze your food intake for 1 week using the Personal Assessments at the end of this chapter.
- Develop a plan to modify your food intake patterns to make them agree with recommended guidelines.
- Explore ways in which you can balance the need for healthful meals with having an occasional fast-food meal.
- Practice judging portion sizes accurately.
- Experiment with alternative dietary patterns, such as semivegetarianism or ovolactovegetarianism.
- List any dietary supplements you take on a regular basis, and discuss this practice with your physician to determine whether they are necessary for your good health.
- Limit your intake of convenience foods, particularly those that are high in sugar and saturated fat.

Eye on the Media

Buying Dietary Supplements on the Internet

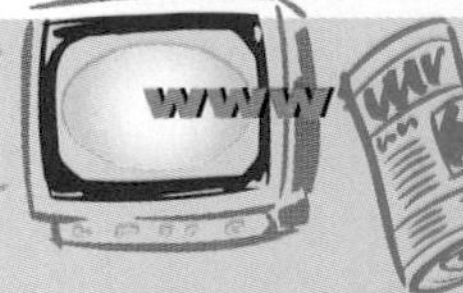

During the 1999 World Series, more TV advertising was purchased by Internet companies than by beer and automobile companies. This was the first time that had happened, and this change reflects the increasing importance of the Internet in U.S. commerce.

Today, virtually every product and service is available through the Internet, including dietary supplements. If you're thinking about buying such products through the Internet, you should understand that you will encounter differences from buying at the pharmacy, grocery store, or discount store.

Convenience: If you have easy access to the Internet and feel comfortable using this technology, shopping for dietary supplements on the Internet will be more convenient than driving to a store.

Selection: Like most stores, many Internet companies carry both nationally recognized and private brands. Some offer only private-label products. In general, the Internet offers a wider array of brands than you could find by going from store to store.

Eye on the Media *continued*

Expertise: Internet vendors argue that their staff members have more experience and a stronger background in supplement use than those who work in the typical grocery or shopping mall store. Some Internet vendors even provide hyperlinks to referenced information for particular dietary supplements and their potential effectiveness. Mall store managers contend that their staffs offer an equal or greater level of expertise and that they can access the same referenced information through their corporate homepages. Whether or not your local pharmacist would be willing or able to give detailed advice about supplement selection and use is open to question.

Cost: On-line vendors of dietary supplements say that their products are much less expensive than those sold in the typical retail store. Except for some nationally recognized brand-name products, they contend that most of their products are 30% to 40% less expensive (excluding shipping costs) than those sold in stores. Most of these Internet purchases are received within 2 to 3 days at a cost of approximately $4 for shipping. Large orders (over $50) may be shipped free, and overnight shipping may be as low as $10 for small orders.

Product Effectiveness: Since there is no FDA-required research on the effectiveness of dietary supplements, consumers are limited to the information in health magazines, newspaper or magazine articles, and various trade books to determine the value of a particular supplement. Internet companies contend that this is where they have a clear advantage over the typical retail store because they have established message boards where reports from satisfied customers can be posted. However, such reports are based on the opinions of individual consumers, not on scientific information about the product.

Protection: Many people feel uncomfortable using credit cards for purchases because they worry that their card number will be used inappropriately by the salesperson. This risk exists for all purchases made by credit card—whether in a retail store or via the Internet. If you shop at your local retail store, you can avoid this potential problem by using cash. However, using cash is not an option if you are making purchases on the Internet. If you don't want your name sold as part of a customer list, keep in mind that this risk is somewhat lower at the local retail level than on the Internet.

As a consumer, it's up to you to consider the pros and cons of buying dietary supplements on the Internet. Consider your experiences with traditional retail shopping and any other Internet shopping you may have done. Use common sense, a reasonable degree of caution, and your preferences to guide you.

From the prenatal period throughout life, sound dietary practices are needed to maintain high-level health. Food provides the body with the **nutrients** required to produce energy, repair damaged tissue, promote tissue growth, and regulate physiological processes.

Physiologically, these nutrients—carbohydrates, fat, protein, vitamins, minerals, dietary fiber, and water—are essential in adequate quantity. In addition, the production, preparation, serving, and sharing of food enriches our lives in other ways (see Exploring Your Spirituality).

TYPES AND SOURCES OF NUTRIENTS

Let's discuss the familiar nutrients first: carbohydrates, fats, and proteins. These three nutrients provide our bodies with **calories.*** Calories are used quickly by our bodies in energy metabolism, or they are stored in the form of glycogen or adipose (fatty) tissue. The other nutrient groups, which are not sources of energy for the body, will be discussed later.

*The term "calorie" is used here to mean kilocalorie (kcal), which is the accepted scientific expression of the energy value of a food.

Carbohydrates

Carbohydrates are various combinations of sugar units, or saccharides. The body uses carbohydrates primarily for energy. Each gram of carbohydrate contains 4 calories. Since the average person requires approximately 2000 calories per day and about 60% of our calories come from carbohydrates, roughly 1200 calories per day come from carbohydrates.[1]

Key Terms

nutrients
Elements in foods that are required for the energy, growth, and repair of tissues and regulation of body processes.

calories
Units of heat (energy); specifically, one calorie equals the amount of heat required to raise the temperature of 1 gram of water by 1°C.

carbohydrates
Chemical compounds composed of sugar units; the body's primary source of energy.

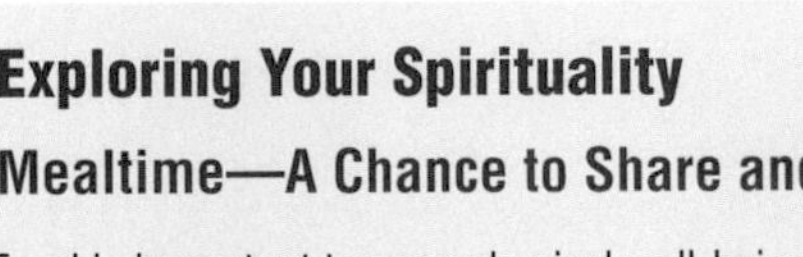

Exploring Your Spirituality

Mealtime—A Chance to Share and Bond

Food is important to your physical well-being—for energy, growth, repair, and regulation of your body and its function. But it's also important to the well-being of your spirit. The sharing of food nourishes our spiritual sense of community. This happens through the type of foods selected, the method of preparation, the uniqueness of presentation, and the people involved. From a spiritual perspective, the sharing of food can be a highly satisfying activity.

No closer sense of community exists than in the family. When food is shared in the company of those who care about us in the deepest and most personal ways, we experience a sense of value and well-being that is rarely found elsewhere. The simple act of being together and engaged in a familiar and comfortable practice is reassuring. It reminds us that we are valued in this setting. Meals that involve the extended family, especially dinners for special occasions or important holidays, are particularly rewarding.

Food is often at the center of the celebration of special occasions. Weddings, birthdays, anniversaries, graduations, promotions, retirements, and funerals take on a special meaning when people come together to share food and drink. From the first birthday cake through the retirement dinner to the lunch provided by neighbors after the funeral of a loved one, food reminds us that these events are benchmarks in our passage through life.

Whether it's an unexpected gift certificate for your favorite restaurant, your favorite dinner prepared at home, an invitation to order anything you'd like from a menu, or a catered banquet, food is often used to recognize a special achievement. This reminds us—in a spiritually uplifting way—that people value us and have chosen to be a part of our success story.

Friends are among the most important resources we have in our quest for self-validation. The sharing of food provides an opportunity for us to have important and meaningful exchanges with our friends. It's also a way of introducing new friends into our lives. New and valuable friendships begin in residence hall dining rooms, on outdoor benches shared on a pleasant autumn day, at a restaurant when someone is invited to join a group at their table, and at picnics at the home of a coworker. Without food, these opportunities might not exist.

Finally, food is the focus of many religious practices and observations. It may be a symbol in a religious service, a means of expressing religious values, or a way of unifying the congregation in times of joy and sorrow.

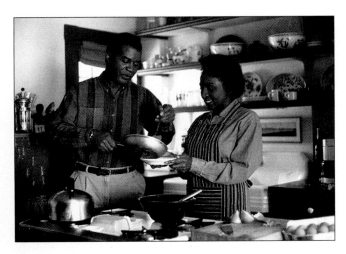

The shared preparation and serving of nourishing meals enhances your overall well-being.

Carbohydrates occur in three forms, depending on the number of saccharide (sugar) units that make up the molecule. Those that contain only one saccharide unit are classified as *monosaccharides* (glucose, or blood sugar), those with two units are *disaccharides* (sucrose, or table sugar), and those with more than two units are *polysaccharides* (starches).

Americans now consume about 125 pounds of sugar (sucrose) each year—usually in colas, candies, and pastries, which offer few additional nutritional benefits.[2] For years, excess sugar intake was blamed for a number of serious health problems, including obesity, mineral deficiencies, behavioral disorders, dental cavities, diabetes mellitus, and cardiovascular disease. However, with the exception of dental cavities, current scientific data do not confirm that sugar itself directly causes any of these health problems. However, the inability of some people to digest milk sugar (lactose) is well documented. Lactose-intolerant people lack an enzyme needed to digest this simple sugar. Today, it is recommended that no more than 10% of our total calories come from simple sugars.

Much of the sugar we consume is hidden. For example, it is an ingredient in foods such as ketchup, salad dressings, cured meat products, and canned vegetables and fruits. High-fructose corn syrup, often found in these items, is a highly concentrated sugar solution.

Starches are complex carbohydrates composed of long chains of sugar units. However, these starches should not be confused with the adjective "starchy." When people talk about starchy foods, they usually mean complex carbohydrates, or "heavy" foods. True starches are among the most important sources of dietary carbohydrates. Starches are found primarily in vegetables, fruits, and grains. Eating

Learning from Our Diversity

Do You Eat Real Ethnic Food?

The typical diets in many other countries tend to contain more high-carbohydrate foods and fewer foods high in animal fats than the common American diet. Moreover, when ethnic foods are prepared in the United States, especially in restaurants, they are often "Americanized" by inclusion of larger portions of meat and cheese, and addition of extra sauces. The examples below describe some traditional, high-carbohydrate ethnic foods and their higher-fat Americanized versions. Which version of these ethnic foods do you tend to eat?

Chinese
- *Traditional:* Large bowl of steamed rice with small amounts of stir-fried vegetables, meats, and sauces as condiments.
- *Americanized:* Several stir-fried or batter-fried entrees in sauces, with a small bowl of fried rice on the side.

Japanese
- *Traditional:* Large bowl of steamed rice with broth-based soups containing rice noodles, vegetables, and small amounts of meat.
- *Americanized:* Tempura (batter-fried vegetables and shrimp), teriyaki chicken, oriental chicken salad with oil-based dressing.

Italian
- *Traditional:* Large mound of pasta with tomato-based sauce containing small amounts of meat or meatballs on the side, served with crusty Italian bread or pizza with an extra-thick crust and a mere sprinkle of tomato sauce, herbs, and cheese.
- *Americanized:* Less pasta, more creamy sauces, and more meat, served with buttery garlic toast or pizza with a thick crust, pepperoni, sausage, olives, and extra cheese.

Mexican
- *Traditional:* Mostly rice, beans, warmed tortillas, and lots of hot salsa and chiles.
- *Americanized:* Crispy fried tortillas, extra ground beef, added cheese, sour cream, and guacamole (avacado dip).

German
- *Traditional:* Large portions of potatoes, rye and whole-grain breads, stew with dumplings, and sauerkraut.
- *Americanized:* Fewer potatoes and less bread, more sausage and cheese.

Middle Eastern
- *Traditional:* Pita bread (round bread), pilaf (rice dish), hummus (chick pea dip), shaved slices of seasoned meat, diced vegetables, and yogurt-based sauces, all seasoned with garlic.
- *Americanized:* Meat kebobs, salads drenched in olive oil, less bread and pilaf.

true starches is overall very nutritionally beneficial because most starch sources also contain much-needed vitamins, minerals, plant protein, and water. Many types of ethnic foods are high in carbohydrates and quite nutritious (see Learning from Our Diversity).

Fats

Fats (lipids) are an important nutrient in our diets. They provide a concentrated form of energy (9 calories per gram) and help give our foods high **satiety value**. Fat also helps give food its pleasing taste, or *palatability.* Fats carry the fat soluble vitamins A, D, E, and K. Without fat, these vitamins would quickly pass through the body. Fat also insulates our bodies to help us retain heat.

Dietary sources of fat are often difficult to identify. The visible fats in our diet, such as butter, salad oils, and the layer of fat on some cuts of meat, represent only about 40% of the fat we consume. Most of the fat we eat is hidden in food.

At the grocery store, the fat content of some foods is expressed as a percentage of the product's weight. For example, the different types of milk available include skim milk (no fat), low-fat milk (1/2%), reduced-fat milk (1% to 2%), and whole milk (3% to 4%). The labeling term "reduced-fat" for 1% and 2% milk was introduced in 1997 to indicate that these types of milk are no longer considered "low-fat."

The current recommendation is that no more than 25% to 30% of our calories come from fat (see the Star Box on p. 92). Complete the Personal Assessment on p. 113 to see whether you eat too many fatty foods. The Changing for the Better box on p. 92 offers information on the proper balance of fats in your diet. Children under 2 years of age, however, need a certain amount of fat in their diets for growth.[3] Check with your doctor before restricting the amount of fat in a young child's diet.

All dietary fat is made up of a combination of three forms of fat: saturated, monounsaturated, and polyunsaturated, based on chemical composition. Paying attention to

Key Term

satiety (suh TIE uh tee) value
A food's ability to cause a feeling of fullness.

Choosing Fats: A Balancing Act

Current dietary recommendations suggest that no more than 30% of a person's total calories (600 calories from the benchmark 2000 calorie/day intake) should come from fat. But what balance should there be among the three forms of dietary fat?

Current guidelines specify that no more than 8% to 10% of total calories (160 to 200 calories/day) should be supplied by saturated fat, such as butter. Nonunsaturated fat sources, such as olive oil, should be relied on for 15% of total calories (300 calories/day), with a maximum of 10% of daily calories derived from polyunsaturated fats. Individuals with elevated LDL cholesterol levels (see Chapter 10) should reduce their intake of saturated fat to 7% or less of their total caloric intake.

Changing *for the Better*

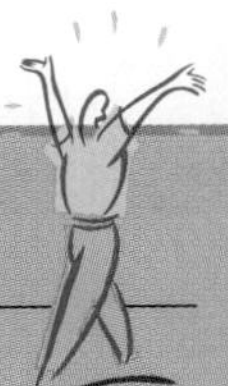

Tips for Reducing the Fat Content of Meals

Now that I'm sharing an apartment with friends, I'm eating more fatty foods than ever. How can I keep the fat content of my diet down?

- Become familiar with today's food labels, and use the information provided to reduce the fat content of your meals.
- Cut away and discard skin from meats such as chicken.
- When eating out, don't order foods with cream-based sauces, such as fettuccine alfredo.
- Trim all visible fat from meat—both within the cut and along the edges.
- Layer vegetables over baked potatoes to reduce any tendency to add butter, margarine, or sour cream.
- Request salad dressing and other condiments on the side so that you can control the amount you use.
- Eat more vegetables, fruits, and breads in place of meats and cheeses.
- Use jelly and apple butter in place of butter and margarine on toast, bread, and bagels.

the amount of each type of fat in our diet is important because of the known link to heart disease (see Chapter 10). **Saturated fats,** including those found in animal sources and vegetable oils to which hydrogen has been added (hydrogenated), becoming *trans-fatty acids,* need to be carefully limited in a healthy diet.

Concern over the presence of trans-fatty acids (an altered form of a normal vegetable oil molecule) is associated with changes detrimental to the cell membrane, including those cells lining the artery wall. Among the changes being suggested is an increase in calcium deposits.[4] This could result in a rough surface, leading to plaque formation (see Chapter 10).

Concern over the presence of trans-fatty acids in margarines has been strong, and the result has been changes to food labels that indicate the presence of these acids and their relationship to cardiovascular disease. The amount of trans-fatty acids in the diet can be reduced by using liquefied margarines rather than the solid-stick forms.

Tropical oils

Although all cooking oils (and fats such as butter, lard, margarine, and shortening) have the same number of calories by weight (9 calories per gram), some oils contain high percentages of saturated fats. All oils and fats contain varying percentages of saturated, monounsaturated, and polyunsaturated fats. However, the tropical oils—coconut, palm, and palm kernel—contain much higher percentages of saturated fats than do other cooking oils. Coconut oil, for example, is 92% saturated fat. Tropical oils can still be found in some brands of snack foods, crackers, cookies, nondairy creamers, and breakfast cereals, although they have been removed from most national brands. Do you check for tropical oils on the ingredients labels of the foods you select?

Cholesterol

A high blood level of **cholesterol** may be a risk factor for the development of cardiovascular disease (see Chapter 10). Cholesterol is necessary in all animal tissue and is manufactured by our bodies. Evidence first reported more than three decades ago suggests that increased intake of saturated fats may increase serum (blood) cholesterol levels. But the relationship between intake of dietary cholesterol and serum cholesterol levels remains unclear.[5]

Currently, a dietary intake of 200 mg (certainly less than 300 mg/day) is recommended in combination with a reduction in total fat and saturated fat intake and regular exercise. High-cholesterol foods include whole milk, shellfish, animal fat, and egg yolks. Only foods of animal origin contain cholesterol. Thus labels that appear on foods such as peanut butter and margarine saying "cholesterol free" are merely stating the obvious.

Two new food products hold promise for assisting in the management of cholesterol. In 1999 the FDA approved for marketing two unique forms of margarine, Benecol and Take Control.[6,7] In carefully controlled clinical studies in Finland, when stanol margarines were consumed on a reg-

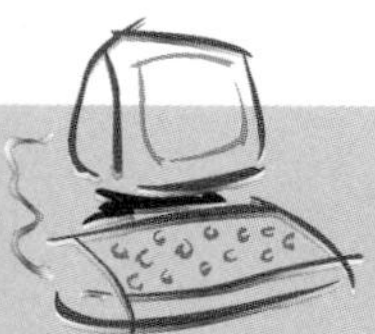

OnSITE/InSIGHT

Learning to Go: Health

Tired of giving up all your favorite foods when dieting? Click on the Motivator icon to see what tips on nutrition the following lessons offer:

Lesson 15: Aim to eat for health.
Lesson 16: Design a healthy, balanced diet.
Lesson 17: Make smart fast-food choices.
Lesson 18: Try a meat-free diet.
Lesson 19: Minimize the fat in your diet.

STUDENT POLL

Are you an organic food eater or a fast-food junkie? Go to the Online Learning Center at **www.mhhe.com/hahn6e** and focus on your nutritional habits. Click on Student Resources to find the Student Poll. There you can answer the following questions and then see how others responded.

1. Is having a well-balanced diet important to you?
2. Does your cultural background affect what you eat?
3. Do you use the nutritional information on food labels?
4. Are you a vegetarian?
5. Do you follow the USDA Food Guide Pyramid?
6. Do you drink several glasses of water daily?
7. Do you often watch TV while eating a meal?
8. Do you eat organic foods on a regular basis?
9. Do you often try different foods?
10. Is eating a social activity to you?
11. Has your diet changed noticeably since you started college?
12. Do you eat a lot of fast food?
13. Do you usually eat three meals a day?
14. Are you a calorie counter?
15. Is taking time to cook important to you?

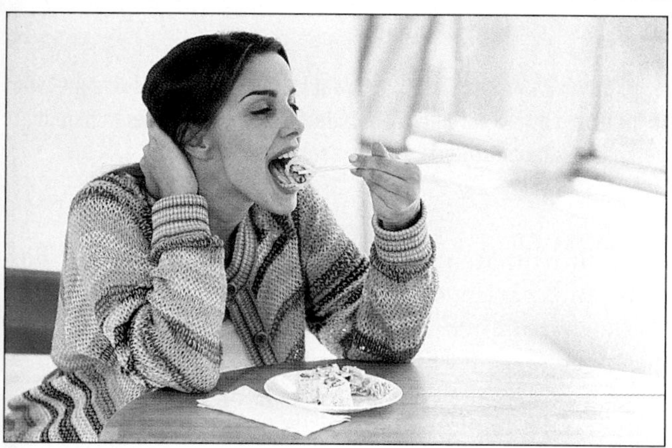

Low-fat, vitamin-rich foods are part of a healthy diet.

ular basis, they were shown to lower total cholesterol by 10% and the low-density lipoprotein (LDL) fraction by 15% (see Chapter 10).[8] In comparison to regular margarine, these products are more expensive because of processing costs; however, retail prices are becoming lower.

Low-fat foods

The fat-free, low-fat, and reduced-fat food items that have appeared in stores and restaurants in recent years reflect our growing concern about how dietary fats are related to many health problems. Nutritionists believe, however, that this trend could weaken as the fast-food industry puts less emphasis on low-fat items. Consumers seem to favor good taste over the long-term health benefits of weight maintenance and reduced incidence of heart disease. It's important to remember that low-fat foods are often high in calories and so should not be consumed in large amounts.

Proteins

Proteins are found in every living cell. They are composed of chains of **amino acids.** Of the twenty naturally occurring amino acids, the body can synthesize all but *nine essential amino acids** from the foods we eat. A food that contains all nine essential amino acids is called a *complete protein* food. Examples are animal products, including milk, meat, cheese, and eggs. A food source that

*Eight additional compounds are sometimes classified as amino acids, so some nutritionists believe that there are more than twenty amino acids.

Key Terms

saturated fats
Fats that promote cholesterol formation; they are in solid form at room temperature; primarily animal fats.

cholesterol
A primary form of fat found in the blood; lipid material manufactured within the body and derived from dietary sources.

proteins
Compounds composed of chains of amino acids; the primary components of muscle and connective tissue.

amino acids
The chief components of protein; can be manufactured by the body or obtained from dietary sources.

does not contain all nine essential amino acids is called an *incomplete protein* food. Vegetables, grains, and *legumes* (peas or beans—including chickpeas, butter beans, soybean curd [tofu], and peanuts) are principal sources of incomplete protein. For some people, including vegan vegetarians (see p. 106 and the Focus on box on p. 117), people with limited access to animal-based food sources, or those who have significantly limited their meat, egg, and dairy product consumption, it is important to understand how essential amino acids can be obtained from incomplete protein sources. This requires the careful selection of plant foods in combinations that will provide all of the essential amino acids, as shown in the following list:

- Sunflower seeds/green peas
- Navy beans/barley
- Green peas/corn
- Red beans/rice
- Sesame seeds/soybeans
- Black-eyed peas/rice and peanuts
- Green peas/rice
- Corn/pinto beans

When even one essential amino acid is missing from the diet, a deficiency can develop.

Protein primarily promotes growth and maintenance of body tissue. However, when caloric intake falls, protein is broken down and converted into glucose. This loss of protein can impede growth and repair of tissue. Protein also is a primary component of enzyme and hormone structure. It helps maintain the *acid-base balance* of our bodies and is a source of energy (4 calories per gram consumed). Nutritionists recommend that 12% to 15% of our caloric intake be from protein, particularly that of plant origin.

Vitamins

Vitamins are organic compounds that are required in small amounts for normal growth, reproduction, and maintenance of health. Vitamins differ from carbohydrates, fats, and proteins because they do not provide calories or serve as structural elements for our bodies. Vitamins are *coenzymes.* By facilitating the action of **enzymes,** vitamins help initiate a wide variety of body responses, including energy production, use of minerals, and growth of healthy tissue.

Vitamins can be classified as *water soluble* (capable of being dissolved in water) or *fat soluble* (capable of being dissolved in fat or lipid tissue). Water soluble vitamins include the B-complex vitamins and vitamin C. Most of the excess of these water soluble vitamins is eliminated from the body in the urine. The fat soluble vitamins are vitamins A, D, E, and K. Excessive intake of these vitamins causes them to be stored in the body in the adipose (fat) tissue. It is therefore possible to consume and retain too many of these vitamins, particularly vitamins A and D. Because excess fat soluble vitamins are stored in the body's fat, organs that contain fat, such as the liver, are primary storage sites.

Because water soluble vitamins dissolve quickly in water, it's important not to lose them during the preparation of fresh fruits and vegetables. One method is not to overcook fresh vegetables. The longer vegetables are steamed or boiled, the more water soluble vitamins will be lost. Some people save the water in which vegetables were boiled or steamed and use it for drinking or cooking.

To ensure adequate vitamin intake, a good approach is to eat a variety of foods. Unless there are special circumstances, such as pregnancy, lactation, infancy, or an existing health problem, nearly everyone who eats a reasonably well-rounded diet consumes enough vitamins to prevent deficiencies.

TALKING POINTS • What would you say to someone who is following a low-carbohydrate/high-fat weight loss diet to help that person see the nutritional weaknesses of the diet?

Unfortunately, not all people eat a balanced diet based on a variety of foods. Recent studies suggest that a somewhat higher intake of vitamins A, C, and E for adults might reduce the risk of developing cancer, atherosclerosis, and depressed levels of high-density lipoprotein (HDL) cholesterol; however, several unanswered questions remain, including the amounts needed for effectiveness (see Chapter 10).[9]

Consuming an adequate amount of folic acid before and during pregnancy has been shown to reduce the incidence of birth defects. To ensure adequate folic acid intake (400 micrograms/day), in 1997 the Food and Drug Administration (FDA) began to require that bread and cereal products be supplemented with folic acid. The goal of this requirement is for pregnant women and women of childbearing age to receive at least 140 micrograms/day through dietary intake. Taking a daily multivitamin before and during pregnancy would easily provide the remaining amount of folic acid necessary to promote fetal neural tube closure (thus preventing spina bifida). Folic acid is also considered important in the prevention of cardiovascular disease.[10]

TALKING POINTS • How would you convince a pregnant friend of the importance of including folic acid in her diet?

At the same time that many health experts are recommending some vitamin supplementation, the FDA has prohibited manufacturers of food supplements, including vitamins, from making *unsubstantiated claims* for the cure and prevention of disease. Supplement manufacturers fought against the implementation of this regulation by suggesting to the public that vitamins might become available only by prescription. This did not happen. Today, manufacturers of folic acid supplements may make claims about the product's ability to prevent neural tube defects in infants.

Minerals

Nearly 5% of the body is composed of inorganic materials, the *minerals.* Minerals function primarily as structural elements (in teeth, muscles, hemoglobin, and hormones). They are also critical in the regulation of body processes, including muscle contraction, heart function, blood clotting, protein synthesis, and red blood cell formation. Approximately twenty-one minerals have been recognized as essential for good health.

Major minerals are those that exist in relatively high amounts in our body tissues. Examples are calcium, phosphorus, sulfur, sodium, potassium, and magnesium. Examples of **trace elements,** minerals seen in relatively small amounts in body tissues, include zinc, iron, copper, selenium, and iodine. Trace elements are required only in small quantities, but they are essential for good health. As with vitamins, the safest, most appropriate way to prevent a mineral deficiency is to eat a balanced diet. However, calcium, a major mineral, can be taken as a supplement to help prevent osteoporosis.

Water

Water may well be our most essential nutrient, since without water most of us would die from the effects of **dehydration** in less than 1 week. We could survive for weeks or even years without some of the essential minerals and vitamins, but not without water. More than half our body weight comes from water. Water provides the medium for nutrient and waste transport, controls body temperature, and functions in nearly all of our body's biochemical reactions.

Most people seldom think about the importance of an adequate intake of water and fluids. Adults require about six to ten glasses a day, depending on their activity level and environment. People who drink beverages that tend to dehydrate the body (tea, coffee, and alcohol) should increase their water consumption. Needed fluids are also obtained from fruits, vegetables, fruit and vegetable juices, milk, and noncaffeinated soft drinks. Excessive water consumption by infants, however, can dilute sodium stores in the body to dangerously low levels, possibly causing death.[11] Also, dentists are increasingly concerned about the abnormally high number of dental caries (cavities) seen in children who have consumed bottled water rather than fluoridated tap water.[12]

Fiber

Although not considered a nutrient by definition, **fiber** is an important component of sound nutrition. Fiber consists of plant material that is not digested but moves through the digestive tract and out of the body. Cereal, fruits, and vegetables all provide us with dietary fiber.

Fiber can be classified into two large groups on the basis of water solubility. *Insoluble* fibers are those that can absorb water from the intestinal tract. By absorbing water, the insoluble fibers give the stool bulk and decrease the time it takes the stool to move through the digestive tract. In contrast, *soluble* fiber turns to a "gel" in the intestinal tract and binds to liver bile, to which cholesterol is attached. Thus the soluble fibers may be valuable in removing cholesterol, which lowers blood cholesterol levels. Also, since foods that are high in soluble fiber are generally low in sugar and saturated fats, fiber may indirectly contribute to keeping the blood sugar level low and reduce the risk of colon cancer associated with diets high in saturated fat.

In recent years, attention has been given to three forms of soluble fiber—oat bran, psyllium (from the weed plantain), and rice bran—because of their ability to lower blood cholesterol levels. Psyllium can be obtained by using laxatives, such as Metamucil, Konsyl, Fiberall fiber wafers, and Perdiem Fiber.

Key Terms

vitamins
Organic compounds that facilitate the action of enzymes.

enzymes
Organic substances that control the rate of physiological reactions but are not themselves altered in the process.

trace elements
Minerals present in very small amounts in the body; micronutrient elements.

dehydration
The abnormal depletion of fluids from the body; severe dehydration can be fatal.

fiber
Plant material that cannot be digested; found in cereal grains, fruits, and vegetables.

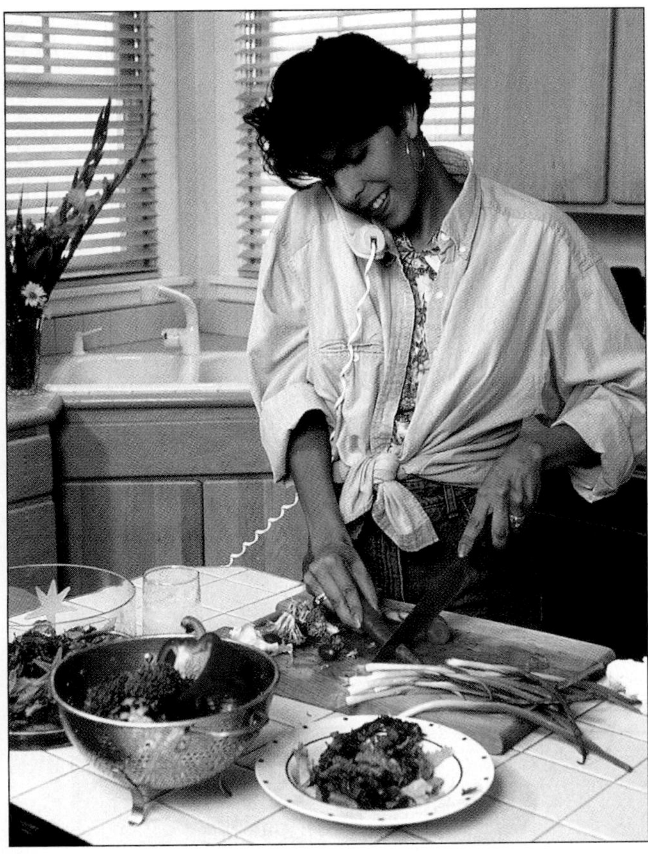

Vegetables provide vitamins, complex carbohydrates, and fiber and help prevent some types of cancer. Are you eating three to five servings a day?

Although earlier studies were contradictory regarding the effectiveness of soluble fiber in lowering cholesterol levels, now it appears that oat bran can lower cholesterol levels by five to six points in people whose initial cholesterol levels are moderately high. To accomplish this reduction, a daily consumption of oat bran equal to a large bowl of cold oat bran cereal or three or more packs of instant oatmeal would be necessary. Oatmeal can also be eaten as a cooked cereal or used in other foods, such as hamburgers, pancakes, or meatloaf.

THE FOOD GROUPS

The most effective way to take in adequate amounts of nutrients is to eat a **balanced diet**—one that includes a wide variety of foods from different food groups. Over the past several decades, various methods of grouping foods have been used, identifying five, seven, four, and now (again) five food groups from which selections are to be made. Today, the U.S Department of Agriculture (USDA) Food Guide Pyramid outlines five groups for which recommendations have been established and an additional group (fats, oils, and sweets) for which no specific recommendations exist (Figures 5-1 and 5-2). Table 5-1 summarizes the major nutrients that each food group supplies, and Table 5-2 shows the adult recommended dietary allowances (RDAs). To determine whether you are eating a healthful diet balanced with choices from each food group, complete the Personal Assessment on p. 115.

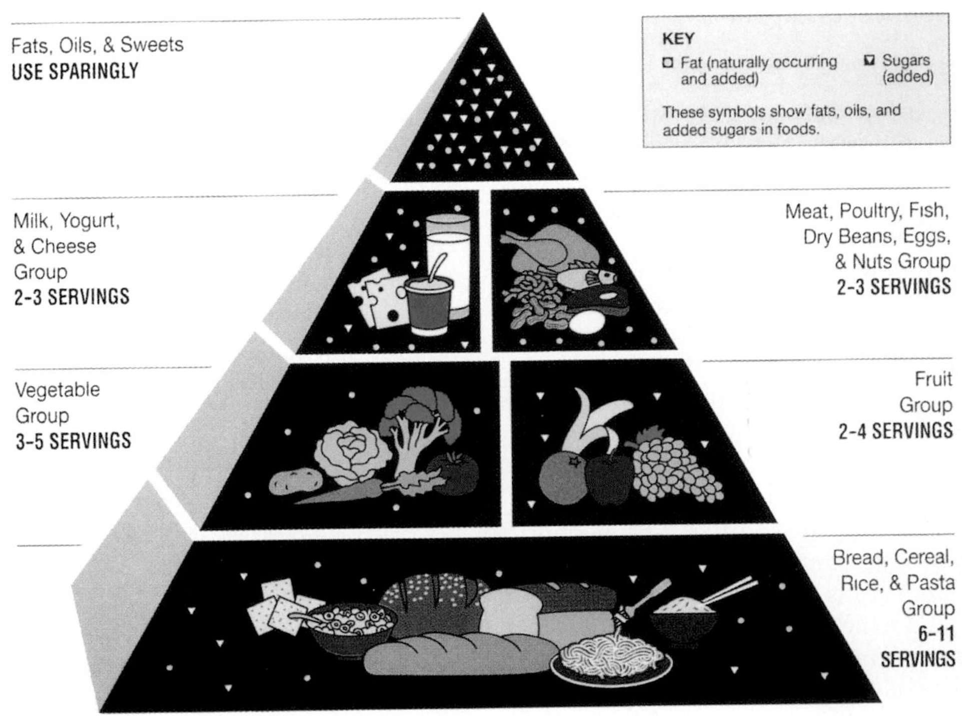

Figure 5-1 The USDA Food Guide Pyramid.

USDA-recommended daily servings for 2- to 6-year olds

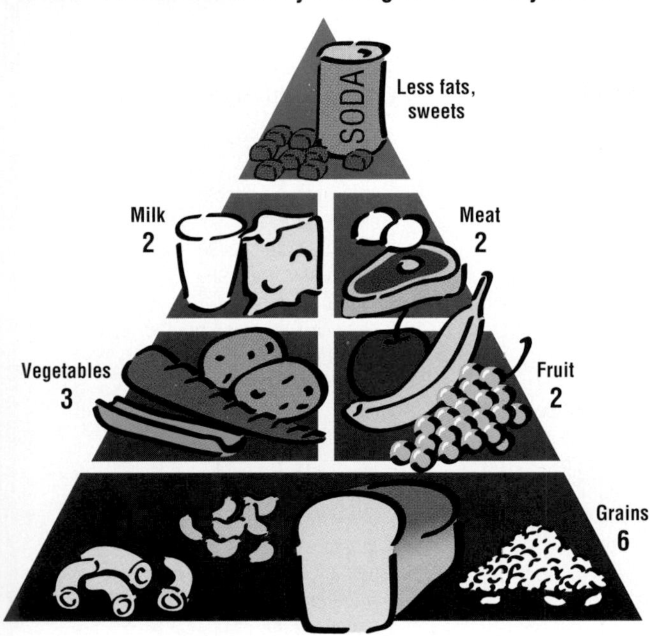

Figure 5-2 Children's nutritional requirements are different from those of adults, but they do need to eat a variety of nutrient-dense foods. This pyramid shows what the USDA recommends for 2- to 6-year olds.

Fruits

Two to four daily servings from the fruit group are recommended for an adult. The important functions of this group are to provide vitamin A, vitamin C, complex carbohydrates, and fiber in our diets. At least one serving high in vitamin C should be eaten daily.

Vegetables

Three to five servings from the vegetable group are recommended for an adult. As with the fruit group, the important functions are to provide vitamin A, vitamin C, complex carbohydrates, and fiber. Foods included in this group are dark-green, yellow, and orange vegetables, canned or cooked vegetables, and tossed salads. **Cruciferous vegetables,** such as broccoli, cabbage, brussels sprouts, and cauliflower, may be especially important in the prevention of certain forms of cancer.[13]

Milk, Yogurt, and Cheese

This group contributes two primary nutritional benefits: high-quality protein and calcium (required for bone and tooth development). Foods included in this group are whole milk, reduced-fat milk, low-fat milk, fat-free milk, yogurt, cheese, and ice cream. The adult recommendation is 2 to 3 cups of milk or two to three equivalent servings from this group each day. Premenopausal women should consume three to four daily servings from this group to provide maximal protection from osteoporosis.

Because of the general concern about saturated fat, cholesterol, and additional calories, low-fat and fat-free milk products are recommended in place of high-fat milk products. The Changing for the Better box on p. 102 shows the differences in calories (per cup), fat content (in grams), and % Daily Value among types of milk currently available. Aside from differences in fat content, all forms of milk offer similar nutritional benefits.

Meat, Poultry, Fish, Dry Beans, Eggs, and Nuts

It's essential to make daily selections from the protein-rich group because of our daily need for protein, iron, and the B vitamins. Meats include all red meat (beef, pork, and game), fish, and poultry. Meat substitutes include eggs, cheese, dried peas and beans (legumes), and peanut butter. Eggs can also be used as meat substitutes; however, using only the separated egg whites provides excellent protein without the accompanying fat (including cholesterol). The current recommendation for adults is 4 ounces total per day, preferably in two to three servings.

The fat content of meat varies considerably. Some forms of meat yield only 1% fat, but others may be as high as 40% fat. Poultry and fish are usually significantly lower in overall fat than red meat. The higher the grade of red meat, the more fat will be marbled throughout the muscle fiber and thus the higher will be its caloric value.

Bread, Cereal, Rice, and Pasta

The nutritional benefit from this group lies in its contribution of B-complex vitamins and energy (in the form of calories) to our diets. Some nutritionists believe that eating foods from this group also promotes protein intake, since many of them are prepared with foods in other groups and thus become complete-protein foods, such as macaroni and cheese, cereal and milk, and bread and meat sandwiches. Six to eleven

Key Terms

balanced diet
A diet featuring food selections from each of the lower levels of the Food Guide Pyramid.

cruciferous vegetables
Vegetables whose plants have flowers with four leaves in the pattern of a cross, such as broccoli.

Table 5-1 Guide to Daily Food Choices

Food Group	Serving	Major Contributions	Foods and Serving Sizes*
Milk, yogurt, and cheese	2 (adult†) 3 (children, teens, young adults, and pregnant or lactating women)	Calcium Riboflavin Protein Potassium Zinc	1 cup milk 1½ oz cheese 2 oz processed cheese 1 cup yogurt 2 cups cottage cheese 1 cup custard/pudding 1½ cups ice cream
Meat, poultry, fish, dry beans, eggs, and nuts	2–3	Protein Niacin Iron Vitamin B_6 Zinc Thiamin Vitamin B_{12}‡	2–3 oz cooked meat, poultry, fish 1–1½ cups cooked dry beans 4 T peanut butter 2 eggs ½–1 cup nuts
Fruits	2–4	Vitamin C Fiber	¼ cup dried fruit ½ cup cooked fruit ¾ cup juice 1 whole piece fruit 1 melon wedge
Vegetables	3–5	Vitamin A Vitamin C Folate Magnesium Fiber	½ cup raw or cooked vegetables 1 cup raw leafy vegetables
Bread, cereal, rice, and pasta	6–11	Starch Thiamin Riboflavin§ Iron Niacin Folate Magnesium‖ Fiber‖ Zinc‖	1 slice of bread 1 oz ready-to-eat cereal ½–¾ cup cooked cereal, rice, or pasta
Fats, oils, and sweets		Foods from this group should not replace any from the other groups. Amounts consumed should be determined by individual energy needs.	

This is a practical way to turn the RDA into food choices. You can get all essential nutrients by eating a balanced variety of foods each day from the food groups listed here. Eat a variety of foods in each food group, and adjust serving sizes appropriately to reach and maintain desirable weight.

*May be reduced for children's servings.
†≥ 25 years of age.
‡Only in animal food choices.
‖Whole grains especially.
§enriched.

servings daily from this group are recommended. Several daily servings of any **enriched** or whole-grain bread or cereal are recommended.

Fats, Oils, and Sweets

Butter, candy, colas, cookies, chips, and pastries fit into this food group. Such foods contribute little to healthful nutrition. Since they provide additional calories (generally from table sugar) and large amounts of salt and fat; they should be consumed in moderation. It's important to remember that cookies, crackers, and desserts called "fat free" or "low fat" may be high in sugar and calories. Many of the foods at the top of the food pyramid are known collectively as *junk foods.*

Table 5-2 Adult Recommended Dietary Allowances[1]

		Weight[2]		Height[2]			Fat Soluble Vitamins			
Category	Age (years)	(kg)	(lb)	(cm)	(in)	Protein (g)	Vitamin A (μg RE)[3]	Vitamin D (μg)[4]	Vitamin E (μg α-TE)[5]	Vitamin K (μg)
Males	15–18	66	145	176	69	59	1000	10	10	65
	19–24	72	160	177	70	58	1000	10	10	70
	25–50	79	174	176	70	63	1000	5	10	80
	51+	77	170	173	68	63	1000	5	10	80
Females	15–18	55	120	163	64	44	800	10	8	55
	19–24	58	128	164	65	46	800	10	8	60
	25–50	63	138	163	64	50	800	5	8	65
	51+	65	143	160	63	50	800	5	8	65
Pregnant						60	800	10	10	65
Lactating	1st 6 Months					65	1300	10	12	65
	2nd 6 Months					62	1200	10	11	65

Water Soluble Vitamins							Minerals						
Vitamin C (mg)	Thiamin (mg)	Riboflavin (mg)	Niacin (mg NE)[6]	Vitamin B_6 (mg)	Folate (μg)	Vitamin B_{12} (μg)	Calcium (mg)	Phosphorus (mg)	Magnesium (mg)	Iron (mg)	Zinc (mg)	Iodide (μg)	Selenium (μg)
60	1.5	1.8	20	2.0	200	2.0	1200	1200	400	12	15	150	50
60	1.5	1.7	19	2.0	200	2.0	1200	1200	350	10	15	150	70
60	1.5	1.7	19	2.0	200	2.0	800	800	350	10	15	150	70
60	1.2	1.4	15	2.0	200	2.0	800	800	350	10	15	150	70
60	1.1	1.3	15	1.5	180	2.0	1200	1200	300	15	12	150	50
60	1.1	1.3	15	1.6	180	2.0	1200	1200	280	15	12	150	55
60	1.1	1.3	15	1.6	180	2.0	800	800	280	15	12	150	55
60	1.0	1.2	13	1.6	180	2.0	800	800	280	10	12	150	55
70	1.5	1.6	17	2.2	400	2.2	1200	1200	320	30	15	175	65
95	1.6	1.8	20	2.1	280	2.6	1200	1200	355	15	19	200	75
95	1.6	1.7	20	2.1	260	2.6	1200	1200	340	15	16	200	75

[1]The allowances, expressed as average daily intakes over time, are intended to provide for individual variations among most normal people as they live in the United States under usual environmental stresses. Diets should be based on a variety of common foods to provide other nutrients for which human requirements have been less well defined. See text for detailed discussion of allowances and of nutrients not tabulated.

[2]Weights and heights of reference adults are actual medians for the U.S. population of the designated age, as reported by NHANES II. The use of these figures does not imply that the height-to-weight ratios are ideal.

[3]Retinol equivalents. 1 retinol = 1 μg retinol or 6 μg β-carotene.

[4]As cholecalciferol. 10 μg cholecalciferol = 400 IU of vitamin D.

[5]α-Tocopherol equivalents. 1 mg d-α tocopherol = 1 α-TE.

[6]1 NE (niacin equivalent) is equal to 1 mg of niacin or 60 mg of dietary tryptophan.

HEALTH PYRAMID ALTERNATIVES

The USDA Food Guide Pyramid has its critics, and alternatives have been proposed. The Healthy Weight Pyramid,[14] introduced by the Mayo Clinic in 2000, emphasizes unlimited fruits and vegetables, lots of whole grains, and exercise as a central element. The Healthy Eating Pyramid,[15] proposed by Dr. Walter Willett and colleagues of Harvard, has exercise and weight control at its base. Whole grains, plant oils, vegetables, and fruits are prominent; red meat is strictly limited. These pyramids can be viewed at: www.mhhe.com/hahn6e.

FAST FOODS

Fast foods deliver a high percentage of their calories from fat, often associated with their method of preparation

Key Term

enriched

The process of returning to foods some of the nutritional elements (B vitamins and iron) removed during processing.

Table 5-3 Fast Food: Fast, Convenient, Affordable—But Fattening

Menu Item	Calories	Calories from Fat	% Calories from Fat
Burgers			
McDonald's Hamburger	260	81	31%
Wendy's Jr. Hamburger	270	90	33%
Jack in the Box Hamburger	280	108	36%
Hardee's Hamburger	270	99	37%
McDonald's Cheeseburger	320	117	38%
Wendy's Jr. Cheeseburger	320	117	38%
Wendy's Plain Single Hamburger	360	144	39%
Jack in the Box Cheeseburger	330	135	42%
Burger King Cheeseburger	380	171	45%
Wendy's Jr. Bacon Cheeseburger	380	171	45%
McDonald's Quarter Pounder	420	189	45%
Wendy's Plain Double Hamburger	560	261	46%
McDonald's Big Mac	560	279	50%
McDonald's Quarter Pounder w/Cheese	530	270	51%
Hardee's Works Burger	530	270	51%
Burger King Double Cheeseburger	600	324	53%
Burger King Whopper	640	351	55%
Burger King Whopper with Cheese	730	414	56%
Jack in the Box Jumbo Jack	560	324	57%
Burger King Double Whopper	870	504	57%
Hardee's Monster Burger	1060	711	67%
Jack in the Box Ultimate Bacon Cheeseburger	1150	801	70%
Chicken Sandwiches			
Boston Market Plain Chicken Sandwich	430	45	9%
Chick-Fil-A Chargrilled Chicken Sandwich	280	27	11%
McDonald's Plain Grilled Chicken Deluxe	300	45	15%
Wendy's Grilled Chicken Sandwich	310	72	23%
Chick-Fil-A Chicken Sandwich	290	81	28%
Hardee's Grilled Chicken Sandwich	350	99	29%
Hardee's Chicken Fillet Sandwich	480	162	33%
Wendy's Breaded Chicken Sandwich	440	162	36%
KFC Original Recipe Chicken Sandwich	497	198	40%
McDonald's Crispy Chicken Deluxe	500	225	44%
Burger King Broiler	550	261	47%
Jack in the Box Chicken Sandwich	450	234	51%
Burger King Chicken Sandwich	710	387	55%
Jack in the Box Chicken Supreme	680	405	59%
Sub Sandwiches (6″)			
Subway Veggie Delite	237	27	11%
Blimpie Roast Beef	340	45	12%
Subway Turkey Breast	289	36	12%

(e.g., frying in saturated fat). **Fat density** is a serious limitation of fast foods (Table 5-3). In comparison with the recommended standard (25% to 30% of total calories from fat), 40% to 50% of the calories in fast foods come from fats. Although many fast food restaurants are now using vegetable oil instead of animal fat for frying (to reduce cholesterol levels), this change has not lowered the fat density of these foods. One average fast food meal supplies over one-half the amount of fat needed in a day. In addition, fast foods are often high in sugar and salt.

During the early 1990s, the fast food industry made an effort to offer alternatives to its fat-dense menu items by offering pasta, whole-wheat rolls, and lighter dressing. Unfortunately, this limited effort has nearly disappeared because many customers prefer large serving sizes (at low cost) and fat-dense foods. Today, supersize burgers, packing nearly 1,000 calories each, and pizza by the foot are popular choices among 18- to 35-year-old customers. The Changing for the Better box on p. 102 offers advice for choosing healthful foods when you're eating out.

Table 5-3 Fast Food: Fast, Convenient, Affordable—But Fattening

Menu Item	Calories	Calories from Fat	% Calories from Fat
Blimpie Grilled Chicken	400	81	20%
Subway Steak & Cheese	398	90	23%
Blimpie Ham & Swiss	400	117	30%
Subway Cold Cut Trio	378	117	31%
Subway Meatball	419	144	34%
Blimpie Steak & Cheese	550	234	42%
Blimpie Tuna	570	288	51%
Subway Tuna	542	288	53%
French Fries			
Hardee's Medium	350	135	37%
Hardee's Small	240	90	38%
Dairy Queen Large	390	162	41%
Jack in the Box Regular	360	153	42%
Jack in the Box Jumbo	430	180	42%
McDonald's Super Size	540	234	43%
McDonald's Small	210	90	43%
Wendy's Biggie	460	207	43%
McDonald's Large	450	198	44%
Wendy's Small	260	117	46%
Burger King Medium	370	180	49%
Jack in the Box Seasoned Curly	420	216	52%
Jack in the Box Chili Cheese Curly	650	369	57%
Tacos, Burritos, Pitas (and related items)			
Taco Bell Bean Burrito	380	108	29%
Taco Bell Steak Soft Taco	200	63	30%
Wendy's Chicken Caesar Pita	490	153	33%
Taco Bell Gordita Fiesta (steak)	270	90	33%
Wendy's Garden Veggie Pita	390	135	36%
Taco Bell Burrito Supreme	440	162	39%
Wendy's Classic Greek Pita	430	171	40%
Taco Bell Beef Burrito Supreme	520	207	40%
Taco Bell Steak Fajita Wrap	460	189	41%
Long John Silver's Salsa Chicken Wrap	690	288	42%
Long John Silver's Tartar Fish Wrap	730	315	42%
Long John Silver's Cajun Chicken Wrap	730	324	44%
Taco Bell Gordita Santa Fe (beef)	380	180	47%
Jack in the Box Taco	190	99	53%
Taco Bell Taco Supreme	220	117	55%
Jack in the Box Monster Taco	290	162	55%
Taco Bell BLT Soft Taco	340	207	62%

PHYTOCHEMICALS

Certain physiologically active components are believed to deactivate carcinogens or function as antioxidants. Among these are the carotenoids (from green vegetables), polyphenols (from onions and garlic), indoles (from cruciferous vegetables), and the allyl sulfides (from garlic, chives, and onions). These *phytochemicals* may be important agents in reducing the risk of cancer in people who consume a large quantity of particular fruits and vegetables. At this time, however, the exact mechanisms through which the various phytochemicals reduce the formation (or elimination) of cancer cells is not understood.[16] Although it is generally agreed that these foods

Key Term

fat density
The percentage of a food's total calories that are derived from fat; above 30% is considered to be a high fat density.

Changing *for the Better*

Milk Fat—Less Is More

I've been drinking whole milk for years, and I enjoy it. Would changing to one of the lower-fat types really make a health difference?

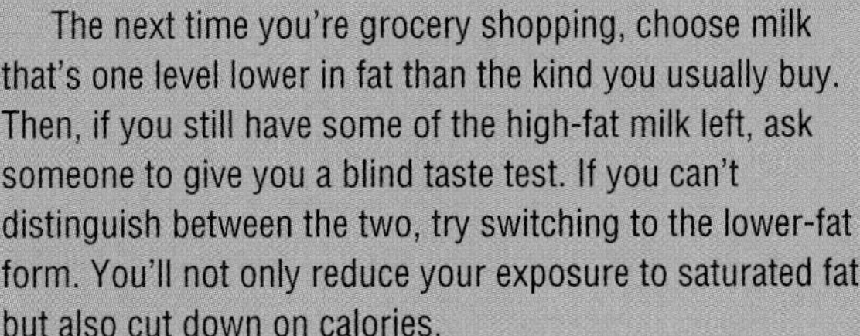

The next time you're grocery shopping, choose milk that's one level lower in fat than the kind you usually buy. Then, if you still have some of the high-fat milk left, ask someone to give you a blind taste test. If you can't distinguish between the two, try switching to the lower-fat form. You'll not only reduce your exposure to saturated fat but also cut down on calories.

Milk's New Names

Old Name	Possible New Names	Total Fat [per cup] Grams	% Daily Value	Calories per cup
Milk	Milk	8.0 g	12%	150
Low-fat 2% milk	Reduce fat or less fat milk	4.7 g	7%	122
Not on the market	Light milk	4.0 g or less	6% or less	116 or less
Low-fat 1% milk	Low-fat milk	2.6 g	4%	102
Skim milk	Fat-free, skim, zero-fat; no-fat or nonfat milk	less than 0.5 g	0%	80

As you can see from the information above, the names assigned to various types of milk have recently undergone a big change.

Changing *for the Better*

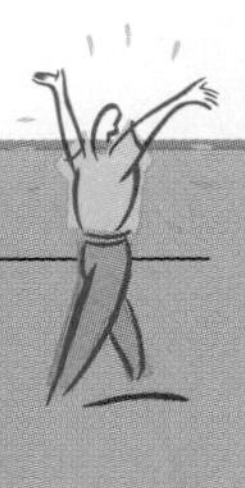

Eating Healthfully Away from Home

I've got a full load of classes and a part-time job, too, so I'm always in a time crunch. I buy a lot of my meals at fast-food restaurants. Is there a way to eat nutritiously while eating on the run?

- Choose nutritious foods, such as salads, baked potatoes, and whole-grain breads, instead of french fries.
- At a salad bar, choose the plain vegetables. Avoid mayonnaise-based salads, and limit your use of cheese, croutons, and salad dressings.
- Order a plain hamburger without condiments. When you add your own, you can control the amounts.
- Add lettuce and tomato to hamburgers to add vitamins, not calories.
- Order plain chicken; it has fewer calories than beef.
- Avoid breaded and fried foods.
- Choose skim milk, low-fat milk, juice, or water, not soda or shakes.
- For dessert, bring a piece of fresh fruit with you.
- Eat a small, nonfat, low-calorie snack at 10 AM and another at 2 PM. This kind of "grazing" can be healthier than gulping down one big fat-filled meal at noon.

are important in planning food selections, no precise recommendations regarding the amounts of various phytochemical-rich plants have been made.

FUNCTIONAL FOODS

At the forefront of healthful nutrition is the identification and development of foods intended to affect a particular health problem or to improve the functional capability of the body. **Functional foods** contain not only recognized nutrients but also new or enhanced elements that impart medicine-like properties to the food. Alternative labels also exist for various subclasses of functional foods, such as *nutraceuticals,* or food elements that may be packaged in forms appearing more like medications (for example, pills or capsules), and *probiotics,* or foods that improve the microbial flora that reside within the human digestive tract.[17]

Examples of functional foods include garlic (believed to lower cholesterol), olive oil (thought to prevent heart disease), foods high in dietary fiber (which prevent constipation and lower cholesterol), and foods rich in calcium (which prevent osteoporosis). In addition, foods that contain high levels of vitamins A, C, and E—primarily fruits and vegetables—and provide the body with natural sources of antioxidants are functional foods.

Other functional foods are those that contain or are enriched with folic acid. These vitamin B–family foods aid in the prevention of spina bifida and other neural tube defects and the prevention of heart disease. Foods that are rich in selenium are sometimes categorized as functional foods because of selenium's potential as an agent in cancer prevention. Most recently, the FDA has approved a "heart healthy" label for foods that are rich in soy protein.[18] All of the functional foods discussed here are approved to carry **health claims** on the basis of current FDA criteria.[19]

One category of functional foods being researched is vegetables that are genetically engineered to produce a specific biological element that is important to human health. An example is tomatoes that are high in lycopene. Another example, as described earlier, is a new type of margarine that can lower the level of and change the properties of blood cholesterol. Food technologists are interested in expanding the functional food family to include a greater array of health-enhancing food items.

TALKING POINTS • What would you say to convince your congressional representative to support a bill funding increased research on the effectiveness of functional foods?

FOOD ADDITIVES

Today many people believe that the food they consume is unhealthy because of the 2,800 generally recognized as safe (GRAS) **food additives** that can be put into food during production, processing, and preparation. But should these additives be banned?

Today's food manufacturers add chemical compounds to the food supply for several reasons, which they believe consumers support: (1) to maintain the nutritional value of the food; (2) to maintain the food's freshness by preventing changes in its color, flavor, and texture; (3) to contribute to the processing of the food by controlling its texture, acidity, and thickness; and (4) to make the food more appealing to the consumer by enhancing its flavor and standardizing its color. Market research indicates that consumers will continue to accept these alterations, regardless of what consumers say about not wanting them. Apparently, many people recognize that living in urban areas, working outside the home, and having foods available at all times during the year are worth the "price" of food additives.

FOOD LABELS

Since 1973, the FDA has required food manufacturers to provide nutritional information (labels) on products to which one or more nutrients have been added or for which some nutritional claim has been made. Originally, there was concern about whether the public could understand the labels and whether additional information would be required. So the FDA, in consultation with individual states and public interest groups, developed new labeling regulations. Revised labels began appearing on food packages in May 1993. The currently used label is shown in Figure 5-3. Specific types of information contained on this label are highlighted. (See also the HealthQuest Activities box on the right.)

Foods that were not initially covered by the 1993 food labeling guidelines are gradually being assigned labels. For example, many single-ingredient meats are now being labeled. Processed meat, fish, and poultry products, such as hot dogs and chicken patties, must bear labels. Fresh fruits and vegetables are not required to be labeled, but many stores do so voluntarily.

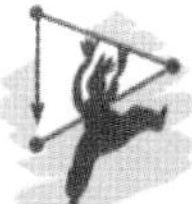

HealthQuest Activities

- One of the most valuable consumer skills you can acquire is the ability to read and interpret food labels. The Food Labeling activity in the Nutrition and Weight Control module demonstrates the purpose and importance of food labels. A tutorial outlines the steps in reading a food label, explains the terms used on food labels, and helps you evaluate health claims. The activity also lets you plan a meal and have it critiqued, using food labels as resources to guide you. Choose a food not listed in the activity, and do a nutritional comparison of five different labels for that food. Compare the ingredients on each label to determine where the differences in nutrient content may be. Research the ingredients to find out their sources, other foods or substances that contain the ingredients, and the purpose for including each ingredient.

Recent additions to the 1993 requirements include the labeling of fruit juices for pasteurization (unpasteurized juices can be a source of *Escherichia coli [E. coli]* contamination), the identification of milk from cows whose food has been enhanced with bovine growth hormone, and the issuing of specific criteria for legal use of the term "organic." Some supermarkets also label fresh and frozen poultry and seafood with information about how it was prepared and stored. This point-of-purchase labeling is voluntary. Additionally, some restaurant menus now state the nutritional content of some selections and provide cautionary notes about their safe cooking.

DIETARY SUPPLEMENTS

In 1998 it was estimated that 60 million Americans spent 9.8 billion dollars on a wide array of over-the-counter (OTC) products known collectively as *dietary*

Key Terms

functional foods
Foods capable of contributing to the improvement/prevention of specific health problems.

health claims
Liable statements attesting to a food's contribution to the improvement/prevention of specific health problems.

food additives
Chemical compounds intentionally added to our food supply to change some aspect of the food, such as its color or texture.

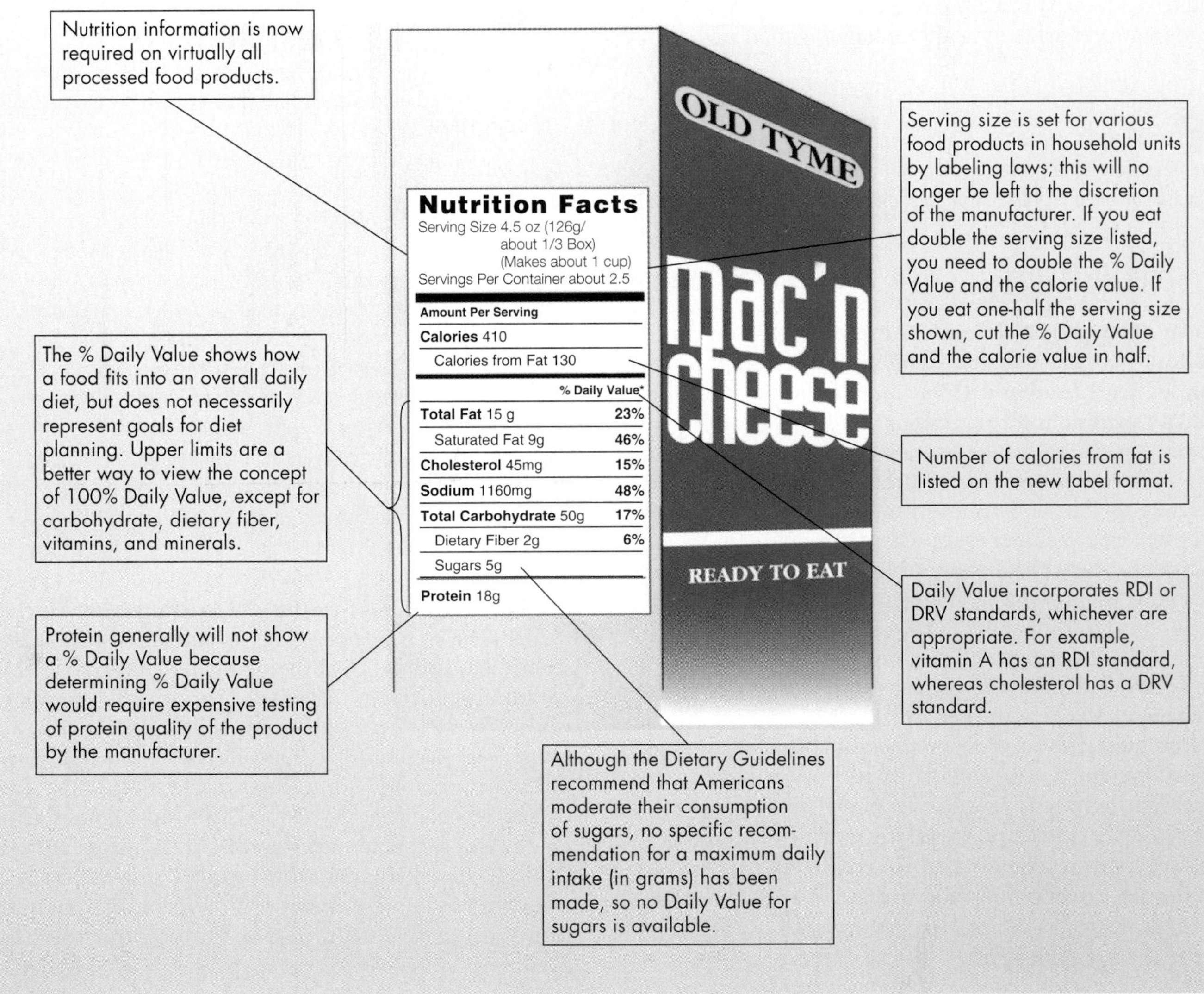

Nutrition information is now required on virtually all processed food products.
OLD TYME
mac'n cheese
READY TO EAT
Nutrition Facts
Serving Size 4.5 oz (126g/ about 1/3 Box) (Makes about 1 cup)
Servings Per Container about 2.5
Amount Per Serving
Calories 410
Calories from Fat 130
% Daily Value*
Total Fat 15 g 23%
Saturated Fat 9g 46%
Cholesterol 45mg 15%
Sodium 1160mg 48%
Total Carbohydrate 50g 17%
Dietary Fiber 2g 6%
Sugars 5g
Protein 18g
Serving size is set for various food products in household units by labeling laws; this will no longer be left to the discretion of the manufacturer. If you eat double the serving size listed, you need to double the % Daily Value and the calorie value. If you eat one-half the serving size shown, cut the % Daily Value and the calorie value in half.
The % Daily Value shows how a food fits into an overall daily diet, but does not necessarily represent goals for diet planning. Upper limits are a better way to view the concept of 100% Daily Value, except for carbohydrate, dietary fiber, vitamins, and minerals.
Number of calories from fat is listed on the new label format.
Daily Value incorporates RDI or DRV standards, whichever are appropriate. For example, vitamin A has an RDI standard, whereas cholesterol has a DRV standard.
Protein generally will not show a % Daily Value because determining % Daily Value would require expensive testing of protein quality of the product by the manufacturer.
Although the Dietary Guidelines recommend that Americans moderate their consumption of sugars, no specific recommendation for a maximum daily intake (in grams) has been made, so no Daily Value for sugars is available.

Figure 5-3 The Nutrition Facts panel on a current food label.

supplements. These nonprescription products are legally described as:[20]

- Products (other than tobacco) that are intended to supplement the diet, including vitamins, amino acids, minerals, glandular extracts, herbs, and other plant products such as fungi
- Products that are intended for use by people to supplement the total daily intake of nutrients in the diet
- Products that are intended to be ingested in tablet, capsule, softgel, gelcap, and liquid form
- Products that are not in themselves to be used as conventional foods or as the only items of a meal or diet

Unlike prescription medications (see Chapter 15), dietary supplements have been available in the marketplace for years almost without restriction. However, dietary supplements now must be deemed safe for human use on the basis of information supplied to the FDA by the manufacturers. In addition, the labels on these products cannot make a direct claim, with the exception of calcium and folic acid supplements, that they can cure or prevent illnesses. However, other materials with such claims may be displayed close to the dietary supplements themselves. Further, the labels on dietary supplements must remind consumers that the FDA has not required these products to undergo the rigorous research required of prescription medications and so the FDA cannot attest to their effectiveness. Beyond this, consumers are left to themselves to decide whether to purchase and use dietary supplements.

Easily accessible to anyone, dietary supplements can be purchased in grocery stores, drugstores, and discount stores, through mail-order catalogs, and over the Internet (see the Eye on the Media box on p. 88). Because of the great demand for these products, major pharmaceutical companies are now entering the dietary supplement field. Whether this trend leads to the development of more effective products, or to a greater effort on the part of the FDA to demand proof of effectiveness, remains to be seen. By definition, supplements are not foods, but simply "supplements." Therefore they remain free from requirements to substantiate their claims of effectiveness (as now required for functional foods).

TALKING POINTS • Several of your friends take multiple dietary supplements on a daily basis. What potential disadvantages of this practice would you point out to them?

TECHNOLOGICAL DEVELOPMENTS IN THE FOOD INDUSTRY

Technological advances in food manufacture and processing have done much to assure that the food we eat is fresh and safe. Yet there is growing concern that certain recent developments may also produce harmful effects on humans. For example, irradiation of foods, genetic engineering of foods, and the use of growth-enhancement agents for food animals are currently at the center of increasing controversy.

Irradiation of Food

In the 1990s, several recalls of meat and meat products were necessary because of bacterial contamination. As a result, the meat industry has been considering irradiation as a way to significantly reduce this problem. Current estimates are that nearly 99% of all bacteria in both processed and fresh meat could be killed by exposure to radiation.

Opponents of this approach argue that the use of radiation would make the meat industry less likely to use other antibacterial processes before the meat arrives at the processing plant. Then radiation would be the only technological procedure protecting the American consumer. Others fear that the damaging effect that radiation has on the structure of all cells, both microorganisms and the muscle cells of meat, might alter the meat in some harmful way.

Genetically Modified Foods

The success of American agriculture, in terms of food quality and marketability, has been based on the ability to genetically alter food sources to improve yield, reduce production costs, and introduce new food characteristics. Today, however, genetic technology is so sophisticated that changes are being introduced faster than scientists can fully evaluate the effects of these changes. Concerned individuals and agencies in the United States and abroad called for more extensive longitudinal research into safety issues and stricter labeling requirements for genetically modified foods. In January of 2001, the FDA determined that food companies did not need to label foods as having genetically modified components, although they could inform consumers that they are "derived through biotechnology." They had argued that without these measures consumers would have been at risk for unrecognized problems.

Growth Enhancement in Meat Production

The use of powerful growth stimulants and antibiotics by U.S. meat producers has already resulted in international political disagreements. In Europe, the import of U.S. meat products is being restricted because of safety concerns. In response to these actions, the U.S. government has restricted the import of a variety of European consumer products. Many overseas consumers would like access to these products, despite these safety concerns. Diplomatic efforts could resolve this issue at any time, but currently it remains the basis for strained relationships between the United States and some of its closest allies.

GUIDELINES FOR DIETARY HEALTH

Although dietary guidelines have been issued on many occasions, the Dietary Guidelines for Americans are the most current and widely used guidelines. The newest version appeared in June 1, 2000 as the fifth edition of *Nutrition and Your Health: Dietary Guidelines for Americans.*[21] These guidelines are directed to healthy Americans 2 years of age and older and to the health professional, who can influence public dietary practices. Information contained in these guidelines came from a variety of sources, including the Surgeon General's Report on Nutrition and Health. The most recent dietary guidelines are shown in the Star Box on p. 106.

Table 5-4 shows how healthful dietary changes can lead to reduced chances of developing certain major diseases. Notice that a reduction in fat and better control of caloric intake are important factors in reducing the likelihood of chronic illness.

Table 5-4 Recommended Dietary Changes to Reduce the Risk of Diseases and Their Complications

Change in Diet:	Reduce Fats	Control Calories	Increase Starch* and Fiber	Reduce Sodium	Control Alcohol
Reduce risk of:					
Heart disease	√	√		√	
Cancer	√	√	√		√
Stroke	√	√		√	√
Diabetes	√	√	√		
Gastrointestinal disease†	√	√	√		√

*Starch refers to complex carbohydrates provided by fruits, vegetables, and whole-grain products.

†Primarily gallbladder disease (fat), diverticular disease (fiber), and cirrhosis (alcohol).

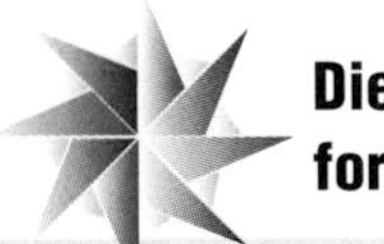

Dietary Guidelines for Americans

- Aim for healthy weight.
- Exercise at least 30 minutes each day.
- Make food choices based on the U.S. Department of Agriculture *"food pyramid"* diagram.
- Eat a variety of grains daily, especially whole grains.
- Eat a variety of fruits and vegetables daily.
- Keep food safe to eat.
- Choose a diet that is low in saturated fat and cholesterol and moderate in total fat.
- Choose beverages and foods to moderate your intake of sugars.
- Choose and prepare foods with less salt.
- Drink alcoholic beverages in moderation.

Almost all Americans could make changes that would bring them closer to meeting these guidelines. The Changing for the Better box on p. 109 presents recommendations for making healthful food choices.

VEGETARIAN DIETS

During the college years, many students follow some kind of nontraditional diet. Vegetarian diets, weight-reduction diets, and overreliance on fast foods represent some of these nontraditional dietary approaches. Most nutritionists believe that these diets do not need to be discontinued or avoided; instead, they should be undertaken with care and insight because of their potential nutritional limitations.

A *vegetarian diet* relies on plant sources for all or most of the nutrients needed by the body. This approach includes a range of diets from those that allow some animal sources of nutrients to those that exclude animal sources and are also restrictive in terms of plant sources. Three types of vegetarian diets, beginning with the least restrictive, are summarized below.

TALKING POINTS • If you and your friends have various dietary practices, how can you choose a restaurant that will accomodate everyone's needs and preferences?

Ovolactovegetarian Diet

Depending on the particular pattern of consuming eggs (*ovo*) and milk (*lacto*) or using one but not the other, an **ovolactovegetarian diet** can be a very sound approach to healthful eating for adults (see Figure 5-4 for an Ovolactovegetarian Food Guide Pieramid.) Ovolactovegetarian diets provide the body with the essential amino acids and limit the high intake of fats involved in more conventional diets. The exclusion of meat as a protein source lowers the total fat intake, and the consumption of milk or eggs allows an adequate amount of saturated fat to remain in the diet. The consistent use of vegetable products as the primary source of nutrients complies with the current dietary recommendations for an increase in overall carbohydrates, complex carbohydrates, and fiber.

Lactovegetarian Diet

People who include dairy products in their diet but no other animal products, including eggs, are *lactovegetarians.* As with the ovolactovegetarian diet, there is little risk associated with this dietary pattern.

Vegan Vegetarian Diet

A **vegan vegetarian diet** is one in which not only meat but also other animal products, including milk, cheese, and eggs, are not part of the diet. When compared with the ovolactovegetarian diet, the vegan diet requires greater nutritional knowledge and planning to avoid malnourishment.

When plants are the body's only source of nutrients, some difficulties can arise. The novice vegan needs to be particularly alert for these problems. One potential difficulty is obtaining all the essential amino acids. Since a single plant source does not contain all the essential amino acids, the vegan must learn to consistently use a

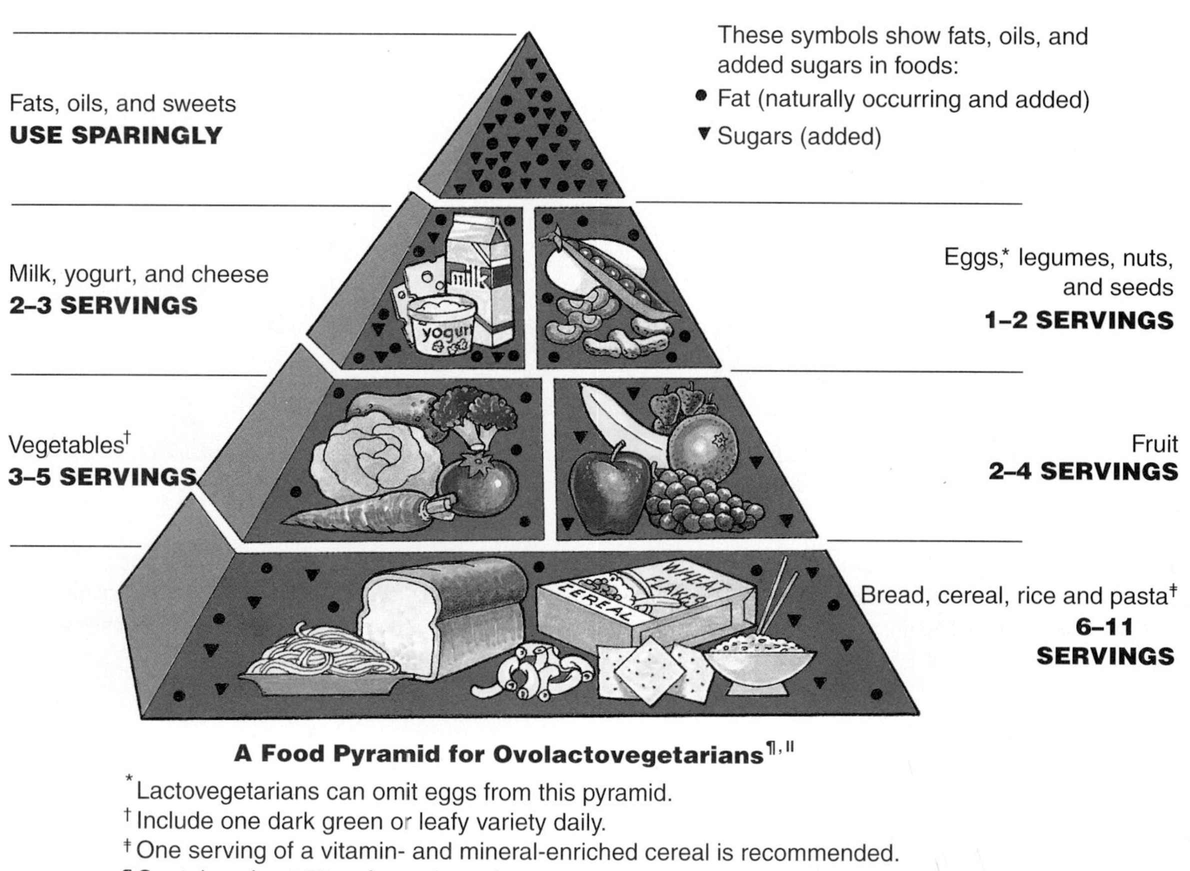

Figure 5-4 A food pyramid for ovolactovegetarians (vegetarians who include eggs and dairy products in their diet).

complementary diet. By carefully combining various grains, seeds, and legumes, amino acid deficiency can be prevented. This diet probably should not be used by pregnant women and **lactating** mothers.

In addition, the vegan could have difficulty maintaining the necessary intake of vitamin B_{12}, iron, zinc, and calcium. Vitamin D deficiencies also can occur.

Because of the nutritional limitations of the vegan vegetarian diet, many nutritionists do not recommend it. This diet should be followed only for reasons related to ecological, philosophical, or animal rights beliefs, since the total exclusion of animal products seems to accomplish little—from a nutritional point of view—that cannot be accomplished through ovolactovegetarianism. The American Dietetic Association currently says that a vegan diet is appropriate for infants and children as long as necessary supplements are provided.[22] Many people have adopted *semivegetarian* diets, in which meat consumption is significantly reduced but not eliminated (see the Focus on box on p. 117).

NUTRIENT DENSITY

For many college students, the issue of nutrient density may prompt certain dietary adjustments. The *nutrient density* of a food relates to its ability to supply proportionally more of the recommended daily allowance (RDA) for select vitamins and minerals than for daily

Key Terms

ovolactovegetarian diet
A diet that excludes all meat but does include the consumption of eggs and dairy products.

vegan vegetarian diet
A vegetarian diet that excludes all animal products, including eggs and dairy products.

lactating
Breastfeeding, nursing.

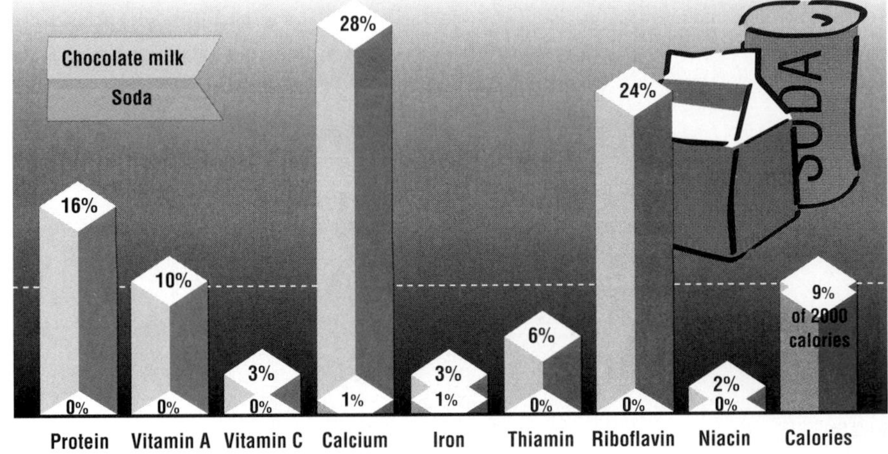

Figure 5-5 A comparison of the nutrient density of chocolate milk with that of soda. The bars that represent protein, vitamin A, calcium, and riboflavin in chocolate milk are all taller than the calorie bar, showing that chocolate milk is nutrient dense for these nutrients. All of the nutrient bars for soda are shorter than the calorie bar, illustrating that soda has a low nutrient density relative to the number of calories it supplies.

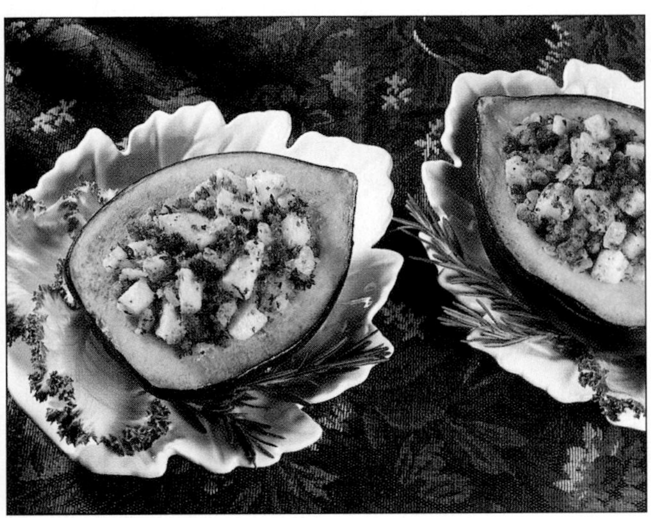

Vegetarian foods are delicious as well as healthful.

calorie requirements. Foods with a high nutrient density are better choices than those that supply only *empty calories* (Figure 5-5). For example, a bag of potato chips or a bottle of beer has a much lower nutrient density than either a serving of lightly steamed mixed vegetables or a 3-ounce serving of broiled skinless chicken breast. Choosing foods with a high nutrient density is especially important for people who are trying to limit their caloric intake.

NUTRITION AND THE OLDER ADULT

Nutritional needs change as adults age. Age-related changes to the structure and function of the body are primarily responsible for such altered nutritional requirements. These changes can involve the teeth, salivary glands, taste buds, oral muscles, gastric acid production, and peristaltic action. In addition, chronic constipation resulting from changes in gastrointestinal tract function can decrease the older adult's interest in eating.

The progressive lowering of the body's basal metabolism is another factor that will eventually influence the dietary patterns of older adults. As energy requirements fall, the body gradually senses the need for less food. In addition a tendency to decrease activity levels also occurs with aging. Because of this decreased need for calories, nutrient density—the nutritional value of food relative to calories supplied—is an important consideration for the elderly.

Psychosocial factors also alter the role of food in the lives of many older adults. Social isolation, depression, chronic alcohol consumption, loss of income, transportation limitations, and housing are lifestyle factors that can lessen the ease and enjoyment associated with the preparation and consumption of food. Consequently, a person's food intake might decrease.

Changing *for the Better*

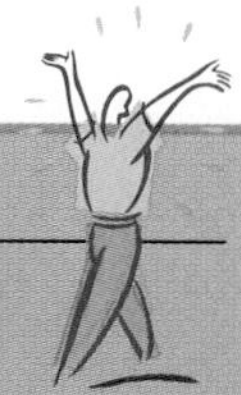

Ways to Improve Your Nutritional Health

Two of my relatives had heart attacks in middle age. I'm only in my twenties, but I know I've got to do what I can now to lower my risk for heart disease. Where do I start?

It's very likely that you can improve your dietary health and reduce the risk of developing heart disease and cancer by implementing the following practices.

Eat More High-Fiber Foods

- Choose dried beans, peas, and lentils more often.
- Eat whole-grain breads, cereals, and crackers.
- Eat more vegetables—raw and cooked.
- Eat whole fruit in place of drinking fruit juice.
- Try other high-fiber foods, such as oat bran, barley, brown rice, or wild rice.

Eat Less Sugar

- Avoid regular soft drinks. One 12-ounce can has nine teaspoons of sugar!
- Avoid eating table sugar, honey, syrup, jam, jelly, candy, sweet rolls, fruit canned in syrup, regular gelatin desserts, cake with icing, pie, and other sweets.
- Choose fresh fruit or fruit canned in natural juice or water.
- If desired, use sweeteners that don't have any calories, such as saccharin or aspartame, instead of sugar.

Use Less Salt

- Reduce the amount of salt you use in cooking.
- Try not to salt your food at the table.
- Eat fewer high-salt foods, such as canned soups, ham, sauerkraut, hot dogs, pickles, and foods that taste salty.
- Eat fewer convenience and fast foods.

Eat Less Fat

- Eat smaller servings of meat. Eat fish and poultry more often. Choose lean cuts of red meat.
- Prepare all meats by roasting, baking, or broiling. Trim off all fat. Be careful of added sauces or gravy. Remove skin from poultry.
- Avoid fried foods. Avoid adding fat when cooking.
- Eat fewer high-fat foods, such as cold cuts, bacon, sausage, hot dogs, butter, margarine, nuts, salad dressing, lard, and solid shortening.
- Drink skim or low-fat milk.
- Eat less ice cream, cheese, sour cream, cream, whole milk, and other high-fat dairy products.

INTERNATIONAL NUTRITIONAL CONCERNS

Nutritional concerns in the United States are centered on overnutrition, including fat density and excessive caloric intake. In contrast, in many areas of the world the main concern is the limited quantity and quality of food. Reasons for these problems are many, including the weather, the availability of arable land, religious practices, political unrest, war, social infrastructure, and material and technical shortages. Underlying nearly all of these factors, however, is unabated population growth.

To increase the availability of food to countries whose demand for food outweighs their ability to produce it, a number of steps have been suggested, including the following:

- Increase the yield of land currently under cultivation.
- Increase the amount of land under cultivation.
- Increase animal production on land not suitable for cultivation.
- Use water (seas, lakes, and ponds) more efficiently for the production of food.
- Develop unconventional foods through the application of technology.
- Improve nutritional practices through education.

Little progress is being made despite impressive technological breakthroughs in agriculture and food technology (such as a wide array of genetically modified seeds and soybean-enhanced infant foods), the efforts of governmental programs, and the support of the Food and Agricultural Organization of the United Nations and the U.S. Department of Agriculture. Particularly in Third World countries, where fertility rates are two to four times higher than those of the United States, annual food production needs to increase between 2.7% and 3.9% to keep up with population needs. With the world population now at 6.1 billion, and projected to reach 9 billion by 2070 before dipping to 8.4 billion in 2100,[23] food production in the coming decades may need to be increased beyond these estimates.

SUMMARY

- Carbohydrates, fat, and protein supply the body with calories.
- Carbohydrates differ on the basis of their molecular makeup, with sugars being the least complex and starches the most complex.
- Fat is important for nutritional health beyond serving as the body's primary means of storage of excess calories.
- Saturated fats, including trans-fatty acids, should be carefully limited because of their association with chronic diseases.
- Dietary intake of cholesterol should be limited through careful monitoring of food choices.
- Two new brands of margarine have proved effective in lowering cholesterol levels.
- Protein supplies the body with amino acids needed to construct its own protein.
- When few foods of animal origin are consumed, incomplete protein sources must be carefully balanced to provide complete protein in the diet.
- Vitamins serve as catalysts for body responses and are found in water soluble and fat soluble forms.
- The use of vitamin supplements is desirable for some people, but extensive use of food supplements can be dangerous.
- Minerals are incorporated into various tissues of the body and participate in regulatory functions within the body.
- An adequate amount of water and other fluids is required by the body daily and is obtained from a variety of food sources, including beverages.
- Fiber is undigestible plant material and has two forms, water soluble and water insoluble.
- Foods are currently classified into six groups, although recommendations regarding the needed number of daily servings have been given for only five of them.
- Fat-free or low-fat foods can be more calorie dense than anticipated.
- Fast foods should play only a limited role in daily food intake because of their high fat density and their high levels of sugar and sodium.
- Phytochemicals, capable of protecting the body from carcinogens or free radicals, are now being identified in many types of vegetables.
- Functional foods are capable of assisting in the prevention of specific health conditions.
- Food additives enhance the overall quality and convenient use of our food supply.
- New food labels provide considerably more information for the consumer than labels used previously.
- Dietary supplements are taken by millions of Americans, although their effectiveness is uncertain.
- Controversy exists about the application of new food technologies such as irradiation, genetic engineering, and the use of growth stimulants.
- Current dietary recommendations focus on the role of fat, saturated fat, starch, and sodium in health and disease.
- Ovolactovegetarianism, lactovegetarianism, and vegan vegetarianism are different forms of vegetarianism. Semivegetarianism is similar in some important ways to other forms of vegetarianism.
- Nutrient density plays an important role in the management of caloric intake for people of all ages, particularly older adults.
- A variety of factors contribute to malnourishment in many areas of the world.

REVIEW QUESTIONS

1. Which nutrients supply the body with calories?
2. How do sugars differ structurally from starches?
3. What is the function of fat in nutritional health besides serving as the body's primary means of storage for excess calories? What is the basis of our current concern about saturated fats, cholesterol, and trans-fatty acids?
4. What is the principal role of protein in the body? How can complete protein be obtained by people who eat few or no animal products?
5. Which vitamins are water soluble and which are fat soluble? What is the current perception regarding the need for vitamin supplementation? Which vitamins are regarded as antioxidants?
6. What functions do minerals have in the body? What is a trace element?
7. What are the two principal forms of fiber, and how does each of them contribute to health?
8. How many glasses of water per day are currently recommended?
9. What method of grouping foods is now used?
10. What are the current dietary recommendations regarding fat, saturated fat, starch, and sodium intake?
11. How can fat-free or low-fat foods be both low in nutritional density and high in caloric density?
12. What are functional foods, and how are they different from dietary supplements? Which has been empowered by the FDA to make health claims?

13. What information can be obtained from our current food labels?
14. If additives were eliminated from our food, what lifestyle adjustments would the public be forced to make?
15. What are an ovolactovegetarian diet and semivegetarianism, and how do they differ from a vegan diet?
16. What is nutrient density, and how does it relate to the aging process?

THINK ABOUT THIS . . .

- Is it more economical to buy a generic brand of cereal and take a generic multivitamin than to buy a highly supplemented but more expensive brand-name cereal?
- What nutrients are missing from your diet?
- Do your roles in parenting, employment, school, or home management compromise your ability to eat healthfully?
- Analyze your diet in terms of the recommendations made by *Nutrition and Your Health: Dietary Guidelines for Americans.*
- Consider your own dietary practices and those of your friends. Are you/they following sound nutritional guidelines?
- Would you say that you live to eat or eat to live?
- What are the most immediate changes that need to be made in your diet?
- In your opinion, what is the role of diet in both the cause and prevention of chronic disease? Are we currently too concerned about the role of food in preventing disease and enhancing health?

REFERENCES

1. Wardlaw GM, Kessel M: *Perspective in nutrition,* ed 5, 2002, McGraw-Hill.
2. Wardlaw GM: *Contemporary nutrition: issues and insights,* 1999, McGraw-Hill.
3. *Caring for your school-age child: 5–12,* 2001, American Academy of Pediatrics.
4. Kummerow FA, Zhou Q, Mahfouz MM: Effect of trans-fatty acids on calcium influx into human arterial endothelial cells, *Am J Clin Nutr* 70(5):832–838, 1999.
5. U.S. Department of Health and Human Services: *The surgeon general's report on nutrition and health,* DHHS Pub No 88-50210, 1988, U.S. Government Printing Office.
6. FDA letter clears way for revolutionary new Benecol spreads, *Johnson & Johnson News Letter,* May 1999.
7. Take Control: In the media, Unilever, April 30, 1999.
8. Law M: Plant sterol and stanol margarines and health, *Br Med J* 320(7238):861–864, 2000.
9. Greenberg ER, Sporn MB: Antioxidant vitamins, cancer, and cardiovascular disease, *N Engl J Med* 334(18):1189–1190, 1996.
10. Jacques PF, et al: The effect of folic acid fortification on plasma folate and total homocysteine concentrations, *N Engl J Med* 340(19):1449–1454, 1999.
11. Scariati PD, et al: Water supplementation of infants in the first month of life, *Arch Pediatr Adolesc Med* 151(8):830–832, 1997.
12. Children, water, and fluoride: AAPD parent information, American Academy of Pediatric Dentistry.
13. American Cancer Society: *Cancer facts and figures—2001,* 2001, The Association.
14. New Mayo Clinic Healthy Weight Pyramid helps you lose weight and keep it off! *Mayo Clin Rochester News,* Nov 21, 2000.
15. Willet W, Skerrett PJ, Giovannucci EL: *Eat, drink, and be healthy: the Harvard Medical School guide to healthy eating,* 2001, Simon & Schuster.
16. Waladkhani AR, Clemens MR: Effect of dietary phytochemicals on cancer, *Int J Mol Med* 1(4): 747–753, 1998.
17. Fransworth ER: What we are trying to do? *Medicinal Food News* 1(1):1–6, 1999.
18. FDA approves new health claim for soy protein and coronary heart disease [FDA talk paper], U.S. Food and Drug Administration Center for Food Safety and Applied Nutrition, October 20, 1999.
19. Kurtzweil P: Staking a claim to good health, *FDA Consumer,* November–December 1998.
20. Dietary Supplement Health and Education Act of 1994, U.S. Food and Drug Administration, Center for Food Safety and Applied Nutrition, 1 December 1995.
21. U.S. Department of Agriculture, U.S. Department of Health and Human Services. June 2000.
22. Mangels AR, Messina V: Considerations in planning vegan diets: infants, *J Am Diet Assoc* 101(6):670–677, 2001.
23. Lutz W, Sanderson W, Scherbov S: The end of the world population growth, *Nature* 412(6846):543–545, 2001.

SUGGESTED READINGS

Duyff R: *The American Dietetic Association's complete food and nutrition guide,* 1998, John Wiley & Sons.

This 600-page book blends nutritional theory with advice about the day-to-day need for a varied and balanced diet. It's written in a very understandable style. Using the newest nutritional recommendations as a basis, the author strongly supports adherence to the current USDA-recommended Food Pyramid. Because of this, however, the book will not appeal to readers interested in alternative diets, such as the currently popular low-carbohydrate/high-fat diets.

Kraus B: *Calories and carbohydrates,* ed 13, 1999, Signet.

For whatever reason readers—lay and professional alike—want to know about the caloric and carbohydrate composition of individual food items. This book is the time-honored standard. The author presents information about more than 8,550 food items, including familiar American food choices, such as pizza, fast food items, and various snack foods. Special attention is given to portion size, an aspect of sound nutritional practice that has proven difficult to master, particularly when today's food industry promotes foods in large amounts.

Margen S: *Wellness encyclopedia of food and nutrition,* 1999, Rebus.

The author, a retired professor from the University of California, Berkeley, and an editor of that institution's highly regarded *Wellness Letter,* takes readers through the theory and practices of healthful eating. Included are topics as diverse as food selection in the supermarket, the preparation, serving, and storage of food, and the role of diet in the cause and prevention of several health problems. Information pertaining to over 500 separate food items, each listed in alphabetical order, is visually supported through the use of over 80 color photographs. This book is very highly regarded by nutritionists for both its content and presentation.

Martinez Z: *The food and life of Oaxaca: traditional recipes from Mexico's heart,* 1997, IDG Books Worldwide.

If you want to learn more about one of Mexico's most unique cultural regions, and the equally unique food of its indigenous people, this book is highly recommended. The author, Zarela Martinez, a New York restaurant owner, visually depicts both the people and their foods, while providing instructions for how to prepare several of their famous sauce-based dishes.

As we go to Press...

In the past, small studies have suggested a protective relationship between a diet that includes high levels of fruits and vegetables and certain types of cancer, such as breast and colorectal cancer. Recently, however, a meta-analysis of eight studies that assessed the health behaviors of 351,825 women from North America and Europe failed to demonstrate a clear protective role for consumption of fruits and vegetables in the prevention of breast cancer. Although the segment of the study population that consumed the highest level of fruits and vegetables (4.5 to 10 servings/day) did have 7% less cases of breast cancer than those who consumed fewer servings, the difference was not found to be statistically significant. On a positive note, however, high levels of consumption of fruits and vegetables are associated within improved heart health, an extremely important factor in achieving a longer life.

Name ______________________ **Date** __________ **Section** __________

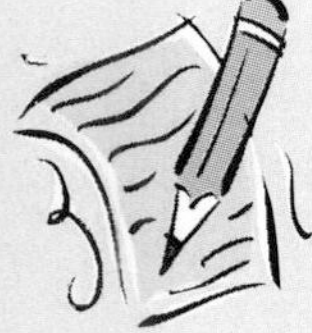

Personal Assessment

Do You Have Fatty Habits?

Fat has earned a bad reputation because of the health problems to which it contributes when we eat too much of it. The questionnaire below will help you think about the amounts and types of fat that you generally eat. For each general type of food or food habit, circle the response category that is most typical for you. If you never or almost never eat any items of a particular food type, just skip that type.

Food Type/Habit	High Fat	Medium Fat	Low Fat
Chicken	Fried with the skin	Baked, broiled, or barbecued with the skin	Baked, broiled, or barbecued without the skin
Fat present on meats	Usually eat	Sometimes eat	Never eat
Fat used in cooking	Butter, lard, bacon grease, chicken fat	Margarine, oil	Nonstick cooking spray or no fat used
Additions to rice, bread, potatoes, vegetables, etc.	Butter, lard, bacon grease, chicken fat, coconut oil, cream cheese	Margarine, oil, peanut butter	Butter-flavored granules or no fat used
Pizza toppings	Sausage, pepperoni, extra cheese, combination	Canadian bacon	Vegetable
Sandwich spreads	Mayonnaise or mayonnaise-type dressing	Light mayonnaise, oil and vinegar	Mustard, fat-free mayonnaise
Milk and milk products (e.g., yogurt)	Whole milk and whole-milk products	Reduced fat and low-fat milk and milk products	Skim milk and milk products
Sandwich side orders	Chips, potato salad, macaroni salad with creamy dressing	Coleslaw, pasta salad with clear dressing	Vegetable sticks, pretzels, pickle
Salad dressings	Blue cheese, Ranch, Thousand Island, other creamy type	Oil and vinegar, clear-base dressing	Oil-free dressing, lemon juice, flavored vinegar
Typical meat portion eaten	6–8 ounces or more	4–5 ounces	2–3 ounces
Sandwich fillings	Beef or pork hot dogs, salami, bologna, pepperoni, cheese, tuna, or chicken salad	Turkey hot dogs, 85% fat-free lunch meats, corned beef, peanut butter, hummus (chickpea paste)	95% fat-free lunch meats, roast turkey, roast beef, lean ham
Ground meats	Regular ground beef, sausage meat, ground meat, ground pork (about 30% fat)	Lean ground beef, ground chuck, turkey sausage meat (20%–25% fat)	Ground turkey, extra lean ground beef, ground round (about 15% fat)
Deep-fried foods (e.g., french fries, onion rings, fish or chicken patties, egg rolls, tempura)	Eat every day	Eat once a week	Eat once a month or never
Bread for sandwiches	Croissant	Biscuit	Whole wheat, French, tortilla, pita or pocket bread, bagel, sourdough, or English muffin

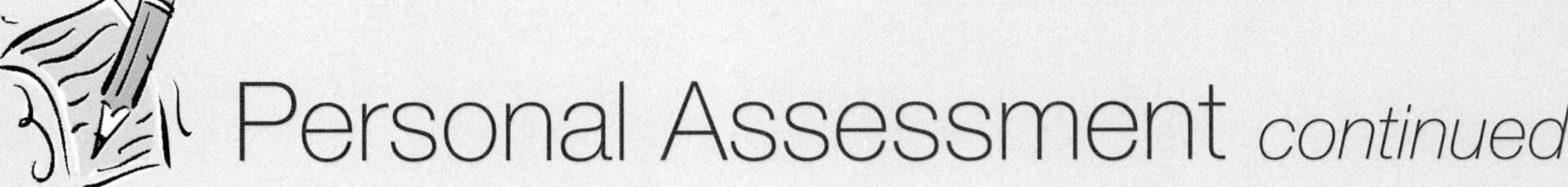

Personal Assessment *continued*

Food Type/Habit	**High Fat**	**Medium Fat**	**Low Fat**
Cheeses	Hard cheeses (e.g., cheddar, Swiss, provolone, Jack, American, processed)	Part skim mozzarella, part skim ricotta, low-fat and reduced fat cheeses	Nonfat cheeses, nonfat cottage cheese, no cheese
Frozen desserts	Premium or regular ice cream	Ice milk or low-fat frozen yogurt	Sherbet, Italian water ice, nonfat frozen yogurt, frozen fruit whip
Coffee lighteners	Cream, liquid or powdered creamer	Whole milk	Low-fat or skim milk
Snacks	Chips, pies, cheese and crackers, nuts, donuts, microwave popcorn, chocolate, granola bars	Muffins, toaster pastries, unbuttered commercial popcorn	Pretzels, vegetable sticks, fresh or dried fruit, air-popped popcorn, bread sticks, jelly beans, hard candy
Cookies	Chocolate coated, chocolate chip, peanut butter, filled sandwich type	Oatmeal	Ginger snaps, vanilla waters, graham crackers, animal crackers, fruit newtons

SCORING: (____________ × 2) + (____________ × 1) + (____________ × 0) =

TOTAL SCORE ____________

Once you have completed the questionnaire count the number of circles in each column and calculate your score as follows: multiply the number of choices in the left-hand (high fat) column by 2 and multiply the number of choices in the middle by 1. Any number of choices in the right-hand column will equal 0.

Less than 10 = Excellent fat habits

10 to 20 = Good fat habits

20 to 30 = Need to trim some fat

Over 30 = Very high fat diet

If your score is 20 or above, try to substitute more foods from the middle (medium fat) column or, better still, the right (low fat) column for foods in the left-hand (high fat) column.

Name ______________________ Date __________ Section __________

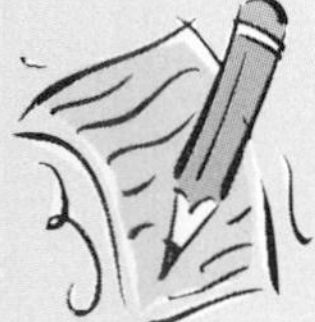

Personal Assessment

Rate Your Plate

Take a closer look at yourself—your current food decisions and your lifestyle. Think about your typical eating pattern and food decisions.

Do You . . .

	Usually	Sometimes	Never
Consider nutrition when you make food choices?	❑	❑	❑
Try to eat regular meals (including breakfast), rather than skip or skimp on some?	❑	❑	❑
Choose nutritious snacks?	❑	❑	❑
Try to eat a variety of foods?	❑	❑	❑
Include new-to-you foods in meals and snacks?	❑	❑	❑
Try to balance your energy (calorie) intake with your physical activity?	❑	❑	❑

Now for the Details

Do You . . .

	Usually	Sometimes	Never
Eat at least 6 servings* of grain products daily?	❑	❑	❑
Eat at least 3 servings* of vegetables daily?	❑	❑	❑
Eat at least 2 servings* of fruits daily?	❑	❑	❑
Consume at least 2 servings* of milk, yogurt, or cheese daily?	❑	❑	❑
Go easy on higher-fat foods?	❑	❑	❑
Go easy on sweets?	❑	❑	❑
Drink 8 or more cups of fluids daily?	❑	❑	❑
Limit alcoholic beverages (no more than 1 daily for a woman or 2 for a man)?	❑	❑	❑

Score Yourself
Usually = 2 points
Sometimes = 1 point
Never = 0 points

If you scored . . .
24 or more points—Healthful eating seems to be your fitness habit already. Still, look for ways to stick to a healthful eating plan—and to make a "good thing" even better.

16 to 23 points—You're on track. A few easy changes could help you make your overall eating plan healthier.
9 to 15 points—Sometimes you eat smart—but not often enough to be your "fitness best."
0 to 8 points—For your good health, you're wise to rethink your overall eating style. Take it gradually—step by step!

Whatever your score, make moves for healthful eating. Gradually turn your "nevers" into "sometimes" and your "sometimes" into "usually."

Adapted from *The American Dietetic Association's Monthly Nutrition Companion: 31 Days to a Healthier Lifestyle,* Chronimed Publishing, 1997.

Sample Serving Sizes
Bread, cereals, rice, and pasta group—6 to 11 servings daily:
1 slice (1 oz.) enriched or whole-grain bread
½ hamburger roll, bagel, English muffin, or pita
½ cup cooked rice or pasta
1 ounce (1 cup) ready-to-eat cereal

Vegetable group 1—3 to 5 servings daily:
½ cup chopped raw, non-leafy vegetables
½ cup cooked vegetables
1 small baked potato (3 ounces)
¾ cup vegetable juice

Fruit group—2 to 4 servings daily:
1 medium fruit (apple, orange, banana, peach)
¾ cup fruit juice
½ cup canned, frozen, or cooked fruit

Milk, yogurt, and cheese group—2 to 3 servings daily:
1 cup milk, buttermilk, or yogurt
1½ ounces natural cheese (cheddar, mozzarella, Swiss)
1 cup frozen yogurt

Meat, poultry, fish, beans, eggs, and nuts group—2 to 3 servings daily:
2 to 3 ounces cooked lean meat, poultry, or fish
½ cup cooked legumes (equals 1 ounce meat)
1 egg (equals 1 ounce meat)

Fats, oils, and sweets—use sparingly:
sugars
salad dressings
oils
cream
butter
soft drinks

*Serving sizes vary depending on the food and food group

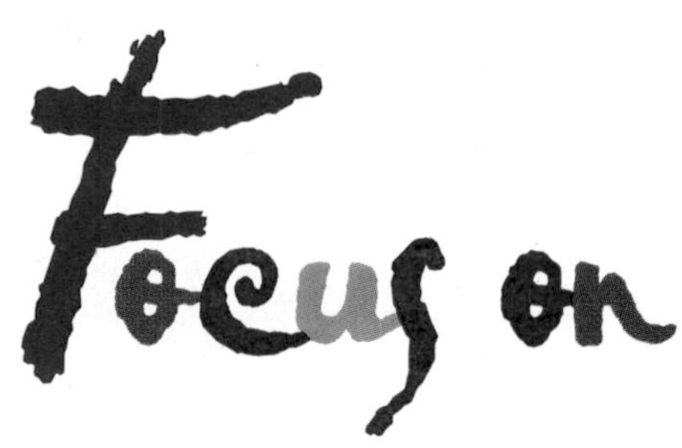

FOLLOWING A SEMIVEGETARIAN DIET

People become vegetarians for many reasons. Some shun meat and animal products for ethical reasons. Others choose vegetarianism for health reasons. Often it seems that vegetarians are viewed in opposition to those who eat meat and that the two lifestyles are not compatible. In recent years, however, some people are choosing a "middle ground" between the two eating styles. These semivegetarians are increasing their intake of vegetables and cutting back greatly on their meat consumption.

There are several types of vegetarians. *Vegans* are the most restrictive with their diets, eating only fruits, grains, and vegetables. *Lactovegetarians* consume milk products along with fruits, vegetables, and grains. *Ovolactovegetarians* include both eggs and milk products in their diets. *Semivegetarians* add occasional servings of fish and poultry to the ovolactovegetarian diet, and some even eat red meat on occasion.

Benefits of Vegetarianism

Semivegetarianism is the most popular option among the 12 million Americans who consider themselves to be vegetarians.[1] Although many vegetarians choose this lifestyle for health reasons, some people do so for ethical reasons. They cite the inhumane conditions in which factory farm animals are raised and processed as reasons to boycott the eating of animal products. This attitude is often associated with vegans, lactovegetarians, or ovolactovegetarians rather than with semivegetarians.

The health benefits of vegetarianism are many. Cutting meat consumption can decrease the risk of heart attacks, and eating more vegetables in place of meat may decrease the risk of some types of cancer.[2] In addition, vegetarianism avoids the possible negative health effects associated with growth-stimulating hormones and antibiotics given to food animals. A vegetarian diet can also aid in weight loss and prevention of obesity.

However, there are some potential risks associated with following a purely vegetarian diet. Protein in plants is generally of lower quality than protein found in animal products, so those on a vegetarian diet must be careful to eat a variety of plant foods to get all of the essential amino acids. Eliminating meat altogether may also lead to a deficiency of vitamin B_{12}, which can affect nervous system function. Eating foods fortified with this vitamin, such as cereals, or taking vitamin supplements can ward off B_{12} deficiency. Vitamin D, which is needed for bone and tooth development, may be lacking in vegetarian diets. Vegans must make sure that they get enough vitamin D by eating fortified foods or getting enough sunlight exposure to promote vitamin D production in the body. Vegetarians should eat plant foods that are high in iron to prevent deficiency. Calcium supplements may also be necessary, since vegan diets may make calcium difficult to absorb.[3]

Is Semivegetarianism Really Vegetarian?

There is some controversy over whether the semivegetarian diet (also referred to as a plant-rich diet) truly qualifies as "vegetarian." Many people on a strict vegetarian diet do not consider the semivegetarian diet to be vegetarian. To them, any consumption of meat products is considered a compromise to vegetarian principles. Likewise, there are debates over the appropriate use of dairy products and eggs among the various vegetarian groups. Some semivegetarians even acknowledge that they are not "real" vegetarians. To some vegetarians, the use of the term "semivegetarian" is not acceptable.

The debate over whether semivegetarians should be categorized as vegetarians revolves around ethical questions concerning treatment of animals. Many vegans especially denounce the eating of any meat or animal products, since animals must be exploited to obtain these foods. They are therefore morally opposed to semivegetarianism. Cutting back, however, may at least cause a decrease in demand for meat and animal products, and some semivegetarians view this as a moral justification for their dietary changes. Although the semivegetarian diet may not effectively address the ethical questions raised by animal rights activists, it has become an acceptable approach for many people who want to eat more healthfully.

There is little doubt that the semivegetarian diet is much healthier than the typical meat-laden Western diet, and its health benefits are well documented.[4] An increased support of vegetarian dietary practices, in all of their forms, including semivegetarianism, is reflected by the current position taken by the American Dietary Association.[5]

Becoming Semivegetarian

The semivegetarian diet is considered advantageous by some people because consuming at least some meat products makes it easier to obtain the required daily nutrients and it is a healthier approach to eating than the typical American diet. If you want to adopt a semivegetarian diet, however, don't try to make the change overnight.[6] Since the sudden elimination of most meat and other animal products may be too drastic of a change to adhere to, it's a good idea to cut back on these foods gradually.

One approach to gradually cutting back your meat consumption is to keep track of how much meat you consume per day. Then begin reducing the amount slowly until you have tapered off to about 4 ounces a day. Meat can be used as a condiment (such as chicken strips on a salad) instead of as a main course, and fish can be substituted for red meat. Try new vegetarian foods at each meal, and keep track of your likes and dislikes. Adding more fruit to your meals can also increase the variety of your diet.

Arlene Spark, a nutrition expert from New York Medical College, has developed a vegetarian food pyramid to help non–meat eaters and semivegetarians to follow a healthful diet (see the inside back cover of this textbook). This pyramid is similar to the USDA Food Guide Pyramid (see Figure 5-1), but it replaces the meat, poultry, fish, dry beans, eggs, and nuts group with a meat/fish substitutes group. It also includes special recommendations for vegans. The pyramid advises vegetarians of all types to eat 6 to 11 servings of grains or starchy vegetables, at least 3 servings of other vegetables, 2 to 4 servings of fruit, and 2 to 4 servings of milk or milk substitutes per day.[7] Legumes can be used as a substitute for meats for obtaining iron, calcium, protein, and zinc, but keep in mind that vitamin B_{12} is not found in plant foods. Semivegetarians can obtain some vitamin B_{12} from the limited meats they consume, but they should be careful not to decrease vitamin B_{12} intake too much. For people changing to vegetarian dietary practices from a meat-rich diet, carefully considered fast-food meals may offer convenience and can be eaten occasionally.[8]

Children can also be involved in the change to a semivegetarian diet, but consult your pediatrician first to be safe.[6] Making dietary changes a "family affair" can make the adjustment easier. Getting kids involved in meal planning, cooking, and label reading can make this new way of eating more interesting to them. Since dietary changes can be a difficult adjustment for kids, be flexible with their restrictions. This approach may help parents and children avoid arguments over meals and keep meals an enjoyable experience for everyone.

A semivegetarian diet may be an acceptable alternative if you want to cut back significantly on meat consumption but don't want to give up meat altogether. Check with your doctor to see if such a diet offers advantages for you. This is especially important if you're pregnant or nursing or have health problems.

For Discussion . . .

Is semivegetarianism more ethically sound than the typical Western diet, or is there no difference between eating meat occasionally and eating it often? Should semivegetarians be considered vegetarians? Is the ethical treatment of animals a consideration for you in the food choices you make? Is health a concern for you in your diet?

References

1. Springer I: Are you ready to go vegetarian? *Cosmopolitan* 219(4), October 1995.
2. Adlercreutz H, Mazur W: Phyto-oestrogens and Western disease, *Ann Med* 29(2):95–120, 1997.
3. Wardlaw G: *Perspective in nutrition,* ed. 4, 1999, McGraw-Hill.
4. Dwyer J: Convergence of plant-rich and plant-only diets, *Am J Clin Nutr* 70(3 suppl):620S–622S, 1999.
5. Position of The American Dietetic Association: Vegetarian diets, 1997. **www.eatright.org/adap1197.html**
6. Messina V: *The vegetarian way: total health for you and your family,* 1996, Crown Publishing.
7. Vegetarian pyramid, *Better Homes and Gardens,* October, 1994.
8. Messina V: *The convenient vegetarian,* 1999, IDG Books Worldwide.

chapter 6

Maintaining a Healthy Weight

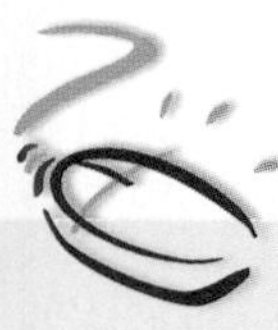

Online Learning Center Resources

www.mhhe.com/hahn6e

Log on to our Online Learning Center (OLC) for access to these additional resources:

- Chapter key terms and definitions
- Learning objectives
- Additional behavior change objectives
- Student interactive question-and-answer sites
- Self-scoring chapter quiz

The OLC also offers web links for study and exploration of health topics. Here are some examples of what you'll find:

- **http://vm.cfsan.fda.gov/~lrd/nutguide.txt** Check out the current edition of the *Dietary Guidelines for Americans.*
- **www.mirror-mirror.org/eatdis.htm** Look here for a wealth of information on eating disorders—signs and symptoms, complications, and getting help.
- **www.caloriecontrol.org** Have fun counting calories on this delightfully interactive site.

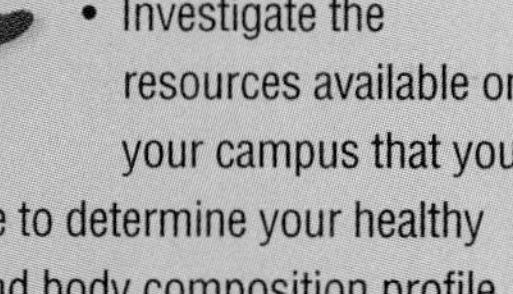

Taking Charge of Your Health

- Investigate the resources available on your campus that you could use to determine your healthy weight and body composition profile.
- Evaluate your eating behaviors to find out if you are using food to cope with stress. If you are, develop a plan to use nonfood options, such as exercise or interaction with friends or family members, to deal with stress.
- Formulate a realistic set of goals for altering your weight and body composition in a time frame that allows you to do so in a healthful way.
- Establish a daily schedule that lets you make any necessary dietary and physical activity adjustments.
- Keep a daily journal of your weight-management efforts.
- Monitor your progress toward meeting your weight-management goals.
- Design a reward system for reaching each goal.

Eye on the Media

TV Zooms In on Body Image

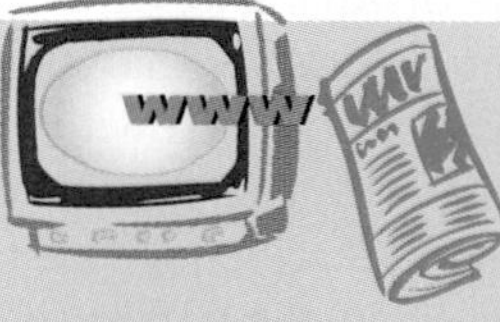

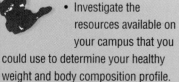

What's on TV tonight? A minute of channel surfing tells you that it's bodies—bodies conditioned through athletics or dance, grotesque bodies hardened through training (and drug enhancement), and bodies thinned to anorexic proportions to show off fashions. Tune in to the cable medical channel and watch a liposuction procedure being done to remove unsightly fat. Or choose a documentary that details, with technical accuracy and human compassion, the struggles experienced by some obese people as they try to lose weight. It's all there—from the sensational to the educational.

A recent prime-time program focused on litigation stemming from the use of the fenfluramine-phentermine (fen-phen) weight-loss regimen and the resulting cases of heart valve damage. Another show featured the popular weight-loss aid Metabolife, raising questions about its safety and effectiveness.

Commercials for weight-loss programs and products are common on television. But you need to look carefully for the small-print disclaimers that say "results may vary widely." Ads for new prescription medications for weight loss are designed to prompt

Eye on the Media *continued*

viewers to ask their doctors about these aids. It's only at the end of such ads that the long list of possible side effects and the caution that these drugs are intended for the most obese people are quickly flashed on the screen.

Prime-time sitcoms send powerful messages about thinness, obesity, and muscularity through their characters and story lines. The women characters on *Friends,* for example, are all thin and have well-toned muscles. For many teenage girls and young women, the message is that they should try to look like these characters on TV. *The Drew Carey Show* makes jokes about the main character being overweight but steers clear of the health/happiness issues involved. After all, this is a comedy.

Critics of TV programming are asking some important questions. How reliable is the medical information we're getting? Can a 30-second feature give a balanced view of the dangers and benefits of a new drug? Is learning about liposuction on TV a good basis for deciding to have that procedure yourself? If the actors on *Friends* look good on TV (which "adds pounds"), are they much too thin in real life? What do you think?

Obesity is a serious health concern. Approximately 60% of all adults in the United States are above their healthy weight, and 26% of adults are classified as obese.[1] In a society that has an abundance of high-quality food and a wide variety of labor-saving devices, being an overweight adult is almost the rule rather than the exception.

When the body is supplied with more energy than it can use, the result is an excess of energy (or a **positive caloric balance**) stored in the form of fat. This continuous buildup of fat can eventually lead to obesity. In the past, the prevailing feeling was that, in terms of medical risk, being only mildly overweight was not dangerous. Today, however, information suggests otherwise. In fact, in a recent study conducted by the RAND Institute, it was found that in terms of chronic conditions, obesity is a more powerful risk factor than poverty, heavy drinking, or smoking.[2]

Regardless of this issue, few experts question the real dangers to health and wellness from obesity.[3] Among the health problems caused by or complicated by obesity are increased surgical risk, hypertension, various forms of heart disease, stroke, type II diabetes mellitus, several forms of cancer, deterioration of joints, complications during pregnancy, gallbladder disease, and an overall increased risk of mortality[4] (see Star box on p. 121). Obesity is so closely associated with these chronic conditions that medical experts now recommend that obesity itself be defined and treated as a chronic disease.

BODY IMAGE AND SELF-CONCEPT

Although physicians focus on obesity, in our image-conscious society, being overweight is also a problem. The media tell people that being overweight is undesirable and that they should conform to certain ideal body images (such as being tall, thin, and "cut" with muscular definition). For example, the average actress and model is thinner than 95% of the female population and weighs 23% less than the average woman. Today's lean but muscular version of perfection is a very demanding standard for both women and men to meet (see Exploring Your Spirituality).

People may become dissatisfied and concerned about their inability to achieve these ideals. The scope of this dissatisfaction is evident in a study of over 800 women, which revealed that nearly half were unhappy with their weight, muscle tone, hips, thighs, buttocks, and legs.[5] When this type of dissatisfaction exists, people begin to question their attractiveness. For some, their self-concept changes and their self-esteem declines. Growing older lessens, but does not eliminate, this dissatisfaction.

In comparison with being overweight, little media attention has been paid to being underweight (see Focus on . . . , p. 147). However, the body image problems experienced by some extremely thin people can be equally distressing.

OVERWEIGHT AND OBESITY DEFINED

What's the difference between overweight and obesity? Nutritionists have traditionally said that obesity is present when fat accumulation produces a body weight that is more than 20% above an ideal or **desirable weight.** People are said to be overweight if their weight is between 1% and 19% above their desirable weight. As weight increases above the 20% level, the label *obese* is routinely applied. An exception is excessive weight caused by extreme muscularity, such as that of many football players.

The term *obesity* requires further refinement. When people are between 20% and 40% above desirable weight, they are described as having *mild obesity* (about 90% of all obese people). Excessive weight in the range of 41% to 99% above desirable weight is defined as *moderate obesity* (9%). Weight of 100% or more above desirable weight is defined as *severe, gross,* or *morbid obesity* (<1%).

Some clinicians and laymen continue to use standard height-weight tables to determine when weight is excessive and to classify obesity as mild, moderate, or severe. However, more precise techniques to determine body composition are currently available. Several of

Health Risks of Obesity

Each of the diseases listed below is followed by the percentage of cases for which obesity is a contributing factor:

Colon cancer 10%
Breast cancer 11%
Hypertension 33%
Heart disease 70%
Diabetes (type II, non–insulin-dependent) 90%

As these statistics show, being obese greatly increases your risk of many serious, and even life-threatening, chronic conditions.

these techniques, including waist-to-hip ratio (*healthy body weight*), body mass index, "BOD POD" assessment electrical impedance, skinfold measurements, and hydrostatic weighing, are described in the following section.

DETERMINING WEIGHT AND BODY COMPOSITION

Some of the techniques used to determine overweight and obesity are common and are routinely used by the general public. Others are expensive and of limited availability.

Height-Weight Tables

Height and weight tables were originally developed to assist people in determining the relationship between their weight and desirable standards. Nearly every version of these tables has come under criticism for not considering variables such as gender, age, frame size, and body composition. Some versions were thought to be too rigorous in establishing cutoff points for desirable or ideal weight, and others were deemed too generous. Although still available, these tables are being gradually replaced by other assessment techniques.

Healthy Body Weight

You can determine your **healthy body weight** by using the weight guidelines (Table 6-1) found in the *Dietary Guidelines for Americans*.[6] This assessment involves converting two body measurements, the waist and the hip circumferences, into a waist-to-hip ratio (WHR) that can then be applied to weight ranges for people of particular ages and heights. Among people who have an acceptable WHR, female healthy weight is near the lower end of each weight range, and male healthy weight is at the higher end of each weight range.

Table 6-1 Healthy Weight: Recommended Guidelines

	Weight*	
Height+	**19–34 years**	**35 years and over**
5′	97–128	108–138
5′1″	101–132	111–143
5′2″	104–137	115–148
5′3″	107–141	119–152
5′4″	111–146	122–157
5′5″	114–150	126–162
5′6″	118–155	130–167
5′7″	121–160	134–172
5′8″	125–164	138–178
5′9″	129–169	142–183
5′10″	132–174	146–188
5′11″	136–179	151–194
6′	140–184	155–199
6′1″	144–189	159–205
6′2″	148–195	164–210
6′3″	152–200	168–216
6′4″	156–205	173–222
6′5″	160–211	177–228
6′6″	164–216	182–234

*Without clothes.
+Without shoes.
Note: The higher weights in the ranges generally apply to men, who tend to have more muscle and bone mass; the lower weights more often apply to women, who generally have less muscle and bone mass.

TALKING POINTS • If a friend or close family member were dangerously overweight or obese, how would you express your concern?

To make a WHR determination, follow these steps:

1. Measure around your waist near your navel while you stand relaxed (not pulling in your stomach).
2. Measure around your hips, over the buttocks where the hips are largest.
3. Divide the waist measurement by the hip measurement.

Key Terms

positive caloric balance
Caloric intake greater than caloric expenditure.

desirable weight
The weight range deemed appropriate for people of a specific gender, age, and frame size.

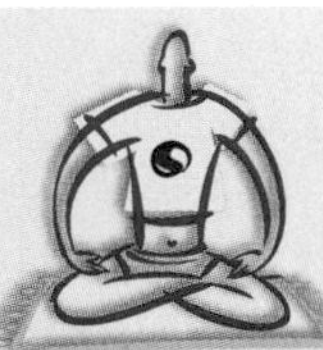

Exploring Your Spirituality

Want to Be Fashion-Model Thin?

Do fashion magazines influence readers' sense of self-worth and self-esteem? Do some readers actually question their human value because they don't look fashion-model thin? Critics say that fashion magazines such as *Cosmopolitan* and *Glamour* actually do have this kind of power. They argue that the publishers knowingly promote body images that their readers, mostly young women, probably can never attain. Recently, it was reported that models appearing in *Seventeen* were perceived by 70% of readers as being ideal, even though these models were thinner than over 80% of the readers. Other studies have reported that those who read such magazines regularly are more dissatisfied with their bodies than those who do not.

Boys and men are also affected by these images. Ask a friend to describe his ideal date, and the answer may sound a lot like the fashion-model type. Some men also identify with (or wish they looked like) the male models featured in fashion ads.

The disparity between ideal body image and reality can affect an individual's spiritual health—at least among vulnerable adolescents and young adults. For those who believe that all people should love and respect themselves because they are created in the image of a higher being or that each person is uniquely valuable, the conflict between the fashion industry's portrayal of the ideal body and the reality of not measuring up presents a spiritual dilemma.

One response is to try to conform to the unrealistic ideal through strict dieting or purging. But at what price? What happens if you continue to fail—after more time spent in the weight room, tougher calorie restriction, or an expensive surgical procedure? How would you feel about yourself then?

An alternative approach is to search within yourself for other types of self-validation, such as undiscovered interests and untapped capabilities. Or you can look outward, into the real world, where you can make a positive difference by giving your talent, time, support, and personal faith to others. If you choose one of these approaches, the power of the fashion magazine will fade. By drawing on your deepest spiritual resources, you can put these images into perspective and strengthen your feelings of self-worth and self-esteem.

For example, a woman with a 25-inch waist and 36-inch hips has a WHR of .69, which is well within the healthful range. Women with a WHR of less than .85 generally have a body weight that falls within the healthy range for their age and height; men with a WHR of less than 1.00 will also probably fall within the range considered healthy for their age and height. Any person whose WHR is equal to or greater than the recommended ratio should attempt to lose weight. Weight loss should occur no faster than ½ to 1 pound per week.

This new system was developed because of the growing concern over the relationship between the amount of fat located around the waist (the spare tire) and the development of several serious health problems. As a point of interest, the *Dietary Guidelines for Americans* do not use WHR as a clinical marker for the treatment of obesity; instead they use only waist circumference (40 or more inches for men and 35 inches or more for women).

Body Mass Index

Another method for assessing healthy body weight is the **body mass index (BMI).** The BMI indicates the relationship of body weight (expressed in kilograms) to height (expressed in meters) for both men and women.[7] The BMI does not reflect body composition (fat versus lean tissue) or consider the degree of fat accumulated in the central body cavity; nor is it adjusted for age. Yet it is widely used in determining obesity. A BMI of 25 to 29.9 indicates overweight, while a BMI of 30 or above represents obesity.

An alternative method of determining the BMI is to use a **nomogram,** such as that shown in Figure 6-1. Like the BMI, the nomogram requires information about both weight and height.

Once the BMI has been obtained, its relationship to a desirable BMI for persons of various ages can be determined by using Table 6-2.

BOD POD (Body Composition System)

The newest method of determining body composition involves the use of the BOD POD, an egg-shaped chamber in which a subject is briefly enclosed to determine how much air he or she displaces in the chamber. Once the amount of displaced air is known, a mathematical formula is used to calculate the subject's body density. Body density can then be used to determine the percentage of the subject's body that is composed of fat. Additional techniques in which highly accurate but expensive technology is used to determine body composition, including *computed tomography (CT) scans, magnetic resonance imaging (MRI), infrared light transmission,* and *neutron activation,* may become common ways of measuring body composition in the future.

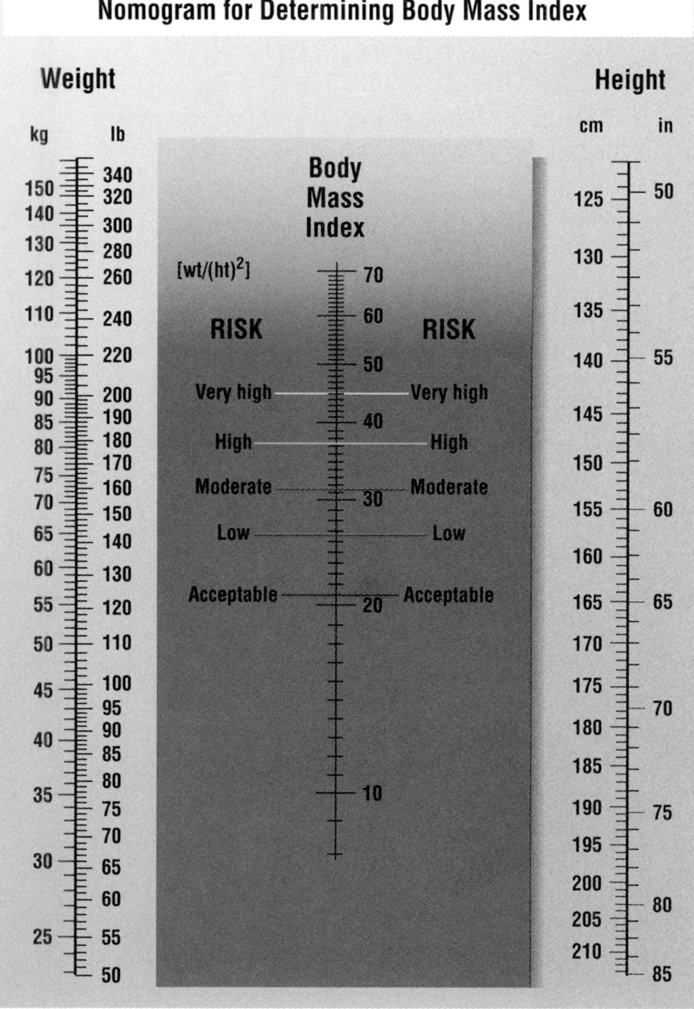

Figure 6-1 To use this nomogram, place a ruler or other straight edge between the body weight in kilograms or pounds (without clothes) located on the left-hand column and the height in centimeters or in inches (without shoes) located on the right-hand column. The BMI is read from the middle of the scale and is in metric units.

Skinfold Measurements

Skinfold measurements are a relatively precise and inexpensive indicator of body composition. In this assessment procedure, constant-pressure **calipers** are used to measure the thickness of the layer of fat beneath the skin's surface, the *subcutaneous fat layer.* These measurements are taken at key places on the body. Through the use of specific formulas, skinfold measurements can be used to calculate the percentage of body fat. The percent body fat value can also be used in determining desirable weight.

Table 6-2 Desirable Body Mass Index in Relation to Age

Age Group (years)	BMI (kg/m^2)
19–24	19–24
25–34	20–25
35–44	21–26
45–54	22–27
55–65	23–28
>65	24–29

Young adult men normally have a body fat percentage of 10% to 15%. The normal range for young adult women is 20% to 25%. When a man's body fat is higher than 20% and a woman's body fat is above 30%, they are considered to be obese. The higher percentage of fat typically found in women is related to preparation for pregnancy and breastfeeding.

Hydrostatic Weighing

Hydrostatic (underwater) *weighing* is another precise method of determining the relative amounts of fat and lean body mass that make up body weight. A person's percentage of body fat is determined by comparing the underwater weight with the body weight out of water. The need for expensive facilities (a tank or pool) and experienced technicians make the availability and cost of this procedure limited to small-scale application, such as a large research university or teaching hospital.

Key Terms

healthy body weight
Body weight within a weight range appropriate for a person with an acceptable waist-to-hip ratio.

body mass index (BMI)
A numerical expression of body weight based on height and weight.

BOD POD
Body composition system used to measure body fat through air displacement.

nomogram
Graphic means for finding an unknown value, such as body mass index.

calipers
A device used to measure the thickness of a skinfold, from which percent body fat can be calculated.

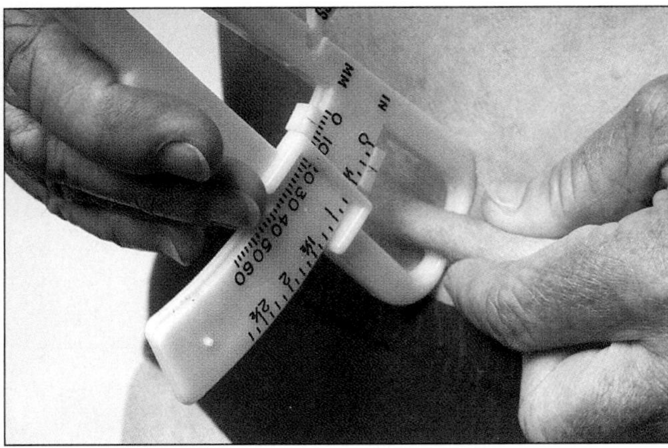

Body fat determination using skinfold calipers. Skinfold measurements are used in equations that calculate body fat density and percent body fat.

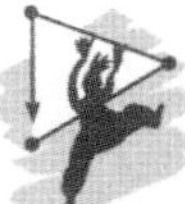

HealthQuest Activities

- The *Stages of Change* activity in the Nutrition and Weight Control module assesses your readiness to follow a diet containing appropriate levels of fats, carbohydrates, and proteins. It outlines concrete steps you can take to maintain healthy intake levels of these nutrients. The feedback for this activity is provided separately for each of these three dietary areas. You may address all three areas or choose among them. Develop a strategy for overcoming unhealthful eating habits, and keep an ongoing account of your progress. Record your mood, activity level, schedule, and any other factors that may affect your eating behavior. Then write down several ways to lessen the effects of such events on your eating behavior.

ORIGINS OF OBESITY

Experts continue to investigate the origins of obesity. Many theories focus on factors within the individual and from the environment. If the definitive cause of obesity is ever identified, it will probably have a complex basis that includes strong genetic and **neurophysiological** factors.

A great deal remains unknown about the causes of obesity. However, some basic explanations can be made about why some people gain weight easily.

Appetite Centers

In the early twentieth century, the growing prevalence of obesity lead researchers to speculate about the body's ability (or inability) to recognize feelings of hunger, as well as to note feelings of satiety, or fullness. By the 1940s, research directed toward finding the body's "appetite center(s)" showed that both the hunger and satiety centers were located in the thalamic and hypothalamic areas of the brain. Subsequent research indicated that these centers controlled food intake by monitoring the levels of various materials in the blood, particularly glucose and various amino acids. They also recognized hormonal signals coming from endocrine glands and nervous stimuli arising both from within and outside the body. These signals informed the centers about the need to adjust eating behavior. Once these centers were identified, drugs capable of influencing their function were developed. Some of these drugs already exist and are described later in the chapter.

Set Point Theory

The **set point** theory focuses on the central nervous system's ability or inability to fine tune resting energy expenditure, or the basal metabolic rate (BMR). Central to this theory is the contention that the appetite control centers of the brain are programmed with an awareness of the body's most physiologically desirable weight. When functioning properly, the appetite centers act as thermostats to adjust resting energy expenditure, or BMR, up or down to accommodate an excessive or inadequate caloric intake. By burning more energy or storing excessive energy as fat, the body maintains its best weight. This adjusting of the brain's energy expending/storing capability is referred to as **adaptive thermogenesis.**

It has been suggested that if excessive energy is stored easily, the body prevents planned weight loss (dieting) by adjusting the set point to a lower level. This change keeps already-stored fat from being used as fuel. In addition, according to this theory, to prevent further episodes of "starvation," a newer and even lower set point is established; once normal eating patterns return, lost weight is regained to a level above that of the initial set point. Every time the dieter tries to lose weight, he or she will "yo-yo" between weight loss and weight gain.

Today, evidence suggests that the **yo-yo syndrome,** explained by set point readjustment, may not be accurate. According to some researchers, the weight gain that follows a period of failed dieting occurs because food intake has increased subtly in comparison to the intake level before dieting was started; so the lost weight is regained and more weight is added. Many dieters still contend that they gain weight every time they go on and off a diet.[8]

There has been a renewed interest in the body's *brown fat* (most fat is white). Unlike white fat cells, which are designed to store excess calories as triglycerides, brown fat cells can convert stored fat into heat, which subsequently dissipates from the body. These brown fat cells are particularly prominent in infants; they may constitute as much as 6% of the infant's total body weight[9] and are thought to augment its underdeveloped temperature regulation system. As children age, however, the brown fat stores become less prominent, and by adulthood they are virtually nonexistent. So adults lose the ability to disperse excess calories as heat, and white fat cells may begin to store large quantities of surplus energy as liquefied fat. Recently, in rodents a gene has been identified whose protein may relate to the functioning of brown fat. Such a gene may exist in humans.[10]

Genetic Basis of Obesity

Throughout the last half of the twentieth century, the issue of faulty genetic mechanisms has been the focus of weight management, including obesity. In fact, today it is estimated that 70% of obesity can be directly attributed to genetic causes.[11]

The initial clues to how inherited tendencies are involved in obesity resulted from the study of identical twins who, having been reared apart, demonstrated very similar body weights when reunited as adults. Today about thirty genetic markers for obesity have been identified.[11] These genes, when normally configured, communicate important information about hunger and satiety, allowing dietary intake, caloric expenditure, and fat storage to occur in a way that sustains healthy weight. When faulty genes are present, either through inheritance or mutation, people are predisposed to gain excessive weight when caloric intake exceeds caloric expenditure.

Central to the genetic theory of obesity is the recent discovery of faulty genes involved in the production and recognition of the protein leptin, which is critical in terminating food consumption. Leptin levels were first found to be in low in mice genetically bred for obesity, and so researchers were able to reverse obesity in these mice by injecting leptin. Most recently, small, carefully controlled studies involving the injection of leptin into obese humans produced modest weight loss.[12] Researchers remain optimistic that eventually leptin (or some related hormone) can be delivered to the brain in amounts sufficient to stimulate additional weight loss.[13]

Body Type

An inheritance basis for obesity could involve the interplay of *somatotype* (body build) and other unique energy-processing characteristics passed on from parents to their children.

The classic work of Sheldon is credited with establishing the now-familiar body types: *ectomorph, mesomorph,* and *endomorph.* In an ectomorph, the tall, slender body seems to protect the individual from excessive weight. Ectomorphs usually have difficulty maintaining normal weight for their height.

The shorter, more muscular, athletic body of the mesomorph represents a genetic middle ground. During childhood, adolescence, and adulthood, as long as activity levels are maintained, mesomorphic people appear to be "solid" without seeming to be obese. For well-conditioned mesomorphs, scale weight may suggest obesity, but the excessive weight is more likely the result of heavy muscularity. Mesomorphs have their greatest difficulty with obesity during adulthood when eating patterns fail to adjust to declining physical activity.

Endomorphs have body types that tend to be round and soft. Many endomorphs have excessively large abdomens and report having had weight problems since childhood.

Sheldon was interested in the personality traits and temperament of people with each body type. However, the relationship of body type to inheritance, body weight, and weight management is strong. Sheldon's work simply gives us labels to use in discussing our observations.

TALKING POINTS • How would you advise a friend who complains that she is failing at another diet?

Infant and Adult Eating Patterns

Obesity can be categorized according to eating patterns. Two general feeding patterns are related to two forms of obesity: hypercellular obesity and hypertrophic obesity.

The first of these patterns involves infant feeding. Many researchers believe that the number of fat cells a person has will be determined during the first two years of life. Babies who are overfed will develop a greater number of fat cells than babies who receive a balanced diet of appropriate, infant-sized portions. Overfed babies, especially those with a family history of obesity, will tend to develop **hypercellular obesity.** When these children reach adulthood, they will have extra fat cells.

Key Terms

neurophysiological
Pertaining to nervous system functioning; processes through which the body senses and responds to its internal and external environments.

set point
A genetically programmed range of body weight beyond which a person finds it difficult to gain or lose additional weight.

adaptive thermogenesis
Physiological response of the body to adjust its metabolic rate to the presence of food.

yo-yo syndrome
The repeated weight loss followed by weight gain experienced by many dieters.

hypercellular obesity
A form of obesity seen in people who possess an abnormally large number of fat cells.

Late childhood and adolescence are also times when excessive weight gain may result in the formation of additional fat cells. For adults, substantial weight gain can also stimulate an increase in the number of fat cells and thus foster hypercellular obesity.

A second type of obesity with its origin in eating patterns is called **hypertrophic obesity.** It is related to a long-term positive caloric balance during adulthood. Over a period of years, existing fat cells increase in size to accommodate excess calorie intake.

Hypertrophic obesity is generally associated with excessive fat around the waist and is thought to contribute to conditions such as diabetes mellitus (type II, non–insulin-dependent diabetes), high levels of fat in the blood, high blood pressure, and heart disease. In our society, hypertrophic obesity shows itself during middle age—a time when physical activity generally declines but food intake remains the same.

Endocrine Influence

For many years, people believed that obesity was the result of glandular problems. Often the thyroid gland was said to be underactive, preventing the person from burning up calories. Until recently it was believed that only a few obese people have an endocrine dysfunction that would cause obesity. Today, however, renewed interest in thyroid dysfunction is appearing.

Decreasing Basal Metabolic Rate

The body's requirement for energy to maintain basic physiological processes falls steadily with age. This change reflects the loss of muscle tissue that occurs as both men and women age. On a short-term basis, little adjustment needs to be made to maintain weight. However, if adjustments are not made, weight gain can become a problem over time. A gradual decrease in food intake combined with an increase in exercise can be effective in preventing the gradual onset of obesity.

Family Dietary Practices

Food preferences and eating practices are strongly influenced by the family. In some families lessons about eating are taught as though they were from a nutrition textbook. Other families encourage unhealthy food choices, which can lead to a lifetime of malnourishment, including obesity. For example, between-meal snacking on high-sugar or high-fat foods, large serving sizes, multiple servings, and high-calorie meals are poor lessons taught by some families.

Inactivity

When weight management experts are asked to identify the single most important reason for obesity in today's society, they point to inactivity. People of all ages tend to do less and therefore burn fewer calories than their ancestors did only a few generations ago. Automation in the workplace, labor-saving devices in the home, the inactivity associated with watching television, and a general dislike of exercise are a few of the reasons for this inactivity.

Most important, however, is the sedentary lifestyle of many of today's children. Researchers believe that aggressive restrictions on television, videos, and video game use, as well as prohibiting meal eating while watching TV, may be necessary to halt their slide into lifelong obesity.[14]

CALORIC BALANCE

Any calories consumed in excess of those that are used by the body are converted to fat. We gain weight when our energy input is greater than our energy output. On the other hand, we lose weight when our energy output is greater than our energy input (Figure 6-2). Weight remains constant when caloric input and output are identical. In such situations, our bodies are said to be in *caloric balance.*

ENERGY NEEDS OF THE BODY

What are our energy needs? How many calories should we consume (or burn) to achieve a healthy weight? Although there are rough estimates for college-aged men (2500 to 3300 calories daily) and women (approximately 2500 calories daily), we all vary in our specific energy needs. These needs are based on three factors: (1) activity requirements, (2) basal metabolic rate (also referred to as resting energy expenditure, or REE), and (3) the thermic effect of food.

Activity Requirements

Each person's caloric *activity requirements* vary directly according to the amount of their daily physical activity. For example, sedentary office workers require a smaller daily caloric intake than construction workers, lumberjacks, or farm workers do.

Physical activity that occurs outside the workplace also increases caloric needs. Sedentary office workers may be quite active in their recreational pursuits. Active employees may spend their off hours lounging in front of the TV. It's important to closely examine the total amount of work or activity an individual engages in to accurately estimate that person's caloric requirements. Physical activity uses 20% to 40% of caloric intake. See Table 6-3 for a breakdown of caloric expenditures for various recreational pursuits.

TALKING POINTS • A good friend is clearly underweight. She is trying, with little success, to gain weight by increasing her food consumption. How would you counter your friend's claim that the last thing she needs is increased physical activity?

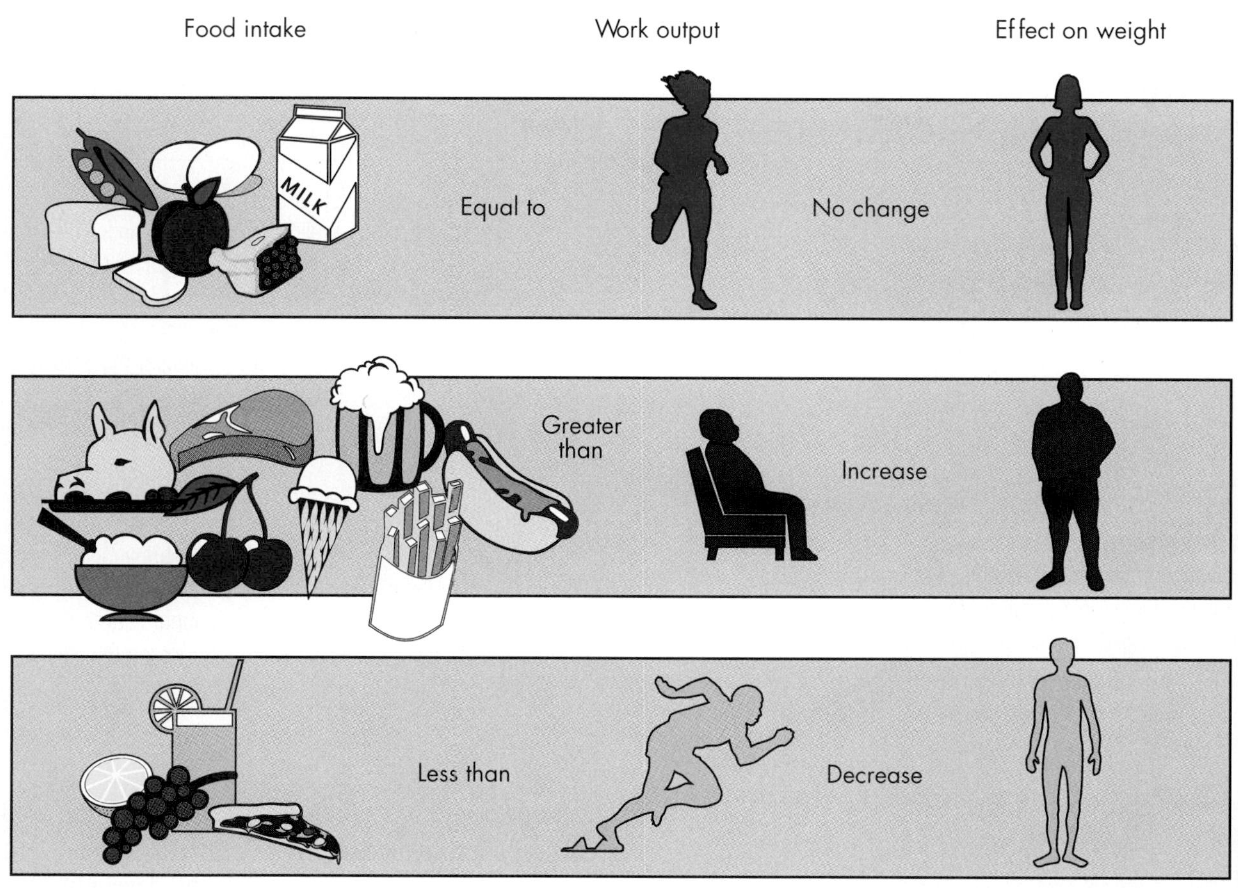

Figure 6-2 Caloric balance: energy input equals energy output, some of which comes from physical activity.

Basal Metabolism

Of the three factors that determine energy needs, basal metabolism uses the highest proportion (50% to 70%) of the total calories required by each person. Expressed as a **basal metabolic rate (BMR),** basal metabolism reflects the minimum amount of energy the body requires to carry on its vital functions, such as blood circulation and glandular activity. Even when a person is totally relaxed or sleeping, these vital body functions continue to expend calories.

Basal metabolism changes as people age. For both males and females, the BMR is relatively high at birth and continues to increase until the age of 2. Except for a slight rise at puberty, the BMR will then gradually decline throughout life.[15] If people fail to recognize that their BMR decreases as they grow older (2% per decade), they might also fail to adjust their food intake and activity level accordingly. Thus they will gradually put on unwanted pounds as they grow older.

Thermic Effect of Food

Formerly called the *specific dynamic action* of food, or *dietary thermogenesis,* the thermic effect of food represents the energy our bodies require for the digestion, absorption, and transportation of food. This energy breaks the electrochemical bonds that hold complex food molecules together, resulting in smaller nutrient units that can be distributed throughout the body. This energy requirement is in addition to activity needs and basal metabolic needs. The thermic effect of food is estimated to represent about 10% of total energy needs. Some nutritionists now consider the thermic effect of food merely one component of overall basal metabolism.

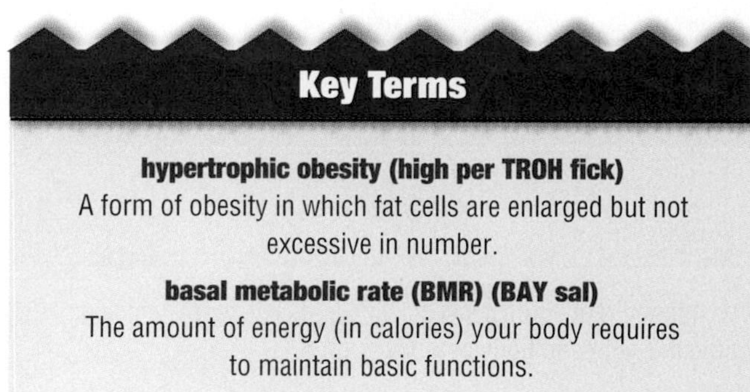

Key Terms

hypertrophic obesity (high per TROH fick)
A form of obesity in which fat cells are enlarged but not excessive in number.

basal metabolic rate (BMR) (BAY sal)
The amount of energy (in calories) your body requires to maintain basic functions.

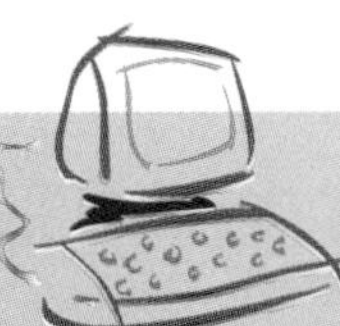

OnSITE/InSIGHT

Learning to Go: Health

Having trouble maintaining a healthy weight? Click on the Motivator icon and check out the following lessons on weight management:

Lesson 20: Discover your weight and body composition.
Lesson 21: Maintain your healthy weight.
Lesson 22: Choose the right weight-loss plan for you.
Lesson 23: Identify eating disorders.

STUDENT POLL

Are you affected by weight issues and body image concerns? Go to the Online Learning Center at **www.mhhe.com/hahn6e**. Click on Student Resources to take part in a poll that asks the following questions. Then find out how other students responded.

1. Are you comfortable with the appearance of your body?
2. Have you ever gained or lost a lot of weight?
3. Are you on a diet to reach or maintain a specific weight?
4. Do you feel pressured to weigh a certain amount?
5. Do people make negative comments about your weight?
6. Do you envy people who are thinner than you?
7. When choosing friends, do you consider the person's weight?
8. Are you influenced by what the media says you should look like?
9. Do you usually eat alone?
10. Have you ever participated in a weight-loss program?
11. Have you ever taken dietary pills or supplements?
12. Do you often try fad diets?
13. Have you ever suffered from an eating disorder?
14. Is portion control a part of your approach to eating?
15. Have you ever thought of having liposuction?

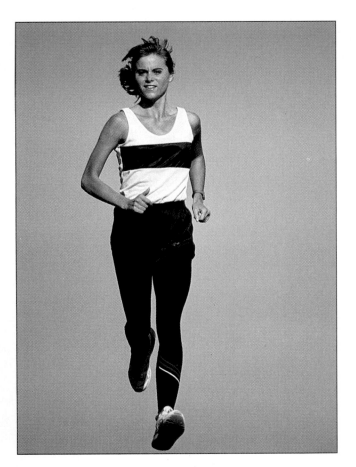

Engaging in regular physical activity is the key to maintaining optimal weight and body composition.

Pregnancy

During a normal pregnancy, about 75,000 additional calories are required to support the development of the fetus and the formation of maternal supportive tissues and to fuel the mother's BMR. In addition, the typical pregnant woman will develop about 9 extra pounds of fat tissue to be used as an energy source during breastfeeding. In total, the typical woman, under competent medical supervision, gives birth having gained, on average, 28 pounds (normally ranging from 19.8 lbs to 33 lbs).[16]

After the birth of the baby, the woman will ideally have a weight gain of only 2 to 3 pounds over her prepregnancy weight. This small amount of additional weight will normally be lost by the end of the sixth to eighth month after childbirth.

In spite of the modest (and short-term) additional weight a woman carries in the first few months following giving birth, some women may assume that pregnancy is a significant contributor to adult obesity. Although excessive weight gain does occur during pregnancy for some women, early competent medical management, emphasizing sound nutritional practices and regular physical activity, should largely eliminate this concern. Overly aggressive restrictions on weight gain, however, are potentially harmful to fetal development.[17]

TALKING POINTS • A friend confides in you that she would like to have a child but does not want to become pregnant because she fears gaining weight. How would you respond?

Table 6-3 Calories Expended During Physical Activity

To determine the number of calories you have spent in an hour of activity, simply multiply the *calories per hour per pound* column by your weight (in pounds). For example after an hour of archery a 120-pound person will have expended 209 calories; a 160-pound person, 278 calories; and a 220-pound person, 383 calories.

Activity	Calories/hour/pound	Activity	Calories/hour/pound
Archery	1.74	Marching (rapid)	3.84
Basketball	3.78	Painting (outside)	2.10
Baseball	1.86	Playing music (sitting)	1.08
Boxing (sparring)	3.78	Racquetball	3.90
Canoeing (leisure)	1.20	Running (cross-country)	4.44
Climbing hills (no load)	3.30	Running	
Cleaning	1.62	11 min 30 sec per mile	3.66
Cooking	1.20	9 min per mile	5.28
Cycling		8 min per mile	5.64
5.5 mph	1.74	7 min per mile	6.24
9.4 mph	2.70	6 min per mile	6.84
Racing	4.62	5 min 30 sec per mile	7.86
Dance (modern)	2.28	Scrubbing floors	3.00
Eating (sitting)	0.60	Sailing	1.20
Field hockey	3.66	Skiing	
Fishing	1.68	Cross-country	4.43
Football	3.60	Snow, downhill	3.84
Gardening		Water	3.12
Digging	3.42	Skating (moderate)	2.28
Mowing	3.06	Soccer	3.54
Raking	1.44	Squash	5.76
Golf	2.34	Swimming	
Gymnastics	1.80	Backstroke	4.62
Handball	3.78	Breaststroke	4.44
Hiking	2.52	Free, fast	4.26
Horseback riding		Free, slow	3.48
Galloping	3.72	Butterfly	4.68
Trotting	3.00	Table tennis	1.86
Walking	1.14	Tennis	3.00
Ice hockey	5.70	Volleyball	1.32
Jogging	4.15	Walking (normal pace)	2.16
Judo	5.34	Weight training	1.90
Knitting (sewing)	0.60	Wrestling	5.10
Lacrosse	5.70	Writing (sitting)	0.78

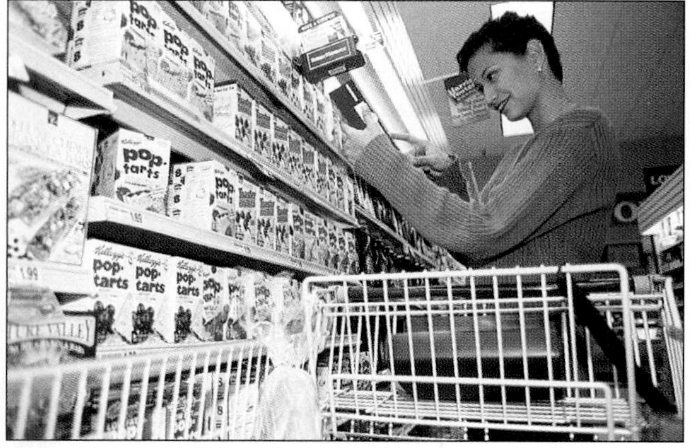

Successful lifelong weight management involves making informed food choices.

Lifetime Weight Control

Obesity and frequent fluctuation in weight are thought to be associated with higher levels of morbidity and mortality. So it is highly desirable to maintain your weight and body composition at or near optimum levels. Although this may be a difficult goal to achieve, it is not unrealistic when begun early in life and from a starting point at or near optimum levels. The following are some keys to success:

- *Exercise:* Caloric expenditure through regular exercise, including cardiovascular exercise and strength training, is a key to maintaining optimum weight and body composition (see Chapter 4 and Learning from Our Diversity, p. 131).

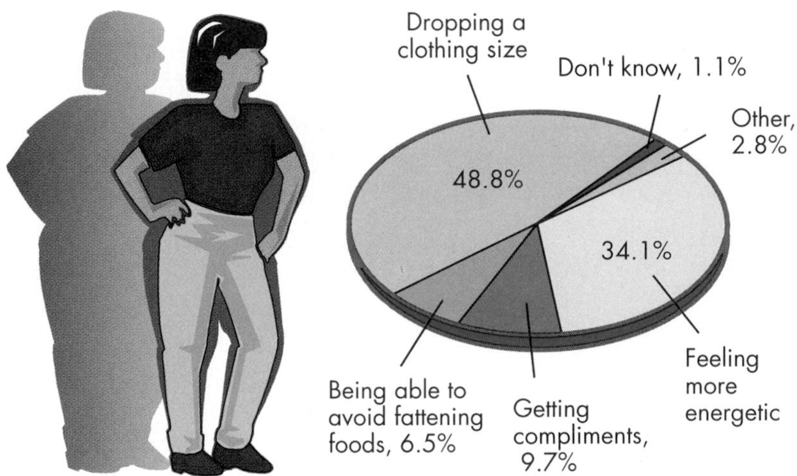

Figure 6-3 How do Americans measure success when it comes to losing weight? Most say dropping a clothing size is the best indicator that their diet is working.

- *Dietary modification:* Plan meals around foods that have moderate levels of fat and are low in total fat and saturated fat and high in complex carbohydrates. Many nutritionists are concerned about the safety of high-fat diets and ultra-low-fat diets for long-term weight management.
- *Lifestyle support:* In addition to committing yourself to a lifestyle that features regular physical activity and careful food choices, build a support system that will nurture your efforts. Inform your family, friends, classmates, and coworkers that you intend to rely on them for support and encouragement.
- *Problem solving:* Reevaluate your current approaches to dealing with stressors. Replace any reliance on food as a coping mechanism with nonfood options, such as exercise or talking with friends or family members.
- *Redefinition of health:* Think about health and wellness in terms of proactivity (see Chapter 2) and involvement, rather than simply focusing on not becoming sick or incapacitated.

If you have an acceptable weight and body composition at this time, these suggested lifestyle choices will make a significant contribution to preventing a weight problem later.

WEIGHT-MANAGEMENT TECHNIQUES

If you're already overweight, you may need to take specific measures to reduce your weight that are different from the total lifestyle approach just described. Once you reach a more healthful weight and body composition, maintaining that status will depend on adopting the lifestyle changes described on p. 129–130. Figure 6-3 depicts ways, other than scale weight, through which people define whether their weight loss program has been successful.

Weight loss occurs when the amount of energy taken into the body is less than that demanded by the body for maintenance and activity. The Personal Assessments at the end of this chapter will help you evaluate your food habits in relation to healthy weight (p. 143) and decide if you're a candidate for a weight-loss program (p. 145).

Dietary Alterations

A diet that reduces caloric intake is the most common approach to weight loss. The choice of foods and the amount of food are the two factors that distinguish the wide range of diets currently available. It's important to note, however, that dieting alone usually does not result in long-term weight loss. In fact, whether individuals manage their diets by themselves or follow a recognized weight-loss program, most dieters regain at least two-thirds of the weight they lost within 2 years of the initial loss. A study of successful dieters conducted by the National Weight Control Registry demonstrated that people in this select group relied on balanced diets and exercise, rather than restrictive diets and medication, to lose weight and maintain that loss[18] (see Changing for the Better on p. 132).

Balanced diets supported by portion control

For nutritional health, a logical approach to weight loss and subsequent weight maintenance is to establish a nutritionally sound balanced diet (moderately-low in fat, low in saturated fat, and high in complex carbohydrates) that controls portions. Most people have difficulty controlling portion sizes. The labels of many packaged foods provide nutrition information for a single serving, yet the package

Learning from Our Diversity

Pyramid Power—Mediterranean Style

In Chapter 5 we explored the components of the USDA Food Guide Pyramid, which is designed to help Americans make healthful food choices in appropriate quantities. As you'll recall, we're encouraged to enjoy relatively more servings of bread, cereal, rice, pasta, fruits, and vegetables (located on the first and second levels of the pyramid), while eating fewer servings of meat and dairy products and restricting our intake of fats, oils, and sweets (which occupy the narrower top levels of the pyramid).

Did you know there's another food pyramid that points the way to nutritious food selections that are essential to successful weight control? It's called the Mediterranean Pyramid, and some nutritionists believe it offers the best diet for good health (see the illustration below). Like the USDA Food Guide Pyramid, the Mediterranean Pyramid emphasizes a diet based on grains, fruits, and vegetables. The Mediterranean Pyramid recommends eating red meat just a few times a month and allows generous amounts of olive oil. The USDA Pyramid likewise calls for limited consumption of lean read meat, but it urges sparing consumption of all fats, including olive oil. Another important difference between these two pyramids is that the Mediterranean Pyramid calls for limited consumption of alcohol, which may reduce the risk of coronary heart disease; the USDA Pyramid makes no such recommendation.

Here are some of the other reasons many nutritionists advocate a diet based on Mediterranean favorites:

Greens: Dark leafy greens are rich in antioxidant vitamins, which may help guard against cancer and heart disease and possibly prevent damage to the eyes. Greens are also excellent sources of calcium, iron, and the B vitamin folic acid, which research shows can reduce the risk of neural tube (spinal cord) defects in fetuses. Folic acid may also reduce the risk of heart disease and stroke.

Legumes: Like dark leafy greens, legumes such as garbanzo beans (chick peas), cannellini beans, and red kidney beans are rich in folic acid and iron. What's more, they're high in protein, making them low-fat, no-cholesterol alternatives to meat. And they're great sources of soluble fiber, which can help reduce levels of blood cholesterol.

Garlic: Also shown to be effective in lowering blood cholesterol even when eaten in small quantities, garlic is a traditional staple of Mediterranean cuisine that adds flavor without contributing either fat or sugar.

Olive oil: For centuries, olive oil has been the fat of choice in Mediterranean cooking. Unlike butter and lard, animal products that are loaded with saturated fat, olive oil is a monounsaturated fat, which some studies suggest may reduce the risk of atherosclerosis.

Do you know any students of Mediterranean descent, such as those of Italian, Greek, or Turkish ancestry, who follow a diet based on the Mediterranean Pyramid? If so, what foods do they typically eat? Using the pyramid structure, make a diagram of your current food choices, with those you consume the most at the bottom and those you eat least at the top. How close is your diet to that recommended by the USDA Food Guide Pyramid? The Mediterranean Pyramid?

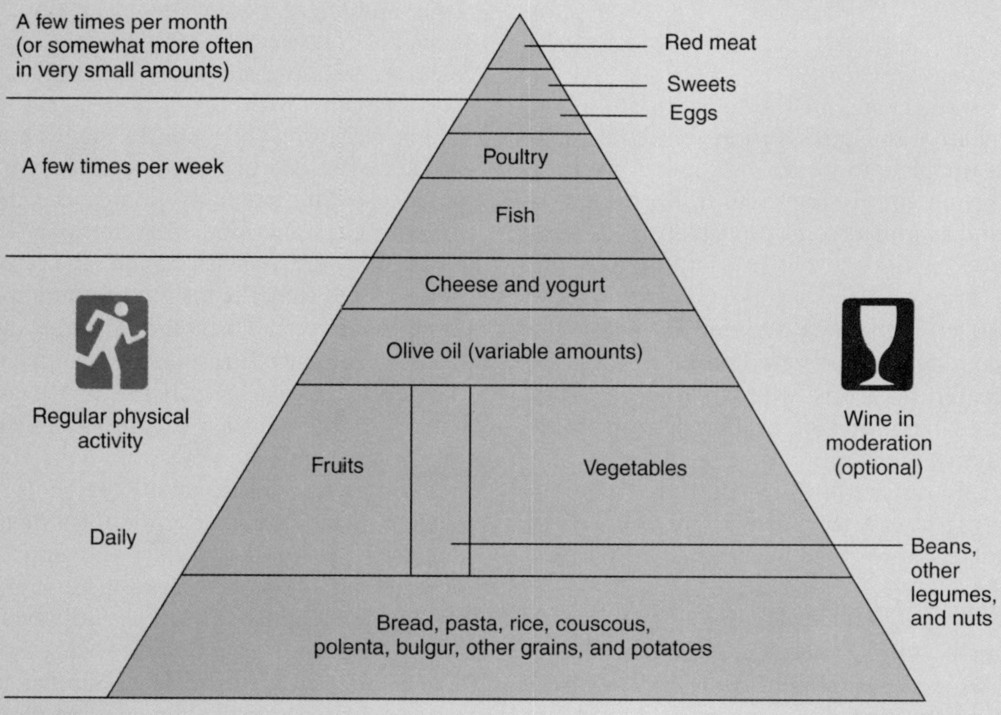

The Mediterraneon Food Pyramid.

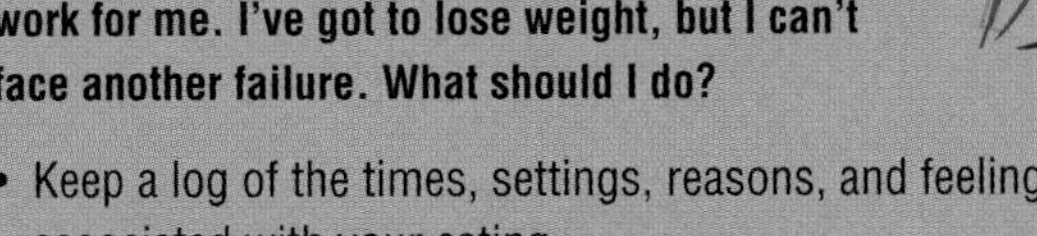

Changing *for the Better*

Tips for Losing Weight Successfully

I've tried all kinds of diets, and nothing seems to work for me. I've got to lose weight, but I can't face another failure. What should I do?

- Keep a log of the times, settings, reasons, and feelings associated with your eating.
- Set realistic long-term goals (for example, loss of 1 pound a week instead of 5 pounds per week).
- Don't completely deprive yourself of enjoyable foods (occasionally reward yourself with a small treat).
- Realize that the sacrifices you're making are important for your health and happiness.
- Eat slowly. It takes about 20 minutes for your brain to recognize satiety signals from your body.
- Put more physical activity into your daily routine (take stairs instead of elevators or park in the distant part of a parking lot, for example).
- Reward yourself when you reach your goals (with new clothes, sporting equipment, a vacation trip).
- Share your commitment to weight loss with your family and friends so that they can support your efforts.
- Keep careful records of your daily food consumption and weekly weight change.
- Be prepared to deal with occasional plateaus and setbacks in your quest for weight loss.
- Remember that moderately-low fat, low saturated fat, and high–complex carbohydrate meals in combination with regular physical activity are the basis for these strategies.

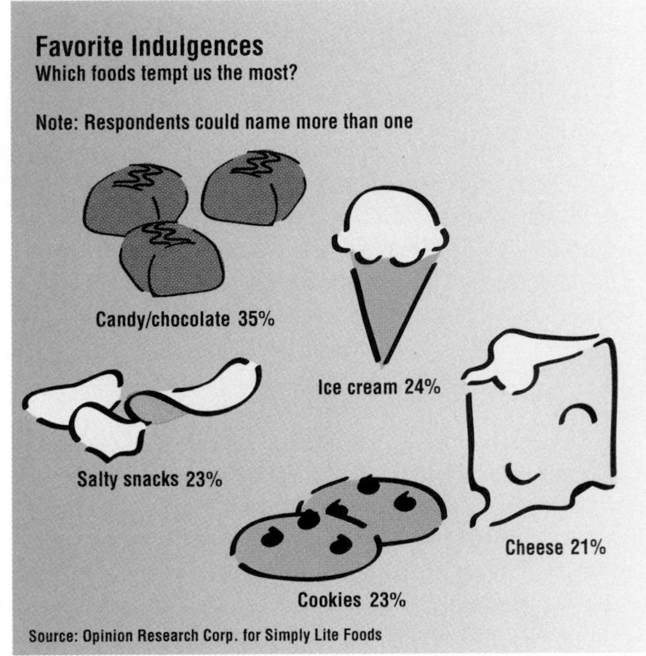

Figure 6-4 Late night kitchen raids and too many daytime snacks can compromise a healthy diet. Which foods are the most difficult for you to resist?

often contains two servings of the food. In addition, restaurants rarely serve standard portion sizes, preferring to heap food on the plate to justify high menu prices. A balanced diet/portion control approach to weight loss is nutritionally sound and offers some probability of success.

Fad diets

Many people use fad diets in an attempt to lose weight quickly. These popular diets are often promoted in best-selling books written by people who claim to be nutrition experts (see Changing for the Better on p. 135). With few exceptions, these approaches are both ineffective and potentially unhealthful. In addition, some involve significant expense. A brief assessment of a variety of popular diet plans is presented in Table 6-4.

High-protein/low-carbohydrate diets

Currently, the most popular diets are those that reduce carbohydrate intake to an extremely low level, while permitting an almost unlimited consumption of animal protein (meat), with its accompanying moderately high to high fat content. As indicated in Table 6-4, these diets, such as *Dr. Atkin's New Diet Revolution, Mastering the Zone,* and *Sugar Busters,* involve potential problems, particular if followed for long periods. However, they do generate an impressive initial weight loss.

The central theory underlying these diets is the "short-circuiting" of insulin's role as a facilitator of fat storage when the body has to deal with excessive levels of glucose. This situation occurs easily in sedentary people who consume foods that are high in carbohydrates, particularly simple sugars. When the carbohydrate intake is greatly reduced, the insulin response is minimal. In addition, as noted in Chapter 5, the body does not consider dietary protein to be a preferred source of calories, thus the body turns aggressively to stored fat as fuel for muscular activity. When fat becomes the principal source of calories, as happens in these diets, metabolic waste products are produced that acidify the body. Additionally, the need to metabolize large amounts of dietary protein produces a strain on the kidneys and an accompanying loss of water. Finally, stored protein (muscle) is broken down to replace the glucose normally supplied by dietary carbohydrates and needed for nervous system operation. The overall effect of the diet is similar to the metabolic state of people with undiagnosed or poorly managed di-

Table 6-4 Advantages and Disadvantages of Selected Diets

Type of Diet	Advantages	Disadvantages	Examples
Limited food choice diets	Reduce the number of food choices made by the users Limited opportunity to make mistakes Almost certainly low in calories after the first few days	Deficient in many nutrients, depending on the foods allowed Monotonous—difficult to adhere to Eating out and eating socially are difficult Do not retrain dieters in acceptable eating habits Low long-term success rates No scientific basis for these diets	Banana and milk diet Fitonics for Life Diet Kempner rice diet The New Beverly Hills Diet Fit for Life
Restricted-calorie, balanced food plans	Sufficiently low in calories to permit steady weight loss Nutritionally balanced Palatable Include readily available foods Reasonable in cost Can be adapted from family meals Permit eating out and social eating Promote a new set of eating habits May employ a point system	Do not appeal to people who want a "unique diet" Do not produce immediate and large weight losses	Weight Watchers Diet Prudent Diet (American Heart Association) Eating Thin for Life Take Off Pounds Sensibly (TOPS) Overeaters Anonymous Jenny Craig
Fasting starvation diet	Rapid initial loss	Nutrient deficient Danger of ketosis >60% loss is muscle <40% loss is fat Low long-term success rate	ZIP Diet 5-Day Miracle Diet
High-carbohydrate diet	Emphasizes grains, fruits, and vegetables High in bulk Low in cholesterol	Limits milk, meat Nutritionally very inadequate for calcium, iron, and protein	Quick Weight Loss Diet Pritikin Diet Hilton Head Metabolism Diet
High-protein, low-carbohydrate diets Usually include all the meat, fish, poultry, and eggs you can eat Occasionally permit milk and cheese in limited amounts Prohibit fruits, vegetables, and any bread or cereal products	Rapid initial weight loss because of diuretic effect Very little hunger	Too low in carbohydrates Deficient in many nutrients—vitamin C, vitamin A (unless eggs are included), calcium, and several trace elements High in saturated fat, cholesterol, and total fat Extreme diets of this type could cause death	Dr. Stillman's Quick Weight Loss Diet Calories Don't Count by Dr. Taller Dr. Atkin's New Diet Revolution Scarsdale Diet Air Force Diet The Carbohydrate Addict's Life Span Program Mastering the Zone Diet

Continued

abetes. Also, the fat content of the diet will eventually resupply the body with calories that were initially obtained by breaking down the fat stores.

Controlled fasting

In cases of extreme obesity, some patients are placed on a complete fast in a hospital setting. The patient is maintained on only water, electrolytes, and vitamins. Weight loss is profound because the body is quickly forced to begin **catabolism** of its fat and muscle tissues. Sodium loss, a negative nitrogen balance, and potassium loss are particular concerns.

Today, some people regularly practice unsupervised modified fasting for short periods. Solid foods are removed from the diet for a number of days. Fruit juice,

Key Term

catabolism
The metabolic process of breaking down tissue for the purpose of converting it into energy.

Table 6-4 Advantages and Disadvantages of Selected Diets

Type of diet	Advantages	Disadvantages	Examples
		Impossible to adhere to these diets long enough to lose any appreciable amount of weight Dangerous for people with kidney disease Weight lost, which is largely water, is rapidly regained Expensive Unpalatable after first few days Difficult for dieter to eat out Unattractive side effects (e.g., bad breath) May require potassium and calcium supplements	The Carbohydrate Addict's Diet Sugar Busters Protein Power Get Skinny on Fabulous Food (with modifications)
Low-calorie, high-protein supplement diets Usually a premeasured powder to be reconstituted with water or a prepared liquid formula	Rapid initial weight loss Easy to prepare—already measured Palatable for first few days Usually fortified to provide recommended amount of micronutrients Must be labeled if >50% protein	Usually prescribed at dangerously low calorie intake of 300 to 500 Cal Overpriced Low in fiber and bulk—constipating in short amount of time	Metracal Diet Cambridge Diet Liquid Protein Diet Last Chance Diet Oxford Diet Genesis New Direction
High-fiber, low-calorie diets	High satiety value Provide bulk	Irritating to the lower colon Decreases absorption of trace elements, especially iron Nutritionally deficient Low in protein	Pritikin Diet F Diet Zen Macrobiotic Diet
Protein-sparing modified fats <50% protein: 400 Cal	Safe under supervision High-quality protein Minimize loss of lean body mass	Decreases BMR Monotonous Expensive	Optifast Medifast
Premeasured food plans	Provide prescribed portion sizes—little chance of too small or too large a portion Total food programs Some provide adequate calories (1200) Nutritionally balanced or supplemented	Expensive Do not retrain dieters in acceptable eating habits Preclude eating out or social eating Often low in bulk Monotonous Low long-term success rates	Nutri-System Carnation Plan

water, protein supplements, and vitamins are used to minimize the risks associated with total fasting. However, unsupervised short-term fasting that is done too frequently can be dangerous and is not generally recommended.

Commercial weight-reduction programs

In virtually every area of the country, at least one version of the popular commercial weight-reduction programs, such as TOPS (Take Off Pounds Sensibly), Jenny Craig, Nutri Sure Losers, and Weight Watchers, can be found. These programs generally feature a format consisting of (1) a well-balanced diet emphasizing portion control and moderate fat, low–saturated fat, and high–complex carbohydrate foods, (2) realistic weight loss goals to be attained over a reasonable period of time, (3) encouragement from supportive leaders and fellow group members, (4) emphasis on regular physical activity, and (5) a weight-management program (follow-up program). The Changing for the Better box on p. 136 presents some guidelines for choosing a commercial weight loss program.

Changing *for the Better*

Choosing a Diet Plan

I've been trying to find a good diet plan, but I'm confused by all the promotional materials. How can I recognize a sensible approach to weight loss?

- Make sure the program incorporates a balanced diet, an exercise program, and behavior modification.
- Beware of inflexible plans, such as those that require you to eat certain foods on certain days.
- Avoid plans that allow fewer than 1200 calories a day, the minimum needed to get essential nutrients.
- Make sure the recommended rate of weight loss does not exceed 2 pounds per week.
- Avoid programs that promote vitamins, pills, shots, gimmicks, gadgets, or brand-name diet foods.
- Look for a statement of approval by a reputable nutrition expert or institution.
- Beware of diets that promise fast, easy, or effortless weight loss or "a new secret formula."
- Choose a plan that teaches you how to keep the weight off once you've lost it.

In theory, these programs offer an opportunity to lose weight for people who cannot or will not participate in an activity program. But their effectiveness is very limited. In fact, the limited success of these programs and the difficulty that working people have in attending meetings have resulted in falling enrollment and the development of home-based programs, such as hospital-based wellness programs, YMCA and YWCA programs, and Weight Watchers. All these programs are costly when compared with self-directed approaches, especially when the program markets its own food products.

Diet and physical activity

Most Americans attempting to lose weight fail to include a physical activity component in their dietary approach. Recent research strongly encourages 150 minutes or more of increased activity per week to maximize success in losing weight and maintaining that loss.[19] Additionally, using home exercise equipment may be an important part of the success of programs that incorporate a structured short-term exercise activity.[20]

Physical Intervention

A second approach to weight loss involves techniques and products designed to alter basic eating patterns. Some are self-selected and self-applied, and others must be administered in an institutional setting by highly trained professionals.

Hunger- and satiety-influencing products

Many overweight people want to lessen their desire to eat or develop a stronger sense of when they have eaten enough. Today, many dieters are confused about the safety of pharmaceutical approaches to weight loss, including both over-the-counter (OTC) and prescription drugs.

Until recently, **phenylpropanolamine (PPA)** was incorporated into many OTC weight-loss products. Discontinuation of its use is based on its adverse effects on conditions such as hypertension, diabetes, glaucoma, and thyroid disease. If found in a medicine cabinet, products contain PPA should be discarded.

The FDA also continues to voice concern about OTC weight-loss and energy-promotion products containing ephedrine (*ma huong* and Chinese ephedra). Ephedrine has been linked to heart attacks and strokes and should be used with caution.

Some prescription medications have been shown to produce serious side effects. Two such medications, phentermine and fenfluramine, have been prescribed for patients who wanted to lose weight. Both drugs affect levels of serotonin, the neurotransmitter associated with satiety. This popular combination, referred to as *phen-fen,* gradually raised concern among health experts because of the side effects it produced in people with angina, glaucoma, and high blood pressure. In addition, reports began to surface that some patients had developed a rare but potentially lethal condition called *pulmonary hypertension.* Still, use of the drugs continued.

During the mid-1990s, a new serotonin-specific weight loss drug, *dexfenfluramine* (Redux), was approved for use in the United States. Results among patients who used the drug, in combination with dietary modification and exercise, seemed impressive during the initial months of its widespread use. However, some patients began to take dexfenfluramine with fenfluramine in an attempt to find a new combination that would be even more effective than phen-fen or Redux used alone, and death resulted in some cases.

Thus, two combinations of three serotonin-specific drugs were in vogue in early 1997. However, by May of 1997, there were reports of weight loss patients with newly diagnosed heart valve damage who had been using these drug combinations. In some cases, damage was correctable only by valve-replacement surgery. Accordingly, in September 1997, the FDA requested voluntary

Key Term

phenylpropanolamine (PPA)
The active chemical compound found in most over-the-counter diet products.

Changing *for the Better*

Choosing the Right Weight-Loss Program

Dieting on my own isn't working for me. I need the guidance and support of a structured program. What things should I be cautious about in choosing a plan?

When checking out commercial weight loss programs, avoid any program that:

- Is not led by qualified specialists, including a registered dietitian
- Promises or encourages quick weight loss
- Does not require a preenrollment physical examination
- Does not warn clients of the risk of developing health problems related to weight loss, such as ketosis and diabetes-related complications
- Claims that an unusually high percentage of its clients are successful in achieving and maintaining weight loss
- Requires you to buy its products, such as foods or nutritional supplements
- Does not encourage lifestyle changes, including an exercise program
- Does not provide follow-up support after you reach your weight loss goal

withdrawal of fenfluramine and dexfenfluramine from the market.[21] Manufacturers responded by ceasing all distribution of the drugs. Phentermine remains on the market and is used in combination with various antidepressants, such as Prozac, Zoloft, and Paxil.

Soon after reports of the initial concern over the use of phentermine and fenfluramine, the FDA approved another serotonin-specific obesity drug, sibutramine (Meridia). Sibutramine functions as a serotonin reuptake inhibitor, as did fenfluramine and dexfenfluramine, thus enhancing satiety. Unlike dexfenfluramine, however, sibutramine does not cause excessive production of serotonin in other areas of the nervous system. In addition, sibutramine retards the reuptake of norepinephrine, a second neurotransmitter that influences eating behavior. When used in its approved form, sibutramine appears to have few serious side effects.[22]

A non–serotonin-influencing drug, *orlistat* (Xenical), has recently been approved. Unlike the serotonin-specific drugs, orlistat reduces fat absorption in the small intestine by about 30%. The drug is intended for use among people who are 20% or more above ideal weight. It could cause a 10% loss of body weight without significant dietary restriction. Some concern exists about the lack of absorption of fat soluble vitamins among people taking the drug. Additionally, anal leakage may accompany the drug's use, particularly following meals with high fat content.

Surgical Measures

When a person is morbidly obese and weight loss is imperative, surgical intervention may be considered. A *gastric resection* is a major operation in which a portion of the small intestine is bypassed in an attempt to decrease the body's ability to absorb nutrients. Although this procedure can produce a major weight loss, it is associated with many unpleasant side effects (including diarrhea and liver damage) and various nutritional deficiencies.

Gastroplasty (stomach stapling) is a surgical procedure that involves sealing off a sizable portion of the stomach with surgical staples or recently approved adjustable implanted stomach bands. The resulting reduced capacity of the stomach decreases the amount of food that can be processed at any one time. Patients feel full more quickly after eating a small meal. This procedure carries the general risks associated with surgery, involves the expense of a major surgical procedure, and is nonreversible.

Liposuction

Another form of surgical weight loss management is *liposuction,* or *lipoplasty.* In this procedure, a physician inserts a small tube through the skin and vacuum aspirates away fat cells. This method is generally used for stubborn, localized pockets of fat and is usually appropriate for people under the age of 40.

Liposuction is basically a cosmetic procedure. Possible infection, pain and discomfort, bruising, swelling, discoloration, abscesses, and unattractive changes in body contours are possible outcomes of liposuction. Therefore people considering this procedure should carefully investigate all its aspects, including the training and experience of the surgeon, to determine whether it is appropriate for them.

Body wraps

Although not a surgical procedure or a weight loss technique, *body wrapping* is another form of body contouring. In this procedure, various areas of the body are tightly wrapped with 6-inch strips of materials soaked in a solution of amino acids, which is claimed to draw toxins out of the underlying tissue, shrink fatty deposits, diminish cellulite, lighten stretch marks, and, most important, eliminate inches of fat. Once the wrapping is removed, the newly-contoured body area may remain this way for at least 4 to 10 weeks. Although the secret to the success of a particular spa's body wrapping approach is supposed to lie in its uniquely formulated soaking solution, the contouring effect probably results from dehydration of underlying tissue and redistribution of extracellular fluids through pressure from the wrapping.

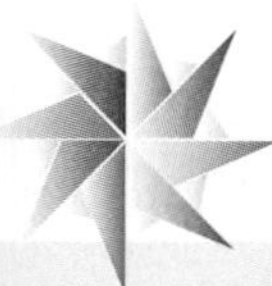

Recognizing Anorexia and Bulimia

The American Psychological Association uses the following diagnostic criteria to identify anorexia nervosa and bulimia:

Anorexia
- 15% or more below desirable weight
- Fear of weight gain
- Altered body image
- Three or more missed menstrual periods; in young adolescents, no onset of menstruation

Bulimia
- Binge eating two or more times a week for 3 months
- A lack of control over binging
- Purging
- Concern about body image

Characteristic symptoms include the following. However, it is unlikely that all the symptoms will be evident in any one individual.

Anorexia
- Looks thin and keeps getting thinner
- Skips meals, cuts food into small pieces, moves food around plate to appear to have eaten
- Loss of menstrual periods
- Wears "layered look" in an attempt to disguise weight loss
- Loss of hair from the head
- Growth of fine hair (lanugo) on face, arms, and chest
- Extreme sensitivity to cold

Bulimia
- Bathroom use immediately after eating
- Inconspicuous eating
- Excessive time (and money) spent food shopping
- Shopping for food at several stores rather than one store
- Menstrual irregularities
- Excessive constipation
- Swollen and/or infected salivary glands, sore throat
- Bursting blood vessels in the eyes
- Damaged teeth and gums
- Dehydration and kidney dysfunction

EATING DISORDERS

Some people have medically identifiable, potentially serious difficulties with body image, body weight, and food selection. Among these disorders are two that are frequently seen among college students—anorexia nervosa and bulimia. In addition, compulsive exercising, compulsive eating, and disorders involving anorexic and/or bulimic practices are also found in college populations. These topics are included in this chapter because most eating disorders begin with dieting. However, most eating disorders also involve inappropriate food choices and deep emotional needs (discussed in Chapters 2 and 5).

Anorexia Nervosa

A young woman, competitive and perfectionistic by nature, determines that her weight (and appearance) is unacceptable. She begins to disregard her appetite, and her food consumption virtually ceases. This young woman may be seen by her friends as active and intelligent and simply dieting and exercising with an unusual degree of commitment. Eventually, however, they observe that her food consumption has nearly stopped. Her weight loss has continued beyond the point that is pleasing—at least to others. Still, her activity level remains high. When questioned about her weight loss, she says that she still needs to lose more weight.

This person is suffering from a medical condition called **anorexia nervosa** (see the Star Box above). This self-induced starvation is life-threatening in 5% to 20% of cases. The stunning amount of weight that some anorexic people lose—up to 50% of their body weight—eventually leads to failure of the heart, lungs, and kidneys.

Although this condition involves a weight loss orientation, experts believe that the anorexic person is attempting to meet a much deeper need for control. Specifically, in a family setting where much is expected of the individual but little opportunity for self-directed behavior is provided, control over the body becomes a need-fulfilling tool. Eventually, a normal body image is lost, and the condition progresses as described above. Fortunately, psychological intervention in combination with

Key Term

anorexia nervosa
A disorder of emotional origin in which appetite and hunger are suppressed and marked weight loss occurs.

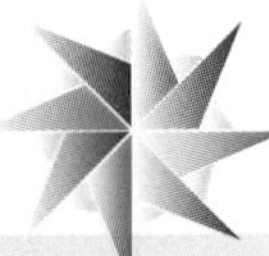

Resources for Anorexia and Bulimia Treatment

Local Resources

- College or university health centers
- College or university counseling centers
- Comprehensive mental health centers
- Crisis intervention centers
- Mental health associations

Organizations and Self-Help Groups

American Anorexia/Bulimia Association, Inc.
165 W. 46th St., Suite 1108, New York, NY 10036
www.aabainc.org

Anorexia Nervosa and Associated Disorders, Inc.
P.O. Box 7, Highland Park, IL 60035
(847) 831-3438

Anorexia Nervosa and Related Eating Disorders, Inc.
P.O. Box 5102, Eugene, OR 97405
(541) 344-1144

Bulimia Anorexia Nervosa Association
300 Cabana Road, East, Windsor, Ontario, Canada N9G 1A3
(519) 969-2112

Eating Disorders Awareness and Prevention, Inc.
www.edap.org

Laureate Eating Disorders Program
P.O. Box 470207
Tulsa, OK 74147
(800) 322-5173
www.laureate.org

National Institute of Mental Health
Eating Disorders Information Page
www.nimh.nih.gov/publicat/eatdis.htm

medical and dietary support can return the anorexic person to a more healthful pattern of eating. The anorexic person, and often the family, needs professional help. If you observe this condition in a friend, it is vital to secure immediate assistance for this person.

Bulimia Nervosa

Bulimia nervosa is an eating disorder that involves gorging oneself with food. People who practice a pattern of massive eating followed by **purging** are said to suffer from *bulimarexia,* or *bulimia nervosa* (see the Star Box on p. 137). Most often, however, the term *bulimia* is used to describe this binge-purge pattern. As with anorexia, most people with bulimia are young women, although the incidence in men is growing.

People with bulimia lose or maintain weight not because they stop eating but because they eat and then purge their digestive system by vomiting, using laxatives, or taking syrup of ipecac, a dangerous drug used to stimulate vomiting after an accidental poisoning. They may gorge themselves with food (up to 10,000 calories in a sitting) and then disappear, only to return later seemingly unaffected by the amount of food they ate. Diuretic, or "water pills," may also be used. In the mid-1980s, medical experts estimated that as many as 19% of 18- to 22-year-old women developed all the principal symptoms of bulimia. However, when all of the criteria mentioned in the Star Box on p. 137 are applied, rather than simply reporting "experience" with bulimia-associated behavior, the percentage drops to less than 2%.

In addition to the binge-purge disorder, people who binge but do not purge also suffer from an eating disorder. Whether called *bulimia,* "eating disorder not otherwise specified," or *binge-eating disorder,* this practice also requires intervention and effective treatment.

Compulsive Exercising, Compulsive Eating, and Night-Eating Syndrome

The compulsive nature of some people's exercising or eating patterns suggests slightly different versions of the two principal eating disorders. In compulsive exercise, a desire for control may exist, as in anorexia nervosa. With compulsive eating, food is related to feelings of insecurity and stress. Since dieting may be the starting point for both of these behavior patterns, family members and friends need to be alert to signs of these conditions.

Night-eating syndrome (NES) involves an anorexic eating pattern during the day, followed by food consumption prior to retiring or during the night. Often, the late-night snack exceeds 1000 calories. Noticeable fluctuations in nocturnal levels of cortisol (a stress hormone), melatonin (associated with sleep cycles), and leptin have been noted in individuals with NES in comparison to normal subjects. These changes suggest that a neuroendocrine component is involved in this pattern of food consumption.[23]

Treatment for Eating Disorders

The treatment of eating disorders is complex and demanding. The physical care for a person with anorexia usually begins with hospitalization to stabilize the physical deterioration associated with starvation. Stomach tubes and intravenous feedings are sometimes necessary, particularly when the patient will not (or cannot) eat. In addition, drugs used to treat depression, obsessive-compulsive disorder, and anxiety are often prescribed. Behavior modification, including eating contracts, is used, as is psychotherapy (in both individual and group formats). Nutritional and family counseling complete the therapy.

Treatment for bulimia involves individual, family, and nutritional counseling. Unlike treatment for anorexia, however, the treatment does not involve hospitalization as often. The Star Box on p. 138 lists resources for people with eating disorders.

Although eating disorders are clinical realities to the physicians and psychologists who treat affected patients and can be described with detachment, they are very personal matters to the patients and families involved. Effective treatment must take place within the supportive environment of concerned and knowledgeable friends and family members.

TALKING POINTS • You suspect that a close friend at school is anorexic but has hidden her physical condition from her family by going home infrequently and skillfully layering her clothing. Do you have an obligation to talk to your friend's family about her condition? If so, how would you approach the subject?

UNDERWEIGHT AND UNDERNOURISHED

For some young adults, the lack of adequate body weight is a serious concern. Particularly for those who have inherited an ectomorphic body build (tall, narrow shoulders and hips with a tendency to thinness), attempts to gain weight are routinely undertaken, often with limited success. These people would likely fall into a BMI category (see p. 123) of less than 18.5 and be from 10% to 20% below normal on a standard height-weight table. If these people are to be successful in gaining weight, they must find an effective way to take in more calories than they burn (see Focus on . . . article on p. 147).

Nutritionists believe that the healthiest way to gain weight is to increase the intake of calorie-dense food. These foods are characterized by high fat density resulting from high levels of vegetable fats (polyunsaturated fats). Foods that meet this requirement are dried fruits, bananas, nuts, granola, and cheeses made from low-fat milk. These foods should be consumed later in a meal so that the onset of satiety that quickly follows eating fat-rich foods does not occur. The current recommendation is to eat three calorie-dense meals of moderate size per day, interspersed with two or three substantial snacks. Using the Food Guide Pyramid (see Chapter 5, p. 96) as a guide, underweight people should eat the highest number of recommended servings for each group.

A second component of weight gain for those who are underweight is an exercise program that uses weight-training activities intended to increase muscle mass. As detailed in Chapter 4, the use of anabolic drugs without highly component medical supervision has no role in healthful weight gain. In addition, carefully monitored aerobic activity should be undertaken in sessions that adequately maintain heart-lung health. At the same time, unnecessary activity that expands calories should be restricted. See Chapter 4 to review the female athlete triad and its relationship to underweight.

For those who cannot gain weight, even by using these approaches, a medical evaluation may offer an explanation. If no medical reason can be found, the person must begin to accept the reality of his or her unique body type. The Focus on . . . box on p. 147 further explores the problems of being underweight.

When individuals fall below 80% of their desirable weight on standard height-weight tables and display BMI rates from 16 to 10, it is highly probable that they are not only underweight but, more important, *undernourished*.[24] This condition suggests clinically significant deficiencies in both the quantity of food being consumed and its nutritional value. Whether the undernourishment is associated with anorexia nervosa, other medical conditions characterized by weight loss (such as irritable bowel diseases), or poverty or famine, affected people are in danger of death from starvation.

Key Terms

bulimia nervosa
A disorder of emotional origin in which binge eating patterns are established; usually accompanied by purging.

purging
Using vomiting or laxatives to remove undigested food from the body.

SUMMARY

- Overweight and obesity are the most common forms of malnutrition in the United States.
- Obesity results from an abnormal accumulation of fat.
- The health implications of moderate to severe obesity are clear, but the seriousness of mildly obese or overweight is questioned by some.
- Body image and self-concept can be adversely influenced by obesity.
- Obesity and overweight can be defined in a variety of ways and determined by different methods.
- Maintaining a healthy body weight is desirable because central body cavity obesity is associated with a variety of serious health problems.
- Theories regarding the cause of obesity focus on factors from within the individual and from the environment.
- Many complex theories exist regarding the role of appetite centers, set point, thermogenesis, inheritance, body type, infant feeding patterns, aging, family dietary patterns, and activity patterns.
- Caloric balance influences weight gain, loss, and maintenance.
- The body's energy needs arise from three areas: activity, basal metabolic rate, and the thermic effect of food.
- If well managed, pregnancy should not contribute to excessive weight gain.
- Weight loss can be attempted through dieting, which is the restriction of food intake.
- Drugs, behavior modification, and other techniques, including surgery, can be used to achieve weight loss.
- A combination approach involving moderately-low fat, low–saturated fat, high–complex carbohydrate food, portion-controlled dieting, and exercise may be the most effective way to lose weight.
- Surgical intervention may be required in cases of extreme obesity.
- Body wraps only contour the body in localized areas.
- Although many people can lose some weight through dieting, very few can maintain that weight loss.
- The use of certain prescription medications in various combinations caused serious heart valve damage and other dangerous side effects, leading to removal of these drugs from the market.
- Serious eating disorders usually begin with dieting but are often sustained in an attempt to meet deeper needs.
- Compulsive exercise, compulsive eating, and night-eating syndrome are less common forms of eating disorders.
- Underweight is a condition that may be resolved through the use of calorie-dense foods or by increasing muscle mass.

REVIEW QUESTIONS

1. Why are obesity and overweight considered to be forms of malnutrition and potentially serious health problems?
2. How are obesity and overweight defined? Why is it possible to be overweight without being overfat? What is the set point?
3. In what ways can obesity be determined? What is desirable weight? What is body mass index? What is waist-to-hip ratio? Why is central body cavity obesity of concern to physicians?
4. Describe the function of each of the following in causing obesity: heredity, set point, body type, infant feeding patterns, pregnancy, aging, inactivity, and family eating patterns.
5. What is caloric balance? What are the body's three areas of energy needs? How does aging influence caloric balance? How is exercise involved in both weight loss and long-term weight maintenance?
6. What is the role of surgery, fasting, and fad diets? What advances are being made in the development of drugs that are effective in weight management?
7. How effective is dieting in terms of both immediate success and later weight maintenance?
8. What two techniques are used in a combination approach to weight loss? How should this program be structured to ensure the highest level of success? What is now known about the use of certain medications prescribed in combination to treat obesity?
9. What are the two principal eating disorders found among college students? What is binge-eating disorder? What are compulsive exercise, night eating syndrome, and compulsive eating? How are eating disorders treated?

THINK ABOUT THIS . . .

- What are your attitudes toward people with weight-control problems? Why do you feel this way?
- Do you believe that being underweight is as psychologically traumatic as being overweight?

- If you have a weight problem, do you agree or disagree that you have a responsibility to yourself and to other people to reduce your weight?
- What do you see as your responsibility in dealing with a friend or family member who is displaying signs of an eating disorder?

REFERENCES

1. Morgan K, Morgan S, Quitno N, editors: *Health care state rankings 2000: health care in the 50 United States,* 2000, Morgan Quiton Press.
2. Sturm R, Wells KB: Does obesity contribute as much to morbidity as poverty or smoking?, *Public Health* 115(3):229–235, 2001.
3. Crowley LV: *Introduction to human disease,* ed 4, 1996, Jones & Bartlett.
4. Field AE et al: Impact of overweight on the risk of developing common chronic diseases during a 10-year period, *Arch Intern Med* 161(13):1581–1586, 2001.
5. Cash T, Henry P: Women's body images: the results of national survey in the U.S.A., *Sex Roles: A Journal of Research* 33(1–2):19–29, 1995.
6. *Nutrition and your health: dietary guidelines for Americans,* ed 5th, 2000, Home and Garden Bulletin 232, U.S. Department of Agriculture and U.S. Department of Health and Human Services.
7. Roche AF: Anthropometric methods: new and old, what they tell us, *Int J Obess* 8(5):509–523, 1984.
8. Friedman MA, Schwartz MB, Brownell KD: Differential relation of psychological functioning with the history and experience of weight cycling, *J Consult Clin Psychol* 66(4):646–650, 1998.
9. Saladin KS: *Anatomy and physiology: the unity of form and function,* ed 2, 2001, McGraw-Hill.
10. Kozak LP: Genetic studies of brown adipocyte induction, *J Nutr* 130(12):3132S–3133S, 2000.
11. Yanovski JA, Yanovski SZ: Recent advances in basic obesity research, *JAMA* 282(16):1504–1506, 1999.
12. Heymsfield SB, et al: Recombinant leptin for weight loss in obese and lean adults: a randomized, controlled, dose-escalation trial, *JAMA* 282(16):1568–1575, 1999.
13. Fujioka K, Patane J, Lau D: CSF leptin levels after exogenous administration of recombinant methionyl human leptin (research letter), *JAMA* 282(16):1517–1518, 1999.
14. Robinson TN: Reducing children's television viewing to prevent obesity: a randomized controlled trial, *JAMA* 282(16):1561–1570, 1999.
15. Ganong WF: *Review of medical physiology,* ed 18, 1997, Appleton & Lange.
16. Thorsdottir I, Birgisdottir BE: Different weight gain in women of normal weight before pregnancy: postpartum weight and birth weight, *Obstet Gynecol* 92(3):377–383, 1998.
17. Lederman SA: Pregnancy weight gain and postpartum loss: avoiding obesity while optimizing growth and development of the fetus, *J Am Med Womens Assoc* 56(2):53–58, 2001.
18. What if takes to take off weight (and keep it off), *Tufts University Health and Nutrition Letter* 15(4):4–5, January, 1998.
19. Serdula MK, et al: Prevalence of attempting weight loss and strategies for controlling weight, *JAMA* 282(16):1353–1358, 1999.
20. Jakicic JM, et al: Effects of intermittent exercise and use of home exercise equipment on adherence, weight loss, and fitness in overweight women, *JAMA* 282(16):1554–1559, 1999.
21. FDA announces withdrawal of fenfluramine and dexfenfluramine, News Release # P97-32, September 15, 1997, Center for Drug Evaluation and Research, U.S. Food and Drug Administration.
22. Weissman NJ et al: Natural history of valvular regurgitation 1 year after discontinuation of dexfenfluramine therapy. A randomized, double-blind, placebo-controlled trial, *Ann Intern Med* 134(4):267–273, 2001.
23. Birketvedt GS, et al: Behavioral and neuroendocrine characteristics of the night eating syndrome, *JAMA* 282(7):657–663, 1999.
24. Ferro-Luzzi A, James WP: Adult malnutrition: simple assessment techniques for use in emergencies, *Br J Nutr* 75(1):3–10, 1996.

SUGGESTED READINGS

Keene MS: *Chocolate is my kryptonite: feeding your feelings—how to survive the forces of food,* 1998, Saguaro Publishing.
The author, a psychiatrist and recognized authority on eating disorders, advances an explanation for compulsive eating based on self-medicating with food. She contends that the compulsive eater reduces feelings of depression and irritability by using food to elevate levels of serotonin, a neurotransmitter associated with feelings of arousal and well-being. Once this faulty food consumption pattern has become well established, she claims, only a broadly based intervention program using techniques for managing feelings and reducing cravings, a modified diet, and, if necessary, medications (antidepressants) will stop the binge eating. Many who have tried this multifaceted program credit it with being highly effective.

Mellin L: *The solution: six winning ways to permanent weight loss,* 1998, Regan Books.
This book has been praised by many who have tried diet books only to experience failure. The author takes her readers deep inside to the underlying emotional needs that have been routinely dulled (but not met) by compulsive eating. Presented in a workbook format, this book helps readers move toward more nurturing relationships with themselves and others.

Price DS: *Healing the hungry self: the diet-free solution to lifelong weight management,* 1998, Plume.
Disturbances in the physical, emotional, mental, and spiritual selves that constitute each person are described as the basis of flawed relationships with food. The author, drawing on her expertise in the treatment of eating disorders, uses a workbook format to bring readers into contact with these selves in order to better understand each, thus enhancing their self-esteem and altering their relationship with food.

As we go to Press...

People who are overweight or obese are commonly viewed by others as physically unfit. However, this is not necessarily the case. In a recent study conducted by the Cooper Institute for Aerobic Research, it was reported that overweight and obese people who engage in regular physical activity, including planned exercise programs, experienced a death rate that was 50% lower than that of equally overweight and obese persons who were inactive. According to the study's lead researcher, this finding suggests that body weight per se is not the sole factor affecting mortality. It may also suggest that, among this group of individuals, other aspects of physiological function were substantially improved by regular physical activity, although there was no apparent impact on body weight.

Name ______________________ **Date** __________ **Section** __________

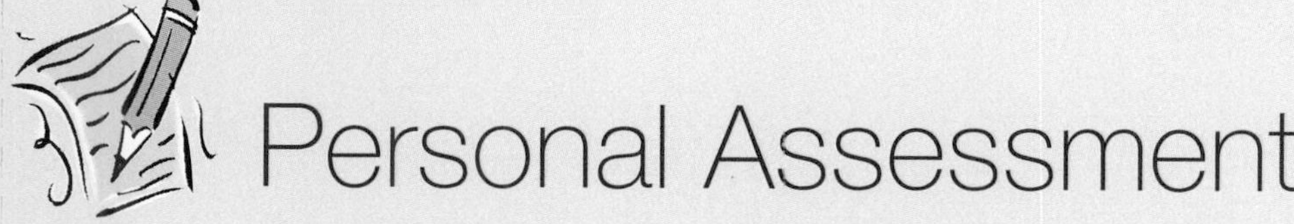

Personal Assessment

Are Your Food Habits Weight-Smart?

To maintain a healthy weight throughout your lifetime, it's important to have healthy food habits. To find out whether your current food practices will work *for* you or *against* you, put them to the test.

For each statement, place a checkmark in the column at the right to indicate how it relates to your own behavior. Follow the Scoring instructions below to find out if you're on the right track or need to start making changes today.

	Always	Generally, but not always	Rarely
1. I shop for food soon after eating.	_____	_____	_____
2. I use a prepared list for food shopping.	_____	_____	_____
3. I store food out of sight.	_____	_____	_____
4. I eat only at scheduled times.	_____	_____	_____
5. I eat in the same area within the home.	_____	_____	_____
6. I use small-size dishes.	_____	_____	_____
7. I take small bites of food.	_____	_____	_____
8. I chew food thoroughly.	_____	_____	_____
9. I put my fork down after each bite of food.	_____	_____	_____
10. I keep serving dishes off the table.	_____	_____	_____
11. I remove dishes promptly after eating.	_____	_____	_____
12. I politely decline unwanted food and beverages.	_____	_____	_____
TOTAL	_____	_____	_____

Scoring

Nine (9) or more answered **Always** reflects a food-related behavior score that is very supportive of effective weight management.

Seven (7) or eight (8) answered **Always** reflects a food-related behavior that will serve as a strong starting point for improvement.

Six (6) or fewer answered **Always** reflects a food-related behavior score that is making weight management much more difficult than it should (or will) be.

Name ______________________ **Date** ____________ **Section** ____________

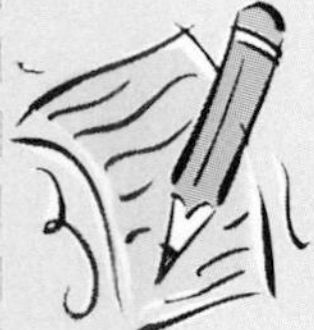

Personal Assessment

Is It Time for a Weight-Loss Program?

Before undertaking a program, it is important to look at your past experiences and feelings about weight loss. Perhaps in doing so, you might decide that you would do better with other alternatives besides dieting.

Answer each of the following items with a "True" or "False" as it applies to you.

_______ 1. I am frustrated about my inability to stick to a diet.
_______ 2. I have less self-control than most dieters.
_______ 3. Most of the times I try to lose weight I lose control and go off my diet.
_______ 4. When I try to develop a habit of regular exercise, something always interferes and I stop.
_______ 5. Exercise seems to be an ordeal to me.
_______ 6. I often feel tired during the day.
_______ 7. My weight has gone up and down several times when I go on and off diets.
_______ 8. My body seems to be getting thicker in the middle over the years.
_______ 9. My weight seems to be increasing over the years.
_______ 10. I find myself thinking about food more than I should.
_______ 11. I find myself thinking about my weight all through the day.
_______ 12. I feel there is probably no hope for my weight problem.
_______ 13. Sometimes I lose control and really binge on food.
_______ 14. I use food to make myself feel better when I am angry, nervous, or depressed.
_______ 15. Some people reject me as a friend because I am too heavy.
_______ 16. My social life is limited because of my weight.
_______ 17. My sex life is limited because of my weight.
_______ 18. Other people think I am unattractive because of my weight.
_______ 19. I put a lot of effort into choosing clothes that tend to cover up my weight problem.

To Carry This Further . . .

For those items that you answered as true, consider these recommendations:

Items 1, 2, and 3: Rather than going on a diet, why not try to reduce your fat intake by avoiding fried food and foods with added fat. Eat more low-fat foods, and make certain that your dairy products are low-fat and your meats are lean.

Items 4, 5, and 6: You need a gradual but regular exercise program. Check around your community, and identify a reputable program that has a proven success rate in helping others who have had a weight problem.

Items 7, 8, and 9: These items indicate the development of a weight problem that could truly be damaging your health. These are reasons for being serious about weight loss that go beyond appearance.

Items 10, 11, 12, 13, and 14: You may be into "living to eat" rather than "eating to live." Now is the time to give serious thought on what is important in your life, other than appearance-related needs.

Items 15, 16, and 17: Work at forming new relationships. Seek out people who are capable of looking beyond your physical appearance for those attributes that they will find to be attractive in you.

Items 18 and 19: As for 15 to 17, assess your current relationships. Put your efforts into relationships with people who seem capable of looking "into" you, rather than only "at" you.

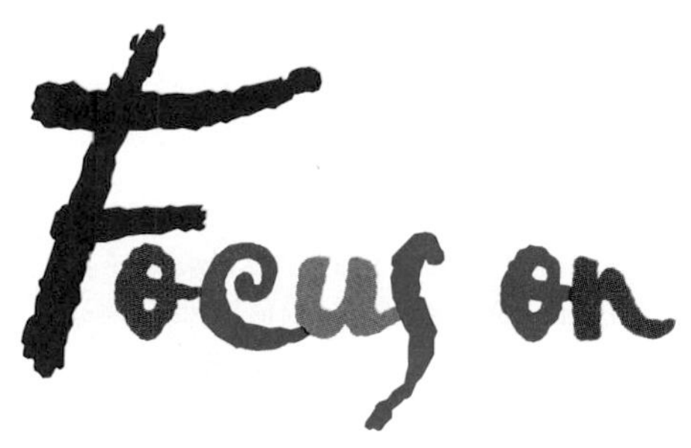

GAINING WEIGHT HEALTHFULLY

"I can't believe how thin you are! It must be so great to eat whatever you want. I wish I had your problem. Of course, it wouldn't hurt you to put on a few pounds. You sure would look healthier!"

"Hey, stick! Do you have anorexia or what? Don't you ever eat?"

These real-life exchanges are examples of how cruel people can be to the underweight. Some observers think that naturally thin people must have an eating disorder because of their appearance; others are envious because they wish they could indulge in high-fat foods without a second thought. Even in a society where thin is in, being too thin can be just as emotionally and physically devastating as being too heavy. Our society has little understanding or sympathy for people who can eat all they want and never gain a pound.

Causes of Being Underweight

The causes of being underweight are multiple. Some people inherit an ectomorphic body type; their unusually high level of metabolism burns excess calories for basic body maintenance. For others, periods of being underweight are associated with chronic illness or injury, long periods of stress, overly aggressive dieting, eating disorders, strenuous physical training (such as that seen among competitive athletes; see Chapter 4 for a discussion of the female athlete triad), and a vegetarian diet. As discussed at the end of this chapter, careful monitoring of food intake and caloric expenditure, as well as appropriate weight training to build muscle mass, can often assist people who are trying to gain or regain weight.

Effects of Being Underweight

For people who are below normal weight, particularly for long periods, being underweight can cause a variety of physical problems. Women who are underweight are at increased risk of amenorrhea, a reproductive system disorder characterized by the complete absence of menstruation. Underweight people tend to have lower bone density than people of normal weight, which may place underweight people at risk for bone fractures and osteoporosis.[1] Being female, over 65, and underweight can increase the risk for hip fractures.[2] Additionally, being underweight is often accompanied by extreme sensitivity to cold and contributes to the discomfort from cold temperatures seen in people with certain diseases.[3] Even in the absence of disease, underweight people often wear layers of additional clothing in weather considered comfortable by people of normal weight.

Being underweight can also cause psychological problems. Anna, a young woman who spent her youth, teenage years, and early twenties as an underweight person, recalls what life was like for her during that time. "It was like a never-ending nightmare. I hated to go to school because the kids made fun of me all the time. They called me names like 'concentration camp victim' and 'twig.' Many nights I would cry myself to sleep because I hated the way I looked so much. I tried everything I could think of to gain weight: eating as much high-calorie food as I could, using commercial weight-gain products, even not exercising in hopes that I'd get fatter. Nothing worked. When I graduated from high school, I was five feet eight inches tall and still weighed 98 lbs. So many people had told me that I was ugly that I believed it must be true. I spent 6 years in therapy trying to get my self-esteem back. Thank God I finally began to gain weight when I graduated from college. I'm actually a little overweight now. If I had to choose between being this way or being the way I was, there's no question in my mind that I'd choose to be like I am now. People say and do things to underweight people that they'd never dream of saying or doing to people who are overweight."[4]

Gaining Weight Safely

For people who are underweight, gaining weight safely is not just a matter of continuously gorging on food. Gaining fat pounds will increase a person's actual weight but will not make him or her any healthier. Diet and exercise plans are available for those who wish to gain weight safely. The first step is to consult a physician to determine the cause of the underweight. If the underweight condition is not due to disease, a combination of diet and exercise can be prescribed to gain lean body mass. Such a weight-gain plan should include a diet that is higher in complex carbohydrates and lower in fat than that described in Chapter 5. One example is a diet that increases carbohydrate intake to 65% of total calories (with a five to one ratio between starches and sugars), reduces fat intake to 20% of total calories, while increasing protein intake to 15% of daily calories.[5]

Underweight people must also exercise to gain muscle mass. The exercise program should be a combination of weight training and endurance training. About 80% of the exercise program should consist of weight training, with the other 20% focusing on endurance exercises such as aerobics. Fairly heavy weights should be used with fewer repetitions to gain lean body mass, since more repetitions with lighter weights will not increase lean body mass as effectively.

Stretching and calisthenics also can be incorporated into the weight training. Weight training can help underweight people (and women in particular) gain upper body strength, which may be lacking. Exercise is also important because it improves cardiovascular fitness and may help prevent osteoporosis.

It's important to remember that these changes in diet and lifestyle must be continued on a long-term basis. It may take 6 to 12 months to see results. If the program is discontinued, any weight gained may be lost again. A lifetime commitment to gaining the weight and keeping it on is required. As always, consult your physician before starting any exercise or diet program.

For Discussion . . .

Why might being underweight be just as dangerous as being overweight? Is it easier to chastise underweight people than overweight people? What are the similarities and differences between people who are thin because of their metabolism and those who are thin as a result of disease (such as anorexia)?

References

1. Leeds MJ: *Nutrition for healthy living,* 1998, McGraw-Hill.
2. Abrams WB, Berkow R, editors: *The Merck manual of geriatrics,* 1990, Merck & Co.
3. Fauci AS, et al, editors: *Harrison's principles of internal medicine (14th ed): companion handbook,* 1998, McGraw-Hill.
4. "Anna," personal interview, 1996.
5. David Pearson, Ph.D., personal interview, 1999, Human Performance Laboratory, Ball State University.

part 3

Preventing Drug Abuse and Addiction

chapter **7**

Making Decisions about Drug Use

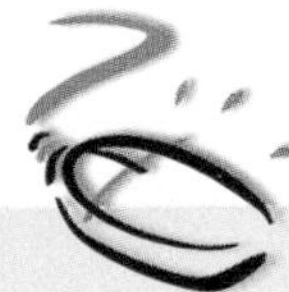

Online Learning Center Resources

www.mhhe.com/hahn6e

Log on to our Online Learning Center (OLC) for access to these additional resources:

- Chapter key terms and definitions
- Learning objectives
- Additional behavior change objectives
- Student interactive question-and-answer sites
- Self-scoring chapter quiz

The OLC also offers web links for study and exploration of health topics. Here are some examples of what you'll find:

- **www.doorway.org** Look here for prevention, education, intervention, and recovery information, and find dozens of links to other sources.
- **www.edc.org/hec** Click on *Effective Prevention* for campus-centered alcohol and other drug information, and check out *Just for Students* for lots of other good stuff.
- **www.habitsmart.com** Take the self-scoring alcohol checkup here if you're curious about your drinking habits.

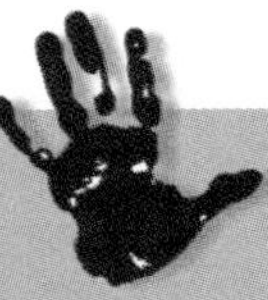

Taking Charge of Your Health

- Assess your knowledge of drug use by completing the Personal Assessment on p. 169.
- Calculate the amount of caffeine you consume daily. If you're using too much caffeine, develop a plan to reduce your overall intake.
- Prepare a plan of action to use if someone you know needs professional assistance with a drug problem.
- Identify five activities that can provide you with a drug-free high.
- Analyze your drug use patterns (if any), and assess the likelihood that you might fail a preemployment drug test.
- Assess your lifestyle for addictive behaviors that do not involve drugs, such as overexercising or watching too much TV. Develop a plan to moderate these activities and achieve more balance in your life.

Eye on the Media

Do Media Scare Tactics Keep People from Using Drugs?

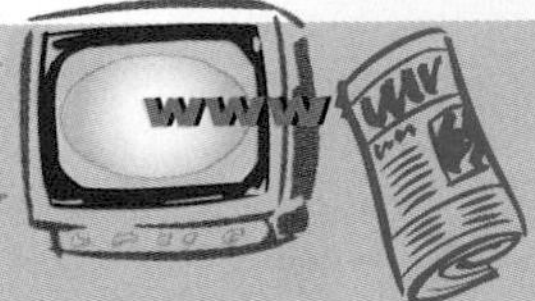

The media has tried to frighten people in many ways to keep them away from unhealthy behaviors. Bloody films showing the aftermath of a prom night car crash have been used to scare teenagers about dangerous drinking and driving behaviors. The classic film *Reefer Madness* was intended to scare people in the 1940s and 1950s about experimenting with marijuana. The late Frank Zappa, founder of the alternative music group the Mothers of Invention, warned young people in the early 1970s not to use stimulants (speed) because doing so would cause them "to turn out like your parents," a frightening thought for many counter-culture youth. More recently, television ads have featured celebrities speaking out against drug use.

Posters produced by both government and private health agencies have depicted cigarette smokers as filthy, wrinkled old men and women. Many of these posters are eye-catching in an almost humorous way. They grab the observer's attention and send the clear message that "this could happen to YOU." Advertisements for drug and

Eye on the Media *continued*

alcohol rehabilitation facilities have shown alcoholics drowning in a sea of alcohol, drug users being confronted by their families, and employees caught by a drug screening test. The message is that miserable life situations can be changed if people are willing to get help.

It's difficult to measure the effectiveness of these approaches to drug prevention. Many people recall these media presentations, so they do make an impression. But, given the many variables involved in drug-taking behavior—family influence, inherited predispositions, life events and situations, drug availability, and peer influence—it's impossible to pinpoint the influence of a single media event. These scare tactics seem to be especially effective among people who have already made the decision not to use drugs. They remind these people how dangerous it is to use drugs. For people who are thinking about starting drug use, these messages may be beneficial, since they portray drug use in a negative light.

For hard-core drug users, though, it's unlikely that scare tactics will be effective. These people tend to lead chaotic lives, may never see the ads, and often remain in denial about their addiction. Nonusers and individuals leaning away from drug use are more likely to be influenced by this approach. Despite the fact that these ad campaigns are highly visible and costly, they seem to have only limited influence in drug prevention.

SOCIETY'S RESPONSE TO DRUG USE

During the last 25 years, society has responded to illegal drug use with growing concern. Most adults see drug abuse as a clear danger to society. This position has been supported by the development of community, school, state, and national organizations directed toward the reduction of illegal drug use. These organizations have included such diverse groups as Parents Against Drugs, Partnership for a Drug-Free America, Mothers Against Drunk Driving (MADD), Narcotics Anonymous, and the U.S. Drug Enforcement Administration. Certain groups have concentrated their efforts on education, others on enforcement, and still others on the development of laws and public policy. Famous people, such as athletes, are also speaking out against drug use (see Learning from Our Diversity on p. 152).

The personal and social issues related to drug abuse are very complex. Innovative solutions continue to be devised. Some believe that only through early childhood education will people learn alternatives to drug use. Starting drug education in the preschool years may have a more positive effect than waiting until the upper elementary or junior high school years. Recently, the focus on reducing young people's exposure to **gateway drugs** (especially tobacco, alcohol, and marijuana) may help slow down the move to other addictive drugs. Some people advocate harsher penalties for drug use and drug trafficking, including heavier fines and longer prison terms.

Others support legalizing all drugs and making governmental agencies responsible for drug regulation and control, as is the case with alcohol. Advocates of this position believe that drug-related crime and violence would virtually cease once the demand for illegal products is reduced. Sound arguments can be made on both sides of this issue. What's your opinion?

In comparison with other federally funded programs, the "war on drugs" is less expensive than farm support, food stamps, Medicare, and national defense. However, it remains to be seen whether any amount of money spent on enforcement, without adequate support for education, treatment, and poverty reduction, can reduce the illegal drug demand and supply. The United States now spends nearly $18 billion annually to fight the drug war.[1] About 70% is spent on law enforcement (supply reduction) and 30% on education, prevention, and treatment (demand reduction).

ADDICTIVE BEHAVIOR

Experts in human behavior view drug use and abuse as just one of the many forms of addictive behavior. Such behavior includes addictions to shopping, eating, gambling, sex, television, video games, and work, as well as to alcohol or other drugs.

TALKING POINTS • How would you tell a friend that her video game playing is becoming an addiction that needs to be controlled?

The Process of Addiction

The process of developing an addiction has been a much-studied topic. Three common aspects of addictive behavior are exposure, compulsion, and loss of control.

Key Term

gateway drug
An easily obtainable legal or illegal drug that represents a user's first experience with a mind-altering drug.

Learning from Our Diversity

Athletes Speak Out Against Drug Use

In the past decade, many public figures have been cautioning youth about the dangers of drug abuse. Politicians, rock stars, and actors have gone public with their antidrug messages. Some of them have admitted to having had drug-abuse problems in their own lives. Their personal accounts have probably influenced some drug abusers to curtail their drug-taking behaviors and seek professional help.

World-class athletes have also taken a public stance against drugs. In Washington, D.C., a group of former Olympians recently kicked off a campaign against the use of performance-enhancing drugs by young people. Gold medal winners Frank Shorter, Jim Ryan, Donna de Varona, Edwin Moses, John Nabor, and Bruce Baumgartner gave their public support to this anti-steroid campaign. The message to youth was that it's possible to achieve remarkable athletic success through hard work, personal sacrifice, and determination. The athletes headlining this campaign came from a variety of sports, so it's likely that their message reached a wide range of young people.

Recently, the mother of basketball superstar Michael Jordan launched a campaign to discourage the use of inhalants by young people. Can you recall other antidrug messages delivered by famous athletes or their families?

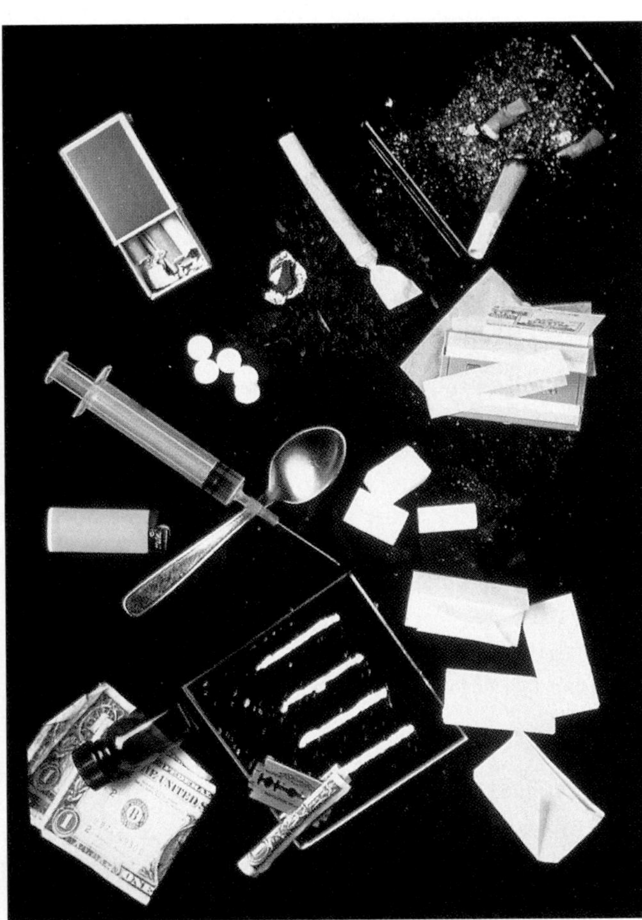

Drug abuse of all types remains a significant problem as we enter the twenty-first century.

Exposure

An addiction can begin after a person is exposed to a drug (such as alcohol) or a behavior (such as gambling) that he or she finds pleasurable. Perhaps this drug or behavior temporarily replaces an unpleasant feeling or sensation. This initial pleasure gradually, or in some cases quickly, becomes a focal point in the person's life.

Compulsion

Increasingly, the person spends more energy, time, and money pursuing the drug use or behavior. At this point in the addictive process, the person can be said to have a compulsion for the drug or behavior. Frequently, repeated exposure to the drug or behavior continues despite negative consequences, such as the gradual loss of family and friends, unpleasant physical symptoms resulting from taking a drug, or problems at work.

During the compulsion phase, a person's normal life often degenerates while she or he searches for increased pleasures from the drug or the behavior. An addicted person's family life, circle of friends, work, or study patterns become less important than the search for more and better "highs." The development of tolerance and withdrawal are distinct possibilities. (These terms are discussed later in the chapter.)

Why some people develop compulsions and others do not is difficult to pinpoint, but addiction might be influenced by genetic makeup, family dynamics, physiological processes, personality type, peer groups, and available resources for help.

Loss of control

Over time, the search for highs changes to a desire to avoid the effects of withdrawal from the drug or behavior. Addicted people lose their ability to control their be-

Changing *for the Better*

Finding Help for Drug Abuse

I have a college friend who may need help for drug abuse. Where can I find information about drug abuse and treatment options?

National Groups

Alcoholics Anonymous
(212) 870-3400
www.alcoholics-anonymous.org

Cocaine Anonymous
(800) 347-8998
www.ca.org

Drug Strategies
(202) 289-9070
www.drugstrategies.org

Narcotics Anonymous
(818) 773-9999
www.na.org

National Clearinghouse for Alcohol and Drug Information
(800) 729-6686
www.health.org

National Inhalant Prevention Coalition
(800) 269-4237 or (512) 480-8953
www.inhalants.org

National Institute on Drug Abuse
(301) 443-1124
www.nida.nih.gov

Partnership for a Drug-Free America
www.drugfreeamerica.org

PRIDE (Parent's Resource Institute for Drug Education)
www.prideusa.org

Substance Abuse and Mental Health Services Administration (SAMHSA)
(800) 662-4357
www.samhsa.gov

Toughlove International
(800) 333-1069
www.toughlove.org

Hot Lines/Other Resources

American Council for Drug Education
(800) 662-HELP
www.drughelp.org

For treatment referral
(800) 821-4357

Go Ask Alice! Columbia University's Health Education Program
www.goaskalice.columbia.edu

havior. Despite overwhelming negative consequences (for example, deterioration of health, alienation of family and friends, or loss of all financial resources), addicted people continue to behave in ways that make their lives worse. The person addicted to alcohol continues to drink heavily, the person addicted to shopping continues to run up heavy debts, and the person addicted to food continues to eat indiscriminately. This behavior reflects a loss of control over one's life. Frequently, a person has addictions to more than one drug or behavior.

Intervention and Treatment

The good news for people with addictions is that help is available. Within the last two decades, much attention has been focused on intervention and treatment for addictive behavior. Many people with drug problems can be helped through programs such as those described in the Changing for the Better box above. These programs often include inpatient or outpatient treatment, family counseling, and long-term aftercare counseling.

It is common for people in aftercare treatment for addictive behavior to belong to a self-help support group, such as Alcoholics Anonymous, Gamblers Anonymous, or Sex Addicts Anonymous. These groups are often listed in the phone book or in the classified section of the newspaper.

DRUG TERMINOLOGY

Before discussing drug behavior, it's important to become familiar with some basic terminology. Much of this terminology originates from the field of *pharmacology,* or the study of the interaction of chemical agents with living material.

What does the word *drug* mean? Each of us may have different ideas about what a drug is. Although a

Changing *for the Better*

Improving Your Mood Without Drugs

It's tempting to reach for a pill when I feel down, but I don't want to get into that habit. What can I do to improve my mood without using drugs?

Talk with a trusted friend. Confide your feelings to a close, trusted friend or family member. By opening up to another person, you'll gain insights into how you can get beyond your negative feelings without resorting to drug use.

Get moving. Go for a walk, ride your bike, or swim a few laps. Physical activity is a natural way to enhance your mood. Nearly every college provides recreation programs such as aerobics, swimming, dancing, or weight lifting.

Give yourself a break. If you're tired, take a quick power nap. If you're overworked, set aside some personal time—just for yourself. Read, watch TV, surf the net, or phone an old friend. Decide what you like to do, and then do it. You'll return to your responsibilities with renewed enthusiasm.

Do volunteer work. One way to feel good is to help others. Teach reading to adults, become a Big Brother or Big Sister, work in a soup kitchen, or drive a van for the elderly in your community.

Reexamine your spiritual health. Many people find comfort by making connections to their spiritual life. Through activities such as meditation, spiritual reflection, and renewal of faith, people often gain reassurance and a sense of calmness.

Restructure your daily activities. If you have one hectic day after another but feel as though you're not accomplishing anything, try reorganizing your daily activities. Experiment with new patterns. Plan to get sufficient sleep, eat regular meals, and set aside specific times for work, family activities, and pleasure. Find out what works best for you.

Seek professional guidance. If you've tried these strategies but your mood still isn't improving, consider seeking professional help. This important first step is up to you. Visit your college health center or counseling center, and talk with people who are trained to help you learn how to become a happier person.

number of definitions are available, we will consider a drug to be "any substance, natural or artificial, other than food, that by its chemical or physical nature alters structure or function in the living organism."[2] Included in this broad definition is a variety of psychoactive drugs, medicines, and substances that many people do not usually consider to be drugs.

Psychoactive drugs alter the user's feelings, behavior, perceptions, or moods. This group includes stimulants, depressants, hallucinogens, opiates, and inhalants. (The Changing for the Better box above suggests ways to improve your mood without resorting to drug use.) Medicines function to heal unhealthy tissue. They are also used to ease pain, prevent illness, and diagnose health conditions. Although some psychoactive drugs are used for medical reasons, as in the case of tranquilizers and some narcotics, the most commonly prescribed medicines are antibiotics, hormone replacement drugs, sulfa drugs, diuretics, oral contraceptives, and cardiovascular drugs. Legal substances not usually considered to be drugs (but which certainly are drugs) include caffeine, tobacco, alcohol, aspirin, and other over-the-counter (OTC) preparations. These substances are used so commonly in our society that they are rarely perceived as true drugs.

For organizational reasons, this chapter primarily deals with psychoactive drugs. Alcohol is covered in Chapter 8. The effects of tobacco are discussed in Chapter 9. Prescription and OTC drugs and medicines are explored further in Chapter 15. Anabolic steroids, drugs used primarily for increasing muscle growth, are discussed in Chapter 4.

Routes of Administration

Drugs generally enter the body through one of four methods: ingestion, injection, inhalation, and absorption. *Ingestion,* or oral administration, is the entry of drugs through the mouth and into the digestive tract. *Injection* refers to the use of a needle to insert a drug into the body. With *inhalation,* the drug enters the body through the lungs. *Absorption* refers to the administration of a drug through the skin or mucous membranes.

Dependence

Psychoactive drugs have a strong potential for the development of **dependence.** When users take a psychoactive drug, the patterns of nervous system function are altered. If these altered functions provide perceived benefits for the user, the drug use may continue, perhaps at increasingly larger dosages. If persistent use continues, the user can develop a dependence on the drug. Pharmacologists have identified two types of dependences: physical and psychological.

A person can be said to have developed a *physical dependence* when the body cells have become reliant on a drug. Continued use of the drug is then required because body tissues have adapted to its presence.[3] The person's body needs the drug to maintain homeostasis, or dynamic balance. If the drug is not taken or is suddenly withdrawn, the user develops a characteristic **withdrawal illness.** The symptoms of withdrawal reflect the attempt by the body's cells to regain normality without the drug. Withdrawal symptoms are always unpleasant (ranging from mild to severe irritability, depression, nervousness, digestive difficulties, and abdominal pain) and can be life-threatening, as in the case of abrupt withdrawal from barbiturates or alcohol. In this chapter the term *addiction* is used interchangeably with physical dependence.

Continued use of most drugs can lead to **tolerance.** Tolerance is an acquired reaction to a drug in which continued intake of the same dose has diminishing effects.[3] The user needs larger doses of the drug to receive previously felt sensations. The continued use of depressants, including alcohol, and opiates can cause users to quickly develop a tolerance to the drug.

For example, college seniors who have engaged in 4 years of beer drinking usually recognize that their bodies have developed a degree of tolerance to alcohol. Many such students can vividly recall the initial and subsequent sensations they felt after drinking. For example, five beers consumed during a freshman social gathering might well have resulted in inebriation, but if these same students continued to drink beer regularly for 4 years, five beers would probably fail to produce the response they experienced as freshmen. Seven or eight beers might be needed to produce such a response. Clearly, these students have developed a tolerance to alcohol.

TALKING POINTS • Some of your friends have started making a contest of beer drinking. How would you tell them you think this is dangerous without sounding preachy?

Tolerance developed for one drug may carry over to another drug within the same general category. This phenomenon is known as **cross-tolerance.** The heavy abuser of alcohol, for example, might require a larger dose of a preoperative sedative to become relaxed before surgery than the average person would. The tolerance to alcohol "crosses over" to the other depressant drugs.

A person who possesses a strong desire to continue using a particular drug is said to have developed a *psychological dependence.* People who are psychologically dependent on a drug believe that they need to consume the drug to maintain a sense of well-being. (The Exploring Your Spirituality box on p. 156 shows how some people have a strong dependence on drugs for social situations.) They crave the drug for emotional reasons despite having persistent or recurrent physical, social, psychological, or occupational problems caused or worsened by the drug use. Abrupt withdrawal from a drug by such a person would not trigger the fully expressed withdrawal illness, although some unpleasant symptoms of withdrawal might be felt. The term *habituation* is often used interchangeably with psychological dependence.

Drugs whose continued use can quickly lead to both physical and psychological dependence are the depressants (barbiturates, tranquilizers, and alcohol), narcotics (the opiates, which are derivatives of the Oriental poppy: heroin, morphine, and codeine), and synthetic narcotics (Demerol and methadone). Drugs whose continued use can lead to various degrees of psychological dependence and occasionally to significant (but not life-threatening) physical dependence in some users are the stimulants (amphetamines, caffeine, and cocaine), hallucinogens (LSD, peyote, mescaline, and marijuana), and inhalants (glues, gases, and petroleum products).

Drug Misuse and Abuse

So far in this chapter we have used the term *use* (or *user*) in association with the taking of psychoactive drugs. At this point, however, it is important to define *use* and to introduce the terms *misuse* and *abuse.*[2] By doing so, we can more accurately describe the ways in which drugs are used.

The term *use* is all-encompassing and describes drug-taking in the most general way. For example, Americans use drugs of many types. The term *use* can also refer more narrowly to misuse and abuse.

Key Terms

psychoactive drug
Any substance capable of altering feelings, moods, or perceptions.

dependence
General term that refers to the need to continue using a drug for psychological and/or physical reasons.

withdrawal illness
Uncomfortable, perhaps toxic response of the body as it attempts to maintain homeostasis in the absence of a drug; also called *abstinence syndrome.*

tolerance
An acquired reaction to a drug; continued intake of the same dose has diminished results.

cross-tolerance
Transfer of tolerance from one drug to another within the same general category.

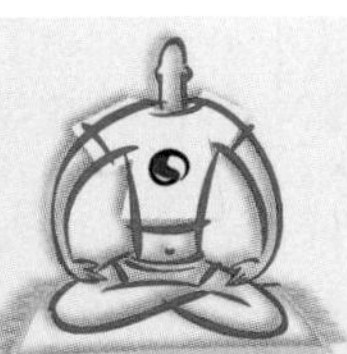

Exploring Your Spirituality

Making Social Connections without Drugs

According to many college and university drug counselors, students who undergo drug counseling often say that they started (or continued) to use drugs because they felt inadequate in social situations. These students believed that they were not attractive, talented, wealthy, or socially skilled enough to start and maintain relationships. In a dating situation, the drug allowed them to be more relaxed and less conscious of their perceived shortcomings. Then, if they did something foolish while socializing, they had an instant excuse—the drug made them act inappropriately.

What are some drug-free strategies you can use to enhance your social relationships? Start by finding people and activities that are free of drug use. Contrary to popular opinion, most college students do not use illegal drugs. More students than ever are supportive of a drug-free lifestyle. So it shouldn't be difficult to find individuals and groups who will be a good match for you. Be aware of all the people around you. Don't get locked into one group too quickly. Keep your options open.

As you explore your inner self and try to connect with people at a deeper level, also consider these approaches:

Be true to yourself. Most people like someone who is genuine, so try to be the person you know yourself to be. Don't present a false image of yourself to others.

Be a good listener. One sure way to discourage a growing relationship is to talk more than you listen. Show others that you're interested in them by hearing what they have to say. Let the other person be the center of attention, at least early in the relationship. By listening carefully, you can evaluate the person or group better and see if you're a good fit.

Be open to new people and ideas. It's good to have firm opinions and ideas, but it's also important to be open to new people and ideas. Take the attitude that the next person you meet or the next group you interact with may change your life forever. Don't limit yourself to a particular group of people or friends. Flexibility can be a real asset to your social life.

Be willing to laugh at yourself. Most surveys indicate that people rate humor as an important quality in people they want to date. Try to find humor in everyday situations. Focusing on the lighter side will make things easier for you and the people around you. Most important—be willing to laugh at yourself sometimes.

Be prepared for setbacks. One sign of social maturity is to recognize that setbacks can happen. Don't be defeated by them. Sometimes it's best for everyone involved when things don't work out. You'll always have another opportunity. Focus on the attitude that things will get better. Don't give in to the idea that drugs will make up for an unsatisfying social life. Seek professional help if things do not improve after a reasonable time.

The term **misuse** refers to the inappropriate use of legal drugs intended to be used as medications. Misuse may occur when a patient misunderstands the directions for use of a prescription or OTC drug or when a patient shares a prescription with a friend or family member for whom the drug was not prescribed. Misuse also occurs when a patient takes the prescription or OTC drug for a purpose or condition other than that for which it was intended or at a dosage other than that recommended.

The term **abuse** applies to any use of an illegal drug or any use of a legal drug when it is detrimental to health and well-being. The costs of drug abuse to the individual are extensive and include absenteeism and underachievement, loss of job, marital instability, loss of self-esteem, serious illnesses, and even death. The Changing for the Better box on p. 157 suggests strategies for coping with family and work stress that can keep you in control of your life and away from drug abuse.

EFFECTS OF DRUGS ON THE CENTRAL NERVOUS SYSTEM

To better understand the disruption caused by the actions of psychoactive drugs, a general knowledge of the normal functioning of the nervous system's basic unit, the **neuron,** is required.

First, stimuli from the internal or external environment are received by the appropriate sensory receptor, perhaps an organ such as an eye or an ear. Once sensed, these stimuli are converted into electrical impulses. These impulses are then directed along the neuron's **dendrite,** through the cell body, and along the **axon** toward the *synaptic junction* near an adjacent neuron. On arrival at the **synapse,** the electrical impulses stimulate the production and release of chemical messengers called *neurotransmitters.*[4] These neurotransmitters transmit the electrical impulses from one neuron to the dendrites of adjoining neurons. Thus neurons function in a coordi-

Changing *for the Better*

Coping with Family and Work Stress

Sometimes the pressures of being a college student, a family member, a parent, and an employee are too much, and I wonder how I'll get through the day. How can I stay healthy and drug-free?

Keep the lines of communication open. Work to communicate effectively with your friends, family members, and employers.

Recognize that trying to escape through drug use only makes situations worse. Realize that using drugs in stressful situations only masks the underlying problems you face.

Discuss your concerns with a trusted friend. Sometimes the person who knows you and your situation best can offer helpful guidance and support during difficult times.

Remember that you are a role model to your children. Because young children look to their parents for guidance, your ability to cope without drugs during stressful times will send an important message to your children.

Seek professional help as soon as possible. Many agencies and support groups are ready to help people who are having personal difficulties with family or work situations. Most large employers have Employee Assistance Programs that can be valuable resources. A campus counseling center or a local mental health association is another good source of assistance. It's up to you, though, to make the decision to seek these services. Don't hesitate to help yourself.

nated fashion to send information to the brain for interpretation and to relay appropriate response commands outward to the tissues of the body.

The role of neurotransmitters is critically important to the relay of information within the system. A substance that has the ability to alter some aspect of transmitter function has the potential to seriously disrupt the otherwise normally functioning system. Psychoactive drugs are capable of exerting these disruptive influences on the neurotransmitters. Drugs "work" by changing the way neurotransmitters work, often by blocking the production of a neurotransmitter or forcing the continued release of a neurotransmitter (see Figure 7-1).

DRUG CLASSIFICATIONS

Drugs can be categorized according to the nature of their physiological effects. Most psychoactive drugs fall into one of six general categories: stimulants, depressants, hallucinogens, cannabis, narcotics, and inhalants (Table 7-1).

Stimulants

In general, **stimulants** excite or increase the activity of the central nervous system (CNS). Also called "uppers," stimulants alert the CNS by increasing heart rate, blood pressure, and the rate of brain function. Users feel uplifted and less fatigued. Examples of stimulant drugs include caffeine, amphetamines, and cocaine. Most stimulants produce psychological dependence and tolerance relatively quickly, but they are unlikely to produce significant physical dependence when judged by life-threatening withdrawal symptoms. The important exception is cocaine, which seems to be capable of producing psychological dependence and withdrawal so powerful that continued use of the drug is inevitable in some users.

Caffeine

Caffeine, the tasteless drug found in chocolate, some soft drinks, coffee, tea, some aspirin products, and OTC "stay-awake" pills, is a relatively harmless stimulant when consumed in moderate amounts. (Visit the Focus on Health website **www.mhhe.com/hahn** for a table listing the caffeine content in some products.) Many coffee drinkers believe that they cannot start the day successfully without the benefit of a cup or two of coffee in the morning.

Key Terms

misuse
Inappropriate use of legal drugs intended to be medications.

abuse
Any use of a legal or illegal drug in a way that is detrimental to health.

neuron (NOOR on)
A nerve cell.

dendrite (DEN drite)
The portion of a neuron that receives electrical stimuli from adjacent neurons; neurons typically have several such branches or extensions.

axon
The portion of a neuron that conducts electrical impulses to the dendrites of adjacent neurons; neurons typically have one axon.

synapse (sinn APS)
The location at which an electrical impulse from one neuron is transmitted to an adjacent neuron; also referred to as a *synaptic junction.*

stimulants
Psychoactive drugs that stimulate the function of the central nervous system.

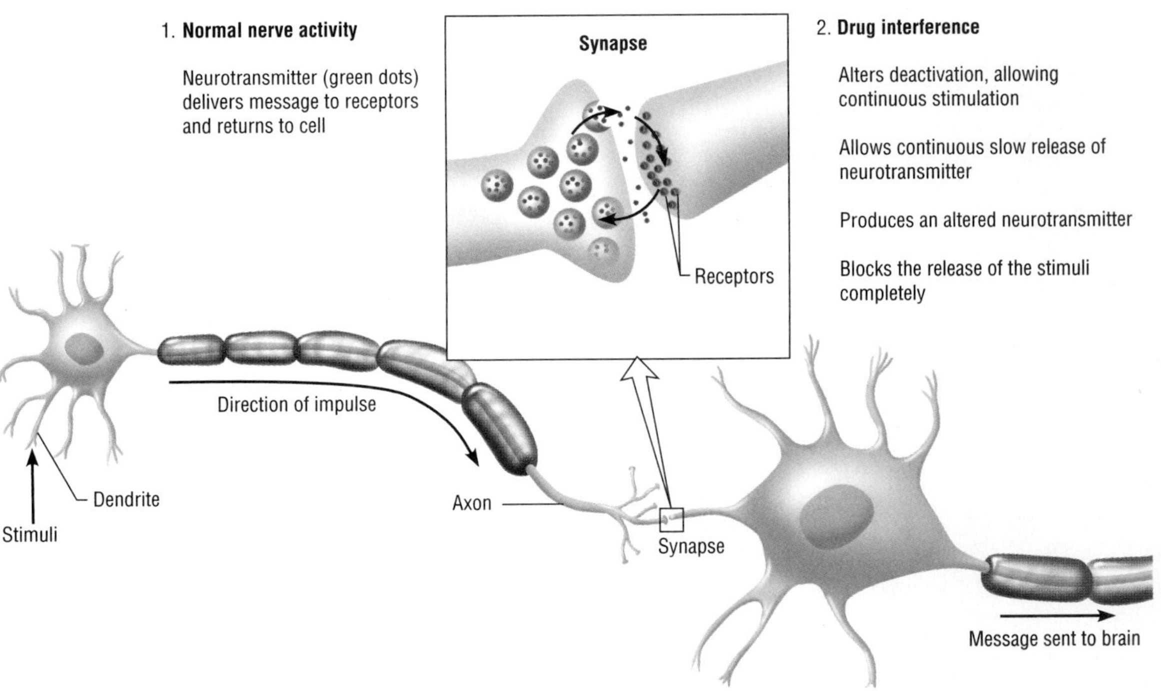

Figure 7-1 This illustration depicts the disruption caused by the action of psychoactive drugs on the central nervous system. Neurotransmitters are chemical messengers that transfer electrical impulses across the synapses between nerve cells. Psychoactive drugs interrupt this process, thus disrupting the coordinating functioning of the nervous system.

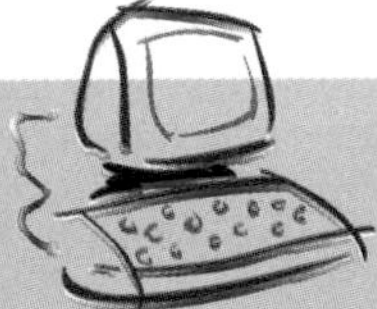

OnSITE/InSIGHT

Learning to Go: Health

Do you take a pill for every ache and pain? Click on the Motivator icon to view the following lessons. You'll find out more about drugs—how they can affect your body and your behavior:

Lesson 24: Unmask addictive behaviors.
Lesson 25: Inform yourself on drug use.

STUDENT POLL

What's your approach to drug use? Access the Online Learning Center at **www.mhhe.com/hahn6e**. Then go to Student Resources to take part in the following poll.

When you're finished, check out how other students responded.

1. Are you currently taking any prescription medications?
2. Do you often use over-the-counter medications?
3. Are you opposed to recreational drug use?
4. Have you ever tried an illegal drug?
5. To have a good time at a party, do you need to take some type of drugs?
6. Do you currently use any illegal drugs?
7. Are you well informed about drugs and their effects?
8. Should marijuana use be legalized?
9. Are public service announcements about drug abuse effective?

For the average healthy adult, moderate consumption of caffeine is unlikely to pose any serious health threat. However, excessive consumption (equivalent to ten or more cups of coffee daily) could lead to anxiety, diarrhea, restlessness, delayed onset of sleep or frequent awakening, headache, and heart palpitations. Pregnant women are advised to consume caffeine sparingly.

Amphetamines

Amphetamines produce increased activity and mood elevation in almost all users. The amphetamines include several closely related compounds: amphetamine, dextroamphetamine, and methamphetamine. These compounds do not have any natural sources and are completely manufactured in the laboratory. Medical use of amphetamines

Table 7-1 Psychoactive Drug Categories

Drugs	Trade or Common Names	Medical Uses	Possible Effects
Stimulants			
Cocaine*	Coke, crack, gin, girlfriend, girl, double bubble, California cornflakes, caballo, bouncing powder, flake, snow	Local anesthetic	Increased alertness, excitation, euphoria, increased pulse rate and blood pressure, insomnia, loss of appetite
Amphetamines	Biphetamine, Delcobese, Desoxyn, Dexedrine, mediatric, methamphetamine (ice), black Mollies, aimies, amps, bam, beans, benz	Hyperactivity, narcolepsy, weight control	
Phendimetrazine	Prelu-2		
Methylphenidate	Ritalin, Methidate		
Other stimulants	Adipex, Bacarate, Cylert, Didrex, Ionamin, Plegine, PreSate, Sanorex, Tenuate, ephedra		
Depressants			
Chloral hydrate	Noctec, Somnos	Hypnotic	Slurred speech, disorientation, drunken behavior without odor of alcohol
Barbiturates	Amobarbital, Butisol, phenobarbital, phenoxbarbital, secobarbital, Tuinal, blockbusters, black bombers	Anesthetic, anticonvulsant, sedative, hypnotic	
Glutethimide	Doriden	Sedative, hypnotic	
Methaqualone	Optimil, Parest, Quaalude, Somnafec, Sopor	Sedative, hypnotic	
Benzodiazepines	Ativan, Azene, Clonopin, Dalmane, diazepam, Librium, Serax, Tranxene, Valium, Verstran	Antianxiety, anticonvulsant, sedative, hypnotic	
GHB	Gamma-hydroxybutyrate (G, liquid ecstasy, Grievous Bodily Harm)	None	Unconsciousness, seizures, vomiting, coma
Other depressants	Equanil, Miltown, Noludar, Placidyl, Valmid	Antianxiety, sedative	
Hallucinogens			
LSD	Acid, microdot, brown dot, cap, California sunshine, brown bomber	None	Delusions and hallucinations, poor perception of time and distance
Mescaline and peyote	Mesc, buttons, cactus, chief	None	
Amphetamine variants (designer drugs)	2,5-DMA, DOM, DOP, MDA, MDMA, PMA, STP, TMA, clarity, chocolate chips, booty juice	None	
Phencyclidine	Angel dust, hog, PCP, AD, boat, black whack, amoeba, angel hair, angel smoke	Veterinary anesthetic	
Phencyclidine analogs	PCE, PCPy, TCP	None	Euphoria, relaxed inhibitions, increased appetite, disorientation
Other hallucinogens	Bufotenin, DMT, DET, ibogaine, psilocybin	None	
Cannabis			
Marijuana	Acapulco gold, black Bart, black mote, blue sage, bobo, butterflowers, cannabis-T, cess, cheeba, grass, pot, sinsemilla, Thai sticks	Under investigation	Euphoria, relaxed inhibitions, increased appetite, disoriented behavior
Tetrahydrocannabinol	THC	Under investigation	
Hashish	Hash	None	
Hashish oil	Hash oil	None	
Narcotics			
Opium	Dover's powder, paregoric, Parapectolin, cruz, Chinese tobacco, China	Analgesic, antidiarrheal	Euphoria, drowsiness, respiratory depression, constricted pupils, nausea
Morphine	Morphine, Pectoal syrup, emsel, first line	Analgesic, antitussive	
Codeine	Codeine, Empirin compound with codeine, Robitussin A-C	Analgesic, antitussive	
Heroin	Diacetylmorphine, horse, smack, courage pills, dead on arrival (DOA)	Under investigation	
Hydromorphone	Dilaudid	Analgesic	Intoxication, excitation, disorientation, aggression, hallucination
Meperidine (pethidine)	Demerol, Pethadol	Analgesic	
Methadone	Dolophine, Methadone, Methadose	Analgesic, heroin substitute	
Other narcotics	Darvon,† Dromoran, Fentanyl, LAAM, Leitine, Levo-Dromoran, Percodan, Tussionex, Talwin,† Lomotil	Analgesic, antidiarrheal, antitussive	
Inhalants			
Anesthetic gases	Aerosols, petroleum products, solvents	Surgical anesthetic	Intoxication, excitation, disorientation, aggression, hallucination, variable effects
Vasodilators (amyl nitrite, butyl nitrite)	Aerosols, petroleum products, solvents	None	

*Designated a narcotic under the Controlled Substances Act.

†Not designated a narcotic under the Controlled Substances Act.

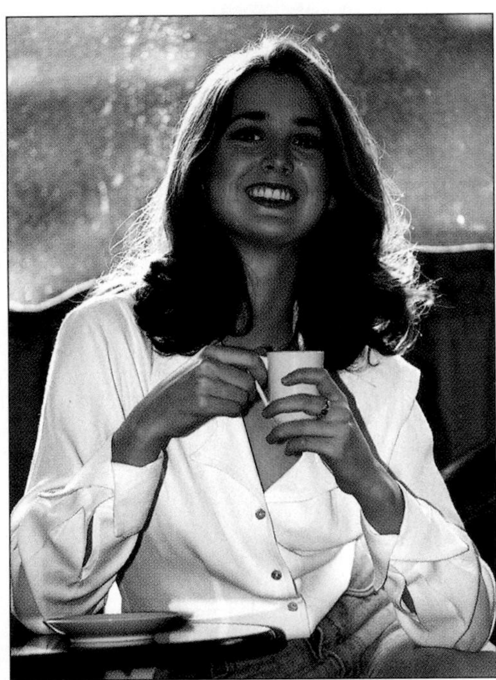

Coffeehouses have become popular places to relax, work, or spend time with friends.

is limited primarily to the treatment of obesity, **narcolepsy,** and **attention deficit hyperactivity disorder** (ADHD).

Amphetamines can be ingested, injected, or snorted (inhaled). At low-to-moderate doses, amphetamines elevate mood and increase alertness and feelings of energy by stimulating receptor sites for two naturally occurring neurotransmitters. They also slow the activity of the stomach and intestine and decrease hunger. In the 1960s and 1970s, in fact, amphetamines were commonly prescribed for dieters. Later, when it was discovered that the appetite suppression effect of amphetamines lasted only a few weeks, most physicians stopped prescribing them. At high doses, amphetamines can increase heart rate and blood pressure to dangerous levels. As amphetamines are eliminated from the body, the user becomes tired.

When chronically abused, amphetamines produce rapid tolerance and strong psychological dependence. Other effects of chronic use include impotence and episodes of psychosis. When use is discontinued, periods of depression may develop.

Today the abuse of amphetamines is a more pressing concern than it has been in the recent past. Underlying this sharp increase in abuse is methamphetamine. Known by a variety of names and forms, including "crank," "ice," "crystal," "meth," "speed," "crystal meth," and "zip," methamphetamine is produced in illegal home laboratories.

Ice. Crystal meth, or ice, is among the most dangerous forms of methamphetamine. Ice is a very pure form of methamphetamine that looks like rock candy. When smoked, the effects of ice are felt in about 7 seconds as a wave of intense physical and psychological exhilaration. This effect lasts for several hours (much longer than the effects of *crack*) until the user becomes physically exhausted. Chronic use leads to nutritional difficulties, weight loss, reduced resistance to infection, and damage to the liver, lungs, and kidneys. Psychological dependence is quickly established. Withdrawal causes acute depression and fatigue but not significant physical discomfort.

Ephedra. Health professionals are warning people about the dangers of using any over-the-counter herbal supplement containing ephedra. Also known as *ma huang,* ephedra is an amphetamine-like drug that can be especially dangerous for people with hypertension or other cardiovascular disease. Presently, ephedra is used in many over-the-counter decongestants and asthma drugs. However, in these products, warning labels indicate possible harmful side effects and drug interactions. In herbal products that contain ephedra, some of which are promoted as weight-control aids, these warnings are not required.[5] At the time of this writing, the FDA was considering restrictions on the use of this drug.

Ritalin. A prescription stimulant drug that has surged in popularity in recent years is Ritalin. This drug is typically prescribed to children and adolescents (and increasing numbers of young adults) to help them focus attention if they are hyperactive or cannot concentrate. Ritalin can be abused when the drug is shared among friends. Critics of Ritalin use argue that it is being over-prescribed to treat a variety of problems, when a preferred course would be to identify and treat root causes of the problems. Supporters respond that Ritalin has enabled youth to succeed in school.

Cocaine

Cocaine, perhaps the strongest of the stimulant drugs, has received much media attention. It is the primary psychoactive substance found in the leaves of the South American coca plant. The effects of cocaine are brief—from 5 to 30 minutes (Figure 7-2). Regardless of the form in which it is consumed, cocaine produces an immediate, near-orgasmic "rush," or feeling of exhilaration. This euphoria is quickly followed by a period of marked depression. Used only occasionally as a topical anesthetic, cocaine is usually inhaled (snorted), injected, or smoked (as *freebase* or crack). There is overwhelming scientific evidence that users quickly develop a strong psychological dependence to cocaine. There is considerable evidence that physical dependence also rapidly develops. However, physical dependence on cocaine does not lead to death upon withdrawal.

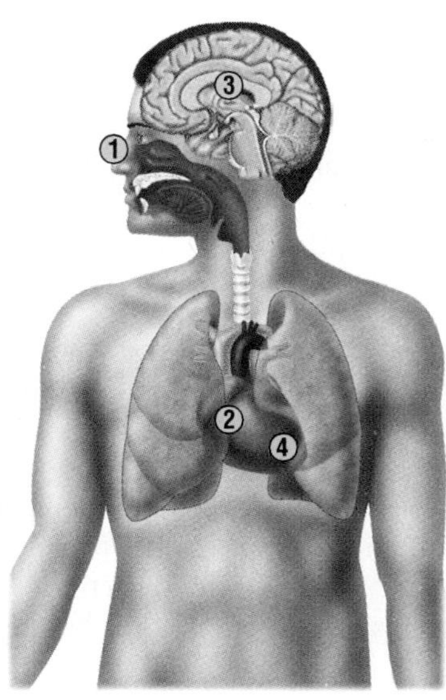

① **The nose:** as cocaine is snorted, nasal vessels immediately constrict and prohibit about 40% of the drug from entering the body. The remaining 60% enters the bloodstream.

② **The heart:** electrical impulses that regulate rhythmic pumping are impaired. Beating becomes irregular (arrhythmia). The heart can no longer supply itself with enough oxygenated blood.

③ **The brain:** dopamine and norepinephrine are released into the brain, producing a feeling of euphoria and confidence. Electrical signals to the heart are distorted, heart rate and pulse increase. A seizure may occur, causing coma and breathing stoppage.

④ **The heart:** blood circulation is out of control. The heart may simply flutter and stop, or it can be pumping so little oxygenated blood to the brain that the brain dies and the heart stops beating.

Figure 7-2 Cocaine's effects on the body.

Freebasing

Freebasing and the use of crack cocaine are the most recent techniques for maximizing the psychoactive effects of the drug. Freebasing first requires that the common form of powdered cocaine (cocaine hydrochloride) be chemically altered (alkalized). This altered form is then dissolved in a solvent, such as ether or benzene. This liquid solution is heated to evaporate the solvent. The heating process leaves the freebase cocaine in a powder form that can then be smoked, often through a water pipe. Because of the large surface area of the lungs, smoking cocaine facilitates fast absorption into the bloodstream.

One danger of freebasing cocaine is the risk related to the solvents used. Ether is a highly volatile solvent capable of exploding and causing serious burns. Benzene is a known carcinogen associated with the development of leukemia. Clearly, neither solvent can be used without increasing the level of risk normally associated with cocaine use. This method of making smokeable cocaine led to a new epidemic of cocaine use, smoking crack.

Crack

In contrast to freebase cocaine, crack is made by combining cocaine hydrochloride with common baking soda. When this pastelike mixture is allowed to dry, a small rocklike crystalline material remains. This crack is heated in the bowl of a small pipe, and the vapors are inhaled into the lungs. Some crack users spend hundreds of dollars a day to maintain their habit.

The effect of crack is almost instantaneous. Within 10 seconds after inhalation, cocaine reaches the CNS and influences the action of several neurotransmitters at specific sites in the brain. As with the use of other forms of cocaine, convulsions, seizures, respiratory distress, and cardiac failure have been reported with this sudden, extensive stimulation of the nervous system.

Within about 6 minutes, the stimulating effect of crack becomes completely expended, and users frequently become depressed. Dependence develops within a few weeks, since users consume more crack in response to the short duration of stimulation and rapid onset of depression.

Intravenous administration has been the preferred route for cocaine users who are also regular users of heroin and other injectable drugs. Intravenous injection

Key Terms

narcolepsy (nar co LEP see)
A sleep disorder in which a person has a recurrent, overwhelming, and uncontrollable desire to sleep.

attention deficit hyperactivity disorder (ADHD)
Above-normal rate of physical movement; often accompanied by an inability to concentrate well on a specified task; also called *hyperactivity.*

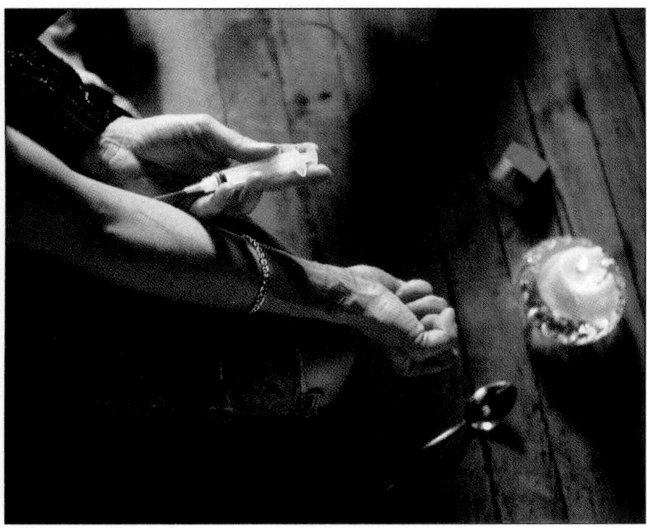

Intravenous injection of cocaine results in an almost immediate high for the user.

results in an almost immediate high, which lasts about 10 minutes. A "smoother ride" is said to be obtained from a "speedball," the injectable mixture of heroin and cocaine (or methamphetamine).[3]

Depressants

Depressants (or sedatives) sedate the user, slowing down CNS function. Drugs included in this category are alcohol (see Chapter 8), barbiturates, and tranquilizers. Depressants produce tolerance in abusers, as well as strong psychological and physical dependence.

Barbiturates

Barbiturates are the so-called sleeping compounds that function by enhancing the effect of inhibitory neurotransmitters. They depress the CNS to the point where the user drops off to sleep or, as is the case with surgical anesthetics, the patient becomes anesthetized. Medically, barbiturates are used in widely varied dosages as anesthetics and for treatment of anxiety, insomnia, and epilepsy.[2] Regular use of a barbiturate quickly produces tolerance—eventually such a high dose is required that the user still feels the effects of the drug throughout the next morning. Some abusers then begin to alternate barbiturates with stimulants, producing a vicious cycle of dependence. Other misusers combine alcohol and barbiturates or tranquilizers, inadvertently producing toxic or even lethal results. Abrupt withdrawal from barbiturate use frequently produces a withdrawal syndrome that can involve seizures, delusions, hallucinations, and even death.

Methaqualone (Quaalude, "ludes," Sopor) was developed as a sedative that would not have the dependence properties of other barbiturates. Although this did not happen, Quaaludes were occasionally prescribed for anxious patients. Today, compounds resembling Quaaludes are manufactured in home laboratories and sold illegally so that they can be combined with small amounts of alcohol for an inexpensive, drunklike effect.

Tranquilizers

Tranquilizers are depressants that are intended to reduce anxiety and to relax people who are having problems managing stress. They are not specifically designed to produce sleep but rather to help people cope during their waking hours. Such tranquilizers are termed *minor tranquilizers,* of which diazepam (Valium) and chlordiazepoxide (Librium) may be the most commonly prescribed examples. Unfortunately, some people become addicted to these and other prescription drugs (see the Focus on . . . box on p. 173).

Some tranquilizers are further designed to control hospitalized psychotic patients who may be suicidal or who are potential threats to others. These *major tranquilizers* subdue people physically but permit them to remain conscious. Their use is generally limited to institutional settings. All tranquilizers can produce physical and psychological dependence and tolerance.

"Date Rape" Depressants. Rohypnol (flunitrazepam) is a minor tranquilizer (a benzodiazepine) that is sold legally as a prescription drug in many countries but not in the United States. When Rohypnol is mixed with an alcoholic drink and then consumed, the drinker (generally an unsuspecting woman) becomes profoundly intoxicated. Hours later, when sober, she is unable to recall what happened to her, including rape. In response to the increased number of cases involving the use of Rohypnol, Congress passed the 1996 Drug-Induced Rape Prevention and Punishment Act. It is now a federal crime to give someone a drug, without the user's knowledge, to aid in sexual assault. The maximum penalty for this crime is 20 years in prison and a $250,000 fine.[2] GHB (G, liquid ecstasy) and ketamine (K, Special K, Cat) are additional depressants that are being used as date rape drugs.[6] These drugs should serve as a reminder to all partygoers to keep an extremely careful watch over any drink in their possession.

Hallucinogens

As the name suggests, hallucinogenic drugs produce hallucinations—perceived distortions of reality. Also known as *psychedelic* drugs or *phantasticants,* **hallucinogens** reached their height of popularity during the 1960s. At that time, young people were encouraged to use hallucinogenic drugs to "expand the mind," "reach an altered state," or "discover reality." Not all of the reality distortions, or "trips," were pleasant. Many users reported "bummers," or trips during which they perceived negative, frightening distortions.

Hallucinogenic drugs include laboratory-produced lysergic acid diethylamide (LSD), mescaline (from the peyote cactus plant), and psilocybin (from a particular genus of mushroom). Consumption of hallucinogens seems to produce not physical dependence but mild levels of psychological dependence. The development of tolerance is questionable. *Synesthesia,* a sensation in which users report hearing a color, smelling music, or touching a taste, is sometimes produced with hallucinogen use.

The long-term effects of hallucinogenic drug use are not fully understood. Questions about genetic abnormalities in offspring, fertility, sex drive and performance, and the development of personality disorders have not been fully answered. One phenomenon that has been identified and documented is the development of *flashbacks*—the unpredictable return to a psychedelic trip that occurred months or even years earlier. Flashbacks are thought to result from the accumulation of a drug within body cells.

LSD

The most well-known hallucinogen is lysergic acid diethylamide. LSD ("acid") is a drug that helped define the counterculture movement of the 1960s. During the 1970s and the 1980s, this drug lost considerable popularity. However, LSD is making a comeback, with some studies showing that about 1 in 10 high school students and 1 in 20 college students has experimented with LSD. Fear of cocaine and other powerful drugs, boredom, low cost, and an attempt to revisit the culture of the 1960s are thought to have increased LSD's attractiveness to today's young people.

LSD is manufactured in home laboratories and frequently distributed in blotter paper decorated with cartoon characters. Users place the paper on their tongue or chew the paper to ingest the drug. LSD can produce a psychedelic (mind-viewing) effect that includes altered perception of shapes, images, time, sound, and body form. Synesthesia is common to LSD users. Ingested in doses known as "hits," LSD produces a 6- to 9-hour experience.

Although the hits today are about half as powerful as those in the 1960s, users still tend to develop high tolerance to LSD. Physical dependence does not occur. Not all LSD trips are pleasant. Hallucinations produced from LSD can be frightening and dangerous. Users can injure or kill themselves accidentally during a bad trip. Dangerous side effects include panic attacks, flashbacks, and occasional prolonged psychosis.

Designer drugs

In recent years, chemists who produce many of the illicit drugs in home laboratories have designed versions of drugs listed on **FDA Schedule 1.** These *designer drugs* are similar to the controlled drugs on the FDA Schedule 1 but are sufficiently different so that they escape governmental control. The designer drugs are either newly synthesized products that are similar to already outlawed drugs but against which no law yet exists, or they are reconstituted or renamed illegal substances. Designer drugs are said to produce effects similar to their controlled drug counterparts.

People who use designer drugs do so at great risk because the manufacturing of these drugs is unregulated. The neurophysiological effect of these homemade drugs can be quite dangerous. So far, a synthetic heroin product (MPPP) and several amphetamine derivatives with hallucinogenic properties have been designed for the unwary drug consumer.

DOM (STP), MDA (the "love drug"), and ecstasy (MDMA or "XTC") are examples of amphetamine-derivative, hallucinogenic designer drugs. These drugs produce mild LSD-like hallucinogenic experiences, positive feelings, and enhanced alertness. They also have a number of potentially dangerous effects. Experts are particularly concerned that ecstasy can produce strong psychological dependence and can deplete serotonin, an important excitatory neurotransmitter associated with a state of alertness. Permanent brain damage is possible.

Phencyclidine

Phencyclidine (PCP, "angel dust") has been classified variously as a hallucinogen, a stimulant, a depressant, and an anesthetic. PCP was studied for years during the 1950s and 1960s and was found to be an unsuitable animal and human anesthetic. PCP is an extremely unpredictable drug. Easily manufactured in home laboratories in tablet or powder form, PCP can be injected, inhaled, taken orally, or smoked. The effects vary. Some users report mild euphoria, although most report bizarre perceptions, paranoid feelings, and aggressive behavior. PCP

Key Terms

hallucinogens
Psychoactive drugs capable of producing hallucinations (distortions of reality).

FDA Schedule 1
A list of drugs that have a high potential for abuse but no medical use.

overdose may cause convulsions, cardiovascular collapse, and damage to the brain's respiratory center.

In a number of cases the aggressive behavior caused by PCP has led users to commit brutal crimes against both friends and innocent strangers. PCP accumulates in cells and may stimulate bizarre behavior months after initial use.

Cannabis

Cannabis (marijuana) has been labeled a mild hallucinogen for a number of years. However, most experts now consider it to be a drug category in itself. Marijuana produces mild effects like those of stimulants and depressants. The implication of marijuana in a large number of traffic fatalities makes this drug one whose consumption should be carefully considered. Marijuana is actually a wild plant (*Cannabis sativa*) whose fibers were once used in the manufacture of hemp rope. When the leafy material and small stems are dried and crushed, users can smoke the mixture in rolled cigarettes ("joints"), cigars ("blunts"), or pipes. The resins collected from scraping the flowering tops of the plant yield a marijuana product called *hashish,* or *hash,* commonly smoked in a pipe.

The potency of marijuana's hallucinogenic effect is determined by the percentage of the active ingredient tetrahydrocannabinol (THC) present in the product. The concentration of THC averages about 3.5% for marijuana, 7% to 9% for higher-quality marijuana (sinsemilla), 8% to 14% for hashish, and as high as 50% for hash oil. Today's marijuana has THC levels that are higher than in past decades.

THC is a fat-soluble substance and thus is absorbed and retained in fat tissues within the body. Before being excreted, THC can remain in the body for up to a month. With the sophistication of today's drug tests, trace **metabolites** of THC can be detected for up to 30 days after consumption in the urine of chronic users of high doses of marijuana.[2] It is possible that the THC that comes from passive inhalation of high doses (for example, during an indoor rock concert) can also be detected for a short time after exposure.

Once marijuana is consumed, its effects vary from person to person. Being "high" or "stoned" or "wrecked" means different things to different people. Many people report heightened sensitivity to music, cravings for particular foods, and a relaxed mood. There is consensus that marijuana's behavioral effects include four probabilities: (1) users must learn to recognize what a marijuana high is like, (2) marijuana impairs short-term memory, (3) users overestimate the passage of time, and (4) users lose the ability to maintain attention to a task.

The long-term effects of marijuana use are still being studied. Chronic abuse may lead to an **amotivational syndrome** in some people. The irritating effects of marijuana smoke on lung tissue are more pronounced than those of cigarette smoke, and some of the over 400 chemicals in marijuana are now linked to lung cancer development. In fact, one of the most potent carcinogens, benzopyrene, is found in higher levels in marijuana smoke than in tobacco smoke. Marijuana smokers tend to inhale deeply and hold the smoke in the lungs for long periods. It is likely that at some point the lungs of chronic marijuana smokers will be damaged.

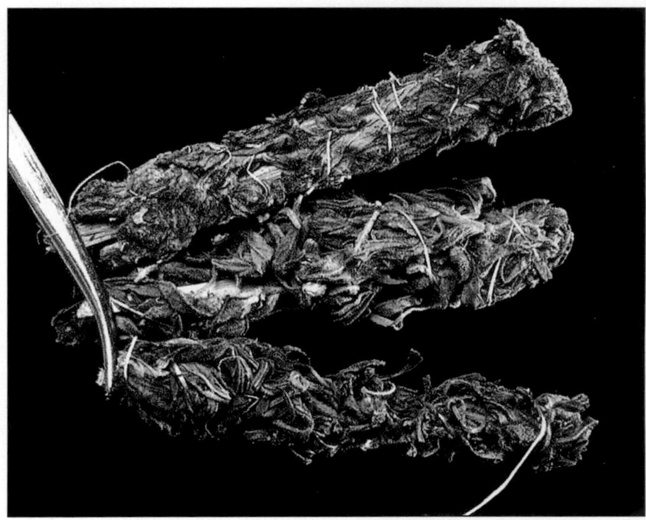

Thai sticks are a potent form of marijuana.

Long-term marijuana use is also associated with damage to the immune system and to the male and female reproductive systems and with an increase in birth defects in babies born to mothers who smoke marijuana. Chronic marijuana use lowers testosterone levels in men, but the effect of this change is not known. The effect of long-term marijuana use on a variety of types of sexual behavior is also not fully understood.

Because the drug can distort perceptions and thus perceptual ability (especially when combined with alcohol), its use by automobile drivers clearly jeopardizes the lives of many innocent people.

The only medical uses for marijuana are to relieve the nausea caused by chemotherapy, to improve the appetite in AIDS patients, and to ease the pressure that builds up in the eyes of glaucoma patients. However, a variety of other drugs, many of which are nearly as effective, are also used for these purposes. In May 2001, the U.S. Supreme Court ruled unanimously against the distribution of marijuana in medical clinics.

TALKING POINTS • How would you comfort a classmate that he is kidding himself when he says he is using marijuana for "medicinal purposes"?

Narcotics

The **narcotics** are among the most dependence-producing drugs. Medically, narcotics are used to relieve pain and induce sleep. On the basis of origin, narcotics can be subgrouped into the natural, quasisynthetic, and synthetic narcotics.z

Natural narcotics

Naturally occurring substances derived from the Oriental poppy plant include opium (the primary psychoactive substance extracted from the Oriental poppy), morphine (the primary active ingredient in opium), and thebaine (a compound not used as a drug). Morphine and related compounds have medical use as analgesics in the treatment of mild to severe pain.

Quasisynthetic narcotics

Quasisynthetic narcotics are compounds created by chemically altering morphine. These laboratory-produced drugs are intended to be used as analgesics, but their benefits are largely outweighed by a high dependence rate and a great risk of toxicity. The best known of the quasisynthetic narcotics is heroin. Although heroin is a fast-acting and very effective analgesic, it is extremely addictive. Once injected into a vein or "skin-popped" (injected beneath the skin surface), heroin produces dreamlike euphoria and, like all narcotics, strong physical and psychological dependence and tolerance.

As with the use of all other injectable illegal drugs, the practice of sharing needles increases the likelihood of transmission of various communicable diseases, including HIV (see Chapter 12). Abrupt withdrawal from heroin use is rarely fatal, but the discomfort during **cold turkey** withdrawal is reported to be overwhelming. The use of heroin has increased during the last decade. The purity of heroin has improved while the price has dropped. Cocaine abusers may use heroin to "come down" from the high associated with cocaine.

Synthetic narcotics

Meperidine (Demerol) and propoxyphene (Darvon), common postsurgical painkillers, and methadone, the drug prescribed during the rehabilitation of heroin addicts, are *synthetic narcotics.* These opiate-like drugs are manufactured in medical laboratories. They are not natural narcotics or quasisynthetic narcotics because they do not originate from the Oriental poppy plant. Like true narcotics, however, these drugs can rapidly induce physical dependence. One important criticism of methadone rehabilitation programs is that in some cases, they merely shift the addiction from heroin to methadone.

Inhalants

Inhalants are a class of drugs that includes a variety of volatile (quickly evaporating) compounds that generally produce unpredictable, drunklike effects in users. Users of inhalants may also have some delusions and hallucinations. Some users may become quite aggressive. Drugs in this category include anesthetic gases (chloroform, nitrous oxide, and ether), vasodilators (amyl nitrite and butyl nitrite), petroleum products and commercial solvents (gasoline, kerosene, plastic cement, glue, typewriter correction fluid, paint, and paint thinner), and certain aerosols (found in some propelled spray products, fertilizers, and insecticides).

Most of the danger in using inhalants lies in the damaging, sometimes fatal effects on the respiratory system. Furthermore, users may unknowingly place themselves in dangerous situations because of the drunklike hallucinogenic effects. Aggressive behavior might also make users a threat to themselves and others.

COMBINATION DRUG EFFECTS

Drugs taken in various combinations and dosages can alter and perhaps intensify effects.

A **synergistic drug effect** is a dangerous consequence of taking different drugs in the same general category at the same time. The combination exaggerates each individual drug's effects. For example, the combined use of alcohol and tranquilizers produces a synergistic

Key Terms

metabolite
A breakdown product of a drug.

amotivational syndrome
Behavioral pattern characterized by lack of interest in productive activities.

narcotics
Opiates; psychoactive drugs derived from the Oriental poppy plant; narcotics relieve pain and induce sleep.

cold turkey
Immediate, total discontinuation of use of a drug; associated withdrawal discomfort.

inhalants
Psychoactive drugs that enter the body through inhalation.

synergistic drug effect (sin er JIST ick)
Heightened, exaggerated effect produced by the concurrent use of two or more drugs.

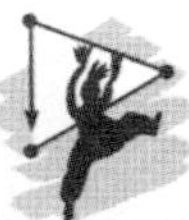

HealthQuest Activities

Drug abuse can occur with illegal drugs or with over-the-counter or prescription drugs. Complete the assessment activity *Drugs: Are You at Risk?* in the Other Drugs module to raise your awareness of the many decisions you make about drugs. What is your overall risk score? Do you think the score is accurate? Do you think your score reflects campuswide drug use? What are the causes of drug abuse, and what can be done to prevent it?

effect greater than the total effect of each of the two drugs taken separately. In this instance a much-amplified, perhaps fatal sedation will occur. In a simplistic sense, "one plus one equals four or five."

When taken at or near the same time, drug combinations produce a variety of effects. Drug combinations have additive, potentiating, or antagonistic effects. When two or more drugs are taken and the result is merely a combined total effect of each drug, the result is an **additive effect.** The sum of the effects is not exaggerated. In a sense, "one plus one plus one equals three."

When one drug intensifies the action of a second drug, the first drug is said to have a **potentiated effect** on the second drug. One popular drug-taking practice during the 1970s was the consumption of Quaaludes and beer. Quaaludes potentiated the inhibition-releasing, sedative effects of alcohol. This particular drug combination produced an inexpensive but potentially fatal drunk-like euphoria in the user.

An **antagonistic effect** is an opposite effect one drug has on another drug. One drug may be able to reduce another drug's influence on the body. Knowledge of this principle has been useful in the medical treatment of certain drug overdoses, as in the use of tranquilizers to relieve the effects of LSD or other hallucinogenic drugs.

DRUG TESTING

Society's response to concern over drug use includes the development and growing use of drug tests. Most of the specimens come from corporations that screen employees for commonly abused drugs. Among these are amphetamines, barbiturates, benzodiazepines (the chemical bases for prescription tranquilizers such as Valium and Librium), cannabinoids (THC, hashish, and marijuana), methaqualone, opiates (heroin, codeine, and morphine), and PCP. With the exception of marijuana, most traces of these drugs are eliminated by the body within a few days after use. Marijuana can remain detectable for weeks after use.

How accurate are the results of drug testing? At typical cutoff standards, drug tests will likely identify 90% of recent drug users. This means that about 10% of recent users will pass undetected. (These 10% are considered false negatives.) Nonusers whose drug tests indicate drug use (false positives) are quite rare. (Follow-up tests on these false positives would nearly always show negative results.) Human errors are probably more responsible than technical errors for inaccuracies in drug tests.

Recently, scientists have been refining procedures that use hair samples to detect the presence of drugs. These procedures seem to hold much promise, although certain technical obstacles remain. Watch for refinements in hair-sample drug testing in the near future.

Most Fortune 500 companies, the armed forces, various government agencies, and nearly all athletic organizations have already implemented mandatory drug testing. Corporate substance abuse policies are being developed, with careful attention to legal and ethical issues.

Do you think that the possibility of having to take a drug test would have any effect on college students' use of drugs?

COLLEGE AND COMMUNITY SUPPORT SERVICES FOR DRUG DEPENDENCE

Students who have drug problems and realize they need help might select assistance based on the services available on campus or in the surrounding community and the costs they are willing to pay for treatment services.

One approach to convince drug-dependent people to enter treatment programs is the use of *confrontation.* People who live or work with chemically dependent people are being encouraged to confront them directly about their addiction. Direct confrontation helps chemically dependent people realize the effect their behavior has on others. Once chemically dependent people realize that others will no longer tolerate their behavior, the likelihood of their entering treatment programs increases significantly. Although effective, this approach is very stressful for family members and friends and requires the assistance of professionals in the field of chemical dependence. These professionals can be contacted at a drug treatment center in your area.

Treatment

Comprehensive drug treatment programs are available in very few college or university health centers. College settings for drug dependence programs are more commonly found in the university counseling center. At such a center the emphasis will probably be not on the medical management of dependence but on the behavioral dimensions of drug abuse. Trained counselors and psychologists who specialize in chemical dependence counseling will work with students to (1) analyze their particular concerns, (2) establish constructive ways to cope with stress, and (3) search for alternative ways to achieve new "highs" (see the Personal Assessment on p. 171).

TALKING POINTS • Do you think that confronting a friend about her cocaine use would prompt her to get help?

Medical treatment for the management of drug problems may need to be obtained through the services of a community treatment facility administered by a local health department, community mental health center, private clinic, or local hospital. Treatment may be on an inpatient or outpatient basis. Medical management might include detoxification, treatment of secondary health complications and nutritional deficiencies, and therapeutic counseling for chemical dependence.

Some communities have voluntary health agencies that deliver services and treatment programs for drug-dependent people. Check your telephone book for listings of drug-treatment facilities. Some communities have drug hot lines that offer advice for people with questions about drugs. (See the Changing for the Better box on p. 153 for a list of anti–drug abuse organizations and hot line numbers.)

Costs of treatment for dependence

Drug-treatment programs that are administered by colleges and universities for faculty and students usually require no fees. Local agencies may provide either free services or services based on a **sliding scale.** Private hospitals, physicians, and clinics are the most expensive forms of treatment. Inpatient treatment at a private facility may cost as much as $1000 per day. Since the length of inpatient treatment averages 3 to 4 weeks, a patient can quickly accumulate a very large bill. However, with many types of health insurance policies now providing coverage for alcohol and other drug dependencies, even these services may not require additional out-of-pocket expenses.

Key Terms

additive effect
The combined (but not exaggerated) effect produced by the concurrent use of two or more drugs.

potentiated effect (poe ten she ay ted)
Phenomenon whereby the use of one drug intensifies the effect of a second drug.

antagonistic effect
Effect produced when one drug reduces or offsets the effects of a second drug.

sliding scale
A method of payment by which patient fees are scaled according to income.

SUMMARY

- Drug abuse has a devastating effect on society.
- Society's response to drug abuse has been widely varied and has included education, enforcement, treatment, testing, and the search for drug-free ways to achieve highs.
- Drug use, drug abuse, tolerance, and dependence are important terms to understand.
- A drug affects the CNS by altering neurotransmitter activity on the neuron.
- Drugs can be placed into six categories: stimulants, depressants, hallucinogens, cannabis, narcotics, and inhalants.
- Drugs enter the body through ingestion, injection, inhalation, or absorption.
- Combination drug effects include synergistic, additive, potentiated, and antagonistic effects.
- Drug testing is becoming increasingly common in our society.

REVIEW QUESTIONS

1. How is the term *drug* defined in this chapter? What are psychoactive drugs? How do medicines differ from drugs?
2. Explain what *dependence* means. Identify and explain the two types of dependence.
3. Define the word *tolerance.* What does *cross-tolerance* mean? Give an example of cross-tolerance.
4. Differentiate between drug misuse and drug abuse.
5. Define the four routes of administration. Select a drug that reflects each of the ways drugs enter the body.
6. Describe how neurotransmitters work.
7. List the six general categories of drugs. For each category, give several examples of drugs and explain the effects they would have on the user. What are designer drugs?

8. What is the active ingredient in marijuana? What are its common effects on the user? What are the long-term effects of marijuana use?
9. Explain the terms synergistic effect, additive effect, potentiated effect, and antagonistic effect.
10. How accurate is drug testing?

REFERENCES

1. Office of National Drug Policy: Federal drug control spending by goal and function, *Summary: FY2002 National Drug Control Budget,* April 2001, U.S. Government Printing Office, p. 9.
2. Ray O, Ksir C: *Drugs, society, and human behavior,* ed 9, 1999, McGraw-Hill.
3. Pinger RR, Payne WA, Hahn DB, Hahn EJ: *Drugs: issues for today,* ed 3, 1998, McGraw-Hill.
4. Shier D, Butler J, Lewis R: *Essentials of anatomy and physiology,* ed 6, 1998, McGraw-Hill.
5. Avoid an herbal supplement containing ephedra, *UC Berkeley Wellness Letter,* 16(1):8, 1999.
6. National Institute on Drug Abuse: *Club drugs,* www.clubdrugs.org, accessed August 21, 2001.

SUGGESTED READINGS

Breggin PR, Cohen D: *Your drug may be your problem: how and when to stop taking psychiatric drugs,* 1999, Perseus Books.

The authors of this book (an MD and a PhD) contend that many people currently using psychiatric drugs, including Prozac and lithium-based medications, might be better off without them. They argue that the side effects of these drugs are dangerous enough, but the drugs also tend to reduce the users' abilities to solve their own difficulties. Much of the book is devoted to showing users how to gradually wean themselves from their medications. This book is controversial, so before starting its recommended program, consult with your physician.

Drummond EH: *Benzo blues: overcoming anxiety without tranquilizers,* 1998, Plume.

Drummond is a physician who believes that too many people are addicted to benzodiazepines ("benzos"), tranquilizers that are frequently prescribed for chronic anxiety. He believes that the problems created by dependence on these tranquilizers can overshadow the original basis for the chronic anxiety. Drummond's approach is to carefully move away from the benzodiazepines and address the core problems. He shows how this can be done successfully.

Marlatt GA: *Harm reduction: pragmatic strategies for managing high-risk behaviors,* 1998, Guilford Press.

This book does an excellent job of discussing harm reduction, the latest approach to treatment of addictions. Instead of focusing on abstinence from high-risk behaviors, harm reduction emphasizes careful management of high-risk activities so that a safe outcome is likely. The author discusses various public health issues, including HIV prevention, in light of this new approach.

West JW: *The Betty Ford Center book of answers: help for those struggling with substance abuse and the people who love them,* New York, 1997, Pocket Books.

This book is written by the former director of the Betty Ford Center, one of the leading alcohol and drug treatment centers in the United States. This authoritative source provides answers to many of the most frequently asked questions about treatment and recovery. It offers comprehensive coverage of drug abuse issues for addicts and their families.

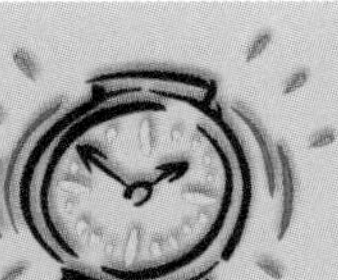

As we go to Press...

Increased attention is being focused on the devastating impact of the use of the prescription narcotic painkiller OxyContin. For cancer patients in severe pain, this agent has been a wonder drug, providing a steady 12-hour release of pain-killing medicine with relatively few side effects. Known as "hillbilly heroin" because of its impact in Appalachian states, OxyContin was linked to nearly 300 recent deaths in an October 2001 federal review of autopsy data by the Drug Enforcement Administration. Law enforcement officials are focusing on criminals who rob pharmacies to get OxyContin and physicians who commit prescription fraud by illegally dispensing OxyContin to otherwise healthy people.

Name ______________________ **Date** __________ **Section** __________

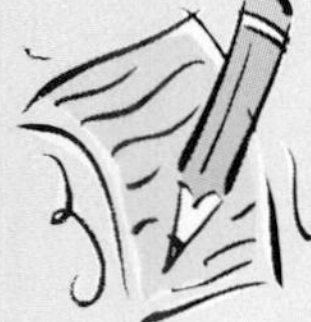

Personal Assessment

Test Your Drug Awareness

1. What is the most commonly used drug in the United States?
   (*a*) heroin
   (*b*) cocaine
   (*c*) alcohol
   (*d*) marijuana

2. Name the three drugs most commonly used by children.
   (*a*) alcohol, tobacco, and marijuana
   (*b*) cocaine, crack, alcohol
   (*c*) heroin, inhalants, marijuana

3. Which drug is associated with the most teenage deaths?
   (*a*) heroin
   (*b*) cocaine
   (*c*) alcohol
   (*d*) marijuana

4. By the eighth grade, how many kids have tried at least one inhalant?
   (*a*) one in one hundred
   (*b*) one in fifty
   (*c*) one in twenty five
   (*d*) one in five
   (*e*) one in two

5. "Crack" is a particularly dangerous drug because it is
   (*a*) cheap.
   (*b*) readily available.
   (*c*) highly addictive.
   (*d*) all of the above.

6. Fumes from which of the following can be inhaled to produce a high?
   (*a*) spray paint
   (*b*) model glue
   (*c*) nail polish remover
   (*d*) whipped cream canisters
   (*e*) all of the above

7. People who have not used alcohol and other drugs before their 20th birthday:
   (*a*) have no risk of becoming chemically dependent.
   (*b*) are less likely to develop a drinking problem or use illicit drugs.
   (*c*) have an increased risk of becoming chemically dependent.

8. A speedball is a combination of which two drugs?
   (*a*) cocaine and heroin
   (*b*) PCP and LSD
   (*c*) valium and alcohol
   (*d*) amphetamines and barbiturates

9. Methamphetamines are dangerous because use can cause
   (*a*) anxiety/nervousness/irritability.
   (*b*) paranoia/psychosis.
   (*c*) loss of appetite/malnutrition/anorexia.
   (*d*) hallucinations.
   (*e*) aggressive behavior.
   (*f*) all of the above.

10. How is marijuana harmful?
    (*a*) It hinders the user's short-term memory.
    (*b*) Students may find it hard to study and learn while under the influence of marijuana.
    (*c*) It affects timing and coordination.
    (*d*) All of the above

Source: *A parent's guide to prevention,* U.S. Department of Education.

Answers to Personal Assessment

1. c
2. a
3. c
4. d
5. d
6. e
7. b
8. a
9. f
10. d

Name ______________________ **Date** __________ **Section** __________

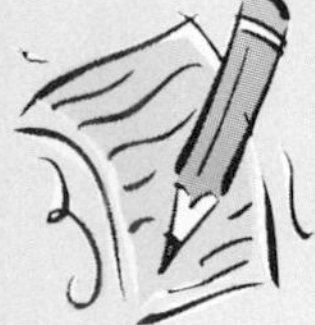

Personal Assessment

Getting a Drug-Free High

Experts agree that drug use provides only short-term, ineffective, and often destructive solutions to problems. We hope that you have found (or will find) innovative, invigorating drug-free experiences that make your life more exciting. Circle the number for each activity that reflects your intention to try that activity. Use the following guide:

1 No intention of trying this activity
2 Intend to try this within 2 years
3 Intend to try this within 6 months
4 Already tried this activity
5 Regularly engage in this activity

1. Learn to juggle	1	2	3	4	5
2. Go backpacking	1	2	3	4	5
3. Complete a marathon race	1	2	3	4	5
4. Start a vegetable garden	1	2	3	4	5
5. Ride in a hot air balloon	1	2	3	4	5
6. Snow ski or water ski	1	2	3	4	5
7. Donate blood	1	2	3	4	5
8. Go river rafting	1	2	3	4	5
9. Learn to play a musical instrument	1	2	3	4	5
10. Cycle 100 miles	1	2	3	4	5
11. Go skydiving	1	2	3	4	5
12. Go rockclimbing	1	2	3	4	5
13. Play a role in a theater production	1	2	3	4	5
14. Build a piece of furniture	1	2	3	4	5
15. Solicit funds for a worthy cause	1	2	3	4	5
16. Learn to swim	1	2	3	4	5
17. Overhaul a car engine	1	2	3	4	5
18. Compose a song	1	2	3	4	5
19. Travel to a foreign country	1	2	3	4	5
20. Write the first chapter of a book	1	2	3	4	5

TOTAL POINTS ______________

Interpretation

61–100 You participate in many challenging experiences

41–60 You are willing to try some challenging new experiences

20–40 You take few of the challenging risks described here

To Carry This Further . . .

Looking at your point total, were you surprised at the degree to which you are aware of alternative activities? What are the top five activities, and can you understand their importance? What activities would you add to this list?

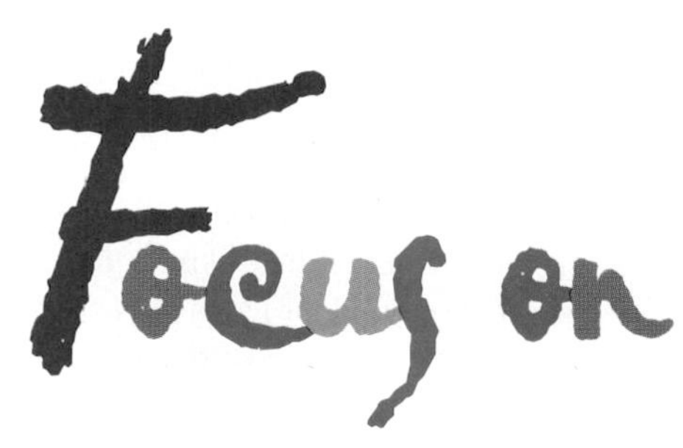

PRESCRIPTION DRUG ABUSE

Lucy, a 35-year-old mother of two, seems like a typical suburban homemaker. She attends church regularly, belongs to the PTA, and volunteers at the local battered women's shelter. Her husband is a well-respected businessman, and her children are honor students at the local high school. Life seems perfect for Lucy and her family, at least on the outside. But Lucy has a secret that few outside her family know about.

Lucy's children and husband regularly come home to a disheveled household, finding Lucy passed out somewhere in the house or on the back porch. Lucy's mood swings are unpredictable. One day, she will be a loving, devoted wife and mother; the next, she will talk rapidly and endlessly to whomever she can get to listen; sometimes, her speech will slur and she will seem incoherent. All this usually occurs whenever a stressful or unpleasant situation comes up in her life with which she cannot cope. Lucy's family never knows what to expect from one day to the next. The children have moved in and out of the home to live with their grandparents dozens of times over the past several years, and Lucy's husband has threatened her with divorce. Lucy has been to inpatient detoxification programs three times, only to "fall off the wagon" whenever a stressful event occurs.

You would probably guess that Lucy is an alcoholic or an illegal drug addict; however, Lucy's drugs of choice are all legal and all readily available to her from any one of a number of reputable physicians she visits. She uses a combination of drugs that range from sedatives to tranquilizers to antidepressants. Lucy is a prescription drug addict. Her suppliers are unwitting physicians who have no idea that she is seeing other doctors.

The reported numbers on the abuse of prescription drugs are alarming.[1] Approximately 245,000 senior citizens are hospitalized each year for abuse of prescription drugs.[2] It is estimated that up to 50% of all prescriptions are used incorrectly.[1,2]

According to the Drug Enforcement Administration, 12 of the top 20 most abused controlled substances are prescription drugs.[1] These drugs fall into the following categories:

- *Opioids.* These drugs are narcotics typically prescribed to relieve acute or chronic pain. Common prescription drugs include Demerol, Darvocet, Vicodin, and drugs with codeine.
- *Stimulants.* These drugs affect the central nervous system and increase mental alertness, decrease fatigue, and produce a sense of well-being. They are usually prescribed for appetite suppression, attention deficit disorder, and narcolepsy. Common prescription drugs include Dexedrine, Ritalin, Fastin, and Cyclert.
- *Sedatives.* These drugs depress the central nervous system and are frequently used to treat anxiety, panic disorder, and insomnia. Some are dispensed for either daytime or nighttime use. Common prescription drugs include Xanax, Valium, Ativan, Dalmane, and Ambien.

Under certain conditions, nearly anybody could wind up abusing a prescription drug, but there are particular groups of people who are at high risk for prescription drug abuse. People with a family history of depression, smokers, and excessive drinkers are more likely to become addicted to prescription drugs, as are those with a history of abusing illegal drugs. Stress from traumatic experiences can also make a person more likely to abuse prescription drugs, and people who are hyperactive, obese, or who suffer from chronic pain are also at risk. Health care professionals are considered to be a high-risk group,[2,3,4] and older people have a greater tendency to abuse prescription drugs.[5]

A patient can become physiologically dependent on a drug, which is considered to be a more manageable condition than addiction. Physiological dependence, involving the body's adaptation to a drug over time, is considered a temporary, benign condition. Physiological dependence is usually treated by gradual reductions in use of the drug, and although there may be withdrawal symptoms during this period, there is not normally a relapse afterward. The gradual reduction in dosage can be handled with medical supervision, and the patient does not normally need to enter a substance abuse program. Addiction involves a continued need to use a drug for psychological effects or mood alteration, and the patient goes to great lengths to obtain the drug even if its effects become harmful. Addiction is considered a chronic, complex problem and is usually handled with specific chemical dependence treatment.[1]

Abuse is often caused or continued because of deliberate deception on the part of the patient, but misuse of a prescription drug can start innocently enough. A patient may be receiving several prescriptions that have the same effect, or a patient may have several doctors prescribing the same medication. Prescription drugs may react with each other and cause different effects than intended. Sometimes communication problems between patient and physician cause errors in prescription dispensation.

The patient may unintentionally use the prescription incorrectly. One of these situations or a combination of factors can start prescription drug abuse.[5] Often a single prescription drug, such as a painkiller or sedative, is enough to start the process of dependence.

Older people are considered at high risk for prescription drug abuse for several reasons. The process of aging or the transition to retirement can leave a person with symptoms of depression or anxiety, and illnesses can also increase as a person gets older. Many people see multiple doctors as they get older and thus may wind up getting several prescriptions for the same drug under different brand names without realizing it. Sometimes physicians give older patients the same dosages as younger patients. Body functions slow and change with age, and when this occurs, the duration and intensity of drug effects can change as well.[5] Such conditions can increase the risk of drug abuse among the elderly.

If addiction starts, older people may then resort to the same tactics as any prescription drug addict. They may begin to "doctor-hop" (moving from one doctor to the next without informing the doctors) to get multiple prescriptions, or they may go to an emergency room to get a quick fix of a particular drug. Patients may also hoard pills or swap pills with friends to cut costs and ensure availability of their drug of choice. In the United States, it is estimated that 2 million older adults are at risk of addiction or are addicted to tranquilizers or sleeping pills.[5]

Health care professionals are also at high risk for prescription drug abuse. Physicians are five times more likely than the general population to take sedatives or tranquilizers without another doctor's supervision. The high stress of the job and the availability of drugs are both believed to be contributing factors to abuse among health care professionals. However, studies suggest that those physicians who are psychologically sound had little problem handling the stress of their jobs and generally resisted the temptation of readily available drugs. Those physicians considered to have psychological problems were more likely to be abusers.[3]

Effects of Abuse

As abuse of a drug continues, the tolerance of the body to that drug increases, which can lead to stronger self-dosing. As use increases, the detoxification process can become more difficult. In some cases, people refuse to believe they are addicted, and older people who are isolated from others do not even realize they are hooked.[5] Physicians may inadvertently promote the abuse by failing or refusing to acknowledge the signs of addiction in a patient.

If a person admits he or she has a problem with a drug, the recovery process can begin, but trying to kick the habit without professional help may only make things worse. If the person tries to cut back or stop use of the drug, withdrawal symptoms may occur. These symptoms include pain, nausea, sleeplessness, nervousness, irritability, hallucinations, and confusion, and can be quite severe. Sometimes other underlying psychological problems (for example, depression) must also be dealt with to prevent a relapse.[5] In short, recovery from prescription drug abuse becomes as difficult as recovery from abuse of illegal drugs. For these reasons, professional help is usually necessary for a full recovery from prescription drug abuse.

If you or someone you know is abusing prescription drugs, help is available. Many hospitals that sponsor detoxification programs for alcoholics and illegal drug addicts also have programs for individuals who are addicted to prescription drugs. Often, insurance will cover the costs of these programs. After detoxification the individual will need to continue recovery through a program such as Alcoholics Anonymous (the principles used for recovery from alcoholism are also applicable to recovery from drug addiction), Narcotics Anonymous, or Benzodiazepine Anonymous. These organizations can be found in the white pages of the phone book.

If the addicted person has family or close friends who are being seriously affected by addiction issues, they may want to try Al-Anon, Alateen, or Adult Children of Alcoholics support groups. Finally, individual or family counseling may be of value in helping to sort out emotional issues that lie behind the addiction. A certified addictions counselor may be the most helpful person to an addict, or the family may choose a psychiatrist, psychologist, or social worker who has knowledge of addiction issues.

You also might wish to get additional information by going on-line to **www.prescriptionabuse.org.** This website was created by a man whose wife was a former prescription drug addict. The site offers education, hope, and recovery approaches for abusers and their families.[6]

Although prescription drug addicts will always be "recovering" rather than "recovered," they can still lead relatively normal lives with proper physical and psychological treatment. However, there are no quick fixes or easy answers. Recovery is an ongoing process for both the addict and his or her family.

For Discussion . . .

Do you know of anyone who has intentionally abused prescription drugs? Have you ever taken a prescription drug in a different way than it was prescribed? Have you ever taken someone else's prescription drug? If so, why did you do it? Can you think of a case where use of another person's prescription drug can be justified?

References

1. Colvin R: *Prescription drug abuse: the hidden epidemic,* 1995, Addicus Books.
2. Colvin R: I tried to be my brother's keeper: one family's battle with prescription drug abuse, *Family Circle,* 108(13), Sep 19, 1995.
3. Vaillant GE: Physician, cherish thyself: the hazards of self prescribing, *JAMA* 267(17), 1992.
4. Dabney D, Heffington TR: The pharmacy profession's reaction to substance abuse among pharmacists: the process and consequences of medicalization, *Journal of Drug Issues* 26(4), Fall 1996.
5. Chastain S: The accidental addict: are you hooked on your prescriptions? *Modern Maturity,* 35(1), Feb–Mar 1992.
6. **www.prescriptionabuse.org** [visited 11/3/99]

chapter **8**

Taking Control of Alcohol Use

Online Learning Center Resources

www.mhhe.com/hahn6e

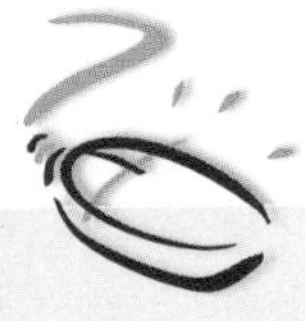

Log on to our Online Learning Center (OLC) for access to these additional resources:

- Chapter key terms and definitions
- Learning objectives
- Additional behavior change objectives
- Student interactive question-and-answer sites
- Self-scoring chapter quiz

The OLC also offers web links for study and exploration of health topics. Here are some examples of what you'll find:

- **www.peele.net/aab/arf.html** Get mileage from this useful research tool provided by the Addiction Research Foundation of Canada.
- **www.alcoholics-anonymous.org** Log on to the homepage of the best known of all alcohol abuse treatment programs, Alcoholics Anonymous.
- **www.niaaa.nih.gov** Check out this indexed site for National Institutes of Health publications and databases, frequently asked questions, and more.

Taking Charge of Your Health

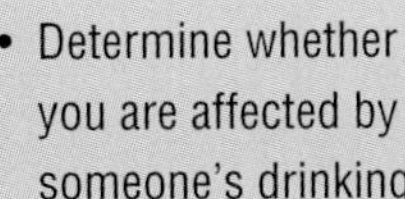

- Determine whether you are affected by someone's drinking by doing the Personal Assessment on p. 199.
- Prepare for a possible alcohol-related emergency by reviewing the signs listed in the Changing for the Better box on p. 183.
- Assess your level of social responsibility by using the Changing for the Better box on p. 189.
- If you think that you are a problem drinker or an alcoholic, join a support group to get help.
- Enter into a "Contract for Life" with your parents or closest friends, a pact that says that you will provide safe transportation for each other if either of you is unable to drive safely after consuming alcohol.
- Make a commitment to responsible alcohol use by joining a campus group that works toward this goal.

Eye on the Media

TV Ads Target Drunk Driving

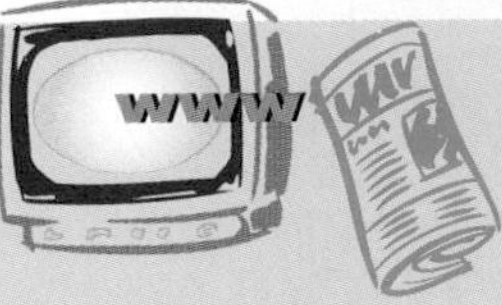

New York City Mayor Rudolph Giuliani needed only a day to do what took decades of advertising to accomplish—focus the public's attention on drunk driving. In the spring of 1999 he confiscated the car of a Queens resident who had a blood alcohol level of 0.19%, almost twice the legal limit of 0.10%. The debate was on—first about the legality of the mayor's action, then about the consequences of drunk driving.

The first successful national campaign against drunk driving, "Designated Driver," began in 1998. Besides targeting specific audiences and using well-timed and strategically placed public service announcements, its developers convinced TV producers and writers to work references to the designated driver into the dialogue of their shows. Gradually, the message got through to young people. It does make sense to plan to have someone else drive if you're not going to be up to it. The designated-driver approach is still considered a good idea on college campuses today.

In contrast, the "Campaign for Alcohol Free Kids," relied heavily on

Eye on the Media *continued*

dramatic graphics, such as grisly photos of car crash scenes on prom night. Although the overall visual impact was powerful, the campaign lacked a practical element. Worse, the ads seemed to be preaching.

The Ad Council's "Friends Don't Let Friends Drive Drunk" is based on the idea that we all have responsibility for each other. If someone is your friend, you want to take care of that person. So don't let your friend do something dangerous. Here the message is practical, not preachy.

The "You Drink & Drive, You Lose" campaign, a part of the National Public Education Campaign, targets two high-risk groups, 21- to 34-year-olds and repeat offenders. The message is simple: Make the right choice—don't drink and drive. The "Don't Lose It!" TV spot focuses on the fact that it's inconvenient to be stopped but the time spent at the checkpoint is for your own safety. It seems to be saying: "Sure, you're in a hurry, but this is important. So be patient." The graphics range from a serious-looking police officer talking to a motorist to hands locked in handcuffs.

What the successful campaigns have in common is a message that is simple, believable, and acceptable. Rather than scolding or preaching, the ads emphasize the fact that you have a choice and ask you to make the right choice.

"Road Predators," an American Public Television special that aired in December 1999, touched off strong contoversy. Funded by the Century Council, a corporation backed by a group of U.S. distillers, the program used tragic accounts of alcohol-related accidents to dramatize the fact that innocent people lose their lives, families are shattered, and billions of dollars are spent because of drunk drivers. The contrast between the life of the featured victim (a good and caring schoolteacher) and that of the drunk driver (an aimless man who spends most of his time drinking) was highlighted.

Beer manufacturers became angry. To them, the show suggested that drinking beer and driving is the problem, not drinking *any* type of alcohol and driving. Why, they wondered, was there no sign of hard liquor in the show? Other critics argued that by focusing on hard-core drinkers, the program implied that the problem of drunk driving is limited to a small group. What about bias? According to *The Wall Street Journal* ("Brewers Attack Drunken-Driving Special," Dec. 14, 1999, p. B8), the special's producer first claimed that the Century Group had had no input into its content but later conceded that it had supplied news clippings as background and had recommended that certain people be interviewed. As for accuracy, the deputy district attorney who tried the case said that it was not true that the drunk driver "very likely won't be required to complete" his 15-year sentence, as the program said. The producer responded that this was probably "a little dramatic license" on the writer's part. The sophisticated and expensive advertising for the special included an elaborate spread in *Newsweek* (Dec. 6, 1999), with an 8-page booklet featuring the drunk driver and the victim.

What is the motivation for an alcohol industry group to fund a campaign to discourage drunk driving? How do such campaigns compare with the tobacco industry's efforts to discourage smoking among teenagers? How effective do you think each kind of ad campaign is?

The push for zero tolerance laws, the tightening of standards for determining legal intoxication, and the growing influence of national groups concerned with alcohol misuse show that our society is more sensitive than ever to the growing misuse of alcohol.

People are concerned about the consequences of drunk driving, alcohol-related crime, and lowered job productivity. National data indicate that per capita alcohol consumption has gradually dropped in the United States since the early 1980s.[1] Alcohol use remains the preferred form of drug use for most adults (including college students), but as a society, we are increasingly uncomfortable with the ease with which alcohol can be misused.

CHOOSING TO DRINK

Clearly, people drink alcoholic beverages for many different reasons. Most people drink alcohol because it is an effective, affordable, and legal substance for altering the brain's chemistry. As **inhibitions** are removed by the influence of alcohol, behavior that is generally held in check is expressed (Figure 8-1). At least temporarily, drinkers become a different version of themselves—more outgoing, relaxed, and adventuresome. If alcohol did not make these changes in people, it would not be consumed as much. Do you agree or disagree?

Key Term

inhibitions
Inner controls that prevent a person from engaging in certain types of behavior.

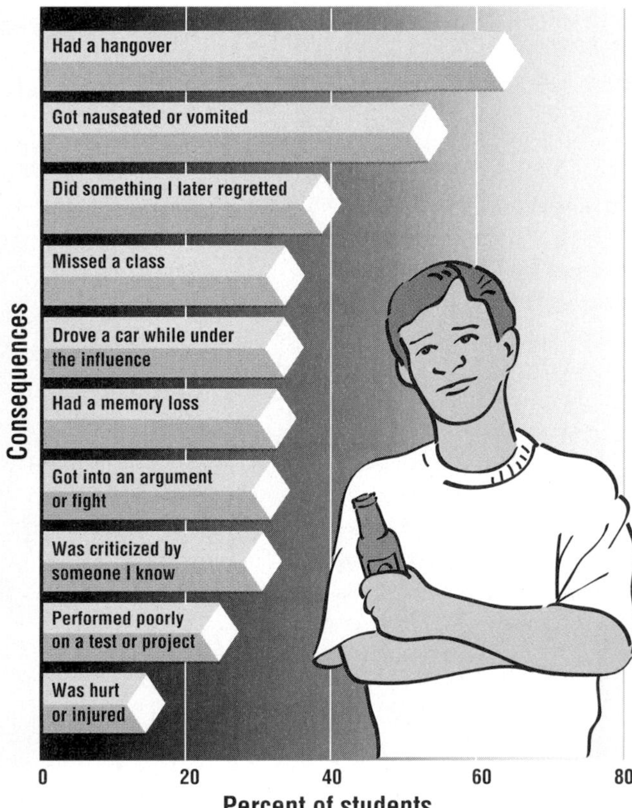

Figure 8-1 Negative consequences of alcohol use as reported by college students. (*Occurred at least once in past year; year 2000 statistics from national sample of over 55,000 undergraduates from 132 colleges in U.S.)

Table 8-1 Criteria for Drinking Classifications

Classification	Alcohol-Related Behavior
Abstainers	Do not drink or drink less often than once a year
Infrequent drinkers	Drink once a month at most and drink small amounts per typical drinking occasion
Light drinkers	Drink once a month at most and drink medium amounts per typical drinking occasion, or drink no more than three to four times a month and drink small amounts per typical drinking occasion
Moderate drinkers	Drink at least once a week and small amounts per typical drinking occasion or three to four times a month and medium amounts per typical drinking occasion or no more than once a month and large amounts per typical drinking occasion
Moderate/ heavy drinkers	Drink at least once a week and medium amounts per typical drinking occasion or three to four times a month and large amounts per typical drinking occasion
Heavy drinkers	Drink at least once a week and large amounts per typical drinking occasion

NOTE: Small amounts = One drink or less per drinking occasion
Medium amounts = Two to four drinks per drinking occasion
Large amounts = Five or more drinks per drinking occasion (binge drinking)
Drink = 12 fluid oz of beer, 4 fluid oz of wine, or 1 fluid oz of distilled spirits

ALCOHOL USE PATTERNS

From magazines to billboards to television, alcohol is one of the most heavily advertised consumer products in the country.[2] You cannot watch television, listen to the radio, or read a newspaper without being encouraged to buy a particular brand of beer, wine, or liquor. The advertisements create a warm aura about the nature of alcohol use. The implications are clear: alcohol use will bring you good times, handsome men or seductive women, exotic settings, and a chance to forget the hassles of hard work and study.

With the many pressures to drink, it's not surprising that most adults drink alcoholic beverages. Two-thirds of all American adults are classified as drinkers. Yet one in three adults does not drink. In the college environment, where surveys indicate that 85% to 90% of all students drink, it's difficult for many students to imagine that every third adult is an abstainer. Although many college students assume that drinking is a natural part of their social life, others are making alternative choices (see Exploring Your Spirituality box on p. 179).

Alcohol consumption figures are reported in many different ways, depending on the researchers' criteria. Various sources support the contention that about one-third of adults 18 years of age and older are abstainers, about one-third are light drinkers, and one-third are moderate-to-heavy drinkers. As a single category, heavy drinkers make up about 10% of the adult drinking population. Students who drink in college tend to classify themselves as light-to-moderate drinkers. It comes as a shock to students, though, when they read the criteria for each drinking classification. According to the combination of quantity of alcohol consumed per occasion and the frequency of drinking, these criteria are established as shown in Table 8-1.

In a recent unpublished survey of our undergraduate health science classes, we found that 39% of the 200 students met the criteria for heavy drinking, 23% met the criteria for moderate drinking, 11% met the criteria for light drinking, 10% were infrequent drinkers, and 17% were abstainers.[3] It's not surprising that many students, faculty, and administrators believe that alcohol abuse is a serious problem on their campuses. If you're worried about a friend's drinking patterns, take the Personal Assessment on p. 199.

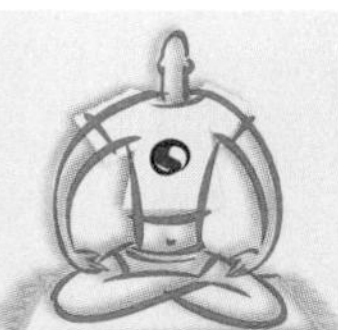

Exploring Your Spirituality

What's a Social Life without Alcohol?

When was the last time you went to a get-together where alcoholic drinks weren't served? It's probably been years. Socializing and drinking are connected in our consciousness in many ways. For instance, it's Friday night after a hard week and your friends ask you to join them for a beer. Why not? It'll be fun. Or you're invited to a party and want to bring something. How about a bottle of wine? That's easy and always appreciated.

Associating drinking with fun is something that many people, including college students, do. For various reasons, though, some college students are choosing to plan their fun around activities that don't involve drinking. Instead of going to a bar for a beer, they find a coffee shop and have a latte. Or they order soda with their pizza (not bad!). Others have discovered that they can get something that tastes great and is actually healthy at a juice bar.

What happens, though, when you go to a party and everyone else seems to be drinking? Choose something nonalcoholic—club soda, juice, soda, or water. (You probably won't be the only one doing this.) If someone gives you trouble about your choice, be firm. Just say that's what you want. You don't need to explain. And you don't have to say "yes" to be nice.

But maybe you want to drink at a party because it loosens you up and makes it easier to talk to people. How will you start a conversation without a drink to relax you? Think about how you talk easily and naturally with the people in your drama group or one of your favorite classes. You've got things in common, so it's easier to do. When you meet someone new at a party, look for common interests. You may feel self-conscious at first. But soon you'll forget about the fact that he or she is a stranger because you'll be involved in what you're talking about. Without that drink, you'll actually be more yourself.

Some students are making the commitment to be active instead of sitting around and drinking. They're going backpacking, joining a cycling group, taking an exercise class, or playing a team sport. What they're discovering is that it feels good—physically and mentally. They're socializing, doing something they enjoy, and getting in better shape. Think about something you've always wanted to try, and get going on it.

Making the choice to have fun without alcohol doesn't mean cutting yourself off from your friends. (If they're real friends, they'll respect your choice.) It's all about deciding what's right for you and making a commitment to that choice.

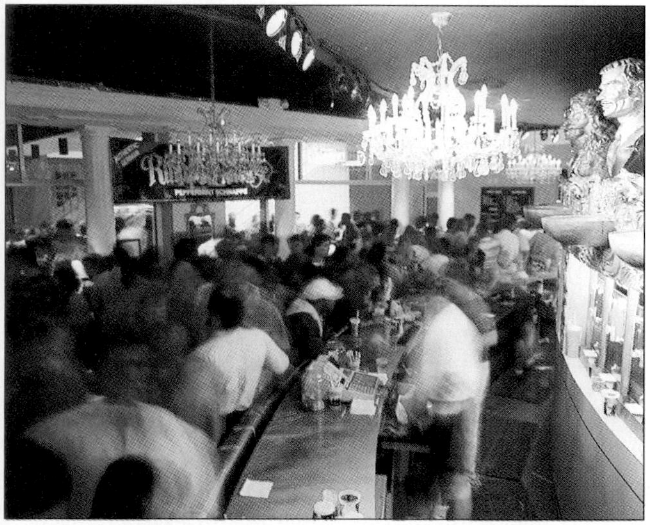

Two-thirds of American adults, including most of those in this Atlanta nightclub, are classified as drinkers. Only one-third choose to abstain from alcohol.

TALKING POINTS • How would you go about telling a friend that you think she has a drinking problem?

Moderate Drinking Redefined

Alcohol Alert, a publication of the National Institute on Alcohol Abuse and Alcoholism (NIAAA), indicates that moderate drinking can be defined as no more than two drinks each day for most men and one drink each day for women.[4] These cutoff levels are based on the amount of alcohol that can be consumed without causing problems, either for the drinker or society. (The gender difference is due primarily to the higher percentage of body fat in women and to the lower amount of an essential stomach enzyme in women.) Elderly people are limited to no more than one drink each day, again due to a higher percentage of body fat.

These consumption levels are applicable to most people. Indeed, people who plan to drive, women who are pregnant, people recovering from alcohol addiction, people under age 21, people taking medications, and those with existing medical concerns should not consume alcohol. Additionally, although some studies have shown that low levels of alcohol consumption may have minor psychological and cardiovascular benefits, the NIAAA does not advise nondrinkers to start drinking.

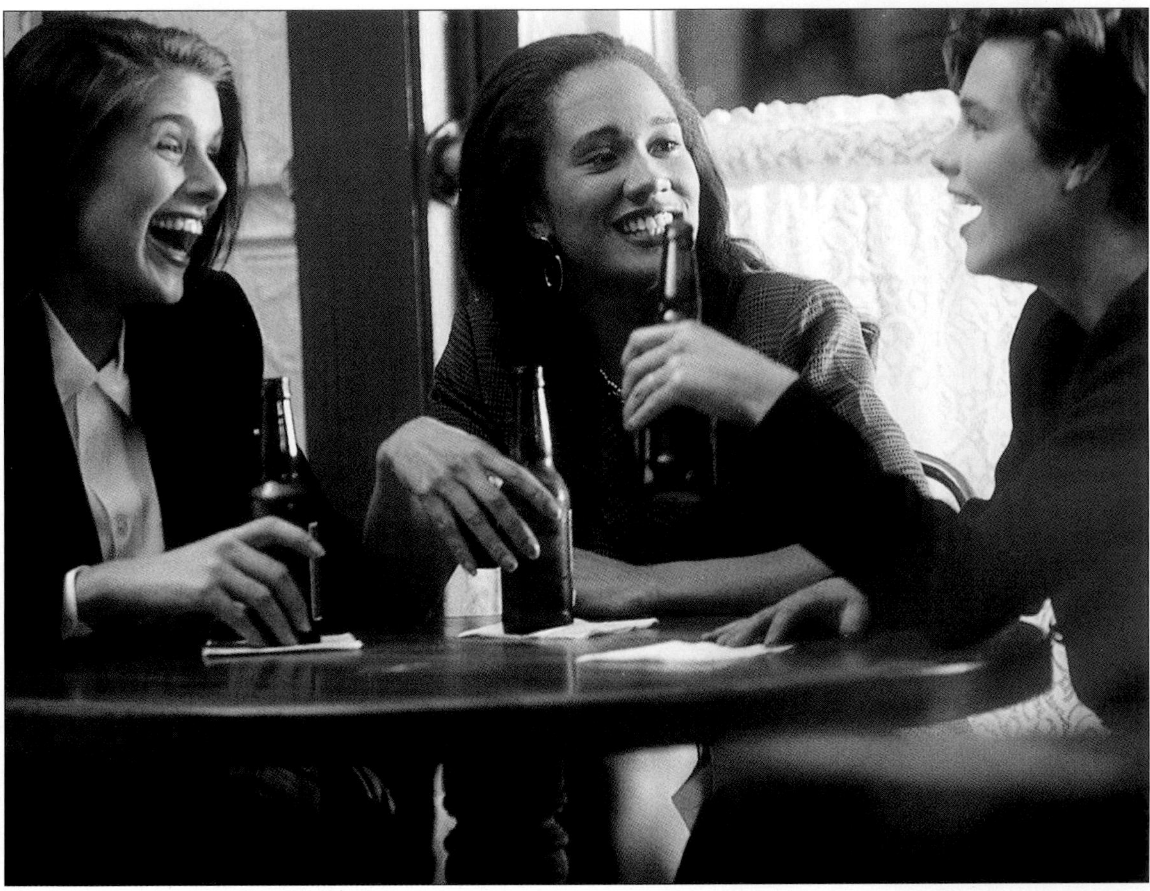

Mature adults know how to enjoy alcohol responsibly and understand how to decline alcohol use when they don't want to drink.

Binge Drinking

Alcohol abuse by college students usually takes place through *binge drinking.* This practice refers to the consumption of five drinks in a row, at least once during the previous 2-week period.[5] College students who fit the category of "heavy drinkers" rarely consume small amounts of alcohol each day but instead binge on alcohol 1 or 2 nights a week. Some students in our classes openly admit that they plan to "get really drunk" on the weekend. They plan to binge drink.

TALKING POINTS • Do you consider it your responsibility to tell a friend that he is binge drinking and explain how dangerous it can be?

Binge drinking can be dangerous. Drunk driving, physical violence, property destruction, date rape, police arrest, and lowered academic performance are all closely associated with binge drinking. The direct correlation between the amount of alcohol consumed and lowered academic performance is clear. Frequently, the social costs of binge drinking are very high, especially when intoxicated people demonstrate their level of immaturity. How common is binge drinking on your campus?

In response to the personal dangers and campus trauma associated with binge drinking, colleges and universities are fighting back. Some colleges are conducting local alcohol education campaigns that feature innovative posters and materials displayed on campus. One large group effort comes from the National Association of State Universities and Land-Grant Colleges (NASULGC). This group of 113 public universities has developed full-page campus newspaper advertisements and created an anti-binge drinking website (**www.nasulgc.org/bingedrink**). NASULGC also has sent campus officials a brochure that shows people how to socialize "without a couple of quarts of liquid courage."[6] In the future, expect to see increasing efforts to reduce binge drinking on your campus to make it a safer environment.

For many students who drink, the college years are a time when they will drink more heavily than at any other

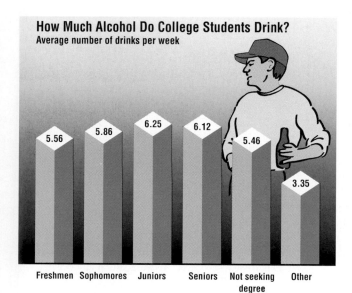

Figure 8-2 Average number of alcoholic drinks consumed by college drinkers (year 2000 statistics from national sample of over 55,000 undergraduates from 132 colleges in U.S.).

time in their life (Figure 8-2). Some will suffer serious consequences as a result (Figure 8-1). These years will also mark the entry into a lifetime of problem drinking for some.

THE NATURE OF ALCOHOLIC BEVERAGES

Alcohol (also known as *ethyl alcohol* or *ethanol*) is the principal product of **fermentation.** In this process, yeast cells act on the sugar content of fruits and grains to produce alcohol and carbon dioxide.

The alcohol concentration in distilled beverages (such as whiskey, gin, rum, and vodka) is expressed by the term *proof,* a number that is twice the percentage of alcohol by volume in a beverage. Thus 70% of the fluid in a bottle of 140 proof gin is pure alcohol. Most proofs in distilled beverages range from 80 to 160. The familiar pure *grain alcohol* that is often added to fruit punches and similar beverages has a proof of almost 200 (see Table 8-2).

The nutritional value of alcohol is extremely limited. Alcoholic beverages produced today through modern processing methods contain nothing but empty calories—about 100 calories per fluid ounce of 100-proof distilled spirits and about 150 calories for each 12-ounce bottle or can of beer.[7] Clearly, alcohol consumption is a significant contributor to the additional pounds of fat that many college students accumulate. Pure alcohol contains only simple carbohydrates; it has no vitamins and minerals and no fats or protein.

"Lite" beer and low-calorie wines have been introduced in response to concerns about the number of calories that alcoholic beverages provide. They are not low-alcohol

Table 8-2 Categories of Alcoholic Beverages*

Alcoholic Beverage	Alcohol Content (%)†	Normal Measure
Beer		
Ale	5	12-oz bottle
Ice beer	5.5	12-oz bottle
Malt liquor	7	12-oz bottle
Lite beer	4	12-oz bottle
Regular beer	4	12-oz bottle
Low-alcohol beer	1.5	12-oz bottle
Wine		
Fortified: port, sherry, muscatel, etc.	18	3-oz glass
Natural: red/white	12	3-oz glass
Champagne	12	4-oz glass
Wine cooler	6	12-oz bottle
Cider (Hard)	10	6-oz glass
Liqueurs		
Strong: sweet, syrupy	40	1-oz glass
Medium: fruit brandies	25	2-oz glass
Distilled Spirits		
Brandy, cognac, rum, scotch, vodka, whiskey	45	1-oz glass
Mixed Drinks and Cocktails		
Strong martini, manhattan	30	3½-oz glass
Medium: old-fashioned, daiquiri, Alexander	15	4-oz glass
Light: highball, sweet and sour mixes, tonics	7	8-oz glass

*In all major alcoholic beverages—beer, table wines, cocktail and dessert wines, liqueurs and cordials, and distilled spirits—the significant ingredient is identical: alcohol. The typical drink, half an ounce of pure alcohol, is provided by a shot of spirits, a glass of fortified wine, a larger glass of table wine, or a bottle of beer.

†In addition, these beverages contain other chemical constituents. Some come from the original grains, grapes, or other fruits; others are produced during the chemical processes of fermentation, distillation, and storage. Some are added as flavoring or coloring. These nonalcohol substances contribute to the effects of certain beverages either by directly affecting the body or by affecting the rates at which alcohol is absorbed into the blood.

Key Term

fermentation
A chemical process whereby plant products are converted into alcohol by the action of yeast cells on carbohydrate materials.

beverages but merely low-calorie beverages. Only beverages marked "low alcohol" contain a lower concentration of alcohol than the usual beverages of that type.

The popular new ice beers actually contain a higher percentage of alcohol than other types of beer. This is due to a production process that chills the fermented mixture sufficiently to allow ice crystals to form. When the ice crystals are removed, the beer contains a higher percentage of alcohol than it had before.

THE PHYSIOLOGICAL EFFECTS OF ALCOHOL

First and foremost, alcohol is classified as a drug—a very strong CNS depressant. The primary depressant effect of alcohol occurs in the brain and spinal cord. Many people think of alcohol as a stimulant because of the way most users feel after consuming a serving or two of their favorite drink. Any temporary sensations of jubilation, boldness, or relief are attributable to alcohol's ability as a depressant drug to release personal inhibitions and provide temporary relief from tension.

Factors That Influence the Absorption of Alcohol

The **absorption** of alcohol is influenced by several factors, most of which can be controlled by the individual. These factors include the following:

- *Strength of the beverage.* The stronger the beverage, the greater the amount of alcohol that will accumulate within the digestive tract.
- *Number of drinks consumed.* As more drinks are consumed, more alcohol is absorbed.
- *Speed of consumption.* If consumed rapidly, even relatively few drinks will result in a large concentration gradient that will lead to high blood alcohol concentration.
- *Presence of food.* Food can compete with alcohol for absorption into the bloodstream, slowing the absorption of alcohol. When alcohol absorption is slowed, the alcohol already in the bloodstream can be removed. Slow absorption favors better control of blood alcohol concentration.
- *Body chemistry.* Each person has an individual pattern of physiological functioning that may affect the ability to process alcohol. For example, in some conditions, such as that marked by "dumping syndrome," the stomach empties more rapidly than is normal, and alcohol seems to be absorbed more quickly. The emptying time may be either slowed or quickened by anger, fear, stress, nausea, and the condition of the stomach tissues.
- *Gender.* A significant study published in the *New England Journal of Medicine* reported that women produce much less alcohol dehydrogenase than men do.[8] This enzyme is responsible for breaking down alcohol in the stomach. As a result, women absorb about 30% more alcohol into the bloodstream than men, despite an identical number of drinks and equal body weight.

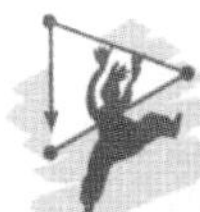

HealthQuest Activities

- The alcohol self-assessment activity in the Alcohol module will help you understand your current drinking behavior and determine how that behavior may affect your health. You can assess your beliefs about alcohol and take a critical look at your ideas about whether alcohol use harms various aspects of your life, such as your friendships, family relationships, and appearance. *HealthQuest* will help you estimate your risk of becoming a problem drinker or alcoholic. After completing the assessment activity, briefly record your answers to the following questions: Do your beliefs about alcohol reflect your own drinking behavior? What factors might cause a person's beliefs and behaviors to be incompatible? What life experiences or influences, such as family, religion, and advertising, have helped form your own beliefs about alcohol? Do you think your beliefs and behavior patterns are fixed, or will they change over time?
- *The Alcohol Decision Maze,* found in the Alcohol module, simulates an evening out with a friend. The activity prompts you to make a variety of choices throughout the evening that may influence whether or how much you drink. First you will choose among several companions for the evening. Then you must decide where to go. At each location, such as a restaurant or sporting event, you can choose from a list of activities to participate in. The choice to buy or drink alcohol comes up often. *HealthQuest* will then provide feedback on the outcome of the evening and estimate your bood alcohol content. Complete this activity several times, making different decisions each time. Does the outcome of the evening relect the drinking behavior you entered? Why or why not?

Three other reasons help explain why women tend to absorb alcohol more quickly than men of the same body weight: (1) Women have proportionately more body fat than men. Since alcohol is not very fat soluble, it enters the bloodstream relatively quickly. (2) Women's bodies have proportionately less water than men's bodies of equal weight. Thus alcohol consumed does not become as diluted as in men. (3) Alcohol absorption is influenced by a woman's menstrual cycle. Alcohol is more quickly absorbed during the premenstrual phase of a woman's cycle. Also, there is evidence that women using birth control pills absorb alcohol faster than usual.[7]

With the exception of a person's body chemistry and gender, all factors that influence absorption can be moderated by the alcohol user.

Blood Alcohol Concentration

A person's **blood alcohol concentration** (**BAC**) rises when alcohol is consumed faster than it can be removed (oxidized) by the liver. A fairly predictable sequence of events takes place when a person drinks alcohol at a rate faster than one drink every hour. When the BAC reaches 0.05%, initial measurable changes in mood and behavior take place. Inhibitions and everyday tensions appear to be released, while judgment and critical thinking are somewhat impaired. This BAC would be achieved by a 160-pound person consuming about two drinks in an hour.

At a level of 0.10% (one part alcohol to 1000 parts blood), the drinker typically loses significant motor coordination. Voluntary motor function becomes quite clumsy. At this BAC, most states consider a drinker legally intoxicated and thus incapable of safely operating a vehicle. Although physiological changes associated with this BAC do occur, certain users do not feel intoxicated or do not outwardly appear to be impaired.

As the BAC rises from 0.20% to 0.50%, the health risk of acute alcohol intoxication increases rapidly. A BAC of 0.20% is characterized by the loud, boisterous, obnoxious drunk person who staggers. A 0.30% BAC produces further depression and stuporous behavior, and the drinker becomes so confused that he or she may not be capable of understanding anything. The 0.40% or 0.50% BAC produces unconsciousness. At this level, a person can die, since the brain centers that control body temperature, heartbeat, and breathing may be virtually shut down.

An important factor influencing the BAC is the individual's blood volume. The larger the person, the greater the amount of blood into which alcohol can be distributed. Conversely, the smaller person has less blood into which alcohol can be distributed, and as a result, a higher BAC will develop.

Sobering Up

Alcohol is removed from the bloodstream principally through the process of **oxidation.** Oxidation occurs at a constant rate (about ¼ to ⅓ ounce of pure alcohol per hour) that cannot be appreciably altered. Since each typical drink of beer, wine, or distilled spirits contains about ½ ounce of pure alcohol, it takes about 2 hours for the body to fully oxidize one typical alcoholic drink.[9]

Although people may try to sober up by drinking hot coffee, taking cold showers, or exercising, the oxidation rate of alcohol is unaffected by these measures. Thus far the FDA has not approved any commercial product that can help people achieve sobriety. Passage of time remains the only effective remedy for diminishing alcohol's effects.

First Aid for Acute Alcohol Intoxication

Not everyone who goes to sleep, passes out, or becomes unconscious after drinking has a high BAC. People who are already sleepy, have not eaten well, are sick, or are bored may drink a little alcohol and quickly fall asleep. However, people who drink heavily in a rather short time may be setting themselves up for an extremely unpleasant, toxic, potentially life-threatening experience because of their high BAC.

Although responsible drinking would prevent **acute alcohol intoxication** (poisoning), it will never be a reality for everyone. As a caring adult, what should you know about this health emergency that may help you save a life—perhaps even a friend's life?

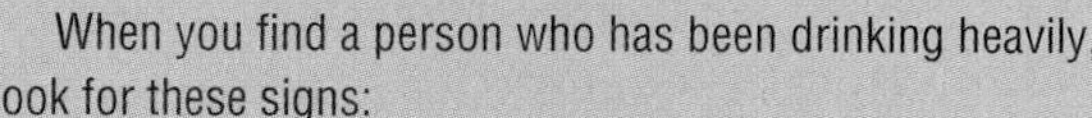

Changing *for the Better*

Are You Ready for an Alcohol-Related Emergency?

How can I recognize and cope with an acute alcohol emergency?

When you find a person who has been drinking heavily, look for these signs:

- Cannot be aroused
- Has a weak, rapid pulse
- Has an unusual or irregular breathing pattern
- Has cool (possibly damp), pale, or bluish skin

Immediately call for emergency help (call 911). Follow their directions. Position the unconscious person on his or her side to avoid choking in case vomiting occurs.

Key Terms

absorption
The passage of nutrients or alcohol through the walls of the stomach or intestinal tract into the bloodstream.

blood alcohol concentration (BAC)
The percentage of alcohol in a measured quantity of blood; BACs can be determined directly through the analysis of a blood sample or indirectly through the analysis of exhaled air.

oxidation
The process that removes alcohol from the bloodstream.

acute alcohol intoxication
A potentially fatal elevation of the BAC, often resulting from heavy, rapid consumption of alcohol.

The first real danger signs to recognize are the typical signs of **shock.** By the time these signs are evident, a drinker will already be unconscious. He or she will not be able to be aroused from a deep stupor. The person will probably have a weak, rapid pulse (over 100 beats per minute). The skin will be cool and damp, and breathing will be increased to once every 3 or 4 seconds. These breaths may be shallow or deep but will certainly occur in an irregular pattern. Skin will be pale or bluish. (In the case of a person with dark skin, these color changes will be more evident in the fingernail beds or in the mucous membranes inside the mouth or under the eyelids.) Whenever any of these signs is present, seek emergency medical help immediately (see the Changing for the Better box on p. 183 for a summary of these signs).

Involuntary regurgitation (vomiting) can be another potentially life-threatening emergency for a person who has drunk too much alcohol. When a drinker has consumed more alcohol than the liver can oxidize, the pyloric valve at the base of the stomach tends to close. Additional alcohol remains in the stomach. This alcohol irritates the lining of the stomach so much that involuntary muscle contractions force the stomach contents to flow back through the esophagus. By removing alcohol from the stomach, vomiting may be a life-saving mechanism for conscious drinkers.

An unconscious drinker who vomits may be lying in such a position that the airway becomes obstructed by the vomitus. This person is at great risk of dying from **asphyxiation.** As a first-aid measure, unconscious drinkers should always be rolled onto their sides to minimize the chance of airway obstruction. If you are with someone who is vomiting, make certain that his or her head is positioned lower than the rest of the body. This position minimizes the chance that vomitus will obstruct the air passages.

It is also important to keep a close watch on anyone who passes out from heavy drinking. Party-goers sometimes make the mistake of carrying these people to bed and then forgetting about them. Monitoring the physical condition of anyone who becomes unconscious from heavy drinking is crucial because of the risk of death. Observe the person at regular intervals until he or she appears to be clearly out of danger. This may mean an evening of interrupted sleep for you, but you could save a friend's life. Are you aware of any recent alcohol-related deaths among U.S. college students?

ALCOHOL-RELATED HEALTH PROBLEMS

The relationship of chronic alcohol use to the structure and function of the body is reasonably well understood. Heavy alcohol use causes a variety of changes to the body that lead to an increase in morbidity and mortality. Figure 8-3 on p. 185 describes these changes.

Research clearly shows that chronic alcohol use also damages the immune system and the nervous system. Thus chronic users are at high risk for a variety of infections and neurological complications.[1] Additionally, many alcoholics suffer from malnutrition, in part because they do not consume a variety of foods. With the deterioration of the liver, stomach, and pancreas, chronic heavy drinkers also have poor absorption and metabolism of many nutrients.

Fetal Alcohol Syndrome and Fetal Alcohol Effects

A growing body of scientific evidence indicates that alcohol use by pregnant women can result in birth defects in unborn children. When alcohol crosses the **placenta,** it enters the fetal bloodstream in a concentration equal to that in the mother's bloodstream. Because of the underdeveloped nature of the fetal liver, this alcohol is oxidized much more slowly than the alcohol in the mother. During this time of slow detoxification, the developing fetus is certain to be overexposed to the toxic effects of alcohol. Mental retardation frequently develops.

This exposure has additional disastrous consequences for the developing fetus. Low birth weight, facial abnormalities (e.g., small head, widely spaced eyes), and heart problems are often seen in such infants (Figure 8-4). This combination of effects is called **fetal alcohol syndrome.** Recent estimates indicate that the full expression of this syndrome occurs at a rate of between 1 and 3 per 1000 births. Partial expression (fetal alcohol effects [FAE]) can be seen in 3 to 9 per 1000 live births. In addition, it is likely that many cases of FAE go undetected.

Is there a safe limit to the number of drinks a woman can consume during pregnancy? Since no one can accurately predict the effect of drinking even small amounts of alcohol during pregnancy, the wisest plan is to avoid alcohol altogether.

Because of the critical growth and development that occur during the first months of fetal life, women who have any reason to suspect they are pregnant should stop all alcohol consumption. Furthermore, women who are planning to become pregnant and women who are not practicing effective contraception must also consider keeping their alcohol use to a minimum.

ALCOHOL-RELATED SOCIAL PROBLEMS

Alcohol abuse is related to a variety of social problems. These problems affect the quality of interpersonal relationships, employment stability, and the financial security of both the individual and the family. Clearly, alcohol's negative social consequences lower our quality of life. In financial terms the annual cost of alcohol abuse and dependence has been estimated at more than $185 billion.

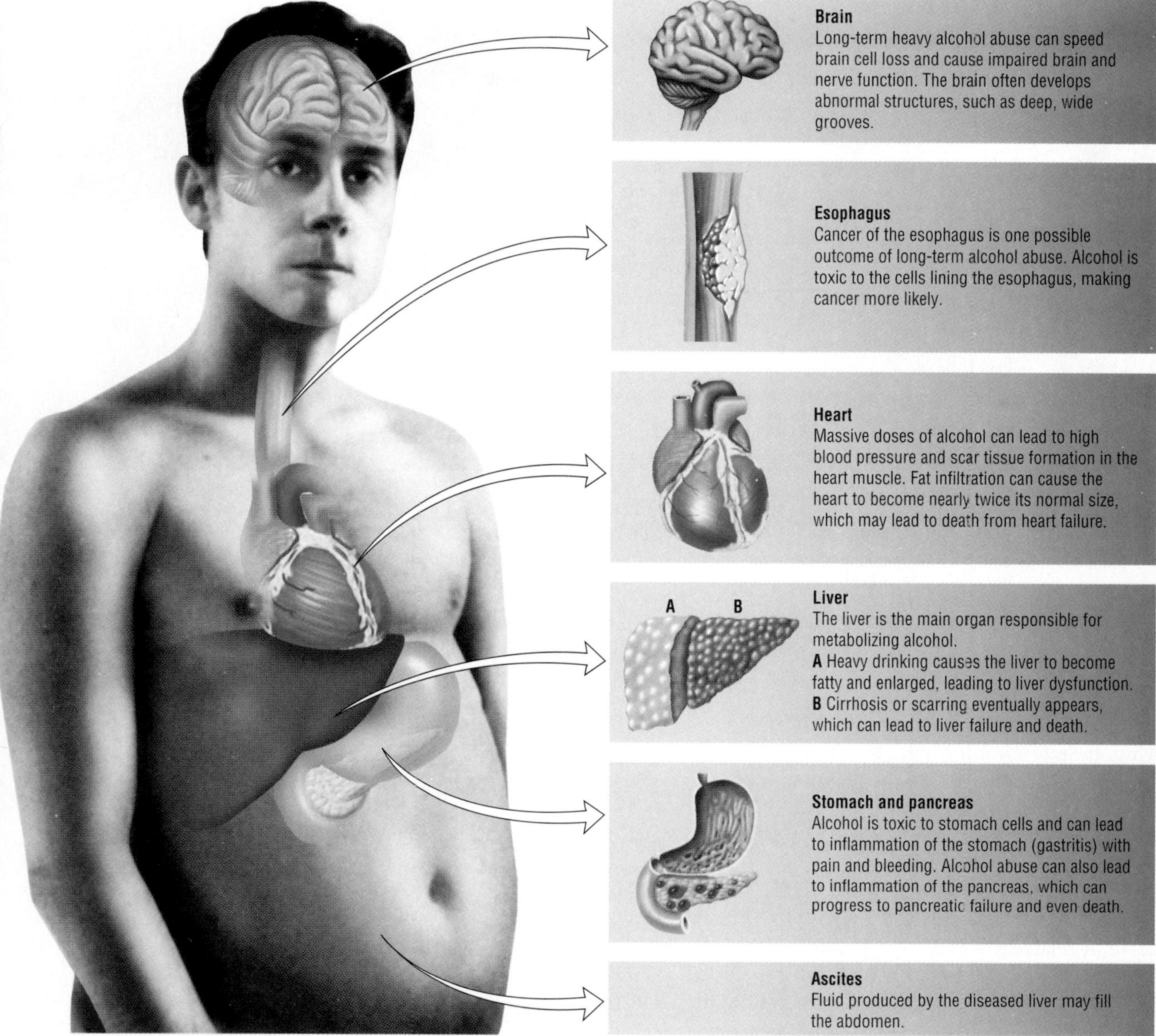

Brain
Long-term heavy alcohol abuse can speed brain cell loss and cause impaired brain and nerve function. The brain often develops abnormal structures, such as deep, wide grooves.
Esophagus
Cancer of the esophagus is one possible outcome of long-term alcohol abuse. Alcohol is toxic to the cells lining the esophagus, making cancer more likely.
Heart
Massive doses of alcohol can lead to high blood pressure and scar tissue formation in the heart muscle. Fat infiltration can cause the heart to become nearly twice its normal size, which may lead to death from heart failure.
Liver
A
B
The liver is the main organ responsible for metabolizing alcohol.
A Heavy drinking causes the liver to become fatty and enlarged, leading to liver dysfunction.
B Cirrhosis or scarring eventually appears, which can lead to liver failure and death.
Stomach and pancreas
Alcohol is toxic to stomach cells and can lead to inflammation of the stomach (gastritis) with pain and bleeding. Alcohol abuse can also lead to inflammation of the pancreas, which can progress to pancreatic failure and even death.
Ascites
Fluid produced by the diseased liver may fill the abdomen.

Figure 8-3 Effects of alcohol use on the body. The mind-altering effects of alcohol begin soon after it enters the bloodstream. Within minutes, alcohol numbs nerve cells in the brain. The heart muscle strains to cope with alcohol's depressive action. If drinking continues, the rising BAC causes impaired speech, vision, balance, and judgment. With an extremely high BAC, respiratory failure is possible. Over time, alcohol abuse increases the risk for certain forms of heart disease and cancer and makes liver and pancreas failure more likely.

Key Terms

shock
Profound collapse of many vital body functions; evident during acute alcohol intoxication and other health emergencies.

asphyxiation
Death resulting from lack of oxygen to the brain.

Key Terms

placenta
The structure through which nutrients, metabolic wastes, and drugs (including alcohol) pass from the bloodstream of the mother into the bloodstream of the developing fetus.

fetal alcohol syndrome
Characteristic birth defects noted in the children of some women who consume alcohol during their pregnancies.

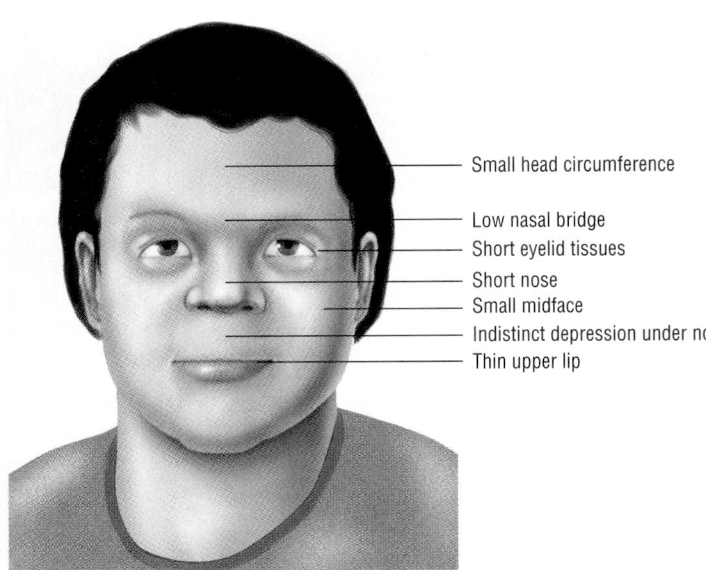

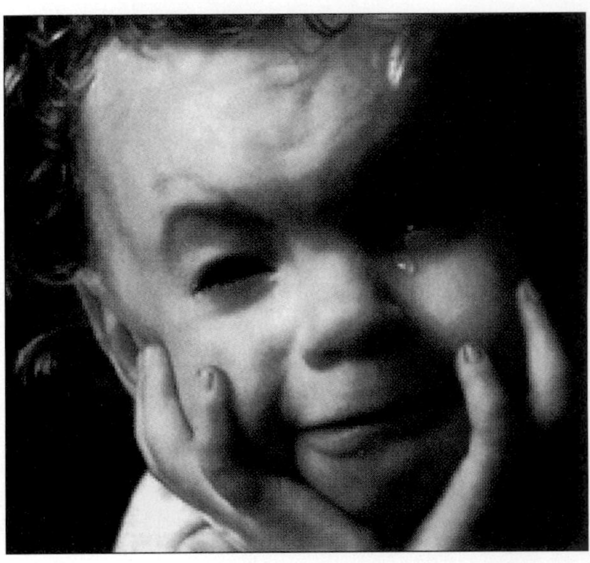

Figure 8-4 Fetal alcohol syndrome. The facial features shown are characteristic of affected children. Additional abnormalities in the brain and other internal organs accompany fetal alcohol syndrome but are not obvious in the child's appearance.

Accidents

The four leading causes of accidental deaths in the United States (motor vehicle collsions, falls, drownings, and fires and burns) have significant statistical connections to alcohol use.

Motor vehicle collisions

Data from the National Highway Traffic Safety Administration (NHTSA) indicate that in 1999 nearly 16,000 alcohol-related vehicular crash deaths occurred. This figure represented 38% of the total traffic fatalities for 1999. Although 16,000 remains an unacceptably high figure, this total represented a 33% reduction from the nearly 24,000 alcohol-related fatalities 10 years earlier, in 1989.[10]

Presently in the United States, an alcohol-related car crash fatality occurs every 33 minutes. Every 2 minutes, an alcohol-related car crash injury happens. An estimated 308,000 people were injured in such crashes in 1999. In 1998, the NHTSA reported that approximately 1.4 million drivers were arrested for drunk driving, reflecting an arrest rate of 1 for every 132 licensed drivers in the United States (To find out what happens to people after they are arrested, read the Star Box on p. 187.)

One response to drunk driving has been for all states to raise the minimum legal drinking age to 21 years. This was accomplished in the mid-1980s. Another response was a federal law that President Clinton signed in October 2000. This law required all states to lower their drunk driving standard to .08% BAC by October 1, 2003 or the states would lose a portion of their federal highway

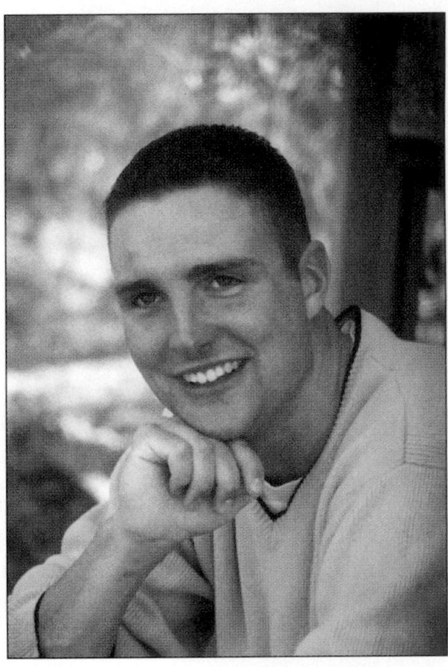

On August 4, 2000, 23-year-old Casey Ray Beaver was driving with two friends along U.S. Highway 71 near Goodman, Missouri, when an oncoming vehicle crossed the center line and collided with his car. Casey, a recent graduate of the University of Kansas, was pronounced dead at the scene, as was the driver of the other vehicle. The offender, who had seven prior convictions of driving under the influence and whose driver's license had been revoked seven years earlier, had a BAC above .10%. Casey was due to begin classes at the Illinois College of Optometry ten days after the accident occurred.

Getting Arrested for Drinking and Driving: The Aftermath

Many college students will admit to having driven a car after drinking alcohol. Some will even admit that they have left a party after drinking and then driven to another location, but could not remember actually driving the car. This behavior reflects an alcoholic blackout. These dangerous activities are serious enough for the driver, the passengers, and anyone else on (or near) the road. For people who get arrested, another drama will unfold—the aftermath of an arrest for drinking and driving.

Although laws vary from state to state, here is the general sequence of events: If you are driving a car and are stopped by a police officer who suspects you may have been driving under the influence of alcohol, you will first be asked to show your driver's license and proof of your car's registration. You may be asked to get out of your car and undergo a field test for sobriety. This test could include tests of motor coordination, such as walking in a line in a heel-to-toe fashion. You may even be given an alcohol breath test on the spot.

If you appear to fail the field test, you could be arrested and frisked, read your Miranda rights, and taken to the local jail. There you will likely be fingerprinted and photographed. A more precise blood alcohol test may be given. Depending on local or state law, you will either spend some hours in jail (until your BAC is lowered) or be immediately eligible for bail (if you, a family member, or a friend can come up with the cash to get you released).

A date for your court appearance will be set. You will be required to face a judge and answer the charges against you. By this time, you probably will have hired an attorney to help you in this process. If you are convicted or decide to plead guilty to misdemeanor charges of driving while intoxicated (DWI) and this is your first offense, a typical scenario will follow. You will receive a fine (perhaps \$200–\$500) and be required to pay court costs (perhaps \$125). You will probably be required to attend alcohol education classes and be placed on probation (for a year). Many states also require a person convicted of DWI to pay a probationer's fee of \$50 plus \$10 each month during the probation period. You will generally be required to see your probation officer once a month, and you may be required to take random drug tests.

Some communities require people convicted of DWI to pay a fee (perhaps \$200) that goes to local drug prevention programs. Finally, some jurisdictions require judges to impose a term of community service hours that you must serve. You will likely lose points on your driver's license and have an official police and court record. The total cost for a simple, first-time conviction can easily reach \$1000 or more, depending on fines and legal fees.

For first-time offenders in jurisdictions in which the courts and jails are overcrowded, "pretrial diversionary programs" may exist. In these programs, lawyers work with local prosecutors to help first-time offenders avoid facing a judge and having a court record. Those arrested agree to pay a set community drug program fine (perhaps \$300–\$500) and attend alcohol education classes. They typically must perform community service and meet with a probation officer each month. (They must also pay the probationer's fees.) At the end of a year, after a positive probationary experience, the arrest record is removed from the police files. Again, the total cost can amount to over \$1000.

The preceding discussion applies to misdemeanor charges. However, if you are arrested and charged with a felony (such as operating a vehicle while intoxicated and you kill or injure someone), the whole ball game changes radically. You will be arrested and put in jail. You may not be able to be bailed out of jail. Almost certainly, you will need an attorney to assist you through a lengthy court process. If you are ultimately convicted of a felony, you are likely to pay a heavy fine and spend time in jail or prison. After a criminal trial, injured people can also pursue a civil suit against you. A civil suit can be quite expensive and time consuming. Indeed, the repercussions of a criminal DWI felony conviction will last for years and will have a significant impact on you, your family, and the lives of others.

Unfortunately, people who drink and drive fail to consider the aftermath of their behavior before it is too late.

dollars. At the time of this writing, nearly thirty states and the District of Columbia had enacted the tougher .08% BAC standard (see Figure 8.5).[11] Do you know if your state has enacted a .08% law? You can search the MADD website at **www.madd.org** to find out current .08% law information.

Other programs and policies are being implemented that are designed to prevent intoxicated people from driving. Many states have enacted **zero tolerance laws** to help prevent underage drinking and driving. Also included

Key Term

zero tolerance laws
Laws that severely restrict the right to operate motor vehicles for underage drinkers who have been convicted of driving under any influence.

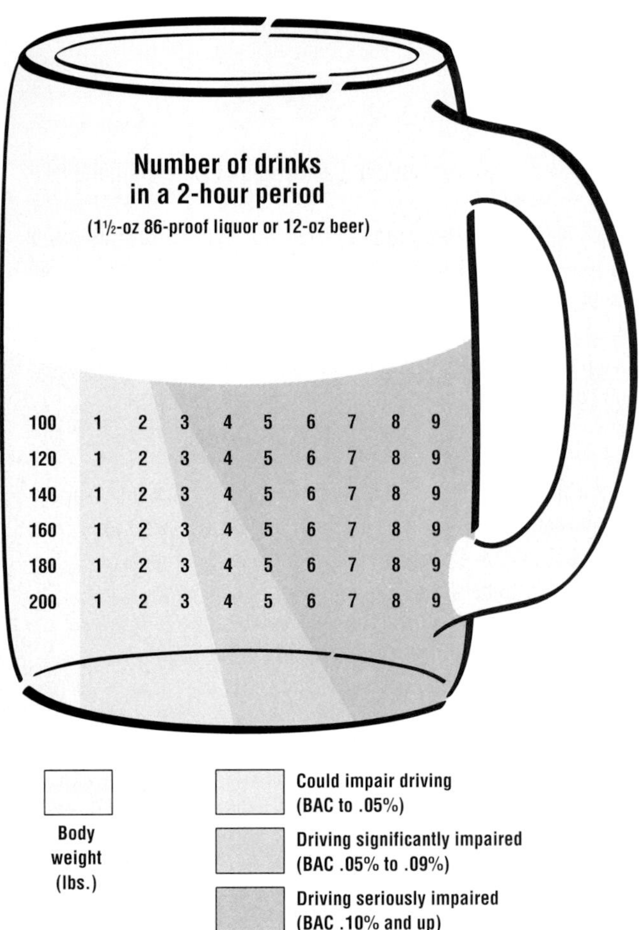

Figure 8-5 For most states, a BAC of .08% constitutes legal intoxication. However, lower BACs can impair functioning enough to cause a serious accident.

have been efforts to educate bartenders to recognize intoxicated customers, to use off-duty police officers as observers in bars, to place police roadblocks, to develop mechanical devices that prevent intoxicated drivers from starting their cars, and to encourage people to use designated drivers.

The use of designated drivers has received some of the credit for the significant reduction in drunk driving deaths mentioned earlier. However, there may be a down side to this solution. Some health professionals are concerned that the use of designated drivers allows the nondrivers to drink more heavily than they might otherwise. In effect, designated drivers "enable" drinkers to be less responsible for their own behavior. The concern is that this freedom from responsibility might eventually lead to further problems for the drinkers. What do you think?

TALKING POINTS • You've heard some of your friends joking about others using the designated-driver approach. How would you introduce this practice in a way that would be acceptable to them?

Falls

Many people are surprised to learn that falls are the second leading cause of accidental death in the United States, with about 13,000 deaths per year. Alcohol use increases the risk for falls. Various studies suggest that alcohol is involved in between 17% and 53% of deadly falls and between 21% and 77% of nonfatal falls.

Drownings

Drownings are the third leading cause of accidental death in the United States. Studies have shown that alcohol use is implicated in approximately 34% of these deaths. High percentages of recreational boaters have been found to drink alcohol while boating.

Fires and burns

Fires and burns are responsible for an estimated 5000 deaths each year in the United States, the fourth leading cause of accidental death. This cause is also connected to alcohol use: studies indicate that half of burn victims have BACs above the legal limit.

Crime and Violence

Have you noticed that most of the violent behavior and vandalism on your campus is related to alcohol use? The connection of alcohol to crime has a long history. Prison populations have large percentages of alcohol abusers and alcoholics: People who commit crimes are more likely to have alcohol problems than are people in the general population. This is especially true for young criminals. Furthermore, alcohol use has been reported in 67% of all homicides, with the victim, the perpetrator, or both found to have been drinking. In rape situations, rapists are intoxicated 50% of the time and victims 30% of the time.[7]

Because of research methodological problems, pinpointing alcohol's connection to family violence is difficult. However, it seems clear that among a large number of families, alcohol is associated with violence and other harmful behavior, including physical abuse, child abuse, psychological abuse, and abandonment.[7] The Focus on . . . article on p. 201 explores the link between alcohol and violence.

Suicide

Alcohol use has been related to large percentages of suicides. Half of all suicides are committed by alcoholics. Between 35% and 40% of the suicides committed by

Changing *for the Better*

Partying 101: How to Party Responsibly

My friends and I are planning a big holiday party. We want to have fun, but we also want to be responsible about alcohol. What guidelines should we follow?

- Provide other social activities as a primary focus when alcohol is served.
- Respect an individual's decision about alcohol if that decision is either to abstain or to drink responsibly.
- Recognize the decision not to drink and the respect it warrants by providing equally attractive and accessible nonalcohol drinks when alcohol is served.
- Recognize that drunkenness is neither healthy nor safe. One should not excuse otherwise unacceptable behavior solely because of "too much to drink."
- Provide food when alcohol is served.
- Serve diluted drinks, and do not urge that glasses be constantly full.
- Keep the cocktail hour before dinner to a reasonable time and consumption limit.
- Recognize your responsibility for the health, safety, and pleasure of both the drinker and the nondrinker by avoiding intoxication and helping others do the same.
- Make contingency plans for intoxication. If it occurs in spite of efforts to prevent it, assume responsibility for the health and safety of guests—for example, by providing transportation home or overnight accommodations.
- Serve or use alcohol only in environments conducive to pleasant and relaxing behavior.
- Discard unattended drinks immediately. This reduces the possibility of someone consuming a drink containing Rohypnol, GHB, ketamine, (see Chapter 7) or other powerful intoxicants.

nonalcoholics are alcohol-related. Also, alcohol use is associated with impulsive suicides rather than with premeditated ones. Drinking is also connected with more violent and lethal means of suicide, such as the use of firearms.[7]

For many of these social problems, alcohol use impairs critical judgment and allows a person's behavior to quickly become reckless, antisocial, and deadly. Because most of us wish to minimize problems associated with alcohol use, acting responsibly when we host a party is a first step in this direction.

HOSTING A RESPONSIBLE PARTY

Some people might say that no party is totally safe when alcohol is served. These people are probably right, considering the possibility of unexpected **drug synergism,** overconsumption, and the consequences of released inhibitions. Fortunately, an awareness of the value of responsible party hosting seems to be growing among college communities. The impetus for this awareness has come from various sources, including respect for an individual's right to choose not to drink alcohol, the growing recognition that many automobile accidents are alcohol-related, and the legal threats posed by **host negligence.**

Responsibly hosting parties at which alcohol is served is becoming a trend, especially among college-educated young adults. The Education Commission of the States' Task Force on Responsible Decisions about Alcohol has generated a list of guidelines for hosting a social event at which alcoholic beverages are served.[12] The list includes the recommendations shown in the Changing for the Better box above.

In addition, using a **designated driver** is an important component of responsible alcohol use. By planning to abstain from alcohol or to carefully limit their own alcohol consumption, designated drivers are able to safely transport friends who have been drinking. Have you noticed an increased use of designated drivers in your community? Would you be willing to be a designated driver?

Key Terms

drug synergism (sin er jism)
Enhancement of a drug's effect as a result of the presence of additional drugs within the system.

host negligence
A legal term that reflects the failure of a host to provide reasonable care and safety for people visiting the host's residence or business.

designated driver
A person who abstains from or carefully limits alcohol consumption to be able to safely transport other people who have been drinking.

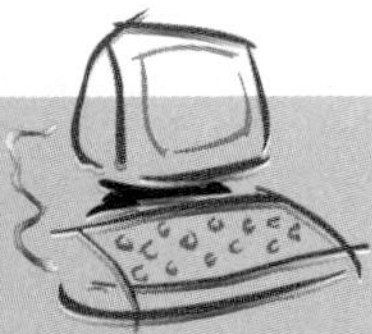

OnSITE/InSIGHT

Learning to Go: Health

Do you drink occasionally or on a daily basis? Click on the Motivator icon to find these lessons, which will put your approach to alcohol use in perspective:

Lesson 26: Know your limits; drink responsibly.
Lesson 27: Recognize the signs of problem drinking.

STUDENT POLL

Is alcohol use an important part of your lifestyle? Go to the Online Learning Center at **www.mhhe.com/hahn6e**. Click on Student Resources to answer the following questions. When you're finished, check the responses of other students.

1. Do you drink alcoholic beverages (either regularly or occasionally)?
2. Is drinking a routine part of your social life?
3. Does your drinking often lead to intoxication?
4. Have you ever driven while under the influence?
5. Do you sometimes feel pressured to drink?
6. Do you often drink alone?
7. Have you ever been to a rehabilitation program for alcohol abuse?
8. Do you belong to an organization that works against drunk driving?
9. Has your alcohol consumption increased now that you're in college?
10. Do you often drink to "escape"?
11. Do you think about the negative health effects of drug abuse?
12. Are your views on drinking influenced by your spiritual values?
13. Does your family background/culture affect your views on alcohol use?
14. Is having a designated driver important to you?
15. Do you look for ways to get a drug-free "high"?

ORGANIZATIONS THAT SUPPORT RESPONSIBLE DRINKING

The serious consequences of the irresponsible use of alcohol have led to the formation of a number of concerned-citizen groups. Although each organization has a unique approach, all attempt to deal objectively with two indisputable facts: Alcohol use is part of our society, and irresponsible alcohol use can be deadly.

Mothers Against Drunk Driving

Mothers Against Drunk Driving (MADD) is a national network of over 600 local chapters in the United States and Canada. This organization attempts to educate people about alcohol's effects on driving and to influence legislation and enforcement of laws related to drunk drivers. For more information about MADD, visit its website at **www.madd.org.**

Students Against Destructive Decisions

Many students have known the acronym *SADD* to stand for the youth group Students Against Driving Drunk. Recently, the group has restructured itself to expand beyond drunk driving to include other high-risk activities that are detrimental to youth, such as underage drinking, drug use, drugged driving, and failure to use seat belts. Founded in 1981, this organization now has millions of members in thousands of chapters throughout the country. Remaining central to the drunk driving aspect of SADD is the "Contract for Life," a pact that encourages students and parents to provide safe transportation for each other if either is unable to drive safely after consuming alcohol. This contract also stipulates that no discussions about the incident are to be started until both can talk in a calm and caring manner. For more information about SADD, visit its website at **www.nat-sadd.org.**

TALKING POINTS • How would you approach asking your parents or friends to join you in signing a "Contract for Life"?

BACCHUS and GAMMA Peer Education Network

BACCHUS (Boost Alcohol Consciousness Concerning the Health of University Students) began in 1975 as an alcohol-awareness organization at the University of Florida. Run by student volunteers, this organization promoted responsible drinking among college students who chose to drink. It was not an anti-alcohol group, but a "harm reduction" group. Over the years, hundreds of chapters were formed on campuses across the country.

When supporters of BACCHUS realized that many students interested in alcohol awareness were from fraternities and sororities, they developed GAMMA (Greeks Advocating Mature Management of Alcohol) to join BACCHUS to form a peer education network. Campuses are now able to choose BACCHUS, GAMMA, or any other acronym or name for their groups.

With the broadening of the original BACCHUS organization has come an expansion of the health issues this group addresses. Originally, the focus was on alcohol abuse and prevention. Now the BACCHUS and GAMMA Peer Education Network confronts a variety of student health and safety issues. For additional information about this organization, check out its website at **www.bacchusgamma.org.**

Other Approaches

Other responsible approaches to alcohol use are surfacing nearly every day. Even among college fraternity organizations, attitudes toward the indiscriminate use of alcohol are changing. Many fraternity rush functions are now conducted without the use of alcohol, and growing numbers of fraternities are alcohol-free.

Another encouraging sign on college campuses is the increasing number of alcohol use task forces. Although each of these groups has its own focus and title, many are meeting to discuss alcohol-related concerns on their particular campus. These task forces often try to formulate detailed, comprehensive policies for alcohol use across the entire campus community. Membership on these committees often includes students (on-campus and off-campus, graduate and undergraduate), faculty and staff members, academic administrators, residence hall advisors, university police, health center personnel, alumni, and local citizens. Does your college have such a committee?

PROBLEM DRINKING AND ALCOHOLISM

Problem Drinking

At times the line separating **problem drinking** from alcoholism is difficult to distinguish (see the accompanying Star Box). There may be no true line, with the exception that an alcoholic is unable to stop drinking. Problem drinking is a pattern of alcohol use in which a drinker's behavior creates personal difficulties or difficulties for other people. What are some of these behaviors? Examples might be drinking to avoid life stressors, going to work intoxicated, drinking and driving, becoming injured or injuring others while drinking, solitary drinking, morning drinking, an occasional **blackout,** high-risk sexual activity, and being told by others that you drink too much. For college students, two clear indications of problem drinking are missing classes and lowered academic performance caused by alcohol involvement. The Changing for the Better box on p. 192 offers suggestions that can help you keep drinking under control.

Problem drinkers are not always heavy drinkers; they might not be daily or even weekly drinkers. Unlike alcoholics, problem drinkers do not need to drink to maintain "normal" body functions. However, when they do drink, they (and others around them) experience problems—sometimes with tragic consequences. It's not surprising that problem drinkers are more likely than other drinkers to eventually develop alcoholism. Are there people around you who show signs of problem drinking?

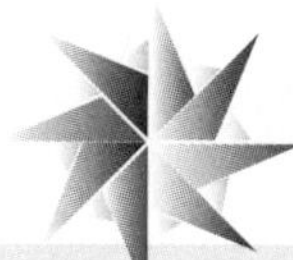

Progressive Stages of Alcohol Dependence

Early
- Escape drinking
- Binge drinking
- Guilt feelings
- Sneaking drinks
- Difficulty stopping once drinking has begun
- Increased tolerance
- Preoccupation with drinking
- Occasional blackouts

Middle
- Loss of control
- Self-hate
- Impaired social relationships
- Changes in drinking patterns (more frequent binge drinking)
- Temporary sobriety
- Morning drinking
- Dietary neglect
- Increased blackouts

Late
- Prolonged binges
- Alcohol used to control withdrawal symptoms
- Alcohol psychosis
- Nutritional disease
- Frequent blackouts

Key Terms

problem drinking
An alcohol use pattern in which a drinker's behavior creates personal difficulties or difficulties for other people.

blackout
A temporary state of amnesia experienced by a drinker; an inability to remember events that occurred during a period of alcohol use.

Changing *for the Better*

Cool, Calm, and Collected: Keeping Your Drinking Under Control

I've watched some of my friends do crazy things while drinking too much at a party. What things should I focus on to avoid overdoing it at parties?

- Do not drink before a party.
- Avoid drinking when you are anxious, angry, or depressed.
- Measure the liquor you put in mixed drinks (use only 1 to 1½ oz).
- Eat ample amounts of food and drink lots of water before and during the time you are drinking.
- Avoid salty foods that may make you drink more than you had planned.
- Drink slowly.
- Do not participate in drinking games.
- Do not drive after drinking; use a designated nondrinking driver.
- Consume only a predetermined number of drinks.
- Stop alcohol consumption at a predetermined hour.

Alcoholism

In the early 1990s a revised definition of **alcoholism** was established by a joint committee of experts on alcohol dependence.[13] This committee defined alcoholism as follows:

> Alcoholism is a primary, chronic disease with genetic, psychosocial, and environmental factors influencing its development and manifestations. The disease is often progressive and fatal. It is characterized by impaired control over drinking, preoccupation with the drug alcohol, use of alcohol despite adverse consequences, and distortions in thinking, most notably denial. Each of these symptoms may be continuous or periodic.

This definition incorporates much of the knowledge gained from addiction research during the last two decades. It is well recognized that alcoholics do not drink for the pleasurable effects of alcohol but to escape being sober. For alcoholics, being sober is stressful.

Unlike problem drinking, alcoholism involves a physical addiction to alcohol. For the true alcoholic, when the body is deprived of alcohol, physical and mental withdrawal symptoms become evident. These withdrawal symptoms can be life threatening.

Uncontrollable shaking can progress to nausea, vomiting, hallucinations, shock, and cardiac and pulmonary arrest. Uncontrollable shaking combined with irrational hallucinations is called *delirium tremens* (DT), an occasional manifestation of alcohol withdrawal.

The complex reasons for the physical and emotional dependence of alcoholism have not been fully explained. Why, when more than 100 million adults use alcohol without becoming dependent on it, are 10 million or more others unable to control its use?

Could alcoholism be an inherited disease? Studies in humans and animals have provided strong evidence that genetics plays a role in some cases of alcoholism. Two forms of alcoholism are thought to be inherited: type I and type II. Type I is thought to take years to develop and may not surface until midlife. Type II is a more severe form and appears to be passed primarily from fathers to sons. This form of alcoholism frequently begins earlier in a person's life and may even start in adolescence.

Genetics may also help protect some Asians from developing alcoholism. About half of all Far East Asians produce low levels of an important enzyme that helps metabolize alcohol. These people cannot tolerate even small amounts of alcohol. Genetic factors pertaining to the absorption rates of alcohol in the intestinal tract have been hypothesized to predispose some Native Americans to alcoholism. It is likely that more research will be undertaken concerning the role of genetic factors in all forms of chemical dependence.

The role of personality traits as conditioning factors in the development of alcoholism has received considerable attention. Factors ranging from unusually low self-esteem to an antisocial personality have been implicated. Additional factors making people susceptible to alcoholism may include excessive reliance on denial, hypervigilance, compulsiveness, and chronic levels of anxiety. Always complicating the study of personality traits is the uncertainty of whether the personality profile is a predisposing factor (perhaps from inheritance) or is caused by alcoholism.

Codependence

Within the last decade, a new term has been used to describe the relationship between drug-dependent people and those around them—**codependence.** This term implies a kind of dual addiction. The alcoholic and the person close to the alcoholic are both addicted, one to alcohol and the other to the alcoholic. People who are codependent often find themselves denying the addiction and enabling the alcohol-dependent person.

Unfortunately, this kind of behavior damages both the alcoholic and the codependent. The alcoholic's intervention and treatment may be delayed for a considerable time. Codependent people often pay a heavy price as well. They often become drug- or alcohol-dependent themselves, or they may suffer a variety of psychological consequences related to guilt, loss of self-esteem, depression, and anxiety. Codependents may be at increased risk for physical and sexual abuse.

Researchers continue to explore this dimension of alcoholism. Many students have found some of the resources identified in this chapter to be especially helpful.

Denial and Enabling

Problem drinkers and alcoholics frequently use the psychological defense mechanism of *denial* to maintain their drinking behavior. By convincing themselves that their lives are not affected by their drinking, problem drinkers and alcoholics are able to maintain their drinking patterns. A person's denial is an unconscious process that is apparent only to rational observers.

Formerly, it was up to alcoholics to admit that their denial was no longer effective before they could be admitted to a treatment program. This is not the case today. Currently, family members, friends, or coworkers of alcohol-dependent people are encouraged to intervene and force an alcohol-dependent person into treatment.

TALKING POINTS • One of your professors is a known alcoholic. You wonder why no one has persuaded her to seek treatment. Would you intervene in any way to make that happen? If so, how?

During treatment, it is important for chemically dependent people to break through the security of denial and admit that alcohol controls their lives. This process is demanding and often time-consuming, but it is necessary for recovery.

For family and friends of chemically dependent people, denial is part of a process known as **enabling.** In this process, people close to the problem drinker or alcoholic inadvertently support drinking behavior by denying that a problem really exists. Enablers unconsciously make excuses for the drinker, try to keep the drinker's work and family life intact, and in effect make the continued abuse of alcohol possible. For example, college students enable problem drinkers when they clean up a drinker's messy room, lie to professors about a student's class absences, and provide class notes or other assistance to a drinker who can't keep up academically.

Alcohol counselors contend that enablers are an alcoholic's worst enemy because they can significantly delay the onset of effective therapy. Do you know of a situation in which you or others have enabled a person with an alcohol problem?

Alcoholism and the Family

Considerable disruption occurs in the families of alcoholics, not only from the consequences of the drinking behavior (such as violence, illness, and unemployment), but also because of the uncertainty of the family's role in causing and prolonging the situation. Family members often begin to adopt a variety of new roles that will allow them to cope with the presence of the alcoholic in the family. Among the more commonly seen roles are the family hero, the lost child, the family mascot, and the scapegoat.[7] Unless family members receive appropriate counseling, these roles may remain intact for a lifetime.

Once an alcoholic's therapy has begun, family members are encouraged to participate in many aspects of the recovery. This participation will also help them understand how they are affected by alcoholism. If therapy and aftercare include participation in Alcoholics Anonymous (AA), family members will be encouraged to become affiliated with related support groups.

Helping the Alcoholic: Rehabilitation and Recovery

Once an alcoholic realizes that alcoholism is not a form of moral weakness but rather a clearly defined illness, the chances for recovery are remarkably good. It is estimated that as many as two-thirds of alcoholics can recover. Recovery is especially enhanced when the addicted person has a good emotional support system, including concerned family members, friends, and employer. When this support system is not well established, the alcoholic's chances for recovery are considerably lower.

AA is a voluntary support group of recovering alcoholics who meet regularly to help each other get and stay sober. Over 51,000 groups exist in the United States, another 5000 in Canada, and nearly 40,000 worldwide.[14] AA encourages alcoholics to admit their lack of power over alcohol and to turn their lives over to a higher power (although the organization is nonsectarian). Members of AA are encouraged not to be judgmental about the behavior of other members. They support anyone with a problem caused by alcohol.

Key Terms

alcoholism
A primary, chronic disease with genetic, psychosocial, and environmental factors influencing its development and manifestations.

codependence
An unhealthy relationship in which one person is addicted to alcohol or another drug and a person close to him or her is "addicted" to the alcoholic or drug user.

enabling
Inadvertently supporting a drinker's behavior by denying that a problem exists.

Al-Anon and Alateen are parallel organizations that give support to people who live with alcoholics. Al-Anon is geared toward spouses and other relatives, and Alateen focuses on children of alcoholics. There are 28,000 Al-Anon groups and 3000 Alateen groups worldwide. Both organizations help members realize that they are not alone and that successful adjustments can be made to nearly every alcoholic-related situation. AA, Al-Anon, and Alateen chapter organizations are usually listed in the telephone book or in the classified sections of local newspapers. You can locate Al-Anon and Alateen on the Web at **www.al-anon.alateen.org.**

For people who feel uncomfortable with the concept that their lives are controlled by a higher power, *secular recovery programs* are becoming popular. These programs maintain that sobriety comes from within the alcoholic. Secular programs strongly emphasize self-reliance, self-determination, and rational thinking about one's drinking. Secular Organizations for Sobriety (SOS) and Rational Recovery are examples of secular recovery programs.

Drugs to Treat Alcoholism

Could there be a medical cure for alcoholism? For nearly 50 years, the only prescription drug physicians could use to help drinkers stop drinking was disulfiram (Antabuse). Antabuse would cause drinkers to become extremely nauseated whenever they used alcohol.

In 1995 the Food and Drug Administration approved the drug naltrexone (ReVia) that works by reducing the craving for alcohol and the pleasurable sensations felt when drinking. Combining naltrexone with conventional behavior modification has shown promising results. Additionally, the use of antidepressants by some alcoholics has been especially helpful during treatment.[1]

CURRENT ALCOHOL CONCERNS

Adult Children of Alcoholic Parents

In recent years a new dimension of alcoholism has been identified—the unusually high prevalence of alcoholism among adult children of alcoholics (ACOAs). It is estimated that these children are about four times more likely to develop alcoholism than children whose parents are not alcoholics. Even the ACOAs who do not become alcoholics may have a difficult time adjusting to everyday living. Janet Geringer Woititz, author of the best-selling book *Adult Children of Alcoholics,*[15] describes thirteen traits that most ACOAs exhibit to some degree (see the Star Box above).

In response to this concern, support groups have been formed to help prevent the adult sons and daughters of alcoholics from developing the condition that afflicted their parents (see the Star Box on p. 195). If a stronger link for an inherited genetic predisposition to alcoholism is found, these groups may play an even greater role in the prevention of alcoholism.

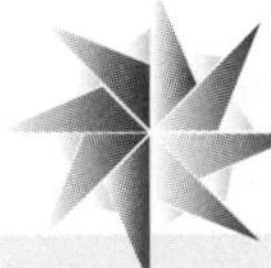

Common Traits of Adult Children of Alcoholics

Adult children of alcoholics may:

- Have difficulty identifying normal behavior
- Have difficulty following a project from beginning to end
- Lie when it would be just as easy to tell the truth
- Judge themselves without mercy
- Have difficulty having fun
- Take themselves very seriously
- Have difficulty with intimate relationships
- Overreact to changes over which they have no control
- Constantly seek approval and affirmation
- Feel that they are different from other people
- Be super-responsible or super-irresponsible
- Be extremely loyal, even in the face of evidence that the loyalty is undeserved
- Tend to lock themselves into a course of action without considering the consequences

Women and Alcohol

For decades, women have consumed less alcohol and had fewer alcohol-related problems than men. At present, evidence is mounting that a greater percentage of women are choosing to drink and that some subgroups of women, especially young women, are drinking more heavily. An increased number of admissions of women to treatment centers may also reflect that alcohol consumption among women is on the rise.[7] Special approaches for women to use for staying sober are discussed in the Learning from Our Diversity box on p. 195.

Studies indicate that currently there are almost as many female as male alcoholics. However, there appear to be differences between men and women when it comes to alcohol abuse: (1) More women than men can point to a specific triggering event (such as a divorce, death of a spouse, a career change, or children leaving home) that started them drinking heavily. (2) Alcoholism among women often starts later and progresses more quickly than alcoholism among men. (3) Women tend to be prescribed more mood-altering drugs than men. So women face greater risk of drug interaction or cross-tolerance. (4) Nonalcoholic men tend to divorce their alcoholic spouses nine times more often than nonalcoholic women divorce their alcoholic spouses. Thus alcoholic women are not as likely to have a family support system to aid them in their recovery attempts. (5) Female alcoholics do not tend to receive as much social support as men in their treatment and recovery. (6) Unmarried, divorced, or single-parent women tend to have significant economic problems that may make

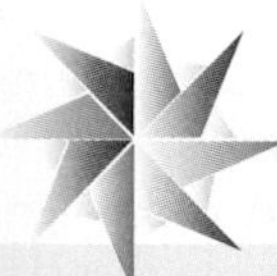

Resources for Adult Children of Alcoholics

Experts agree that adult children of alcoholics who believe they have come to terms with their feelings sometimes face lingering problems. It can prove worthwhile to seek help if you experience the following:

- Difficulty in identifying your needs
- Persistent anger or sadness
- Inability to enjoy your successes
- Willingness to tolerate inappropriate behavior
- Continual fear of losing control

Support groups to contact for more information are listed below:

Al-Anon Family Group Headquarters
1600 Corporate Landing Parkway
Virginia Beach, VA 23454-5617
(757) 563-1600
(888) 4AL-ANON or (888) 425-2666
www.Al-Anon.Alateen.org

Children of Alcoholics Foundation
164 West 74th Street
New York, NY 10023
(212) 595-5810 ext 7760
www.coaf.org

Adult Children of Alcoholics
World Service Organization, Inc.
P.O. Box 3216
Torrance, CA 90510
(310) 534-1815 (message only)
www.adultchildren.org

The Awareness Center
Resources for Adult Children of Alcoholics
(Website of Dr. Janet Woititz)
www.drjan.com

Learning from Our Diversity

Staying Sober: New Pathways for Women

Since 1935, when it was founded by two white American male alcoholics, Alcoholics Anonymous has expanded to encompass millions of members in virtually every region of the world who strive to achieve and maintain sobriety by adhering to AA's well-known 12-step program of recovery. With its strong spiritual orientation emphasizing the acknowledgment of a "higher power," AA offers safety, comfort, and structure to people of all ages and backgrounds, and both sexes. For decades, women as well as men have made AA the cornerstone of their efforts to get sober and stay sober.

Not all women, however, are comfortable with AA's focus on Christian spirituality and the perceived masculine orientation of its chief text, Alcoholics Anonymous (familiarly known as the "Big Book"), and other program literature. These women place an equally high value on sober living as do AA adherents, but they prefer to pursue that goal in other settings. In recent years, alternatives to AA have emerged that offer peer group acceptance and support for recovering alcoholic women, but do so in a nonspiritual, nonsexist context.

One such group, Women for Sobriety, is a mutual aid organization for women with alcohol problems that was founded in 1975 by Dr. Jean Kirkpatrick. The WFS program focuses on improving self-esteem; members achieve sobriety by taking responsibility for their actions and by learning not to dwell on negative thoughts. Another alternative, Rational Recovery, is open to both men and women. RR, which is based on the theories of psychologist Albert Ellis's Rational Emotive Therapy, also uses a cognitive, nonspiritual approach that fosters cohesiveness and provides the emotional support sought by people who seek to gain and maintain sobriety.

Particularly for "marginalized" alcoholic women such as lesbians, racial and ethnic minorities, and those of non-Christian religious backgrounds, alcoholism treatment professionals increasingly are being encouraged to present the full range of support-group options, including but not emphasizing the approach of Alcoholics Anonymous.

If you were seeking help to achieve and maintain sobriety, would you be more inclined to attend a program based on spirituality, or one that offers a rational, cognitive approach? Why?

Kaskutas L: A road less traveled: choosing the "Women for Sobriety" program. *Journal of Drug Issues,* Winter 1996, vol. 26, no. 1, p. 77.

Galanter M and others: Rational Recovery: alternative to AA for addiction? *American Journal of Drug and Alcohol Abuse,* 1993, vol. 19, p. 499.

Hall J: Lesbians' participation in Alcoholics Anonymous: experience of social, personal, and political tensions. *Contemporary Drug Problems,* Spring 1996, vol. 23, no. 1, p. 113.

entry into a treatment program especially difficult. (7) Women seem to be more susceptible than men to medical complications resulting from heavy drinking.[7] In light of the generally recognized educational, occupational, and social gains made by women during the last two decades, it will be interesting to see whether these male-female differences continue. What's your best guess?

Alcohol Advertising

Every few years, careful observers can see subtle changes in the ways the alcoholic beverage industry markets its products. Recently, the marketing push appears to be directed toward minorities (through advertisements for malt liquor and fortified wines), women (through wine and wine cooler ads), and youth (through trendy, young adult-oriented commercials), and spiffy websites.

On the college campus, aggressive alcohol campaigns have used rock stars, beach party scenes, athletic event sponsorships, and colorful newspaper supplements as vehicles to encourage the purchase of alcohol. Critics claim that most of the collegiate advertising is directed at the "below age 21" crowd and that the prevention messages are not strong enough to offset the potential health damage to this population. How do you feel about alcohol advertising on your campus? If you're a nontraditional-age student, do you find the advertising campaigns amusing or potentially dangerous?

SUMMARY

- Alcohol is the drug of choice among college students and the rest of American society.
- Many factors affect the rate of absorption of alcohol into the bloodstream.
- As BAC rises, predictable depressant effects take place.
- People with acute alcohol intoxication must receive first-aid care immediately.
- The health effects of chronic alcohol abuse are quite serious.
- Problem drinking reflects an alcohol use pattern in which a drinker's behavior creates personal difficulties or problems for others.
- Alcoholism is a primary, chronic disease with a variety of possible causes and characteristics.
- Denial, enabling, codependence, ACOAs, and alcohol advertising are current issues related to alcohol abuse in the United States.
- Recovery and rehabilitation programs can be effective in helping alcoholics become sober.
- Antabuse, naltrexone, and antidepressants are drugs prescribed by physicians to help alcoholics in treatment.
- Federal legislation has pushed states to lower the legal BAC standard to .08%.

REVIEW QUESTIONS

1. What percentage of American adults consume alcohol? Approximately what percentage of adults are classified as abstainers? What percentage of college students drink?
2. What is binge drinking?
3. What is meant by the term *proof*?
4. What is the nutritional value of alcohol? How do "lite" and low-alcohol beverages compare?
5. Identify and explain the various factors that influence the absorption of alcohol. Why is it important to be aware of these factors?
6. What is BAC? Describe the general sequence of physiological events that takes place when a person drinks alcohol at a rate faster than the liver can oxidize it.
7. What are the signs and symptoms of acute alcohol intoxication? What are the first-aid steps you should take to help a person with this problem?
8. Describe the characteristics of fetal alcohol syndrome and fetal alcohol effects.
9. Explain the differences between problem drinking and alcoholism.
10. What is codependence? What roles do denial and enabling play in alcoholism?
11. What are some common traits of ACOAs?
12. What unique alcohol-related problems exist for women?
13. Describe the activities undertaken by SADD, MADD, BACCHUS, and GAMMA and by AA, Al-Anon, and Alateen.

THINK ABOUT THIS . . .

- How much is your decision to drink or not drink influenced by those around you?
- This chapter refers to data indicating that over one-third of college drinkers can be considered heavy drinkers. Do you think this is true at your college?
- Do you believe it is your responsibility to make sure friends do not drink and drive?
- Do you think your drinking pattern will change when you are out of college?

REFERENCES

1. U.S. Department of Health and Human Services: *Alcohol and health: tenth special report to the U.S. Congress,* NIH Pub No 00-1583, 2000, U.S. Government Printing Office.
2. U.S. Bureau of the Census: *Statistical abstract of the United States, 1999,* annual ed 119, 2000, U.S. Government Printing Office.
3. Payne WA, Hahn DB: *Alcohol consumption of students in the personal health class,* 1999, unpublished research.
4. U.S. Department of Health and Human Services: *NIAAA alcohol alert: moderate drinking,* No 16 (PH 315), April 1992, U.S. Government Printing Office.
5. U.S. Department of Health and Human Services: *NIAAA alcohol alert: college drinking,* No 29 (PH357), July 1995, U.S. Government Printing Office.
6. Barker O: 113 universities tackle student binge drinking, *USA Today,* p 5D, September 13, 1999.
7. Kinney J: *Loosening the grip: a handbook of alcohol information,* ed 6, 1998, McGraw-Hill.
8. Frezza M et al: High blood alcohol levels in women: role of decreased gastric alcohol dehydrogenase activity and first-pass metabolism, *N Engl J Med* 322(4), 95–99, 1990.
9. Ray O, Ksir C: *Drugs, society and human behavior,* ed 8, 1999, McGraw-Hill.
10. National Highway Safety Traffic Administration: *Traffic safety facts 1999: alcohol,* DOT-HS-809-086, 1999, **www.nhtsa.dot.gov**.
11. MADD: *President Clinton signs federal .08 BAC drunk driving law,* press release, (Oct 23, 2000), **www.madd.org**.
12. Task Force on Responsible Decisions about Alcohol: *Interim report no 2,* undated, Education Commission of the States.
13. Morse RM et al: The definition of alcoholism, *JAMA* 268(8):1012–1014, 1992.
14. Website information, **www.alcoholics-anonymous.org**, November 24, 1999.
15. Woititz JG: *Adult children of alcoholics,* 1990, Health Communications, Inc.

SUGGESTED READINGS

Beattie, M: *Playing it by heart: taking care of yourself no matter what,* 1999, Hazelden Education Information.

This book is a follow-up to the author's highly successful *Codependent no more: how to stop controlling others and start caring for yourself.* Melody Beattie shows readers how to keep focused on yourself as you move between being afraid to trust someone and being absorbed in another's life. The author shows people in recovery that their lives may be challenging but that balance and healing are possible.

Dick B, Seiberling JF: *The Akron genesis of Alcoholics Anonymous,* Newton revised ed, 1998, Paradise Research Publications.

This book traces the fascinating beginning of Alcoholics Anonymous at the Akron, Ohio, home of Dr. Bob Smith, in 1935. The development of the AA spiritual principles is discussed, as well as the activities undertaken in the early meetings of AA in homes and hospitals. The important role of the wives of the early AA members is traced.

Kettelhack G: *First-year sobriety: when all that changes is everything,* 1998, Hazelden Information Education.

This book is an excellent guide for coping with all the changes that take place during the first year of an alcoholic's sobriety. Interacting with family and friends on new levels is one of the many new experiences sober people face during the first year. Additional changes, such as those that occur at work, are also discussed. How to use newly acquired free time effectively is also explored in this book.

Nuwer H: *The wrongs of passage: fraternities, sororities, hazing and binge drinking,* 1999, Indiana University Press.

Binge drinking remains a cornerstone of various Greek activities and rituals, despite the public image displayed by fraternities and sororities. In his serious, critical exploration of the Greek system that exists on many college campuses, Nuwer builds on his 1990 book *Broken pledges: the deadly rite of hazing.* He discusses the continuing problems experienced by young students as they try to fit in with older brothers and sisters. Nuwer places some of the blame on college administrators who fail to acknowledge the continuing problems with alcohol.

Name ______________________ **Date** __________ **Section** __________

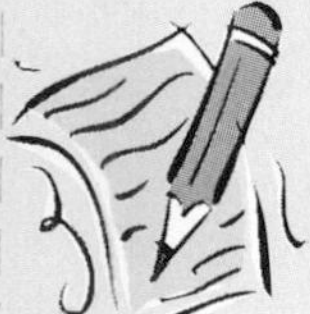

Personal Assessment

Are You Troubled by Someone's Drinking?

The following questions are designed to help you decide whether you are affected by someone's drinking and could benefit from a program such as Al-Anon. Record your number of yes and no responses in the boxes at the end of the questionnaire.

	Yes	No
1. Do you worry about how much someone else drinks?	____	____
2. Do you have money problems because of someone else's drinking?	____	____
3. Do you tell lies to cover up for someone else's drinking?	____	____
4. Do you feel that if the drinker loved you, he or she would stop drinking to please you?	____	____
5. Do you blame the drinker's behavior on his or her companions?	____	____
6. Are plans frequently upset or meals delayed because of the drinker?	____	____
7. Do you make threats, such as: "If you don't stop drinking, I'll leave you?"	____	____
8. Do you secretly try to smell the drinker's breath?	____	____
9. Are you afraid to upset someone for fear it will set off a drinking bout?	____	____
10. Have you been hurt or embarrassed by a drinker's behavior?	____	____
11. Are holidays and gatherings spoiled because of the drinking?	____	____
12. Have you considered calling the police for help in fear of abuse?	____	____
13. Do you search for hidden alcohol?	____	____
14. Do you often ride in a car with a driver who has been drinking?	____	____
15. Have you refused social invitations out of fear or anxiety that the drinker will cause a scene?	____	____
16. Do you sometimes feel like a failure when you think of the lengths to which you have gone to control the drinker?	____	____
17. Do you think that if the drinker stopped drinking, your other problems would be solved?	____	____
18. Do you ever threaten to hurt yourself to scare the drinker?	____	____
19. Do you feel angry, confused, or depressed most of the time?	____	____
20. Do you feel there is no one who understands your problems?	____	____
TOTAL	____	____

Interpretation

If you answered yes to three or more of these questions, Al-Anon or Alateen may be able to help. You can contact Al-Anon or Alateen by looking in your local telephone directory or by writing to Al-Anon Family Group Headquarters, Inc., 1600 Corporate Landing Parkway, Virginia Beach, VA 23454-5617, or you may call (888) 4AL-ANON.

To Carry This Further . . .

Sometimes the decision to seek help from a support group is a difficult one. If you answered yes to any of the questions above, spend a few moments reflecting on your responses. How long have you been experiencing problems because of someone else's drinking? How would sharing your feelings with others—people who have dealt with very similar problems—help you cope with your own situation? Knowing you're not alone can often be a great relief; it's up to you to take the first step.

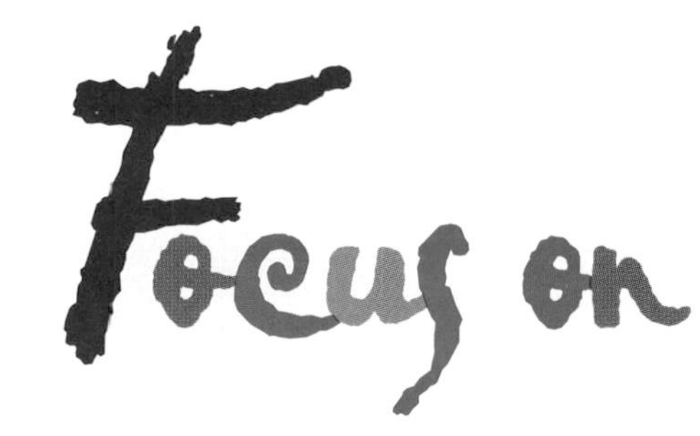

ALCOHOL AND VIOLENCE: A DANGEROUS LINK

In recent years, there has been an increase in public service messages to raise awareness about driving under the influence of alcohol. In fact, the massive campaign against drinking and driving has been quite successful in reducing the number of drunk-driving accidents and fatalities. However, people may think that as long as a person doesn't get behind the wheel, it's okay to drink. But there are other potential dangers to the abuse of alcohol. One particular problem that perhaps has not been stressed enough in the media is the link between alcohol use and violent crime.[1]

Obviously, not everyone who drinks becomes violent, but in many violent crimes at least one person involved has been drinking. Perhaps alcohol by itself is not enough to cause violence, but use of alcohol may be one of several factors that act in combination to cause violent behavior in some instances.[2]

Who is most likely to be involved in an alcohol-related violent crime? A 9-year study of over 4000 Los Angeles homicide victims suggests that men are much more likely to be involved than women. In the study, 51.3% of the male victims had detectable blood alcohol concentrations compared with 25.8% of the female victims.[2] Other studies have shown that young people under age 30 are more likely than older people to be involved in both sexual and nonsexual assault when alcohol is a factor. Data on race and ethnicity are inconclusive; some studies show that whites are more likely to be involved in alcohol-related homicides, whereas others show that African Americans are. In the Los Angeles study, 38.2% of Hispanic homicide victims had detectable blood alcohol concentrations; this places them between the percentage figures for male victims and female victims and thus shows no tendency for or against involvement in alcohol-related violence. Alcohol-related homicides and assaults are more likely to occur on weekends than weekdays in part because more people tend to drink on weekends.[2]

Alcohol and Types of Violent Crime

The risk of a person's perpetrating a violent event is higher among heavy drinkers than light drinkers. Heavy drinkers are also at higher risk of being victims of violent crime and are also more likely to inflict and to receive violent injuries.[3] A Johns Hopkins University study shows that being a victim of sexual abuse or assault is also linked to high rates of alcohol use.[4] An environment where alcohol is prevalent is a risk factor associated with gun injuries, particularly deaths among youths.[5] Alcohol-related violence tends to be more prevalent in urban environments. It is estimated that eliminating the glut of inner city alcohol outlets could cut the U.S. homicide rate by 10% and could save 2000 lives annually.[6]

Alcohol plays a significant role in various types of violent crime. Substantial numbers of sexual-assault victims and offenders were drinking before their crime occurred. Alcohol use is present in over half of all domestic violence cases, and frequency of drunkenness for husbands appears to be associated with spouse abuse.[2] One study estimated that incidences of spouse abuse were almost 15 times higher for households where husbands were described as often drunk as opposed to never drunk. And drinking may also increase the risk of becoming a robbery victim.[2]

Campus Crime and the Effects of Alcohol

Of particular interest to college students are the data linking campus crimes to alcohol use. A *USA Today* study of 13,000 students suggests that as many as 4 out of 5 campus crimes committed by students are related to alcohol or drug use or both. The attitudes of college students may be a contributing factor to alcohol abuse on campus; 85% of freshmen in the survey condoned binge drinking (defined in this study as over five drinks in a continuous period). Victims of violent crime on campus generally reported heavier drinking habits than nonvictims,[7] and this parallels data from the general population.[2] When sexual assaults and rapes were reported, both the perpetrator and the victim had typically been drinking.[7]

Impact of Alcohol on Violent Behavior

So why is alcohol a contributing factor in violent crime? Alcohol acts as a depressant, which can reduce reaction time, impair coordination, and cloud judgment. Such impairment could decrease the chances of avoiding personal injury once a physical altercation begins. Alcohol also decreases inhibitions and may increase aggressive behavior. It also may increase the likelihood of inflicting or receiving a severe injury during a violent act and has been shown to increase the severity of injuries obtained in violent acts. Alcohol impairs cognitive abilities and may increase the chances for miscommunication or misinterpretation during verbal conflicts.[2,3] The fact that many drinkers do not exhibit violent behavior suggests that individual differences in brain chemistry may promote aggressive behaviors in some people but not others.[8]

What You Can Do

Although alcohol alone may not cause violence, when alcohol is introduced into a situation that has the potential to become violent, it can increase the chances that violence will occur. As the number of drunk drivers on the road has decreased, so has the number of drunk-driving accidents and fatalities. It seems logical to assume that if alcohol is kept out of the hands of people who are predisposed to violence, the number of alcohol-related crimes may also decrease. This is not always possible, but it is possible for you to use good common sense when you are drinking or if you are with people who are drinking. Try to avoid potentially violent situations, and avoid people drinking around you who are acting in a reckless or violent manner. Drink in moderation, and help your companions recognize when they have had too much. Perhaps you or one of your companions can remain sober (a "designated thinker") to help avoid potentially dangerous situations and stay safe while partying.

For Discussion . . .

Have you ever encountered an angry drinker? Is there a safe way to handle a person who is drunk and intending to do harm to someone? If you have ever been drunk, do you feel that you could have controlled your actions in a confrontation while you were drunk?

References

1. Jamiolkowski RM: *Drugs and domestic violence,* 1997, Hazelden.
2. Messerschmidt PM: Epidemiology of alcohol-related violence, *Alcohol Health and Research World,* 17(2), 1993.
3. Cherpitel CJ: What emergency room studies reveal about alcohol involvement in violence-related injuries, *Alcohol Health and Research World,* 17(2), 1993.
4. Violence, drugs, alcohol spur decline of youth health across U.S., study says, *Jet,* 88(7), June 26, 1995.
5. Voelker R: Taking aim at handgun violence, *JAMA* 273(22), 1995.
6. Abramson H: Quick fix for violence: cut back on liquor stores, *Nation's Cities Weekly,* 18(3), 1995.
7. Siegel D: What is behind the growth of violence on college campuses? *USA Today Magazine,* 122(2588), May 1994.
8. U.S. Department of Health and Human Services: *NIAAA alcohol alert: alcohol, violence, and aggression,* No. 38-1997, October 1997, U.S. Government Printing Office.

chapter **9**

Rejecting Tobacco Use

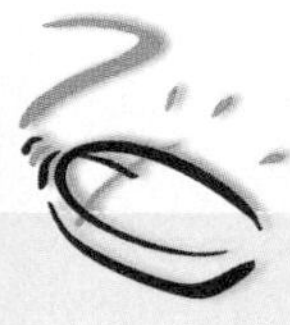

Online Learning Center Resources

www.mhhe.com/hahn6e

Log on to our Online Learning Center (OLC) for access to these additional resources:

- Chapter key terms and definitions
- Learning objectives
- Additional behavior change objectives
- Student interactive question-and-answer sites
- Self-scoring chapter quiz

The OLC also offers web links for study and exploration of health topics. Here are some examples of what you'll find:

- **www.cdc.gov/tobacco** Read all about it here: smoking kills more people than AIDS, alcohol, drug abuse, car crashes, murders, suicides, and fires—combined.
- **www.health.org** Click here for tobacco-related educational and prevention material.
- **www.quitnet.org** Surf this website for help in quitting, including an online support group.

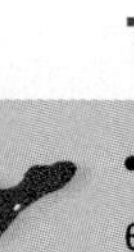

Taking Charge of Your Health

- Commit yourself to establishing a smoke-free environment in the places where you live, work, study, and recreate.
- Support friends and acquaintances who are trying to become smoke-free.
- Support legislative efforts, at all levels of government, to reduce your exposure to environmental tobacco smoke.
- Be civil toward tobacco users in public spaces, but respond assertively if they infringe on smoke-free spaces.
- Support agencies and organizations committed to reducing tobacco use among young people through education and intervention.

Eye on the Media

The Changing Face of Tobacco Ads

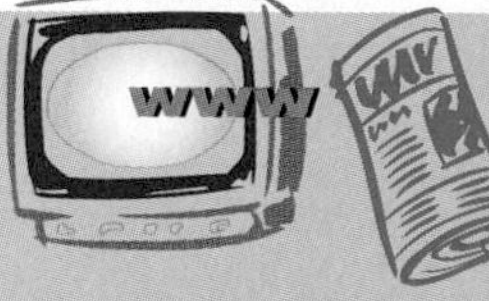

No single consumer product, including automobiles and beer, has had a more complex history in the media than tobacco, particularly cigarettes. This history begins with advertisements for chewing tobacco—still visible along the highways of the Midwest, where old, dilapidated barns show faded ads for Red Man or Mail Pouch tobacco.

From the end of World War I until the introduction of television, magazine advertisements and radio commercials delivered strong messages about the benefits of tobacco use—its wonderful flavor, social sophistication, and "health benefits." Magazine ads showed "physicians" recommending cigarettes to soothe the throat and baseball players attributing their athletic prowess to chewing tobacco.

The most powerful—and harmful—use of the media by the tobacco industry involved the cigarette commercials on television from the early 1950s until 1971. Like beer commercials today, they portrayed a hedonistic lifestyle in which sensual, affluent young adults gathered in an idyllic location to smoke and enjoy each other's company—with no suggestion of the negative effects of smoking.

Eye on the Media *continued*

Television commercials for cigarettes were banned in 1971, when the tobacco industry agreed to discontinue use of this media in exchange for the withdrawal of the highly effective antismoking public service commercials being broadcast by the federal government.

Since then, the tobacco industry has relied on other media to deliver its message of tobacco and "the good life." It sponsors tournaments, special events, and athletic teams, runs full-page ads in magazines, publishes leisure and entertainment magazines sent free to smokers, stages free pop music concerts (at which smoking is permitted), sponsors contests with prizes such as dude ranch vacations, and displays neon signs in stores where tobacco products are sold. When the use of outdoor billboards and murals on buildings for tobacco ads was discontinued, the industry began giving away logo clothing and personal items. However, this practice ended as a part of the settlement of a 1998 class action suit brought by fifty states against the tobacco industry (see p. 205).

The tobacco industry has been skillful in replacing one generation of users—lost because of illness and premature death—with a younger, healthier one. The industry contends that it has no interest in attracting vulnerable adolescents to a lifetime addiction. Instead, it claims to be focusing on challenging brand loyalty by trying to influence people who already smoke to switch to the brand being advertised. Many people question the sincerity of this position. Meanwhile, the millions of dollars being spent on tobacco advertising is having a powerful effect on smokers and potential smokers alike.

Today, the evidence linking tobacco use to impaired health is beyond serious challenge.[1] The regular user of tobacco products, particularly cigarettes, is more likely to become sick, remain sick for extended periods, and die prematurely than is a nonuser. It is estimated that tobacco use, cigarette smoking in particular, resulted in 2 million deaths between 1986 and 2000. Therefore, any contention made by the tobacco industry that tobacco use is not dangerous is groundless and ignores the growing weight of scientific evidence.

TOBACCO USE IN AMERICAN SOCIETY

On the basis of the most recent national data available (1998), cigarette smoking among adults 18 years of age and older is currently at 24.1% and remains relatively constant. Men are more likely to smoke (white men, 26.3%; African American men, 29%) than women (white women, 22.6%; African American women, 21%).[2] Smoking rates among men have fallen steadily since 1964, but rates among women increased until the early 1990s, when they began a gradual decline, that continues today.

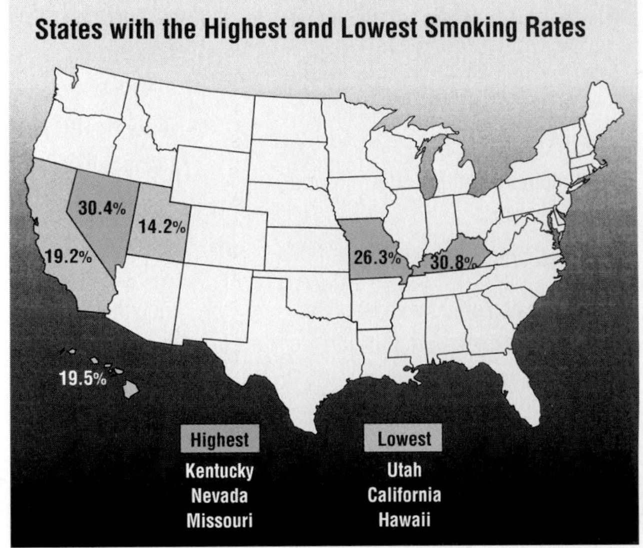

Figure 9-1 Kentucky has the highest smoking rate in the nation. Do you know what the rate is in your state?

The Influence of Education

Until very recently, the rate of cigarette smoking among college graduates was lower than that of people with less education. In fact, the prevalence of smoking among college graduates decreased progressively from 21% in 1964 to 10.9% in 1998.[2] However, an upward trend in cigarette use by college students has been noted, with a recent study finding 30.6% of students smoking at least monthly.[3] In contrast, a downward trend in smoking by twelfth graders was reported in 1998.[4]

The connection between higher levels of education on a lower-than-average incidence of smoking was clearly evident in 1998, when statistics indicated that 34.4% of Americans without a high school diploma were smokers.[2] The reported incidence of smoking on today's college campus brings these two somewhat diverse segments of the population closer together. Today's college students are smoking at about the same level as did people in 1998 with only a high school diploma.

How much do you know about cigarette smoking? Find out by completing the Personal Assessment on p. 223.

Advertising Approaches

In the face of an overall decline in cigarette smoking and overwhelming evidence that tobacco products are life-threatening, the tobacco industry has tried to maintain the loyalty of its consumers. It accomplished this through continuous product development, skilled marketing, aggressive political lobbying, and diversification. These techniques included:

- Shrink-wrapping three-packs of brand-name cigarettes and selling them for the price of two or offering mail-in rebate coupons, making the products more affordable to young and low-income buyers
- Continued marketing of generic brands under the label of "value brands"
- Lowering the price of brand-name cigarettes to compete with value brands
- Carefully targeting advertising, particularly to women, minorities, and less-educated young adults
- Directing advertisements to youths (while simultaneously supporting public policy statements to control minors' access to cigarettes)
- Increased marketing of tobacco products overseas, where health restrictions are less forceful
- Acquiring non–tobacco-related companies (corporate diversification) to minimize the loss of revenues from decreased sales of tobacco products
- Marshalling tobacco users into a "grass roots" effort to counter the political power of antismoking groups

The tobacco industry remains healthy and their products remain life threatening to smokers and nonsmokers.

The Tobacco Industry Under Fire

How much has the tobacco industry known about the addictive and life-shortening nature of its products, particularly cigarettes? This subject has made news almost every day in the last few years. This occurred because the protective wall of denial built by the tobacco industry crumbled in November 1998, when forty-six states joined four other states that had settled with the tobacco industry earlier. The tobacco industry agreed to pay $246 billion (over 25 years) to reimburse the states for Medicaid expenditures associated with treating smoking-related illnesses; to stop advertisements intended to influence tobacco use by children; and to fund antismoking education program development and implementation. In turn, the states agreed not to initiate further class-action lawsuits against the tobacco industry.

Currently, the evidence linking tobacco use to impaired health is beyond challenge. In fact, it has been admitted by the tobacco industry via internal documents released by the Liggett Tobacco Company. These documents (totaling 11 million pages) detail activities by the tobacco industry to disprove, mask, and deny their own knowledge that nicotine is addictive and that cigarette smoking causes cancer and chronic obstructive lung disease and increases the risk of developing cardiovascular disease. They also revealed that concerted marketing efforts were directed toward children and young adolescents to influence them to smoke.

Since the 1999 settlement of the class-action lawsuits brought by states against the tobacco industry for reimbursement of Medicaid monies, efforts to control or monetarily punish the tobacco industry have been escalating. Examples include (1) a renewed effort by individual smokers (or their families) to gain financial compensation for chronic diseases and premature death resulting from long-term smoking that was encouraged by deceptive advertising by the tobacco industry, (2) new class-action efforts by many thousands of smokers to compensate all smokers in a particular area (e.g., the state of Florida) for tobacco-induced illnesses, (3) class-action suits brought by insurance companies seeking redress for the monies spent by that industry in treating smoking-induced illness, (4) suits by states (e.g., Massachusetts) to restrict advertising within their jurisdictions, (5) ordinances in cities and counties to make all food establishments smoke-free, (6) private sector extension of workplace restrictions on smoking beyond the confines of a building to include the outdoor areas located close to building entrances, and (7) a suit by the U.S. Department of Justice against the tobacco industry, on behalf of the federal government, to recoup the $20 billion spent each year to treate smoking-related diseases via the federal and state Medicaid programs.

Pipe and Cigar Smoking

Many people believe that pipe or cigar smoking is a safe alternative to cigarette smoking. However, this is not the case. All forms of tobacco pose health threats.

When compared with cigarette smokers, pipe and cigar smokers have cancer of the mouth, throat, larynx (voice box), and esophagus at the same frequency. Cigarette smokers are more likely than pipe and cigar smokers to have lung cancer, chronic obstructive lung disease (COLD), and heart disease. However, the incidence of respiratory disease and heart disease in pipe and cigar smokers is still greater than that of nonusers of tobacco.[5]

Two recent developments related to the future of cigar smoking in this country have occurred. The first is the possibility that the Federal Trade Commission will require warning labels to be affixed to cigars to inform consumers of the risk they are assuming. Among the warnings being considered are those related to mouth and throat cancer (even when smoke is not inhaled), lung cancer (when smoke is inhaled), and failure of cigars to provide a safe alternative to cigarettes.

The second development is a substantial decline in the 1998–1999 sales of premium cigars. Whether this downturn represents a growing dissatisfaction with cigars as an enjoyable form of tobacco use or reflects adjustments in the import market remains uncertain.

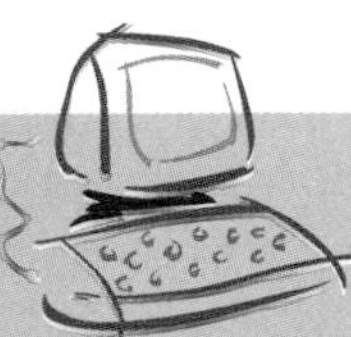

OnSITE/InSIGHT

Learning to Go: Health

Is smoking a part of your everyday life? Click on the Motivator icon to find more information about tobacco in these lessons:

Lesson 28: Adopt a no-smoking rule.
Lesson 29: Keep your lungs healthy.

STUDENT POLL

Whether you're a smoker or not, check to see how other students feel about tobacco use. Go to the Online Learning Center at **www.mhhe.com/hahn6e**. Click on Student Resources to find the Student Poll. Answer the following questions and then find out how other students responded.

1. Are you a nonsmoker?
2. Did you try smoking before age 18?
3. Are you currently a smoker?
4. Are you an ex-smoker who has quit permanently?
5. Have you ever tried smoking a cigar or pipe?
6. Is your generation well educated about the harmful effects of tobacco use?

THE DEVELOPMENT OF DEPENDENCE ON TOBACCO PRODUCTS

Dependence can imply both a physical and a psychological relationship. With cigarettes, *physical dependence* or *addiction,* with its associated *tolerance, withdrawal,* and **titration,** is strongly developed by nearly one-half of all smokers. Most of the remaining population of smokers will experience lesser degrees of physical dependence. The difference in the extent of addiction may reflect a genetic tendency.[6] *Psychological dependence* or *habituation,* with its accompanying psychological *compulsion* and *indulgence,* is frequently seen.

Compulsion is a strong emotional desire to continue tobacco use despite restrictions on smoking and awareness of the health risks. The user is "compelled" to engage in uninterrupted tobacco use by the fear of the unpleasant physical, emotional, and social effects that result from discontinuing its use. In compulsion, indulgence is seen as "rewarding" oneself for aligning with a particular group or behavior pattern. Indulgence is made possible by the reward systems built around tobacco use.

To the great benefit of the tobacco industry, dependence on tobacco is easily established. Many experts believe that physical dependence on tobacco is far more easily established than is dependence on alcohol, cocaine (other than crack), or heroin. Of all people who experiment with cigarettes, 85% develop some type of dependent relationship. This potential for dependence, including addiction, prompted the FDA to request that tobacco products be defined as drug delivery systems, which would allow the FDA to regulate their availability. In 2000 the U.S. Supreme Court ruled that the FDA lacked this authority.

A small percentage of smokers, known as "chippers," can smoke a few cigarettes on a daily basis without becoming dependent. Experts believe that these people have a defective gene that increases the toxic effect of nicotine.[6]

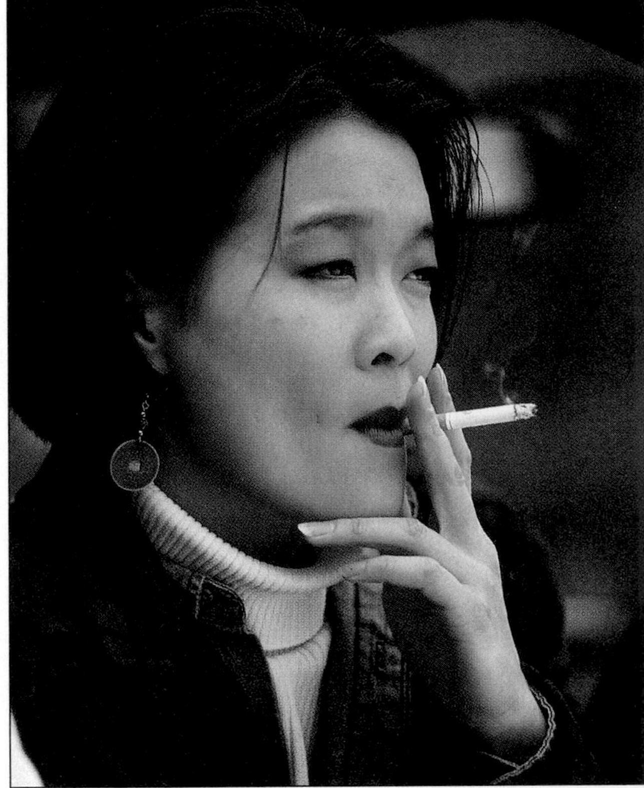

A smoker inhales about 70,000 times during the first year of smoking, resulting in a nicotine addiction that often lasts a lifetime.

Because they enjoy smoking less, chippers smoke fewer cigarettes and do so far less frequently than regular smokers. They may be true "social smokers." Many inexperienced smokers also consider themselves to be only social smokers. Yet, a few months of occasional smoking can lead to a lifetime of dependency.

Physiological Factors

In the brain, **nicotine** stimulates the production of excitatory neurotransmitters, which generate a pleasurable sensation of arousal. To maintain this feeling of arousal, the smoker inhales again and again. Several hundred puffs per day quickly establish the schedule necessary to maintain the desired effect.

Nicotine may also stimulate the release of adrenocorticotropic hormone (ACTH) from the pituitary gland (see Chapter 3). In response to ACTH, beta endorphins (naturally occurring opiate-like chemicals) are produced in specific areas of the brain, leading to mild feelings of euphoria. This stresslike response mechanism involving ACTH may also account for the increased energy expenditure seen in smokers and thus their tendency to maintain lower body weight than nonsmokers.

When these physiological responses are viewed collectively, nicotine may be seen as biochemically influencing brain activity by enhancing the extent and strength of various forms of "communication" between different brain areas. If this is the case, once the smoker is addicted, the functioning of that person's nervous system is greatly altered in comparison with that of a nonsmoker.

Another explanation, called *self-medication,* suggests that nicotine, through the effects of mood-enhancing neurotransmitters, may allow smokers to "treat" feelings of tiredness and lack of motivation. In other words, a smoke lifts the spirits, if only briefly. Eventually, however, smokers become dependent on tobacco as a "medication" to make them feel better. Because tobacco is a legal drug, it becomes preferred over equally effective illegal drugs such as cocaine and stimulants.

For most smokers, the smoking behavior is eventually adjusted to maintain titration and prevent the uncomfortableness of withdrawal. The desire to not experience withdrawal becomes as important as the arousal produced by nicotine.

Nicotine as an Addictive Drug

A great deal of interest and controversy recently existed regarding information about the addictive nature of nicotine contained in documents released by people once inside the tobacco industry. Among these issues were the extent to which the tobacco industry was aware of the addictive nature of nicotine and the appropriateness of studies conducted by the tobacco industry to determine whether young children would become future smokers. Further issues included allegations that the tobacco industry adjusted the pH levels of smokeless tobacco brands to alter nicotine levels and that research was conducted by the industry regarding nicotine enhancement of tobacco products.[7] Many people believe that since tobacco companies knew of the dangers of smoking and still encouraged nicotine addiction, they should compensate smokers or their families for losses resulting from smoking-related illnesses. As a result, hundreds of lawsuits have been filed.

Although these issues are far from resolved, the FDA and various other health organizations remain convinced that tobacco products are, in fact, drug delivery systems intended to deliver a powerfully addictive drug, nicotine. However, since it was determined in 2000 by the Supreme Court that the FDA lacked the authority to regulate the availability of tobacco products, they will continue to be sold as they are now, with tobacco itself under the jurisdiction of the Department of Agriculture. See the Learning from Our Diversity box on p. 208, for another approach toward countering the acceptance of tobacco.

TALKING POINTS • A smoker says that she does not consider smoking to be a form of drug use. She becomes angry at the suggestion that cigarettes are part of a drug delivery system. How would you respond to her position?

For years, ill and dying smokers (and their survivors) have been suing, without success, tobacco companies for damages resulting from tobacco-induced illnesses. The success for the industry in countering these suits has been built around the contention that before 1964, they were unaware of any suspected dangers, and that since 1966, they have warned smokers of the dangers they face when using cigarettes. Smokers were found to be responsible for their own poor judgment, and the tobacco companies were judged to be free of liability because of their compliance with mandates to warn smokers.

With the release of the tobacco industry's internal documents and the successful settlement between all fifty states for Medicaid reimbursement, however, it is anticipated that individual smokers will be increasingly able to use the same documents to bring successful suits against the tobacco industry. Recall, however, from the discussion on page 206, that increasingly, these suits are taking the form of class-action suits involving hundreds of thousands of deceased or former smokers, rather than more expensive individual suits.

Psychosocial Factors

Behavioral scientists suggest that dependence on tobacco can also be explained by psychosocial factors. Both research and general observation support many of the powerful influences these factors have on the beginning smoker.

Key Terms

titration
Particular level of a drug within the body; adjusting the level of nicotine by adjusting the rate of smoking.

nicotine
Physiologically active, dependence-producing drug found in tobacco.

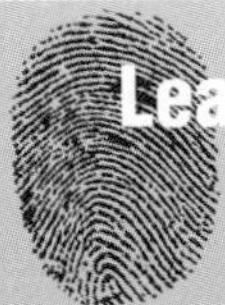

Learning from Our Diversity

World No-Tobacco Day Seeks Support from Athletes and Artists

Sports and smoking seem to make strange bedfellows—but not in the world of advertising. For decades, cigarette manufacturers have worked hand-in-glove with professional athletes and teams, exchanging huge sums of money for endorsements of tobacco products or for the promotion and sponsorship of major sporting events. Although cigarette advertising has been banned from American television for nearly 35 years, the cozy connections continue, with perhaps the most notable example being the women's tennis tournament sponsored by Virginia Slims cigarettes (whose slogan, "You've come a long way, baby," resonated with women of a generation ago but is increasingly quoted in tones ranging from irony to contempt).

A step in the opposite direction is World No-Tobacco Day, promoted annually since 1988 by the World Health Organization (WHO), a unit of the United Nations. On a designated day each year, WHO urges tobacco users to abstain for at least that day— and, ideally, for good. WHO says the annual observance of World No-Tobacco Day "is a unique opportunity to mobilize athletes, artists, and the media, as well as the public in general, in support of the objective of promoting a society and a way of life where tobacco use is no longer an accepted norm."

In sponsoring World No-Tobacco Day, WHO has focused on smoking in public places, on public transportation, in the workplace, and in medical facilities. A recent campaign escalated the stop-smoking effort with a theme of "United Nations and Specialized Agencies Against Tobacco," with the aim of sharply reducing tobacco use worldwide.

As noted earlier, tobacco interests continue to promote many sporting events, as well as some cultural events. As far as sports are concerned, however, WHO officials see reason for encouragement in the recent smoke-free history of the Olympic Games. Beginning with the 1988 Winter Games in Calgary, all Olympic Games—both summer and winter—have been smoke-free.

While a major cigarette manufacturer congratulates its (female) customers on having "come a long way, baby," the World Health Organization is strongly conveying the message that you'll go a lot farther if you don't smoke.

Which tactic do you think is most likely to reduce the rate of tobacco use worldwide: legal bans and restrictions, campaigns of persuasion like World No-Tobacco Day, or a combination of these two approaches?

Modeling

Because tobacco use is a learned behavior, it is reasonable to accept that *modeling* acts as a stimulus to experimental smoking. Modeling suggests that susceptible people smoke to emulate, or model their behavior after, smokers whom they admire or with whom they share other types of social or emotional bonds. Particularly for young adolescents (ages 14 to 17), smoking behavior correlates with the smoking behavior of slightly older peers and very young adults (ages 18 to 22), older siblings, and, to some degree, parents. Is it possible that the very young and attractive models used in tobacco (and beer) advertisements are seen by young adolescents as being closer to their own age than they really are?

Modeling is particularly evident when smoking is a central factor in peer group formation and association; it can lead to a shared behavioral pattern that differentiates the group from others and from adults. When risk-taking behavior and disregard for authority are common to the group, smoking becomes the behavioral pattern that most consistently identifies and bonds the group. Particularly for those young people who lack self-directedness or the ability to resist peer pressure, initial membership in a tobacco-using peer group may become inescapable.

When adolescents have lower levels of self-esteem and are searching for a way to improve their self-image, a role model who smokes is often seen as tough, sociable, and sexually attractive. The last two traits have been played up by the tobacco industry in their carefully crafted advertisements.

Manipulation

Tobacco use may meet the beginning smoker's need to physically manipulate something and provide the manipulative tool necessary to offset boredom, feelings of depression, or social immaturity. Taking out a cigarette or filling a pipe adds a measure of structure and control to situations in which people might otherwise feel somewhat ill at ease. The cigarette becomes a readily available and dependable "friend" to turn to in stressful moments.

Susceptibility to advertising

The images of the smoker's world portrayed in tobacco advertisements can be attractive. For adolescents, women, minorities, and other carefully targeted groups of adults, the tobacco industry associates a better life with the use of their products. Young and potential users are told that using tobacco products offers a sense of power, liberation, affluence, sophistication, and adult

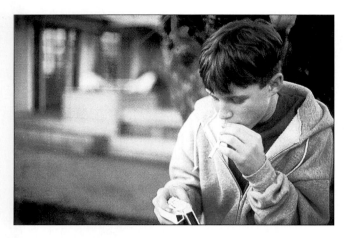

Nine out of ten adult smokers began using tobacco products as kids.

status. The message is that smoking will let them achieve things that most people must work a long time to gain.

Despite the satisfaction of their psychological needs through tobacco use, approximately 90% of adult smokers have, on at least one occasion, expressed a desire to quit, and 80% have actually attempted to become nonsmokers.

Preventing Teen Smoking

Even before the tobacco industry released documents in 1997 confirming that it had targeted adolescents (ages 11 to 14), the federal government stated its intention to curb cigarette advertisements directed at this group. In August 1995 the FDA outlined the specific steps that it wanted to be given authority to implement.[8] These actions, listed below, were intended to discourage cigarette smoking among American teens, resulting in 50% fewer adolescents beginning to smoke in 2002 than in 1995.

1. Limit tobacco advertising in publications that appeal to teens; restrict billboard advertisements to no closer than 1000 feet of schools and playgrounds.
2. Restrict the use of tobacco company logos and other images on nontobacco products, such as towels, T-shirts, and caps.
3. Bar certain sources of access to tobacco products, such as mail-order sales, the distribution of free samples, and vending machines.
4. Prohibit sponsorship of high-visibility sporting events, such as auto racing, in which brand names appear on highly televised surfaces, including hoods, fenders, and uniforms.
5. Require merchants to obtain proof of age when selling tobacco products. (This provision became law in 1997. Merchants are required to validate the age of people whom they suspect to be younger than 27 before selling cigarettes to adults 18 years or older. If found in violation, the salesperson and the store owner will be fined $500 each.)

In spite of the impressive array of restrictions included in this federal proposal, by the end of 1999, Congress had not yet passed the requested legislative package. Congress's failure to pass this legislation was due, in part, to powerful lobbying by the tobacco industry in combination with President Clinton's preoccupation with impeachment proceedings during this period.

Currently, there is some indication that increased protection of younger adolescents may not be as pressing as it was considered in the mid-1990s. This tentative conclusion is based on a December 1999 poll of 165,000 public school students, conducted by *Scholastic* magazine and *The New York Times Upfront,* indicating that 70% of the students interviewed described cigarette smoking as "dumb" and "disgusting" and "not for them." However, will the remaining 30% give in to the peer pressure noted by virtually all of the students interviewed as the reason that some of their classmates had begun smoking?

TOBACCO: THE SOURCE OF PHYSIOLOGICALLY ACTIVE COMPOUNDS

When burned, the tobacco in cigarettes, cigars, and pipe mixtures is a source of an array of physiologically active chemicals, many of which are closely linked to significant changes in normal body structure and function. With each puff of smoke the body is exposed to over 4000 chemical compounds, hundreds of which are known to be physiologically active, toxic, and carcinogenic. The 70,000 plus puffs taken in annually by the one-pack-a-day cigarette smoker result in a regularly occurring environment that makes the most polluted urban environment seem clean in comparison.

Cigarette, cigar, and pipe smoke can be described on the basis of two phases or components: the **particulate phase** and the gaseous phase. The particulate phase includes nicotine, water, and a variety of powerful chemical compounds known collectively as *tar.* Tar includes phenol, cresol, pyrene, DDT, and a benzene-ring group of compounds that includes benzo[*a*]pyrene. As tar is drawn down the airway, the larger particles settle along its length, while the smaller particles reach the alveoli, or small saclike ends of the airway, where air comes in close association with the bloodstream. Most carcinogenic (cancer-causing) compounds are found within the tar.

Key Term

particulate phase
Portion of the tobacco smoke composed of small suspended particles.

The **gaseous phase** of tobacco smoke, like the particulate phase, is composed of a variety of physiologically active compounds, including carbon monoxide, carbon dioxide, ammonia, hydrogen cyanide, isoprene, acetaldehyde, and acetone. At least sixty-nine of these compounds have been determined to be carcinogenic and dozens more may be co-carcinogens.[9] *Carbon monoxide* is the most damaging compound found in this component of tobacco smoke. Its effects are discussed below.

Nicotine

Nicotine is a powerful psychotropic (psychoactive) chemical agent found in the particulate phase of tobacco smoke. When drawn into the lungs, about one-fourth of the nicotine in the inhaled smoke passes into the circulation and to the brain within 10 seconds of inhalation. *Nicotine receptors* within the brain are activated and produce a variety of responses, most of which are stimulating (see the discussion of nicotine addiction on p. 207). High levels of nicotine, however, depress the CNS and result in the relaxation associated with heavy smoking.

The remaining nicotine absorbed into the blood travels throughout the body to nicotinic receptors located in a variety of tissues. Among the presently understood additional effects of nicotine are the reduction of intestinal activity, the release of epinephrine from the adrenal glands, the release of **norepinephrine** from peripheral nerves, an increase in heart rate, the constriction of peripheral blood vessels, and the dilation of airways within the respiratory system.

Nicotine that enters the body by routes other than inhalation produces similar effects but at a much slower rate. Smokeless tobacco, for example, reaches its fullest physiological effect by the end of 20 minutes, nicotine-containing gum within 30 minutes, and transdermal nicotine patches within several hours.

Carbon Monoxide

Burning tobacco forms **carbon monoxide (CO)** gas. Carbon monoxide is one of the most harmful components of tobacco smoke.

Carbon monoxide is a colorless, odorless, tasteless gas that possesses a very strong physiological attraction for hemoglobin, the oxygen-carrying component of each red blood cell. When carbon monoxide is inhaled, it quickly bonds with hemoglobin and forms a new compound, *carboxyhemoglobin.* In this form, hemoglobin is unable to transport oxygen to the tissues and cells where it is needed.

The presence of excessive levels of carboxyhemoglobin in the blood of smokers leads to shortness of breath and lowered endurance. Brain function may be reduced, reactions and judgment are dulled, and cardiovascular function is impaired. Fetuses are especially at risk for this oxygen deprivation because fetal development is so critically dependent on a sufficient oxygen supply from the mother.

ILLNESS, PREMATURE DEATH, AND TOBACCO USE

For people who begin tobacco use as adolescents or young adults, smoke heavily, and continue to smoke, the likelihood of premature death is virtually ensured. Two-pack-a-day cigarette smokers can expect to die 7 to 8 years earlier than their nonsmoking counterparts. Only nonsmoking-related deaths that can afflict both smokers and nonsmokers alike, such as automobile accidents, keep the difference at this level rather than much higher. Not only will smokers, as a group, die sooner, but they also will probably experience painful, debilitating illnesses for an extended time.

Cardiovascular Disease

Cardiovascular disease is the leading cause of death among all adults, accounting for 953,110 deaths annually in the United States.[10] Tobacco use, and cigarette smoking in particular, is clearly one of the major factors contributing to this cause. So important is tobacco use as a contributing factor in deaths from heart disease that cigarette smokers double the risk of experiencing a **myocardial infarction** and increase their risk of **sudden cardiac death** by two to four times. Fully one-third of all cardiovascular disease can be traced to cigarette smoking. The relationship between tobacco use and cardiovascular disease is centered on two major components of tobacco smoke: nicotine and carbon monoxide.

Nicotine and cardiovascular disease

The influence of nicotine on the cardiovascular system occurs when it stimulates the nervous system to release norepinephrine. This powerful stimulant increases the rate at which the heart contracts. The extent to which this is dangerous depends in part on the ability of the heart's own blood supply system to provide blood to the working heart muscle.

In addition to its influence on heart rate, nicotine is also a powerful constrictor of blood vessels throughout the body. As vessels constrict, the pressure within them goes up. Recent research shows that nonreversible atherosclerotic damage to major arteries also occurs with smoking.[11]

Nicotine also increases blood **platelet adhesiveness.** *Platelets* are the component of blood that causes it to clot, or coagulate, after an injury. Nicotine makes these platelets more likely to adhere to one another, or "clump," which can cause blood clots to develop in the arteries. Heart attacks occur when clots form within the coronary arteries (see Chapter 10) or are transported to the heart from other areas of the body.

In addition to other influences on the cardiovascular system, nicotine possesses the ability to decrease the proportion of high-density lipoproteins (HDLs) and to increase the proportion of low-density lipoproteins (LDLs) and very-low-density lipoproteins that make up the body's blood cholesterol. (See Chapter 10 for further information about cholesterol's role in cardiovascular disease.)

Carbon monoxide and cardiovascular disease

Carbon monoxide, a second substance contributed by tobacco, influences the type and extent of cardiovascular disease found among tobacco users. Carbon monoxide interferes with oxygen transport within the circulatory system.

As described previously, carbon monoxide is a component of the gaseous phase of tobacco smoke and readily attaches to the hemoglobin of the red blood cells. Once attached, carbon monoxide makes the red blood cell permanently weaker in its ability to transport oxygen. These red blood cells remain relatively useless during the remainder of their 120-day life. Levels of carboxyhemoglobin in heavy smokers are associated with significant increases in the incidence of heart attack.

When a person has impaired oxygen-transporting abilities, physical exertion becomes increasingly demanding on both the heart and the lungs. The cardiovascular system will attempt to respond to the body's demand for oxygen, but these responses are themselves impaired as a result of the influence of nicotine on the cardiovascular system. If tobacco does create the good life, as advertisers claim, it also decreases the smoker's ability to participate actively in that life.

Cancer

Data supplied by the American Cancer Society (ACS) indicate that during 2001 an estimated 1,268,000 Americans were diagnosed with cancer.* These cases were nearly equally divided between the genders and will eventually result in approximately 553,400 deaths.[12] In the opinion of the ACS, 30% of all cancer cases are heavily influenced by tobacco use. Lung cancer alone accounted for about 169,500 of the new cancer cases and 157,400 deaths in 2001. Approximately 87% of male lung cancer victims were cigarette smokers. Cancer of the respiratory system, including lung cancer and cancers of the mouth and throat, accounted for about 184,600 new cases of cancer and 162,500 deaths.[12] Despite these high figures, not all smokers develop cancer. Perhaps the extent to which the body's cancer suppressor genes are influenced by carcinogenic substances in tobacco smoke makes some smokers at greater risk for tobacco-related cancer than others.

Recall that tobacco smoke has both a gaseous phase and a particulate phase. The particulate phase contains the tar fragment of tobacco smoke. This rich chemical environment contains over 4000 known chemical compounds, hundreds of which are possible carcinogens, or co-carcinogens.

In the normally functioning respiratory system, particulate matter suspended in the inhaled air settles on the tissues lining the airways and is trapped in **mucus** produced by specialized *goblet cells* (Figure 9-2). This mucus, with its trapped impurities, is continuously swept upward by the beating action of hairlike **cilia** of the cells lining the air passages. On reaching the throat, this mucus is swallowed and eventually removed through the digestive system.

When tobacco smoke is drawn into the respiratory system, however, its rapidly dropping temperature allows the particulate matter to accumulate. This brown, sticky tar contains compounds known to harm the ciliated cells, goblet cells, and the *basal cells* of the respiratory lining. As the damage from smoking increases, the cilia becomes less effective in sweeping mucus upward to the throat. When cilia can no longer clean the airway, tar accumulates on the surfaces and brings carcinogenic compounds into direct contact with the tissues of the airway.

Key Terms

gaseous phase
Portion of tobacco smoke containing carbon monoxide and many other physiologically active gaseous compounds.

norepinephrine
Adrenaline-like chemical produced within the nervous system.

carbon monoxide (CO)
Chemical compound that can "inactivate" red blood cells.

myocardial infarction
Heart attack; the death of heart muscle caused by a blockage in one of the coronary arteries.

sudden cardiac death
Immediate death caused by a sudden change in the rhythm of the heart.

platelet adhesiveness
Tendency of platelets to clump together, thus enhancing the speed at which the blood clots.

mucus
Clear, sticky material produced by specialized cells within the mucous membranes of the body; mucus traps much of the suspended particulate matter within tobacco smoke.

cilia
Small, hairlike structures that extend from cells that line the air passages.

*Excluding about 900,000 cases of nonmelanoma skin cancer.

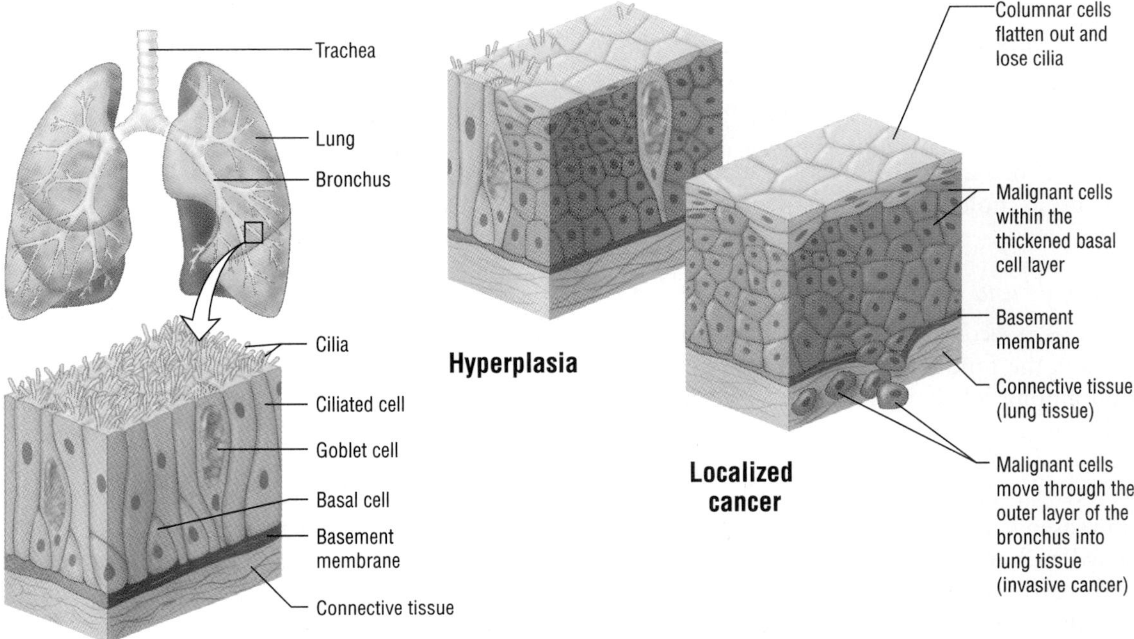

Figure 9-2 Tissue changes associated with bronchogenic carcinoma (lung cancer).

At the same time that the sweeping action of the lining cells is being slowed, substances in the tar are stimulating the goblet cells to increase the amount of mucus they normally produce. The "smoker's cough" is an attempt to remove this excess mucus.

With prolonged exposure to the carcinogenic materials in tar, predictable changes will begin to occur within the respiratory system's *basal cell layer* (see Figure 9-2). The basal cells begin to display changes characteristic of all cancer cells (Figure 9-2). When a person stops smoking, these cells do not repair themselves as quickly as once thought.[13]

By the time lung cancer is usually diagnosed, its development is so advanced that the chance for recovery is very poor. Only 14% of all lung cancer victims survive for 5 years or more after diagnosis.[12] Most die in a very agonizing, painful way.

TALKING POINTS • You're having a discussion with a friend about life insurance and mention that you get a 10% reduction in your annual premium because you're a nonsmoker. Your friend, who is a smoker, becomes annoyed and says that this is just one example of how smokers are penalized. How would you respond?

Cancerous activity in other areas of the respiratory system, including the *larynx,* and the oral cavity (mouth) follows a similar course. With oral cancer, carcinogens found in the smoke and in the saliva are involved in the cancerous changes. Tobacco users, such as pipe smokers, cigar smokers, and users of smokeless tobacco, have a very high rate of cancer of the mouth, tongue, and voice box.

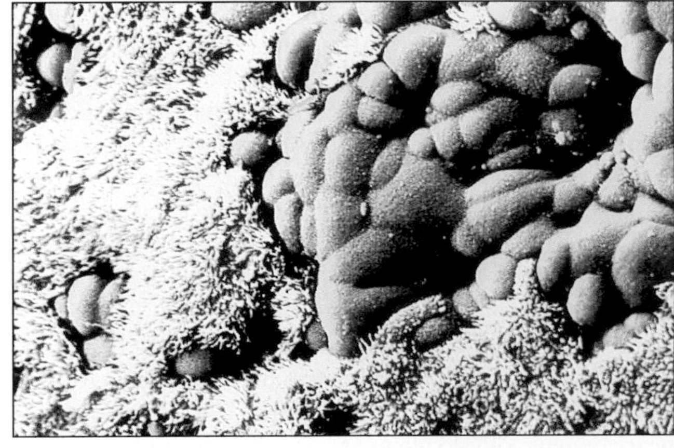

Ciliated lining of a smoker's lung, showing deposits of tar.

In addition to drawing smoke into the lungs, tobacco users swallow saliva that contains an array of chemical compounds from tobacco. As this saliva is swallowed, carcinogens are absorbed into the circulatory system and transported to all areas of the body. The filtering of the blood by the liver, kidneys, and bladder may account for the higher than normal levels of cancer in these organs among smokers.

Chronic Obstructive Lung Disease

Chronic obstructive lung disease (COLD) is a **chronic disorder** in which air flow in and out of the lungs be-

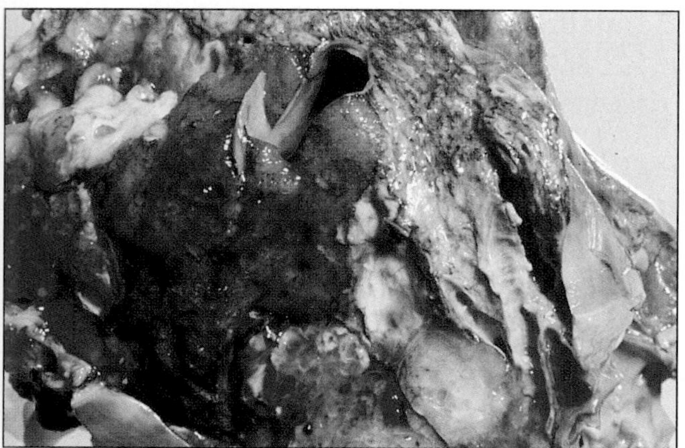

Cancerous lung.

comes progressively limited. COLD is a disease state that is made up of two separate but related diseases: **chronic bronchitis** and **pulmonary emphysema.**

With chronic bronchitis, excess mucus is produced in response to the effects of smoking on airway tissue, and the walls of the bronchi become inflamed and infected. This produces a characteristic narrowing of the air passages. Breathing becomes difficult, and activity can be severely restricted. People who stop smoking can reverse chronic bronchitis.

For college students who have only recently begun smoking, the chronic nature of bronchitis may not yet be in place. However, it is important to realize that the now occasional episodes of airway inflammation and congestion will occur on a more regular basis, and eventually the foundation for COLD will be established.

Pulmonary emphysema causes damage to the tiny air sacs of the lungs, the **alveoli,** that cannot be reversed. Chest pressure builds when air becomes trapped by narrowed air passages (chronic bronchitis), and the thin-walled sacs rupture. Emphysema patients often develop a "barrel chest" as they lose the ability to exhale fully. You have most likely seen people with this condition in shopping malls and other locations as they walk slowly by, carrying or pulling behind them their portable oxygen tanks.

More than 10 million Americans have COLD. It is responsible for a greater limitation of physical activity than any other disease, including heart disease.[14] COLD patients tend to die a very unpleasant, prolonged death, often from a general collapse of normal cardiorespiratory function that results in *congestive heart failure* (see Chapter 10).

Additional Health Concerns

In addition to the serious health problems stemming from tobacco use already described, other health-related changes that are routinely seen include a generally poor state of nutrition, the gradual loss of the sense of smell, and premature wrinkling of the skin. Tobacco users are also more likely to experience strokes (a potentially fatal condition), lose bone mass leading to osteoporosis, experience more back pain and muscle injury, and find that fractures heal more slowly. Further, smokers who have surgery spend more time in the recovery room. Although not perceived as a "health problem" by people who continue smoking to control their weight, smoking does appear to minimize weight gain. In studies using male identical twins, the siblings who smoked were 6 to 8 pounds lighter than their nonsmoking siblings.[15]

SMOKING AND REPRODUCTION

In all of its dimensions the reproductive process is impaired by the use of tobacco, particularly cigarette smoking. Problems can be found in association with infertility, problem pregnancy, breastfeeding, and the health of the newborn.

Infertility

Recent research indicates that cigarette smoking by both men and women can reduce levels of fertility. Among men, smoking adversely affects sperm motility and shape and can also inhibit sperm production. Among women, lower levels of estrogen (a hormone necessary for uterine wall development), a reduced ability to conceive, and a somewhat earlier onset of menopause appear to be related to cigarette smoking.

Problem Pregnancy

The harmful effects of tobacco smoke on the course of pregnancy are principally the result of the carbon monoxide and nicotine to which the mother and her fetus are exposed. Carbon monoxide is carried to the placenta, where it "locks up" fetal hemoglobin. As a result of this exposure to carbon monoxide, the fetus is deprived

Key Terms

chronic disorder
Condition that develops and progresses slowly over an extended period of time.

chronic bronchitis
Persistent inflammation and infection of the smaller airways within the lung.

pulmonary emphysema
Irreversible disease process in which the alveoli are destroyed.

alveoli
Thin, saclike terminal ends of the airways; the sites at which gases are exchanged between the blood and inhaled air.

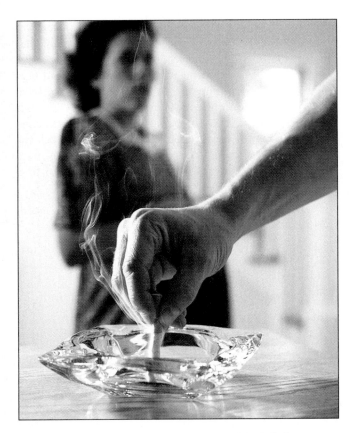

Pregnant women and those around them should refrain from smoking.

of normal oxygen transport, leading to a condition called *hypoxia,* or the abnormally low level of oxygen in tissues throughout the body.

Nicotine also exerts its influence on the developing fetus. Thermographs of the placenta and fetus show signs of marked constriction of blood vessels within a few seconds after inhalation by the mother. This constriction further reduces oxygen supplies. In addition, nicotine stimulates the mother's stress response, placing the mother and fetus under the potentially harmful influence of elevated epinephrine and corticoid levels (see Chapter 3). Any fetus exposed to all of these agents is more likely to be miscarried or stillborn.[16] Children born to mothers who smoked during pregnancy often have low birth weights. Additionally, NNK (4-(methylnitrosamino)-1-(3-pyridyl)-L butanone) can cross the placental barrier, exposing the developing fetus to one of the most powerful carcinogenic agents in tobacco smoke.[17]

Breastfeeding

Women who smoke while they breastfeed their infants will continue to expose their children to the harmful effects of tobacco smoke. Women who stop smoking during pregnancy should be encouraged to continue to refrain from smoking while they are breastfeeding.

Health Problems Among Infants

Babies born to women who smoked during pregnancy will, on average, be shorter and have a lower birth weight than children born to nonsmoking mothers. During the earliest months of life, babies born to mothers who smoke experience an elevated rate of death caused by *sudden infant death syndrome* (SIDS). Statistics also show that these infants are more likely to develop chronic respiratory problems, be hospitalized, and have poorer overall health during their early years of life. Additionally, children exposed to the influences of tobacco prenatally may hold a greater chance of developing *attention deficit disorder* (ADD), and in a recent study it was shown that they may have an increased risk of antisocial behavior extending into adulthood.[18]

Parenting, in the sense of assuming responsibility for the well-being of a child, begins before birth, especially in the case of smoking. A pregnant woman who continues to smoke is disregarding the well-being of the child she is carrying. Other family members, friends, and coworkers who subject pregnant women to cigarette, pipe, or cigar smoke are, in a sense, contributing a measure of their own disregard for the health of the next generation.

ORAL CONTRACEPTIVES AND TOBACCO USE

Women who smoke and use oral contraceptives are placing themselves at a much greater risk of experiencing a fatal cardiovascular accident (heart attack, thrombus, or **embolism**) than oral contraceptive users who do not smoke. This risk of cardiovascular complications is further increased for oral contraceptive users 35 years of age or older. By this age, women who both smoke and use oral contraceptives are four times more likely to die from myocardial infarction (heart attack) than women who only smoke. Because of this adverse relationship, it is strongly recommended that women who smoke not use oral contraceptives.

SMOKELESS TOBACCO USE

As the term implies, smokeless tobacco is not burned; rather, it is placed into the mouth. Once in place, the physiologically active nicotine and other soluble compounds are absorbed through the mucous membranes and into the blood. Within a few minutes, chewing tobacco and snuff generate blood levels of nicotine in amounts equivalent to those seen in cigarette smokers.

Chewing tobacco is taken from its foil pouch, formed into a small ball (called a "wad," "chaw," or "chew"), and placed into the mouth. Once in place, the ball of tobacco is sucked and occasionally chewed but not swallowed. Some users develop great skill at spitting the copious dark brown liquid residue into an empty coffee can, out a car window, or on the sidewalk.

Snuff, a more finely shredded smokeless tobacco product, is marketed in small, round cans. Snuff is formed into a small mass (or "quid"). The quid is "dipped," or placed between the jaw and the cheek; the user sucks the quid and spits out the brown liquid.

Although smokeless tobacco would seem to free the tobacco user from many of the risks associated with smoking, chewing and dipping have their own substantial risks. The presence of *leukoplakia* (white spots) and *erythroplakia* (red spots) on the tissues of the mouth indicate precancerous changes (see the Changing for the Better box on this page). In addition, an increase in **periodontal disease** (the pulling away of the gum from the teeth and later tooth loss), the abrasive damage to the enamel of the teeth, and the high concentration of sugar in processed tobacco all contribute to health problems seen among users of smokeless tobacco.

In addition to the damage done to the tissues of the mouth, the need to process the inadvertently swallowed saliva that contains dissolved carcinogens places both the digestive and urinary systems at risk of cancer.

In the opinion of health experts, the use of smokeless tobacco and its potential for life-threatening disease is presently at the place cigarette smoking was 45 years ago. Consequently, television advertisement has been banned, and one of the following warnings appears on every package of smokeless tobacco:

WARNING: THIS PRODUCT MAY CAUSE MOUTH CANCER.

WARNING: THIS PRODUCT MAY CAUSE GUM DISEASE AND TOOTH LOSS.

WARNING: THIS PRODUCT IS NOT A SAFE ALTERNATIVE TO CIGARETTE SMOKING.

Clearly, smokeless tobacco is a dangerous product. There is little doubt that continued use of tobacco in this form is a serious problem to health in all of its dimensions.

INVOLUNTARY (PASSIVE) SMOKING

The smoke generated by the burning of tobacco can be classified as either **mainstream smoke** (the smoke inhaled and then exhaled by the smoker) or **sidestream smoke** (the smoke that comes from the burning end of the cigarette, pipe, or cigar). When either form of tobacco smoke is diluted and stays within a common source of air, it is referred to as **environmental tobacco smoke.** All three forms of tobacco smoke lead to *involuntary smoking* and can present health problems for both nonsmokers and smokers. As discussed in Exploring Your Spirituality (p. 216), the effects that smoking produces on others are not only physical but also psychological and social.

Surprisingly, mainstream smoke makes up only 15% of our exposure to involuntary smoking. This is because much of the nicotine, carbon monoxide, and particulate matter are retained within the active smokers.

TALKING POINTS • Your 13-year-old brother inadvertently leaves a tin of smokeless tobacco on the desk in his room and you see it. Would you say anything to him about it? If so, what?

Changing *for the Better*

Early Detection of Oral Cancer

I started using smokeless tobacco a few years ago, thinking it was safe. Recently, I read an article about it that was frightening. What are the real danger signs?

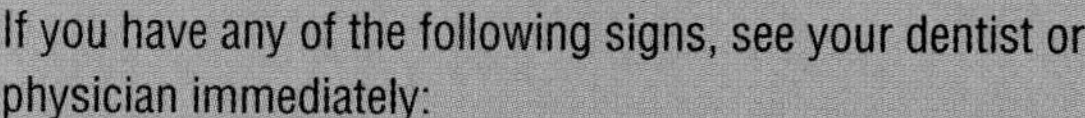

If you have any of the following signs, see your dentist or physician immediately:

- Lumps in the jaw or neck area
- Color changes or lumps inside the lips
- White, smooth, or scaly patches in the mouth or on the neck, lips, or tongue
- A red spot or sore on the lips or gums or inside the mouth that does not heal in 2 weeks
- Repeated bleeding in the mouth
- Difficulty or abnormality in speaking or swallowing

Key Terms

embolism
Potentially fatal condition in which a circulating blood clot lodges itself in a smaller vessel.

periodontal disease
Destruction to soft tissue and bone that surround the teeth.

mainstream smoke
Smoke inhaled and then exhaled by a smoker.

sidestream smoke
Smoke that comes from the burning end of a cigarette, pipe, or cigar.

environmental tobacco smoke
Tobacco smoke that is diluted and stays within a common source of air.

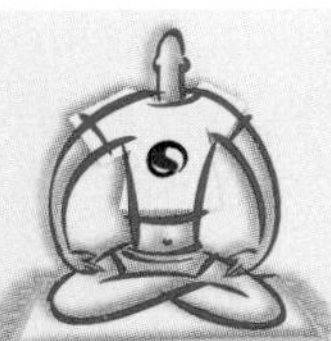

Exploring Your Spirituality

The Hidden Price Tag of Smoking

"I started to hug him but felt myself drawing back. It was almost like a reflex action." Those are the words of a young woman after greeting her brother when he returned home from his first semester at college. The young man had recently become a smoker, and his sister was reacting to the strong smell of smoke in his clothes and hair.

Dramatic as it may sound, smoking does set up barriers between people. First, there's the health issue. Some nonsmokers are adamant about not wanting people they care about to smoke. They also want to protect their children from this danger. And they certainly don't want to breathe in smoke themselves. So, at a family gathering, a smoker may want to have a cigarette after dinner, in the living room with everyone else. But the nonsmokers say no—go outside if you want to smoke. In the process, a birthday dinner or a special holiday is marred by this disagreement.

Whether the person is a family member or a friend, it's difficult to feel close to someone who's doing something you disapprove of—such as smoking. But, from the smoker's point of view, it's hard to feel good about someone who acts superior and doesn't accept you as you are. What do children think about all this? Does a "good" aunt or uncle smoke? If smoking is bad, as a little girl constantly hears at school and at home, why does her favorite uncle smoke?

The physical toll that smoking takes is apparent when the smoker finds himself sitting on the sidelines. A young man wants to play basketball with his buddies, but the last time he tried, he had a coughing fit—very embarrassing. A young woman meets some new people, and they ask her to join them for an "easy hike." Well, easy for them. She needs a break after only 10 minutes and sees what looks like pity in her friends' eyes.

On the job, smoking has gone the way of the three-martini lunch. It's just not politically correct. In fact, many companies have a no-smoking policy. Or smoking is allowed in designated areas only. Ever drive by a big factory or office building and see a group of people standing outside, perhaps huddled under umbrellas? They're not organizing a strike—they're having a smoke (and being reminded of their high school days). Once again, the smoker feels isolated. Just as in the family group, the smoker feels the judgment of others—only now it's her boss or secretary who's frowning.

The price of smoking is hard to measure. The damage to the smoker's health is beyond dispute. But the spiritual and psychological costs are also real. How does it feel to always be the outsider? The unaccepted? Why does the smoker have to take the chance of missing an exciting play in the stadium to go smoke a cigarette? Or feel the resentment of others at work because he leaves to take a smoking break every hour? It's easy for nonsmokers to say: "Just quit." Smokers know it's not that simple. Many who have stopped smoking—often after several attempts—say that they thought about more than their health in deciding to quit. They thought about many situations—involving family, outdoor activities, and work—before they threw away the pack and said: "That was my last cigarette."

Sidestream smoke is responsible for 85% of our involuntary smoke exposure. Because it is not filtered by the tobacco, the filter, or the smoker's lungs, sidestream smoke contains more free nicotine and produces higher yields of both carbon dioxide and carbon monoxide. Much to the detriment of nonsmokers, sidestream smoke has 20 to 100 times the quantity of highly carcinogenic substances (*N*-nitrosamines) that mainstream smoke has.

Current scientific opinion suggests that smokers and nonsmokers are exposed to very much the same smoke when tobacco is used within a common airspace. The important difference is the quantity of smoke inhaled by smokers and nonsmokers. It is likely that for each pack of cigarettes smoked by a smoker, nonsmokers who must share a common air supply with the smokers will involuntarily smoke the equivalent of three to five cigarettes per day. Because of the small size of the particles produced by burning tobacco, environmental tobacco smoke cannot be completely removed from an indoor site by even the most effective ventilation system.

On the basis of reported research, involuntary smoke exposure may be responsible for between 10,000 and 20,000 premature deaths per year among nonsmokers in the United States (other estimates range upward to 53,000 premature deaths).[19] In addition, environmental tobacco smoke is associated with lung cancer, asthma, low birth weight babies, eye irritation, headaches, and coughs in nonsmokers. Most recently, genetic mutations have been found in the newborn children of women exposed to involuntary smoke during pregnancy.[20]

For these reasons, state, local, and private-sector initiatives to restrict smoking have been introduced. Most buildings in which people work, study, play, reside, eat, or shop now have some smoking restrictions. An increasing number have complete smoking bans. Nowhere is smoking more noticeably prohibited than in the U.S. airline industry. Currently, smoking is banned on all domestic plane flights and on all commercial flights to and from the United States. This ban applies to all U.S. and foreign carriers.

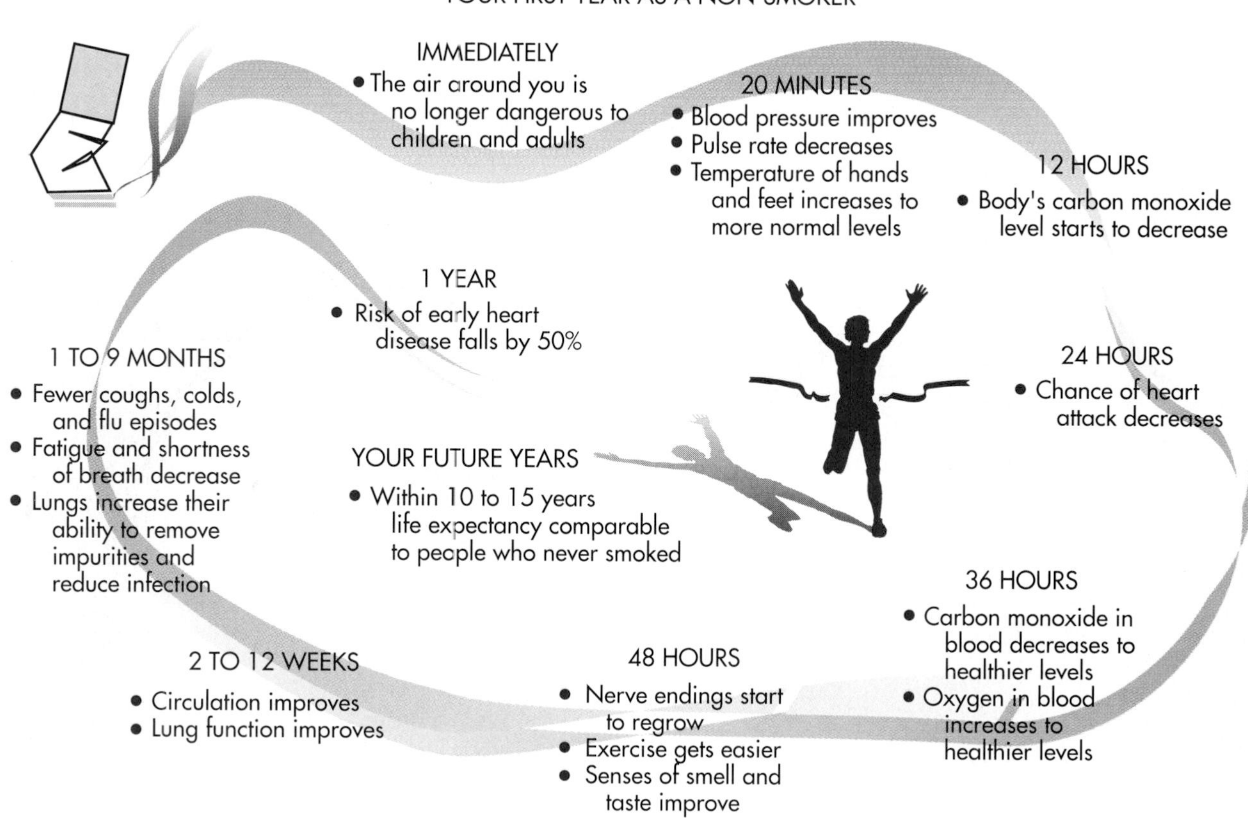
YOUR FIRST YEAR AS A NON-SMOKER
IMMEDIATELY
• The air around you is no longer dangerous to children and adults
20 MINUTES
• Blood pressure improves
• Pulse rate decreases
• Temperature of hands and feet increases to more normal levels
12 HOURS
• Body's carbon monoxide level starts to decrease
1 YEAR
• Risk of early heart disease falls by 50%
1 TO 9 MONTHS
• Fewer coughs, colds, and flu episodes
• Fatigue and shortness of breath decrease
• Lungs increase their ability to remove impurities and reduce infection
24 HOURS
• Chance of heart attack decreases
YOUR FUTURE YEARS
• Within 10 to 15 years life expectancy comparable to people who never smoked
36 HOURS
• Carbon monoxide in blood decreases to healthier levels
• Oxygen in blood increases to healthier levels
2 TO 12 WEEKS
• Circulation improves
• Lung function improves
48 HOURS
• Nerve endings start to regrow
• Exercise gets easier
• Senses of smell and taste improve

Figure 9-3 The health benefits of quitting smoking begin immediately and become more significant the longer you stay smoke-free.

Involuntary smoking poses serious threats to nonsmokers within residential settings. Spouses and children of smokers are at greatest risk from involuntary smoking. Scientific studies suggest that nonsmokers married to smokers are three times more likely to experience heart attacks than nonsmoking spouses of nonsmokers, and they have a 30% greater risk of lung cancer than nonsmoking spouses of nonsmokers.

The children of parents who smoke are twice as likely as children of nonsmoking parents to experience bronchitis or pneumonia during the first year of life. In addition, throughout childhood, these children will experience more wheezing, coughing, and sputum production than children whose parents do not smoke. Also, they will have a higher incidence of middle ear infection.[21] Of course, the impact on children who have two parents who smoke is greater than on children who have only one parent who smokes.

STOPPING WHAT YOU STARTED

As in the case of weight reduction, there are several ways to attempt to stop smoking. Among these are the *cold turkey* approach, a gradual reduction in cigarette use, organized smoking cessation programs, and the use of medically prescribed and OTC drug treatment. For those who fear the discomfort of going cold turkey, a more gradual approach can be attempted. The Changing for the Better box on p. 218 provides several suggestions for quitting smoking or cutting down on tobacco consumption until stopping totally is possible.

Although it is far from easy to stop smoking, most of the 1.3 million people who quit smoking each year do so by throwing their cigarettes away and going cold turkey. After days, weeks, or even months of discomfort, the body will eventually function more effectively (Figure 9-3). Respiratory capacity will return, the ability to taste will return, and, if undertaken soon enough, tissues of the airways will begin returning to a more normal appearance. On a less pleasant note, it may take years before the mental pictures of "smoking pleasures" have faded. For most, some weight will be gained (about 6 to 8 pounds), but this represents a minimal health risk in comparison with the benefits of not smoking. The Changing for the Better box on p. 219 offers tips for avoiding weight gain when you quit smoking.

Changing *for the Better*

Getting Off Tobacco

I started smoking at parties to feel more relaxed. Now I smoke at least a pack a day, and I'm afraid I'm hooked for life. How do I get myself off tobacco?

Instead of reaching for a cigarette, reach out for life and health. The suggestions below, many of which are recommended by the American Cancer Society, will help you make a concerted effort to stop smoking. Are you ready to try?

- Realize how much more independent you could be if you quit smoking. Few smokers can say that they are fully self-directed when they can barely function without their cigarettes.
- Think of one sentence that expresses your personal reason for wanting to quit smoking. Repeat the sentence to yourself often.
- Observe nonsmokers. Note that they are not missing out on anything by not smoking. Recognize that the price you will pay for no longer smoking is not as high as it might have first appeared.
- Pick a quit day, sometime within the next 2 weeks. Plan either to stop cold turkey or to cut down gradually.
- Plan ahead for how you will handle tough times in your first few days off cigarettes.
- Stock up on low-calorie or no-calorie snacks.
- On your quit day, drink a lot of water and keep busy.
- Limit your contact with other cigarette smokers. Keep in mind that once you quit, smokers won't go out of their way to assist you in your efforts.
- Stay clear, as much as possible, of the locations and activities that are now associated with your smoking. Old habits are hard to break, but you don't need to be constantly reminded of them.
- Establish a series of rewards that you will give yourself as you progress through your smoking cessation program.
- Call the American Cancer Society for more information about quitting: self-help, how-to's, and group sessions in your community.

A less effective alternative to total cessation is to reduce your exposure to tobacco. This can be accomplished through one or more of the following approaches:

- Reduce the consumption of your present high-tar and high-nicotine brand by smoking fewer cigarettes, inhaling less often and less deeply, and by smoking the cigarette only halfway down.
- Switch to a low-tar and low-nicotine brand of cigarette. Be careful, though, not to compensate for this change by smoking more cigarettes or by inhaling more deeply and frequently. Instead, try to reduce the number of cigarettes you smoke and the depth and number of inhalations. Smoke only a limited portion of each cigarette.
- Switch to a smokeless form of tobacco, but be prepared for the potential problems that were discussed in this chapter.

Many group-based smoking cessation programs are available. These programs are usually operated by hospitals, universities, health departments, voluntary health agencies, private physicians, and even local churches. Perhaps the best that can be said is that the better programs will have limited success—a 20% to 50% success rate as measured over 1 year—and the remainder will have even poorer levels of success.

Two approaches for weaning smokers from cigarettes to a nontobacco source of nicotine dependency are nicotine-containing chewing gum (Nicorette) and the transdermal nicotine patches (Nicoderm, Habitrol, Prostep) that allow nicotine to slowly diffuse through the skin surface into the body. The chewing gum has been on the market for a number of years and, when used correctly along with smoking cessation counseling, has demonstrated a success rate of 40% or more. Correct use of nicotine-containing chewing gum requires an immediate cessation of smoking, a determination of the initial dosage (4 mg or 2 mg of nicotine per piece), the manner of chewing each piece (rate of chewing and the avoidance of certain foods or beverages), the number of pieces to be chewed each day (usually 9 to 12), and the individual manner of withdrawal from chewing the gum after 2 to 3 months of its use. In 1996 a nonprescription version of Nicorette became available.

In comparison with nicotine-containing chewing gum, the more recently developed transdermal nicotine patches appear to be somewhat less effective than the chewing gum but easier to use. The transdermal nicotine patches, such as Nicoderm, can now be obtained in OTC versions. For these transdermal patches that come in three dosages, a determination must be made about the appropriate initial dosage, the length of time at that dosage and lower dosages, and the manner of withdrawal after the usual 8 to 12 weeks of patch wearing. Recently, nicotine replacement therapies using inhalation and nasal sprays have been approved by the FDA. These new delivery techniques use small pressurized devices that can be easily carried and used. These systems, available by prescription, should prove very effective because of the large surface area of the lungs, which allows rapid absorption of nicotine into the blood.

Changing *for the Better*

Avoiding Weight Gain When You Stop Smoking

I tried to quit smoking once, but I gained weight immediately. How can I avoid this problem next time?

For many smokers, particularly women, an important plus for smoking is weight management. To them, the risks associated with tobacco use are offset by the cigarette's ability to curb their appetite so they can restrict their caloric intake. This fear of weight gain frequently prevents them from seriously trying to stop smoking or lets them lapse back into cigarette use easily.

This fear is well founded. Most people who quit smoking do gain weight during the 10 years after they stop. The amount of weight gain is usually greater than that seen in people who continue smoking or who have never smoked. Still, this weight gain is relatively small and only slightly greater than that experienced by age-mates who smoke or have never smoked. Certainly, the weight gained is a minimal health risk compared with the risks associated with continued smoking.

Success in minimizing weight gain after smoking is centered in two areas: (1) the ability to manage the smoking urges associated with the first several months of being a former smoker without resorting to eating and (2) the willingness to adopt healthy eating and exercise behaviors.

People who are attempting to quit smoking should recognize that smoking urges are powerful but temporary, usually lasting only about 2 minutes. During these periods of intense desire for a cigarette, coping activities such as taking a short walk, drinking water or a diet beverage, or talking with a coworker or family member can be used to distract the mind from a cigarette until the urge has passed. If you must eat during these times, choose healthy low-calorie snacks, such as apple slices.

To minimize weight gain (or actually lose weight) in the years after stopping smoking, it's important to make a commitment to a serious wellness-oriented lifestyle change involving both exercise and diet. Specific information about adult fitness and sound nutrition can be found in Chapters 4 and 5, respectively.

Nicotine replacement products can be used alone or with other therapies. Zyban and Wellbutrin (bupropion) are antidepressant medications that increase the production of dopamine, a neurotransmitter. Dopamine production declines when a smoker quits, creating the craving to smoke. In a recent study, it was found that, when combined, nicotine patches and a sustained-release antidepressant were substantially more effective than the nicotine patch used alone. An antidepressant used alone was, however, nearly as effective as the combination.[22]

In June 2001, the Department of Health and Human Services issued a guideline regarding what is now seen as the most clinically sound and cost-effective means of treatment. It recommends a combination therapeutic approach: 1) first-line pharmacological agents, including antidepressants and nicotine replacement therapies (gum, patches, inhalers, and nasal sprays); 2) second-line pharmacological therapies (clonidine and nortriptyline); and 3) counseling and support.[23] With this guideline, more insurance coverage is likely to become available for smoking cessation efforts. Currently, insurance coverage is minimal. (Figure 9-3 demonstrates the impressive health benefits from quitting smoking.)

TOBACCO USE: A QUESTION OF RIGHTS

Consider these two simple questions about the issues of smokers' vs. nonsmokers' rights:

- To what extent should smokers be allowed to pollute the air and endanger the health of nonsmokers?
- To what extent should nonsmokers be allowed to restrict the personal freedom of smokers, particularly since tobacco products are sold legally?

At this time, answers to these questions are only partially available, but one trend is developing: the tobacco user is being forced to give ground to the nonsmoker. Today, in fact, it is becoming more a matter of when the smoker will be allowed to smoke rather than a matter of when smoking will be restricted. Increasingly, smoking is tolerated less and less. The health concerns of the majority are prevailing over the dependence needs of the minority. See the Focus on . . . box on p. 225 for a fuller explanation of this topic.

IMPROVING COMMUNICATION BETWEEN SMOKERS AND NONSMOKERS

Exchanges between smokers and nonsmokers are sometimes strained, and in many cases, friendships are damaged beyond repair. As you have probably observed, roommates are changed, dates are refused, and memberships in groups are withheld or rejected because of the opposing rights of these two groups.

Recognizing that social skill development is an important task for young adults, the following simple considerations or approaches for smokers can reduce some conflict presently associated with smoking.

- Ask whether smoking would bother others near you.
- When in a neutral setting, seek physical space where you can smoke and in a reasonable way not interfere with nonsmokers' comfort.
- Accept the validity of the nonsmoker's statement that your smoke causes everything and everyone to smell.
- Respect stated prohibitions against smoking.
- If a nonsmoker requests that you refrain from smoking, respond with courtesy, regardless of whether you intend to comply.
- Practice "civil smoking" by applying a measure of restraint when you recognize that smoking is offensive to others. In particular, respect the aesthetics that should accompany any act of smoking—ashes on dinner plates and cigarette butts in flower pots are not appreciated by others.

The suggestions above can become skills for the social dimension of your health that can be applied to other social conflicts. Remember that as a smoker, you are part of a statistical minority living in a society that often makes decisions and resolves conflict based on majority rule.

For those of you who are nonsmokers, the following approaches can make you more sensitive and skilled in dealing with smoking behavior:

- Attempt to develop a feeling for or sensitivity to the power of the dependence that smokers have on their cigarettes.
- Accept the reality of the smoker's sensory insensitivity—an insensitivity that is so profound that the odors you complain about are not even recognized by the smoker.
- When in a neutral setting, allow smokers their fair share of physical space in which to smoke. As long as the host does not object to smoking, you as a guest do not have the right to infringe on a person's right to smoke.
- When asking a person to not smoke, use a manner that reflects social consideration and skill. State your request clearly, and accept a refusal gracefully.
- Respond with honesty to inquiries from the smoker as to whether the smoke is bothering you.

If you are contemplating smoking, consider carefully whether the social isolation that appears to be more and more common for smokers will be offset by the benefits you might receive from cigarettes. Finding satisfaction through social contact may be one of the most important dimensions in a productive and rewarding adult life.

SUMMARY

- Only one quarter of American adults smoke.
- The incidence of adolescent and young-adult smoking increased in recent years but is now leveling off.
- A successful class-action suit exposed the strategies of the tobacco industry and required it to compensate states for Medicaid expenses.
- Dependence, including addiction and habituation, is established quickly through tobacco use.
- Nicotine is the addictive agent in tobacco whose level in tobacco products can be modified.
- Modeling, self-reward, and self-medication play important roles in the development of tobacco dependence.
- The federal government has proposed a broadly based program intended to reduce the use of cigarettes by adolescents.
- Tobacco smoke can be divided into gaseous and particulate phases. Each phase has its unique chemical composition.
- Nicotine, carbon monoxide, and phenol have damaging effects on various body tissues. Several hundred carcinogenic agents are found in tobacco smoke.
- Nicotine has predictable effects on the function of the cardiovascular system.
- Most forms of cancer are worsened by tobacco use. Lung cancer progresses in a predictable fashion.
- Chronic obstructive lung disease (COLD) is a likely consequence of long-term cigarette smoking, with early symptoms appearing shortly after beginning regular smoking.
- Smoking alters normal structure and function of the body, as seen in premature wrinkling, diminished ability to smell, and bone loss leading to osteoporosis.
- Several areas of reproductive health are negatively influenced by tobacco use. Cigarette smoking and long-term use of oral contraceptives are not compatible.
- Smokeless tobacco carries its own health risks, including oral cancer.
- Involuntary smoke carries with it a wide variety of threats to the spouse, children, and coworkers of the smoker.
- Stopping smoking can be undertaken in any one of several ways.
- Smoking cessation therapies are available in a variety of forms, including nicotine gum, transdermal patches, nicotine inhalation devices, and effective antidepressants.
- Both smokers and nonsmokers have certain rights regarding the use of tobacco. Effective communication can be established between smokers and nonsmokers.

REVIEW QUESTIONS

1. What percentage of the American adult population smokes? In what direction has change been occurring? What is the current direction that adolescent smoking is taking? What factors may account for this newly observed trend?
2. In what way do modeling and advertising explain the development of emotional dependency on tobacco? How do self-esteem, self-image, and self-directedness relate to tobacco use?
3. What was the outcome of the massive class-action suit brought against the tobacco industry by state governments in an attempt to recoup Medicaid funds? What is the current status of the federal government's attempt to further control the tobacco industry?
4. What are the principal components of the gaseous and particulate phases of tobacco smoke?
5. What are the specific influences of nicotine and carbon monoxide, on the normal function of the body?
6. In what ways does cigarette smoking contribute to cardiovascular disease? What effect does nicotine have on the cardiovascular system?
7. To what extent is tobacco use a factor in cancer? What specific airway tissues are involved in lung cancer?
8. What is the traditional progression of chronic obstructive lung disease? In what ways does tobacco use impair reproductive health?
9. In what ways is smokeless tobacco equal to smoking in the development of serious health concerns?
10. What is involuntary smoking? Why is there growing concern about the effects of passive smoke on spouses and children?
11. What is the most effective way to stop smoking? What is the average weight gain after stopping smoking? How effective are other approaches to stopping smoking? What are the principal nicotine replacement systems in use today? What is the government's latest guideline for successful smoking cessation?
12. What rights do smokers and nonsmokers have in public places? How can communication be enhanced between smokers and nonsmokers?

THINK ABOUT THIS . . .

- Why has the current generation of college students apparently chosen to disregard the tobacco-related risks understood by earlier generations of college students and graduates?
- If you saw a minor being sold cigarettes, would you feel comfortable mentioning your concern to the merchant?
- If you are among the minority of Americans (including college students) who smoke, do you understand why you will be most likely to die sooner than your classmates if you continue to smoke?
- If you are a smoker, do you understand why some people may feel unappreciative of your presence?

REFERENCES

1. Centers for Disease Control and Prevention: Cigarette smoking: attributable mortality and years of potential life lost, United States, *MMWR* 46:444–450, 1997.
2. *Health, United States, 2000 with adolescent health chartbook,* 2000, National Center for Health Statistics.
3. Institute for Social Research, University of Michigan. Smoking in college increases, as reported in: *USA Today,* August 20, 2001, 15A.
4. National survey results on drug use. From *Monitoring the future study, 1975–1998,* vol 1, Secondary School Students, The University of Michigan Institute for Social Research, U.S. Department of Health and Human Services, Public Health Service, National Institutes of Health, Sept 1999.
5. Satcher D: Cigars and public health, *N Engl J Med* 340(23):1829–1831, 1999.
6. Lerman C et al: Evidence suggesting the role of specific genetic factors in cigarette smoking, *Health Psychol* 18(1):14–20, 1999.
7. Henningfield JE, Radzius A, Cone EJ: Estimation of available nicotine of six smokeless tobacco products, *Tobacco Control* 4:57–61, 1995.
8. Regulations restricting the sale and distribution of cigarettes and smokeless tobacco products to protect children and adolescents, *Federal Register* 60(156):41314–41451, August 11, 1995.
9. Hoffmann D, Hoffmann V, El-Bayoumy K: The less harmful cigarette: a controversial issue, *Chem Res Toxicol* 14(7):767–790, 2001.
10. American Heart Association: *2000 heart and stroke facts: 2000 statistical supplement,* 1999, The Association.

11. Howard G et al: 1989. Cigarette smoking and progression of atherosclerosis, *JAMA* 279(2):119–124, 1998.
12. *Cancer facts & figures–2001,* 2001, American Cancer Association.
13. Wistuba I et al: Molecular damage in the bronchial epithelium of smokers, *J Natl Cancer Inst* 89(18):1366–1373, 1997.
14. Crowley LV: *Introduction to human disease,* ed 4, 1996, Jones & Bartlett.
15. Eisen S et al: The impact of cigarette and alcohol consumption on weight and obesity: an analysis of 1911 monozygotic twin pairs, *Arch Intern Med* 153(21):2457–2463, 1993.
16. Mills JL: Cocaine, smoking, and spontaneous abortion, *N Engl J Med* 340(5):380–381, 1999.
17. Lackmann GM et al: Metabolites of a tobacco-specific carcinogen in urine from newborns, *J Natl Cancer Inst* 91(5):459–465, 1999.
18. Fergusson DM: Prenatal smoking and antisocial behavior, *Arch Gen Psychiatry* 56(3):223–224, 1999.
19. Environmental Protection Agency: *Respiratory health effects of passive smoking: lung cancer and other disorders,* Environmental Protection Agency, Office of Air and Radiation, EPA/600/6–90/006F, 1992.
20. Finette BA et al: Gene mutations with characteristic deletions in cord blood T lymphocytes associated with passive maternal exposure to tobacco smoke, *Nat Med* 4(10):1144–1151, 1998.
21. Adair-Bischoff CE, Sauve RS: Environmental tobacco smoke and middle ear disease in preschool-age children, *Arch Pediatr Adolesc Med* 152(2):127–133, 1998.
22. Jorenby DE et al: A controlled trial of sustained-release bupropion, a nicotine patch, or both for smoking cessation, *N Engl J Med* 340(9):685–691, 1999.
23. Treating tobacco use and dependence: a clinical practice guideline. Department of Health and Human Services, Office of the Surgeon General, 2001.

SUGGESTED READINGS

Gebhardt J: *The enlightened smoker's guide to quitting,* 1998, Element Books.

A smoking cessation program must be tailored to the smoking history of the person attempting to quit. Using a seven-step approach, the author discusses individualizing these components for participants in order to enhance their chance for success. The approach described is frequently used by programs approved by the American Cancer Society.

Hirschfelder AB: *Kick butts: a kid's guide to a tobacco-free America,* 1998, Silver Burdett Press.

The decision to smoke is often made at a surprisingly early age, well before the behavior begins. The author skillfully focuses the information and activities of her book to the children she wants to reach. Her account of the last 100 years of tobacco use is informative to all readers, but the activities described in the latter portion of the book are well suited to young children and will be well received by them. This book is recommended for both parents and teachers.

Orey M: *Assuming the risk: the mavericks, the lawyers, and the whistle-blowers who beat big tobacco,* 1999, Little, Brown & Company.

Michael Orey, a legal journalist for a major national newspaper, uses his expertise and objectivity to describe the tobacco industry's reversal of fortune within the judicial system. Beginning with an obscure 1987 lawsuit on behalf of a poor Mississippi laborer who died of lung cancer and ending with the massive class-action suit brought by the states seeking Medicaid compensation, this is the complete account of how the seemingly impenetrable defenses of the tobacco industry were final bridged.

Tate C: *Cigarette wars: the triumph of the "the little white slaver,"* 1999, Oxford University Press.

This book tells the story of how the cigarette went from being the evil "coffin nail" at the turn of the century to the widely used symbol of personal independence and internationally recognized Americana by mid-century. All the principal players, both against and for the birth and adoption of this "child of the twentieth century," are discussed. This book lays an excellent foundation for Orey's book, described above.

Name ____________________ Date ____________ Section ____________

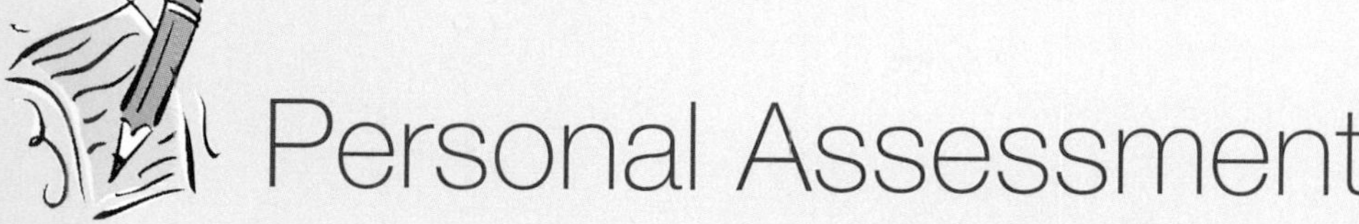

Personal Assessment

How Much Do You Know about Cigarette Smoking?

Are the following assumptions about smoking true or false? Take your best guess, and then read the answer to the right of each statement.

Assumption		Discussion
1. There are now safe cigarettes on the market.	F	Depending on the brand, some cigarettes contain less tar and nicotine; none are safe, however.
2. A small number of cigarettes can be smoked without risk.	F	Even a low level of smoking exposes the body to harmful substances in tobacco smoke.
3. Most early changes in the body resulting from cigarette smoking are temporary.	T	Some changes, however, cannot be reversed—particularly changes associated with emphysema.
4. Filters provide a measure of safety to cigarette smokers.	T	However, the protection is far from adequate.
5. Low-tar, low-nicotine cigarettes are safer than high-tar, high-nicotine brands.	T	Many people, however, smoke low-tar, low-nicotine cigarettes in a manner that makes them just as dangerous as stronger cigarettes.
6. Mentholated cigarettes are better for the smoker than are nonmentholated brands.	F	Menthol simply makes cigarette smoke feel cooler. The smoke contains all of the harmful agents found in the smoke from regular cigarettes.
7. It has been scientifically proven that cigarette smoking causes cancer.	T	Particularly lung cancer and cancers of the larynx, esophagus, oral cavity, and urinary bladder.
8. No specific agent capable of causing cancer has ever been identified in the tobacco used in smokeless tobacco.	F	Unfortunately, smokeless tobacco is no safer than the tobacco that is burned. The user of smokeless tobacco swallows much of what the smoker inhales.
9. The cure rate for lung cancer is so good that no one should fear developing this form of cancer.	F	Approximately 14% of people who have lung cancer will live the 5 years required to meet the medical definition of "cured."
10. Smoking is not harmful as long as the smoke is not inhaled.	F	Because of the toxic material in smoke, even its contact with the tissue of the oral cavity introduces a measure of risk in this form of cigarette use.
11. The "smoker's cough" reflects underlying damage to the tissue of the airways.	T	The cough occurs in response to an inability to clear the airway of mucus as a result of changes in the cells that normally keep the air passages clear.
12. Cigarette smoking does not appear to be associated with damage to the heart and blood vessels.	F	Cigarette smoking is in fact the single most important risk factor in the development of cardiovascular disease.
13. Because of the design of the placenta, smoking does not present a major risk to the developing fetus.	F	Children born to women who smoked during pregnancy show a variety of health impairments, including smaller birth size, premature birth, and more illnesses during the first year of life. Smoking women also have more stillbirths than nonsmokers.
14. Women who smoke cigarettes and use an oral contraceptive should decide which they wish to continue because there is a risk in using both.	T	Women over 35 years of age, in particular, are at risk of experiencing serious heart disease should they continue using both cigarettes and an oral contraceptive.
15. Air pollution is a greater risk to our respiratory health than is cigarette smoking.	F	Although air pollution does expose the body to potentially serious problems, the risk is considerably less than that associated with smoking.
16. Addiction, in the sense of physical addiction, is found in conjunction with cigarette smoking.	T	Dependence, including true physical addiction, is widely recognized in cigarette smokers.

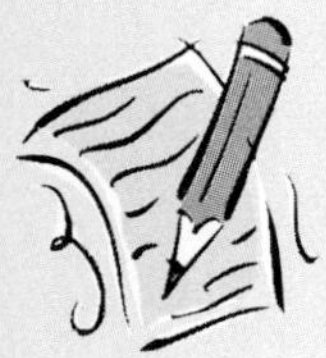

Personal Assessment *continued*

Assumption	Discussion
17. Among the best "teachers" a young smoker has are his or her parents.	T There is a strong correlation between cigarette smoking of parents and the subsequent smoking of their children. Parents who do not want their children to smoke should not smoke.
18. Nonsmoking and higher levels of education are directly related.	T The higher one's level of education, the less likely one is to smoke.
19. About as many women smoke cigarettes as do men.	T Although in the past, more men smoked than did women, the gap is narrowing.
20. Fortunately, for those who now smoke, stopping is relatively easy.	F Unfortunately, relatively few smokers can quit. The best advice is never to begin smoking.

To Carry This Further . . .

Were you surprised at the number of items that you answered correctly? In what areas did you hold misconceptions regarding cigarette smoking? Do you think that most university students are as knowledgeable as you?

Where do you see the general public in terms of its understanding of cigarette smoking? How can the health care community do a better job in educating the public about tobacco use?

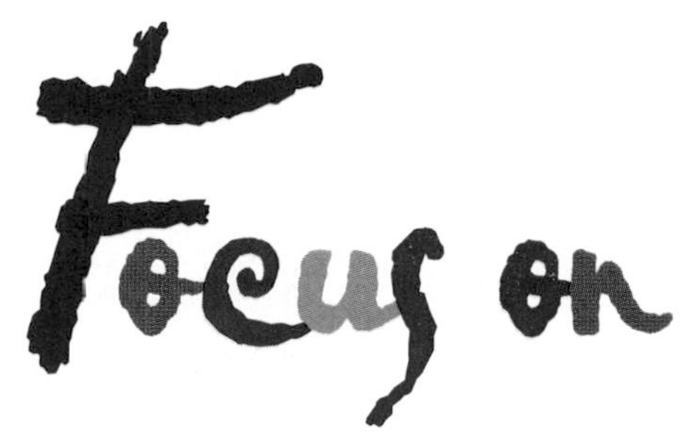

SMOKERS vs. NONSMOKERS: A QUESTION OF RIGHTS

A quiet battle is being waged in the United States over smoking, an activity that was once universally accepted. Within the last decade, regulations restricting smoking have affected stores, restaurants, offices, and public buildings. It is difficult these days to find a place of business in the United States where smoking is totally unrestricted. Some of these restrictions are put in place by law or municipal ordinances; some are placed voluntarily by business management. However, it is clear that the voices of nonsmokers, long silent and largely ignored by society, are finally being heard and are behind the recent increase in restrictions on smoking.

Changing Attitudes

For decades, people smoked whenever and wherever they wished. Smoking was glamorized in the movies, on television, and in print throughout most of the twentieth century. Famous athletes and movie stars were found in cigarette advertisements. Some ads even promoted the "health benefits" of smoking. Although a few people felt that smoking was dangerous, their voices had little effect on society's acceptance of tobacco use. Gradually, these attitudes began to change. As data from medical studies began to accumulate on the dangers of tobacco, antismoking advocates started to achieve some victories in society and in public policy.

Restrictions on Tobacco Use

In the 1980s, restrictions on smoking greatly increased. In 1987, smoking was banned on all domestic airplane flights of less than 2 hours;[1] in 1990, this ban was increased to include all domestic flights of less than 6 hours. Now most international flights ban smoking as well. A growing number of state and local laws curtailing or banning smoking in places of business have been enacted. Many businesses that were not forced by law to restrict smoking did so anyway. Smoking is prohibited on over 80% of Amtrak trains, and 1400 company-owned McDonald's restaurants are now smoke-free.[2] The state of California has even banned smoking in restaurants, bars, and casinos, apparently without affecting profits.[3]

As a result of these restrictions, smoking areas in places of business are shrinking in size or are being eliminated. Congregations of smokers outside office buildings have become a common sight. Some smokers have taken the changes in stride. Others have cut back on smoking or have quit altogether. Many, however, are not happy about having to go outside in all kinds of weather to smoke. They feel ostracized and are speaking out against what they perceive as an outright attack on their personal freedoms.

The Prosmoker Defense

Smokers have started to become organized on a worldwide level and within individual communities and workplaces. They are clearly worried that this trend of restricting tobacco use will not stop until smoking is eliminated everywhere and the use of tobacco becomes illegal.

Groups such as the British-based Freedom Organisation for the Right to Enjoy Smoking Tobacco (FOREST) have actively pushed smokers' rights and have espoused the "benefits" of smoking.[4] They cite controversial scientific studies demonstrating that smokers are less likely to develop Alzheimer's disease and Parkinson's disease and that teen acne is "almost exclusively" a nonsmokers' affliction.

Smokers are also worried about how their smoking activities are perceived by employers and insurers. Companies are growing less tolerant of unhealthy activities by their employees, since they must pay increased insurance costs for treatment. Many fear that insurance companies will begin to refuse treatment to smokers who continue to smoke.

The worst-case scenario for smokers is that their smoking will even be restricted at home. "What if the government starts keeping us from having kids because we smoke?" worries "Earl," a two-pack-a-day smoker. "I've heard tell that we could have our kids taken away because we smoke at home. Do we have to step outside of our own homes to smoke?"[5]

Fighting for Clean Air

Many nonsmokers are just as adamant about their position, saying that smokers have been subjecting them to cancer-causing agents for decades and that the restrictions are long overdue. They are tired of having smoke blown in their faces in public. Antismoking activists find the "individual freedom" argument of smokers objectionable. "What about my right to breathe?" asks "Stan," an office worker who is subjected to smoke from nearby cubicles. "The management, most of whom smoke, have decided that since we don't deal directly with the public, smoking is okay," he complains.[6]

Many nonsmoking activists feel that it is in the public's best interest to restrict exposure to tobacco smoke and cut back on overall tobacco use. They are angered not only because they have to be exposed to smoke, but also because a good portion of their insurance premiums is going toward health care costs from smoking. It is estimated that $65 billion a year goes to treat tobacco-related diseases, roughly one fourth of all money spent on health care in the United States each year.[7] As the data accumulate on the hazards of smoking, many nonsmokers are becoming concerned about their exposure to secondhand smoke. They are also worried about the addictive properties of nicotine and are concerned that their children may get hooked.

Although they have had much success in getting restrictions adopted, antismoking activists have also faced defeat in the legislatures. Municipalities in North Carolina can no longer pass local laws restricting smoking, thanks to a preemptive state law passed on July 15, 1993. As a result, 59% of workers in North Carolina have no legal protection at all from exposure to tobacco smoke.[8]

Even without the health problems posed by tobacco smoke, many nonsmokers feel that smoking should be curtailed simply because of its unpleasant smell. Since smoking is not a self-contained activity, smoke diffuses far away from the smoker, often offending people many feet away. "What good does it do to seat a nonsmoker next to the smoking section in a restaurant?" notes "Irina," an avid antismoking activist.[9] "The smoke just drifts over anyway. It stinks, and not just during the meal. It gets into your clothes and hair and stays with you all day. Why must we tolerate smoke?"

What the Future May Hold

Such arguments may open the door to more restrictions on smoking, a possibility that makes smokers' rights advocates angry. Many are convinced that antismoking forces want nothing less than a total ban on tobacco use—or at least want these bans to be used more aggressively. This might occur, according to smokers' rights advocates, by allowing the courts to use smoking as a factor in determining child custody cases or in defining parental smoking as a form of child endangerment.

Antismoking advocates do not see these regulations as restrictions on individual freedom. They view them as a means of liberation from decades of exposure to smoke with little or no form of legal recourse. Many nonsmokers feel that they should not be forced to breathe in smoke simply because someone wants to light up. Advocates for these regulations claim that tobacco-related illnesses increase health care costs for everyone. They also complain that their tax dollars are being used to subsidize the tobacco industry—in effect, they are paying to be exposed to the smoke of others.

Since smoking, by its very nature, is not a self-contained activity, conflicts are bound to happen. Perhaps some acceptable middle ground can be reached between smokers and nonsmokers, both in law and in society.

For Discussion . . .

Have you ever asked someone not to smoke near you or been asked not to smoke around someone? Should taxpayers be responsible for taking on the burden of those being treated for smoking-related diseases? Are the individual freedoms of smokers being infringed on by smoking regulations? Are the individual freedoms of nonsmokers being violated by smokers? Is smoking at home around your children a form of child endangerment?

References

1. The tyranny of the majority, *The Economist* 313:7626, 1989.
2. Farley CJ, Toufexis A: The butt stops here, *Time* 143(16), Apr 18, 1994.
3. Glantz SA, Smith LR: The effect of ordinances requiring smoke-free restaurants and bars on revenue: a follow-up, *Am J Public Health* 87(10):1687–1693, 1997.
4. Platt S: Ashes to ashes, *New Statesman and Society* 7(289), Feb 11, 1994.
5. Anonymous: Personal communication, January 1996.
6. Anonymous: Personal communication, June 1996.
7. What are they smoking? *FW* 161(5), Mar 3, 1992.
8. Conlisk E et al: The status of local smoking preemption bill, *JAMA* 273(10), 1995.
9. Anonymous: Personal communication, March 1996.

part 4

Preventing Diseases

chapter 10

Reducing Your Risk of Cardiovascular Disease

Online Learning Center Resources

www.mhhe.com/hahn6e

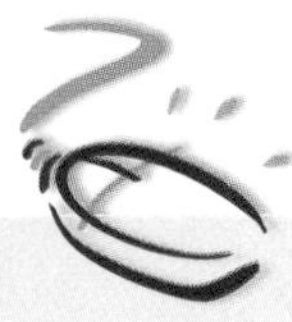

Log on to our Online Learning Center (OLC) for access to these additional resources:

- Chapter key terms and definitions
- Learning objectives
- Additional behavior change objectives
- Student interactive question-and-answer sites
- Self-scoring chapter quiz

The OLC also offers web links for study and exploration of health topics. Here are some examples of what you'll find:

- **www.americanheart.org** Find hundreds of topics related to cardiovascular health and disease, including prevention, nutrition, smoking cessation, and other lifestyle considerations.
- **www.nhlbi.nih.gov/index.htm** Look here if you couldn't find it at the American Heart Association site.
- **www.wellnessweb.com/heart/index.htm** Check out this site to take the Heart IQ Quiz. Also find out more about how your diet affects your heart health.

Taking Charge of Your Health

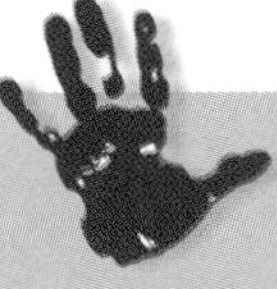

- Complete the Personal Assessment on p. 247 to determine your risk for heart attack and stroke.
- Review the Food Guide Pyramid in Chapter 5 (p. 96), and make changes to your diet so that it is more "heart healthy."
- Begin or continue an aerobic exercise program that is appropriate for your current fitness level.
- If you are a smoker, resolve to quit smoking. Visit your physician to talk about safe and effective approaches. Begin putting your plan into action.
- Develop a plan to lower your dietary intake of fat to keep your blood cholesterol level low.
- Have your blood pressure checked, and review your weight, physical activity, alcohol intake, and salt intake to determine whether you can make changes in any of these areas.
- If you are overweight or obese, develop a plan to combine dietary changes and increased physical activity to lose weight gradually but steadily.

Eye on the Media

How Credible Are Online Health Sites?

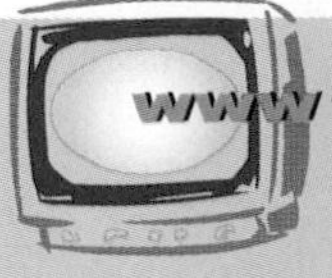

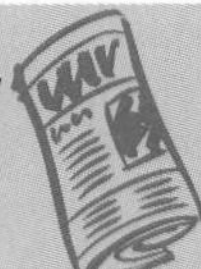

If you're looking for accurate health information on the Internet, make the site's credibility your first priority. Since just about anyone can post information on the web (within legal limits), what you find there ranges from opinion to balanced, carefully researched information. Your challenge is to distinguish between reliable and dubious information.

According to health professionals Kotecki and Chamness,[1] certain key information can help you determine a health information website's credibility. They suggest using the following six criteria: (1) scope, (2) accuracy, (3) authority, (4) currency, (5) purpose, and (6) organization, structure, and design.

If you're looking for information on cardiovascular health, for example, select a popular health information website such as WebMD (**www.webmd.com**). To evaluate this website, search for this topic and ask yourself these questions:

1. Does the website offer adequate *scope?* For example, are many aspects of the topic presented? Is there adequate depth to each topic?

Eye on the Media *continued*

2. How *accurate* is the information? That is, is the information based on scientific data and properly referenced?
3. How much *authority* does the site have? For instance, are the authors identified? Are they recognized experts who are writing in their own field?
4. Is the information *current?* For example, is a date provided to show how recent the information is?
5. Is there a stated *purpose* for the site's existence? That is, do you find a statement of purpose? Are the intended audiences and funding sources identified?
6. Is the site *well-organized* and *well-designed?* For instance, does it include a table of contents that is logical and easy to use? Is the reading level appropriate? Does the site have links to referenced sites?

What you should have found is that **www.webmd.com** does a good job of meeting all six criteria. Its homepage offers a link you can use to read about WebMd's credentials. This provides further assurance that the cardiovascular information it presents is quite accurate and reliable.

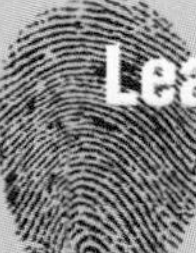

Learning from Our Diversity

Prevention of Heart Disease Begins in Childhood

Youth is one aspect of diversity that is sometimes overlooked. Yet age is important, especially when adults have influence over children's health behavior. Many adults never seriously consider that their health behaviors are imitated by the children around them. When adults care little about their own health, they can also be contributing to serious health consequences in young people. Nowhere is this age diversity issue more pronounced than in the area of cardiovascular health.

For many aspects of wellness, preventive behaviors are often best learned in childhood, when they can be repeated and reinforced by family members and caregivers. This is especially true for preventive actions concerning heart disease. Although many problems related to heart disease appear at midlife and later, the roots of heart disease start early in life.

The most serious childhood health behaviors associated with heart disease are poor dietary practices, lack of physical activity, and cigarette smoking. Unfortunately, the current state of health for America's youth shows severe deficiencies in all three areas. Children's diets lack nutrient density and remain far too high in overall fat. Teenage children are becoming increasingly overweight and obese. Studies consistently show a decline in the amount of physical activity by today's youth, since television and video games have become the after-school companions for many children. In addition, cigarette smoking continues to rise among schoolchildren, especially teenagers.

These unhealthy behaviors are laying the foundation for coronary artery disease, hypertension, and stroke in the future. The focus should be on health measures in childhood that prevent cardiovascular problems rather than treatment of older, already affected people. Parents must make efforts to encourage children to eat more nutritiously and be physically active. Adults should discourage cigarette use by young people. Perhaps the best approach for adults is to set a good example by adopting heart-healthy behaviors themselves. Following the Food Guide Pyramid (p. 95) and exercising regularly are excellent strategies that can be started early in life.

If you're a traditional-age college student, you may have a difficult time realizing the importance of **cardiovascular** health. Unless you were born with a heart problem, it's easy to think that cardiovascular damage will not occur until you reach your 50s or 60s. During your young adult years, you're much more likely to be concerned about cancer and sexually transmitted diseases.

Yet autopsy reports on teenagers and young adults who have died in accidents are now showing that relatively high percentages of young people have developed changes consistent with coronary artery disease; that is, fatty deposits have already formed in their coronary arteries. (See the Learning from Our Diversity box above to discover why these changes have occurred.) Since the foundation for future heart problems starts early in life, cardiovascular health is a very important topic for all college students.

Heart disease continues to be the number one killer of Americans; between 1988 and 1998 the death rates from cardiovascular disease (CVD) declined 20.4%.[2] The

Key Term

cardiovascular
Pertaining to the heart (cardio) and blood vessels (vascular).

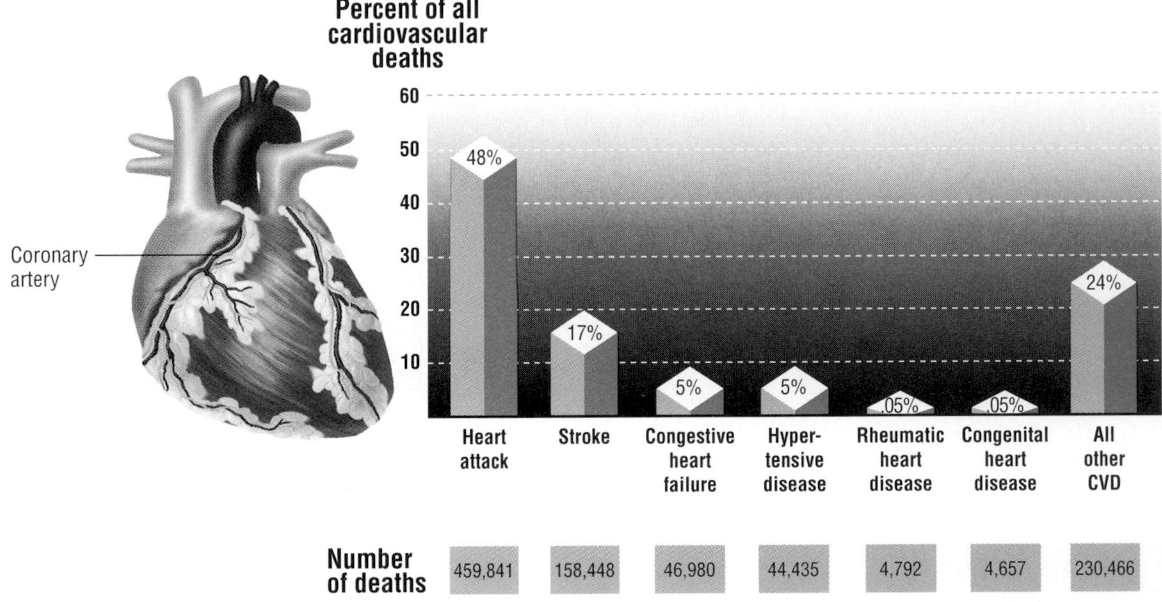

Figure 10-1 Of the 949,619 deaths in the United States in 1998* resulting from cardiovascular diseases, half were attributable to heart attack.[2] (**The most recent year for which statistics are available.*)

American Heart Association, in its 2001 *Heart and Stroke Statistical Update,* credits this reduction to a combination of changing American lifestyles and medical advances in the diagnosis and treatment of CVD.[2]

This chapter explains how the heart works. It also will help you identify your CVD risk factors and suggest ways you can alter certain lifestyle behaviors to reduce your risk of developing heart disease.

PREVALENCE OF CARDIOVASCULAR DISEASE

Cardiovascular diseases are directly related to over 40% of deaths in the United States and indirectly related to a large percentage of additional deaths.[2] Heart disease, stroke, and related blood vessel disorders combined to kill nearly 1 million Americans in 1998 (Figure 10-1).[2] This figure represents more deaths than were caused by cancer, accidents, pneumonia, influenza, lung diseases, diabetes, and AIDS combined. CVD causes one out of every 2.5 deaths in the United States.[2] Indeed, cardiovascular disease is our nation's number one "killer" (see Table 10-1).

Table 10-1 Estimated Prevalence of Major Cardiovascular Diseases*

Coronary heart disease	12,400,000
Hypertension	50,000,000
Stroke	4,500,000
Congenital heart disease	1,000,000
Rheumatic heart disease	1,800,000
Congestive heart failure	4,700,000
TOTAL†	74,400,000

*60,800,000 people total.

†The sum of the individual estimates exceeds 60,800,000 because many people have more than one cardiovascular disorder. For example, many people with coronary heart disease also have hypertension.

NORMAL CARDIOVASCULAR FUNCTION

The cardiovascular or circulatory system uses a muscular pump to send a complex fluid on a continuous trip through a closed system of tubes. The pump is the heart, the fluid is blood, and the closed system of tubes is the network of blood vessels.

The Vascular System

The term *vascular system* refers to the body's blood vessels. Although we might be familiar with the arteries (vessels that carry blood away from the heart) and the veins (vessels that carry blood toward the heart), arterioles, capillaries, and venules are also included in the vascular system. Arterioles are the farther, small-diameter extensions of arteries. These arterioles lead eventually to capillaries, the smallest extensions of the vascular system. At the capillary level, exchanges of oxygen, food, and waste occur between cells and the blood.

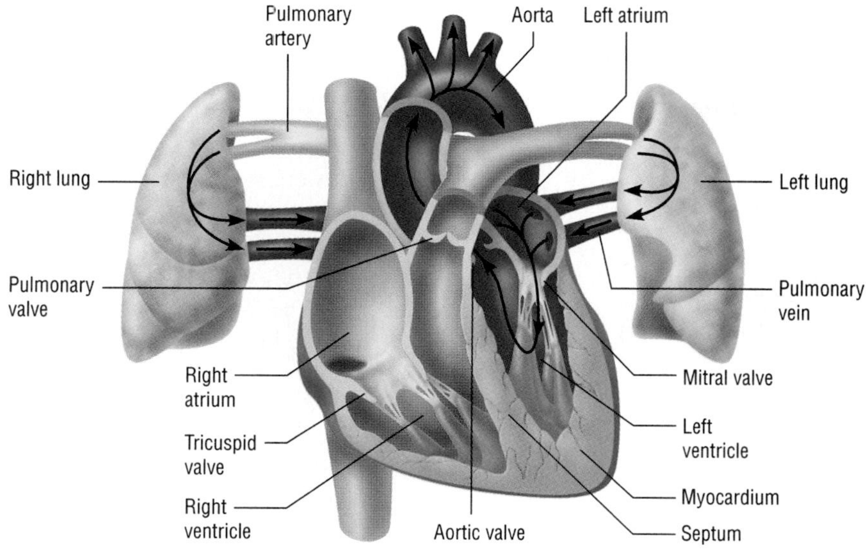

Figure 10-2 The heart functions like a complex double pump. The right side of the heart pumps deoxygenated blood to the lungs. The left side of the heart pumps oxygenated blood through the aorta to all parts of the body. Note the thickness of the walls of the ventricles. These are the primary pumping chambers.

Once the blood leaves the capillaries and begins its return to the heart, it drains into small veins, or venules. The blood in the venules flows into increasingly larger vessels called *veins.* Blood pressure is highest in arteries and lowest in veins, especially the largest veins, which empty into the right atrium of the heart.

The Heart

The heart is a four-chambered pump designed to create the pressure required to circulate blood throughout the body. Usually considered to be about the size of a person's clenched fist, this organ lies slightly tilted between the lungs in the central portion of the **thorax.** The heart does not lie completely in the center of the chest. Approximately two-thirds of the heart is to the left of the body midline, and one third is to the right.

Two upper chambers, called *atria,* and two lower chambers, called *ventricles,* form the heart.[3] The thin-walled atrial chambers are considered collecting chambers, and the thick-walled muscular ventricles are considered the pumping chambers. The right and left sides of the heart are divided by a partition called the *septum.* Use Figure 10-2 to follow the flow of blood through the heart's four chambers.

For the heart muscle to function well, it must be supplied with adequate amounts of oxygen. The two main **coronary arteries** (and their numerous branches) accomplish this. These arteries are located outside the heart (see Figure 10-1). If the coronary arteries are diseased and not functioning well, a heart attack is possible.

Heart stimulation

The heart contracts and relaxes through the delicate interplay of **cardiac muscle** tissue and cardiac electrical centers called *nodes.* Nodal tissue generates the electrical impulses necessary to contract heart muscle.[4] The heart's electrical activity is measured by an instrument called an *electrocardiograph* (ECG or EKG), which provides a printout called an electrocardiogram, which can be evaluated to determine cardiac electrical functioning.

Blood

The average-sized adult has approximately 6 quarts of blood in his or her circulatory system. The functions of blood, which are performed continuously, are similar to

Key Terms

thorax
The chest; portion of the torso above the diaphragm and within the rib cage.

coronary arteries
Vessels that supply oxygenated blood to heart muscle tissues.

cardiac muscle
Specialized smooth muscle tissue that forms the middle (muscular) layer of the heart wall.

the overall functions of the circulatory system and include the following:

- Transportation of nutrients, oxygen, wastes, hormones, and enzymes
- Regulation of water content of body cells and fluids
- Buffering to help maintain appropriate pH balance of body fluids
- Regulation of body temperature; the water component in the blood absorbs heat and transfers it
- Prevention of blood loss; by coagulating or clotting, the blood can alter its form to prevent blood loss through injured vessels
- Protection against toxins and microorganisms, accomplished by chemical substances called *antibodies* and specialized cellular elements circulating in the bloodstream

CARDIOVASCULAR DISEASE RISK FACTORS

As you have just read, the heart and blood vessels are among the most important structures in the human body. By protecting your cardiovascular system, you lay the groundwork for an exciting, productive, and energetic life. The best time to start protecting and improving your cardiovascular system is early in life, when lifestyle patterns are developed and reinforced (see Learning from Our Diversity, p. 229). Of course, it's difficult to move backward through time, so the second best time to start protecting your heart is today. Improvements in certain lifestyle activities can pay significant dividends as your life unfolds. Complete the Personal Assessment on p. 247 to determine your risk for heart disease.

The American Heart Association encourages people to protect and enhance their heart health by examining the ten cardiovascular risk factors related to various forms of heart disease.[5] A *cardiovascular risk factor* is an attribute that a person has or is exposed to that increases the likelihood that he or she will develop some form of heart disease. The first three risk factors are ones you will be unable to change. An additional six risk factors are ones you can change. One final risk factor is one that is thought to be a contributing factor to heart disease.

Risk Factors That Cannot Be Changed

The three risk factors that you cannot change are increasing age, male gender, and heredity.[5] However, your knowledge that they might be an influence in your life should encourage you to make a more serious commitment to the risk factors you can change.

Increasing age

Heart diseases tend to develop gradually over the course of one's life. Although we may know of a few people who experienced a heart attack in their thirties or forties, most of the serious consequences of heart disease are evident in older ages. For example, approximately 85% of people who die from heart diseases are age 65 and older.[2]

Male gender

Young women have lower rates of heart disease than young men. Yet when women move through menopause (typically in their fifties), their rates of heart disease are similar to those of men (see the Star Box on p. 233). It is thought that women are somewhat more protected from heart disease than men because of their natural production of the hormone estrogen during their fertile years.

Heredity

Like increasing age and male gender, heredity cannot be changed. By the luck of the draw, some people are born into families in which heart disease has never been a serious problem; others are born into families in which heart disease is quite prevalent. In this latter case, children are said to have a genetic predisposition (tendency) to develop heart disease as they grow and develop throughout their lives. These people have every reason to be highly motivated to reduce the risk factors they can control.

Race is also a consideration related to heart disease. African Americans have moderately high blood pressure at rates twice that of whites and severe hypertension at rates three times higher than whites (for a detailed discussion of this topic, see the Focus on box on p. 249). Hypertension significantly increases the risk of both heart disease and stroke; however, it can be controlled through a variety of methods. It is especially important for African Americans to take advantage of every opportunity to have their blood pressure measured so that preventive actions can be started immediately if necessary.

Risk Factors That Can Be Changed

There are six cardiovascular risk factors that are influenced largely by our lifestyle choices. These risk factors are cigarette and tobacco smoke, physical inactivity, high blood cholesterol level, high blood pressure, diabetes mellitus, and obesity and overweight. Healthful behavior changes you make for these "big six" risk factors can help you protect and enhance your cardiovascular system.

Tobacco smoke

Although the other five controllable risk factors are important, this one may be the most critical risk factor. Smokers have a heart attack risk that is 2–4 times that of nonsmokers. Smoking cigarettes is the major risk factor associated with sudden cardiac death. In fact, smokers have two to four times the risk of dying from sudden cardiac arrest than nonsmokers.

Cigarette or tobacco smoke also adversely affects nonsmokers who are exposed to environmental tobacco smoke. Studies suggest that the risk of death caused by heart disease is increased about 30% in people exposed

Women and Heart Disease

Is heart disease mainly a problem for men? According to the American Heart Association, the answer is a resounding NO. In fact, data indicate that 53% of all cardiovascular disease deaths occur in women. Cardiovascular disease is the leading cause of death for American women and kills nearly twice as many women as do all forms of cancer combined. Presently, one in five women has some sort of heart or blood vessel disease. Over 60% of stroke deaths occur in women. Also, 38% of women who have heart attacks will die within a year, compared with 25% of men. From age 55, higher percentages of women than men have high blood pressure.[6]

For many years, it was thought that men were at much greater risk than women for the development of cardiovascular problems. Today it is known that young men are more prone to heart disease than young women, but once women reach menopause (usually in their early to middle 50s), their rates of heart-related problems quickly equal those of men.

The protective mechanism for young women seems to be the female hormone estrogen. Estrogen appears to help women maintain a beneficial profile of blood fats. When the production of estrogen is severely reduced at menopause, this protective factor no longer exists. This is one of the reasons that increasing numbers of physicians are prescribing hormone replacement therapy (HRT). However, HRT may not be helpful for all women and poses some possible risks (increase in breast cancer, gallbladder disease, leg blood clots). Women should discuss this option with their physicians.[7]

Young women should not rely solely on naturally produced estrogen to prevent heart disease. The general recommendations for maintaining heart health—good diet, adequate physical activity, monitoring blood pressure and cholesterol levels, controlling weight, avoiding smoking, and managing stress—will benefit women at every stage of life.

to secondhand smoke in the home. Because of the health threat to nonsmokers, restrictions on indoor smoking in public areas and business settings are increasing tremendously in every part of the country.

For years, it was believed that if you had smoked for many years, it was pointless to try to quit; the damage to one's health could never be reversed. However, the American Heart Association now indicates that by quitting smoking, regardless of how long or how much you have smoked, your risk of heart disease declines rapidly. For people who have smoked a pack or less of cigarettes per day, within 3 years after quitting smoking, their heart disease risk is virtually the same as those who never smoked.

This news is exciting and should encourage people to quit smoking, regardless of how long they have smoked. Of course, if you have started to smoke recently, the healthy approach would be to quit now—before the nicotine controls your life and damages your heart. (For additional information about the health effects of tobacco, see Chapter 9.)

TALKING POINTS • A friend complains of not being able to quit smoking after several serious attempts. How could you direct this person toward a new approach?

Physical inactivity

Lack of exercise is a significant risk factor for heart disease. Regular aerobic exercise (discussed in Chapter 4) helps strengthen the heart muscle, maintain healthy blood vessels, and improve the ability of the vascular system to transfer blood and oxygen to all parts of the body. Additionally, physical activity helps lower overall blood cholesterol levels for most people, encourages weight loss and retention of lean muscle mass, and allows people to moderate the stress in their lives.

With all the benefits of physical activity, it amazes health professionals that so many Americans refuse to participate in regular exercise. Some people feel that they don't have enough time or that they must work out strenuously. However, you'll recall from Chapter 4 that only 20 to 60 minutes of moderate aerobic activity three to five times each week can decrease your risk of heart disease. This is not a large price to pay for a lifetime of cardiovascular health. Find a partner and get started! Exploring Your Spirituality (p. 235) discusses how the benefits of physical activity extend into the spiritual dimension of your life.

If you are middle-aged or older and have been inactive, consult with a physician before starting an exercise program. Also, if you have any known health condition that could be aggravated by physical activity, check with a physician first.

TALKING POINTS • You've started exercising many times by yourself, but you can't seem to stick to it. How would you convince a new friend that you can help each other get started on regular physical activity and keep it up?

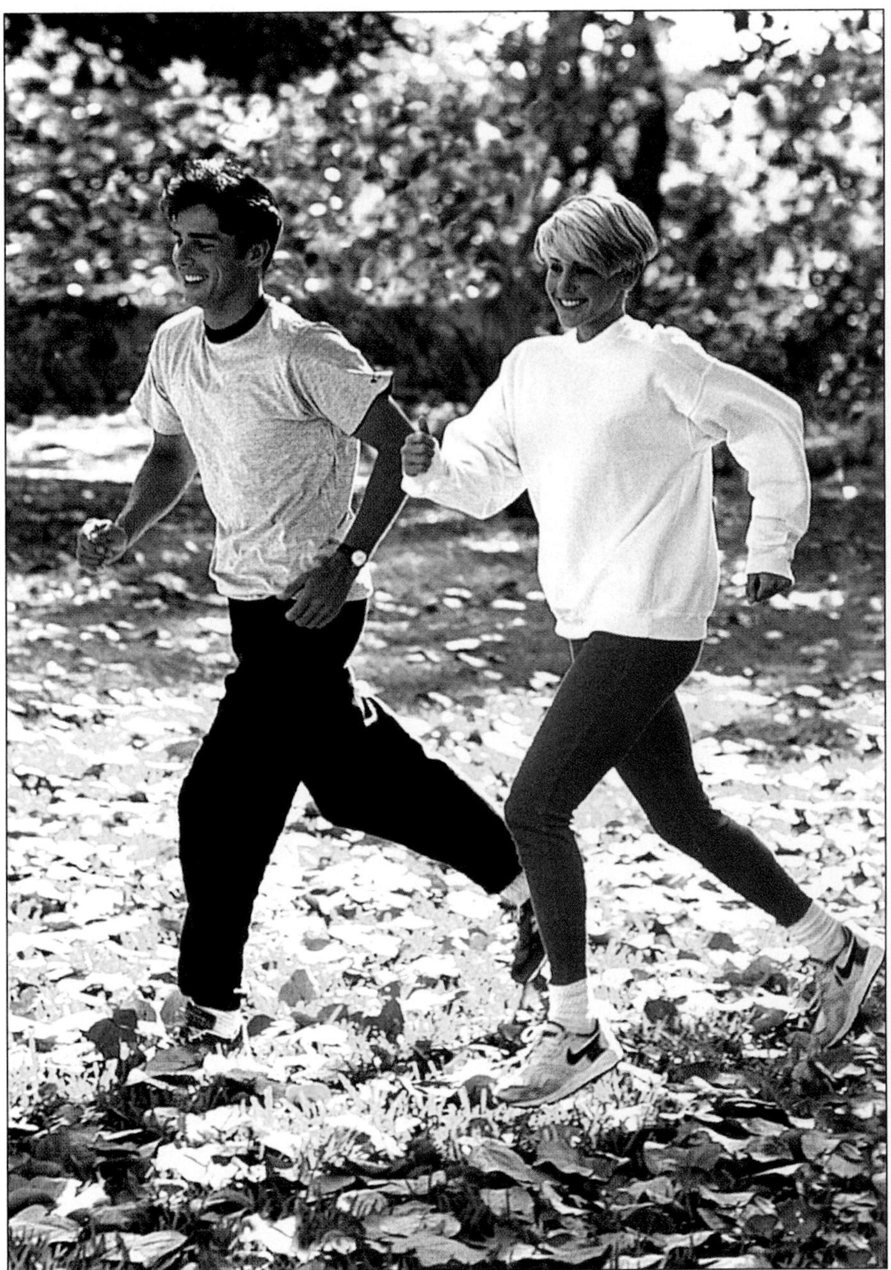

Regular exercise helps strengthen the heart muscle and lower blood cholesterol levels.

High blood cholesterol level

The third controllable risk factor for heart disease is high blood cholesterol level. Generally speaking, the higher the blood cholesterol level, the greater the risk for heart disease. When high blood cholesterol levels are combined with other important risk factors, the risks become much greater.

Fortunately, blood cholesterol levels are relatively easy to measure. Many campus health and wellness centers provide cholesterol screenings for employees and students. These screenings help identify people whose cholesterol levels (or profiles) may be potentially dangerous. Medical professionals have been able to determine the link between a person's diet and his or her cholesterol levels. People with high blood cholesterol levels are encouraged to consume a heart-healthy diet (see Chapter 5) and to become physically active. In recent years a variety of cholesterol-lowering drugs have also been developed that are very effective. Cholesterol will be discussed further later in this chapter.

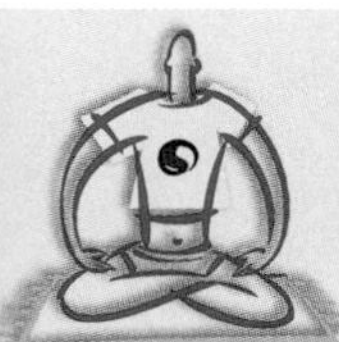

Exploring Your Spirituality

Yoga: Creating Peaceful Time

In a typical college day that includes academic, social, and financial pressures, you can lose the sense of who you really are. Do you ever find yourself wondering why you're making certain choices and what's really important to you? Meditative practices such as yoga offer you the chance to slow down and recapture a sense of yourself.

The word "yoga" comes from a Sanskrit root meaning "union" or "joining," referring to the integration of body, mind, and spirit. Yoga has evolved from ancient beginnings in the Himalayan mountains of India. Accounts of its origin differ, and some suggest that it reaches back 6,000 years. Yoga is practiced by people of all social, economic, and religious backgrounds. Many past yoga masters have been Hindus, but there is no need to embrace or even understand Hinduism if you want to practice yoga.

Yoga is a structured physical and mental discipline, designed to ease tension, improve concentration, and increase mental clarity. Like other meditative disciplines, it emphasizes the benefits of consistent, daily practice. A typical workout, as recommended by the American Yoga Association, lasts 20 minutes: two minutes of breathing exercises, two minutes of warming up, eight minutes of stretching, and eight minutes of meditation. After working out, you can expect to feel relaxed and energized, rather than exhausted.

Each exercise, called an *asan* or *ansana,* has specific effects. The "diamond pose," for example, limbers the lower back, hips, and groin muscles. Specialized workouts—to address pregnancy, sports, weight-loss programs, and other needs—can be created by including carefully selected exercises.

Yoga requires no special equipment and can be practiced in a small space such as a bedroom. Instructors in the United States have worked to make yoga accessible to the American lifestyle by developing special routines that can be pursued during travel, business, or the academic day. Classes are frequently offered on college campuses or in community centers, but any large bookstore stocks books that offer guidance to the beginner who wants to practice alone.

You'll find that most yoga practices offer ethical advice to help you reduce mental and emotional disturbances. Principles include nonviolence, truthfulness, and tolerance, but, again, you don't need to embrace these principles to practice yoga.

Clinical research has not conclusively demonstrated yoga's health benefits, but anecdotal evidence strongly suggests that disciplined practice can offer insight into the self and improve balance in your life.

High blood pressure

The fourth of the "big six" cardiovascular risk factors is high blood pressure, or *hypertension.* You will soon be reading more about hypertension, but for now, suffice it to say that high blood pressure can seriously damage a person's heart and blood vessels. High blood pressure causes the heart to work much harder, eventually causing the heart to enlarge and weaken. It increases the chances for stroke, heart attack, congestive heart failure, and kidney disease.

When high blood pressure is present along with other risk factors, the risk for stroke or heart attack is increased tremendously. Yet this "silent killer" is easy to monitor and can be effectively controlled using a variety of approaches. This is the positive message about high blood pressure.

Diabetes mellitus

Diabetes mellitus (discussed in detail on p. 268) is a debilitating chronic disease that has a significant effect on the human body. In addition to increasing the risk of developing kidney disease, blindness, and nerve damage, diabetes increases the likelihood of developing heart and blood vessel diseases. Over 80% of people with diabetes die of some type of heart or blood vessel disease. The cardiovascular damage is thought to occur when diabetes begins to alter normal cholesterol and blood fat levels. With weight management, exercise, dietary changes, and drug therapy, diabetes can be relatively well controlled in most people. Even with careful management of this disease, diabetic patients are susceptible to eventual heart and blood vessel damage.

TALKING POINTS • How would you show support for a friend who is struggling with the dietary requirements of diabetes?

Obesity and overweight

Even if they have no other risk factors, obese people are more likely than nonobese people to develop heart disease and stroke. Obesity places considerable strain on the heart, and it tends to influence both blood pressure and blood cholesterol levels. Also, obesity tends to trigger diabetes in predisposed people. The importance of maintaining body weight within a desirable range minimizes the chance of obesity ever happening. To accomplish this, maintain an active lifestyle and follow the dietary guidelines in Chapter 5.

TALKING POINTS • How could you tactfully bring up a friend's weight problem to show concern for his or her health?

Contributing Risk Factors

The American Heart Association identifies other risk factors that may contribute to CVD. These include *individual response to stress, sex hormones, birth control pills,* and *drinking too much alcohol.* Unresolved stress can encourage negative health dependencies (for example, smoking, poor dietary practices, underactivity) that lead to changes in blood fat profiles, blood pressure, and heart workload. Female sex hormones tend to protect women from CVD until they reach menopause, but male hormones do the opposite. Birth control pills (see Chapter 14) can increase the risk of blood clots and heart attack, although the risk is small unless the woman also smokes and is over age 35. The consumption of too much alcohol can cause elevated blood pressure, heart failure, and lead to stroke, although moderate drinking (no more than one drink per day for women and two drinks per day for men) is associated with lower risk of heart disease.[2]

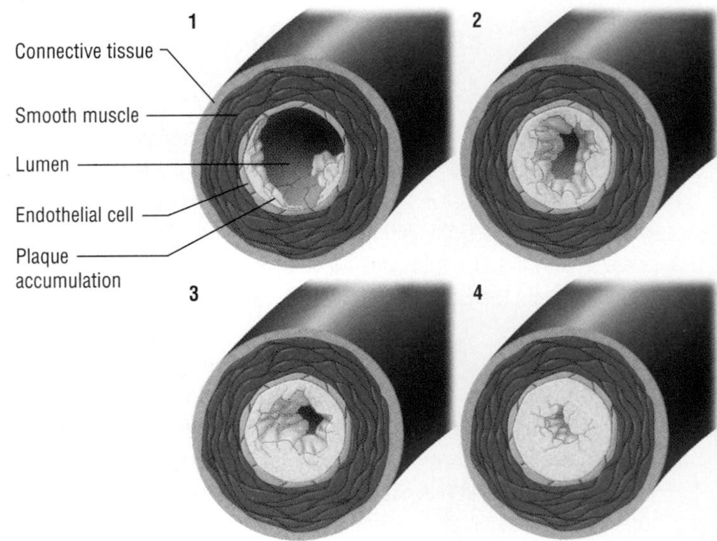

Figure 10-3 Progression of atherosclerosis. This diagram shows how plaque deposits gradually accumulate to narrow the lumen (interior space) of an artery. Although enlarged here, coronary arteries are only as wide as a pencil lead.

FORMS OF CARDIOVASCULAR DISEASE

The American Heart Association describes the six major forms of CVD as coronary heart disease, hypertension, stroke, congenital heart disease, rheumatic heart disease, and congestive heart failure. A person may have just one of these diseases or a combination of them at the same time. Each form exists in varying degrees of severity. All are capable of causing secondary damage to other body organs and systems.

Coronary Heart Disease

This form of CVD, also known as *coronary artery disease,* involves damage to the vessels that supply blood to the heart muscle. The bulk of this blood is supplied by the coronary arteries. Any damage to these important vessels can cause a reduction of blood (and its vital oxygen and nutrients) to specific areas of heart muscle. The ultimate result of inadequate blood supply is a heart attack.

Atherosclerosis

The principal cause for the development of coronary heart disease is atherosclerosis (Figure 10-3). **Atherosclerosis** produces a narrowing of the coronary arteries. This narrowing stems from the long-term buildup of fatty deposits, called *plaque,* on the inner walls of the arteries. This buildup reduces the blood supply to specific portions of the heart. Some arteries of the heart can become so blocked (occluded) that all blood supply is stopped. Heart muscle tissue begins to die when it is deprived of oxygen and nutrients. This damage is known as **myocardial infarction.** In lay terms, this event is called a *heart attack.* The Changing for the Better box on p. 237 explains how to recognize the signs of a heart attack and what to do next.

Cholesterol and lipoproteins. For many years, scientists have known that atherosclerosis is a complicated disease that has many causes. Some of these causes are not well understood, but others are clearly understood. *Cholesterol,* a soft, fatlike material, is manufactured in the liver and small intestine and is necessary in the formation of sex hormones, cell membranes, bile salts, and nerve fibers. Elevated levels of serum cholesterol (200 mg/dl or more for adults age 20 and older, and 170 mg/dl or more for young people below age 20) are associated with an increased risk for developing atherosclerosis[2] (see the Changing for the Better box on p. 238).

About half of American adults age 20 and older exceed the "borderline high" 200 mg/dl cholesterol level. It is estimated that nearly 40% of American youth age 19 and below have "borderline high" cholesterol levels of 170 mg/dl and above. About one out of five American adults has a "high" blood cholesterol level, that is, 240 mg/dl or greater.

Initially, most people can help lower their serum cholesterol level by adopting three dietary changes: lowering their intake of saturated fats, lowering their intake of dietary cholesterol, and lowering their caloric intake to a level that does not exceed body requirements. The aim is to reduce excess fat, cholesterol, and calories in the diet while promoting sound nutrition. By carefully following such a diet plan, people with elevated serum cholesterol levels typically are able to reduce their cholesterol levels by 30 to 55 mg/dl. However, dietary changes do not affect people equally; some will experience greater reductions

Changing *for the Better*

Recognizing Signs of a Heart Attack and Taking Action

I was walking by the track field and saw a runner in distress. I froze and watched as someone else ran to his aid. How could I tell whether or not this person was having a heart attack? What action should I have taken?

Warning Signs of a Heart Attack

- Uncomfortable pressure, fullness, squeezing, or pain in the center of your chest lasting 2 minutes or longer
- Pain spreading to your shoulders, neck, or arms
- Severe pain, dizziness, fainting, sweating, nausea, or shortness of breath

Not all of these warning signs occur with every heart attack. If some start to occur, don't wait. Get help immediately!

What to Do in an Emergency

- Find out which hospitals in your area have 24-hour emergency cardiac care.
- Determine (in advance) the hospital or medical facility that is nearest your home and office, and tell your family and friends to call this facility in an emergency.
- Keep a list of emergency rescue service numbers next to your telephone and in your pocket, wallet, or purse.
- If you have chest discomfort that lasts for 2 minutes or more, call the emergency rescue service.
- If you can get to a hospital faster by going yourself and not waiting for an ambulance, have someone drive you there.

How to Be a Heart Saver

- If you are with someone experiencing the signs of a heart attack and the warning signs last for 2 minutes or longer, act immediately.
- Expect a denial. It is normal for someone with chest discomfort to deny the possibility of something as serious as a heart attack. Don't take "no" for an answer. Insist on taking prompt action.
- Call the rescue service (911), or get to the nearest hospital emergency room that offers 24-hour emergency cardiac care.
- Give CPR (mouth-to-mouth breathing and chest compression) if it is necessary and if you are properly trained.

than others. Some will not respond at all to dietary changes and may need to take cholesterol-lowering medications and increase their physical activity.

Cholesterol is attached to structures called lipoproteins. Lipoproteins are particles that circulate in the blood and transport lipids (including cholesterol).[5] Two major classes of lipoproteins exist: **low-density lipoproteins (LDLs)** and **high-density lipoproteins (HDLs).** A person's total cholesterol level is chiefly determined by the amount of the LDLs and HDLs in a measured sample of blood. For example, a person's total cholesterol level of 200 mg/dl could be represented by an LDL level of 160 and an HDL level of 40, or an LDL level of 140 and an HDL level of 60. (Note that small amounts of additional forms of lipoproteins do exist and may influence the overall distribution percentages in a total cholesterol reading.)

After much scientific study, it has been determined that high levels of LDL are a significant promoter of atherosclerosis. This makes sense because LDLs carry the greatest percentage of cholesterol in the bloodstream. LDLs are more likely to deposit excess cholesterol into the artery walls. This contributes to plaque formation.

For this reason, LDLs are often called the "bad cholesterol."[8] High LDL levels are determined partially by inheritance, but they are also clearly associated with smoking, poor dietary patterns, obesity, and lack of exercise.

On the other hand, high levels of HDLs are related to a decrease in the development of atherosclerosis. HDLs are thought to transport cholesterol out of the bloodstream. Thus HDLs have been called the "good cholesterol." Certain lifestyle alterations, such as quitting smoking, reducing obesity, increasing physical activity, decreasing overall dietary fat intake, and replacing saturated fats with monosaturated fats, help many people increase their level of HDLs.

Key Terms

atherosclerosis
Buildup of plaque on the inner walls of arteries.

myocardial infarction
Heart attack; the death of part of the heart muscle as a result of a blockage in one of the coronary arteries.

low-density lipoprotein (LDL)
The type of lipoprotein that transports the largest amount of cholesterol in the bloodstream; high levels of LDL are related to heart disease.

high-density lipoprotein (HDL)
The type of lipoprotein that transports cholesterol from the bloodstream to the liver, where it is eventually removed from the body; high levels of HDL are related to a reduction in heart disease.

Table 10-2 Classification and Recommended Follow-up Based on Total Cholesterol Level

Total Cholesterol Level	Classification	Recommended Follow-up
<200 mg/dl	Desirable blood cholesterol level	Repeat test within 5 years
200–239 mg/dl	Borderline-high blood cholesterol level	*Without* definite CHD or two other CHD risk factors (one of which may be male gender): dietary modification and annual retesting *With* definite CHD or two other CHD risk factors: lipoprotein analysis; further action based on LDL-cholesterol level
≥240 mg/dl	High blood cholesterol level	Lipoprotein analysis; further action based on LDL-cholesterol level

Changing *for the Better*

Monitoring Your Cholesterol Level

The last time I had a physical exam, I was embarrassed to ask what the cholesterol numbers meant. I thought if there was a problem, the doctor would have notified me. Now I think I should have asked for more information. What should I do next time?

The next time you get your blood cholesterol level checked, try to find out more than just your total cholesterol level. Ask for the following three measurements, and compare them with the desirable measurements for adults, listed below.

Readings for	Your measurement	Desirable measurement
HDL level:	________	Above 45 mg/dl
LDL level:	________	Below 130 mg/dl
Total level:	________	Below 200 mg/dl

How do your measurements compare with the desirable measurements? If they are not satisfactory, refer to Table 10-2 and the discussion on p. 236 to improve your levels.

Reducing total serum cholesterol levels is a significant step in reducing the risk of death from coronary heart disease. For people with elevated cholesterol levels, a 1% reduction in serum cholesterol level yields about a 2% reduction in the risk of death from heart disease. Thus a 10% to 15% cholesterol reduction can reduce risk by 20% to 30%.[9] See Table 10-2 for cholesterol classifications and current recommended follow-up.

Angina pectoris. When coronary arteries become narrowed, chest pain, or *angina pectoris,* is often felt. This pain results from a reduced supply of oxygen to heart muscle tissue. Usually, angina is felt when the patient becomes stressed or exercises too strenuously. Angina reportedly can range from a feeling of mild indigestion to a severe viselike pressure in the chest. The pain may extend from the center of the chest to the arms and even up to the jaw. Generally, the more severe the blockage, the more pain is felt.

Some cardiac patients relieve angina with the drug *nitroglycerin,* a powerful blood vessel dilator. This prescription drug, available in slow-release transdermal patches or small pills that are placed under the patient's tongue, causes the coronary arteries to dilate and allow a greater flow of blood into heart muscle tissue. Other cardiac patients may be prescribed drugs such as **calcium channel blockers** or **beta blockers.**

Emergency response to heart crises

Heart attacks are not always fatal. The consequences of any heart attack depend on the location of the damage to the heart, the extent to which heart muscle is damaged, and the speed with which adequate circulation is restored. Injury to the ventricles may very well prove fatal unless medical countermeasures are immediately undertaken. The recognition of heart attack is critically important (see the Changing for the Better box on p. 237).

Cardiopulmonary resuscitation (CPR) is one of the most important immediate countermeasures that trained people can use when confronted with a victim of heart attack. Programs sponsored by the American Red Cross and the American Heart Association teach people how to recognize, evaluate, and manage heart attack emergencies. CPR trainees are taught how to restore breathing and circulation in persons requiring emergency care. Frequently, colleges offer CPR training through courses in various departments. With revised CPR procedures in place in 2001, we encourage students to take a new course and become certified.

Diagnosis and coronary repair

Once a person's vital signs have stabilized, further diagnostic examinations can reveal the type and extent of damage to heart muscle. Initially an ECG might be taken. This test analyzes the electrical activity of the heart.

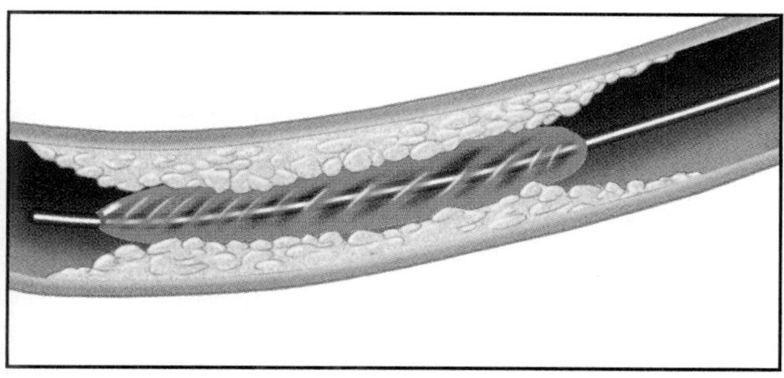
A

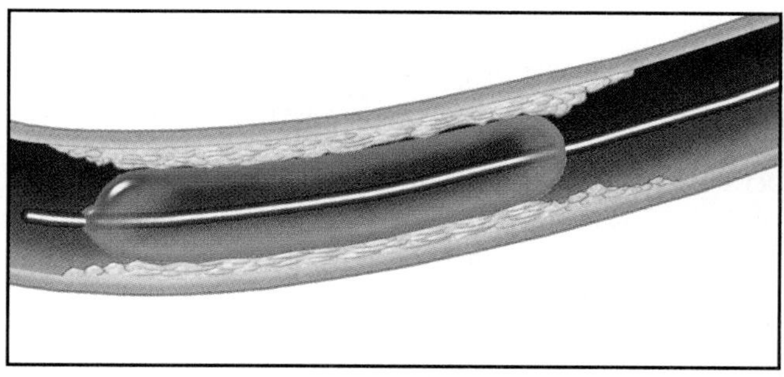
B

Figure 10-4 Angioplasty. **A,** A "balloon" is surgically inserted into the narrowed coronary artery. **B,** The balloon is inflated, compressing plaque and fatty deposits against the artery walls.

Heart catheterization, also called *coronary arteriography,* is a minor surgical procedure that starts with placement of a thin plastic tube into an arm or leg artery. This tube, called a *catheter,* is guided through the artery until it reaches the coronary circulation, where a *radiopaque dye* is then released. X-ray films called *angiograms* record the progress of the dye through the coronary arteries so that areas of blockage can be easily identified.

Once the extent of damage is identified, a physician or team of physicians can decide on a medical course of action. Currently popular is an extensive form of surgery called **coronary artery bypass surgery.** An estimated 553,000 bypass surgeries were performed in 1998.[2] The purpose of such surgery is to detour (bypass) areas of coronary artery obstruction by using a section of a vein from the patient's leg (often the saphenous vein) or an artery from the patient's chest (the internal mammary artery) and grafting it from the aorta to a location just beyond the area of obstruction. Multiple areas of obstruction result in double, triple, or quadruple bypasses.

Angioplasty. *Angioplasty,* an alternative to bypass surgery, involves the surgical insertion of a doughnut-shaped "balloon" directly into the narrowed coronary artery (Figure 10-4). When the balloon is inflated, plaque and fatty deposits are compressed against the artery walls, widening the space through which blood flows. The balloon usually remains in the artery for less than 1 hour. Renarrowing of the artery will occur in about one quarter of angioplasty patients. Balloon angioplasty can be used for blockages in the heart, kidneys, arms, and legs. The decision whether to have angioplasty or bypass surgery can be a difficult one to make. Nearly 540,000 angioplasty procedures were performed in 1998.[2]

The FDA approved a device for clearing heart and leg arteries. This device is called a *motorized scraper.* Inserted through a leg artery and held in place by a tiny inflated balloon, this motor-driven cutter shaves off plaque deposits from inside the artery. A nose cone in the scraper unit stores the plaque until the device is removed.

The use of laser beams to dissolve plaque that blocks arteries has been slowly evolving. The FDA has approved three laser devices for use in clogged leg arteries. In 1992 the FDA approved the use of an excimer laser for use in coronary arteries.

Aspirin. Studies released a decade ago highlighted the role of aspirin in reducing the risk of heart attack in men with no history of previous attacks. Specifically, the studies concluded that for men with hypertension, elevated cholesterol levels, or both, taking one aspirin per day was a significant factor in reducing their risk of heart attack. Aspirin works by making the blood less able to clot. This reduces the likelihood of blood vessel blockages. Presently, there is differing opinion regarding the age at which this preventive action should begin. The safest advice is to check with your physician before starting aspirin therapy. Recent research now indicates that aspirin therapy is also beneficial for women.[10]

Key Terms

calcium channel blockers
Drugs that prevent arterial spasms; used in the long-term management of angina pectoris.

beta blockers
Drugs that prevent overactivity of the heart, which results in angina pectoris.

coronary artery bypass surgery
Surgical procedure designed to improve blood flow to the heart by providing alternative routes for blood to take around points of blockage.

Alcohol. For years, scientists have been uncertain about the extent to which alcohol consumption is related to a reduced risk for heart disease. The current thinking is that moderate drinking (defined as no more than two drinks per day for men and one drink per day for women) is related to a lower heart disease risk. However, the benefit is much smaller than proven risk reduction behaviors such as stopping smoking, reducing cholesterol level, lowering blood pressure, and increasing physical activity. Experts caution that heavy drinking increases cardiovascular risks and that nondrinkers should not start to drink just to reduce heart disease risk.

Heart transplants and artificial hearts. For approximately 30 years, surgeons have been able to surgically replace a person's damaged heart with that of another human being. Although very risky, these transplant operations have added years to the lives of a number of patients who otherwise would have lived only a short time. In 1999, 2,184 heart transplants were performed in the United States.[2]

Artificial hearts have also been developed and implanted in humans. These hearts have extended the lives of many patients, but they have kept them unpleasantly tethered with tubes and wires to large power source machines. However, a major medical breakthrough took place in July 2001, when the world's first self-contained artificial heart was successfully implanted into a 59-year-old patient.

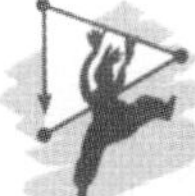

HealthQuest Activities

- The *Heart Attack Risk and Cardiovascular Exploration* activities in the Cardiovascular Health module allow you to assess your risk for cardiovascular disease. In the first of these activities, *Heart Attack Risk,* answer the questions about your health history, behavioral practices, and knowledge about heart disease. *HealthQuest* will then provide the correct answers and point out any health risks indicated by your responses. In the *Cardiovascular Exploration* section, fill out all of the items, and then click on the "Show Me!" button to find out your overall risk. You can get more specific feedback on each risk factor by clicking on the underlined words.
- Many traditional-age college students have difficulty understanding how cardiovascular disease affects quality of life. Heart disease seems only a distant possibility, but for many, it can become all too real. To learn more, read about heart disease among women and minority groups in the *Social Perspectives* section. List several health choices that can increase the likelihood of developing cardiovascular disease, and explain how one's family history can affect the risk. Finally, describe what you would do if you observed someone having a heart attack.

Hypertension

Just as your car's water pump recirculates water and maintains water pressure, your heart recirculates blood and maintains blood pressure. When the heart contracts, blood is forced through your arteries and veins. Your blood pressure is a measure of the force that your circulating blood exerts against the interior walls of your arteries and veins.

Blood pressure is measured with a *sphygmomanometer.* This instrument is attached to an arm-cuff device that can be inflated to stop the flow of blood temporarily in the brachial artery. This artery is a major supplier of blood to the lower arm. It is located on the inside of the upper arm, between the biceps and triceps muscles.

A physician, nurse, or technician using a stethoscope will listen for blood flow while the pressure in the cuff is released. Two pressure measurements will be recorded: the **systolic pressure** is the blood pressure against the vessel walls when the heart contracts, and the **diastolic pressure** is the blood pressure against the vessel walls when the heart relaxes (between heartbeats). Expressed in millimeters of mercury displaced on the sphygmomanometer, blood pressure is recorded in the form of a fraction, for example, 115/82. Because blood pressure drops when the heart relaxes, the diastolic pressure is always lower than the systolic pressure.

Although many people still consider 120/80 as a "normal" or safe blood pressure for a young adult, variations from this figure do not necessarily indicate a medical problem. In fact, many young college women of average weight will indicate blood pressures that seem to be relatively low (100/60, for example), yet these lowered blood pressures are quite "normal" for them. Any wide deviation from 120/80 in your blood pressure should be discussed with a physician.

TALKING POINTS • You're having a regular physical examination, and your doctor remarks that your blood pressure puts you in the category of "borderline hypertension." What questions would you ask about managing this condition?

Hypertension refers to a consistently elevated blood pressure. Generally, concern about a young adult's high blood pressure begins when he or she has a systolic reading of 140 or above or a diastolic reading of 90 or above. Approximately 50 million American adults and children have hypertension. The American Heart Association reports that African Americans, Hispanic Americans, and American Indians have higher rates of high blood pressure than white Americans.[2,5] In contrast, Asian/Pacific Islanders have significantly lower rates of hypertension.[2]

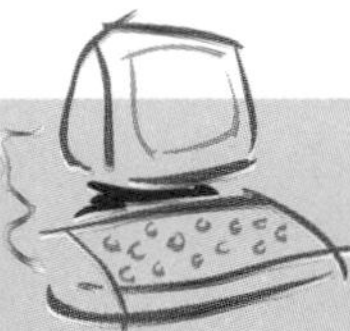

OnSITE/InSIGHT

Learning to Go: Health

Want to keep your heart in good condition? Click on the Motivator icon to find this lesson, which will guide you in how to do just that:

Lesson 33: Plan for a healthy heart.

STUDENT POLL

Are you at risk for developing cardiovascular disease? Go to the Online Learning Center at **www.mhhe.com/hahn6e**. Click on Student Resources to access the Student Poll. Answer the following questions and then find out how other students responded.

1. Does cardiovascular disease run in your family?
2. Are you taking precautions now to avoid heart-related problems in later life?
3. Are men, in comparison with women, more susceptible to heart disease?
4. Do you make heart-healthy food choices?
5. Do you have high blood pressure?
6. Are you a smoker?
7. Do you do an aerobic activity, such as brisk walking or running, on a regular basis?
8. Do you try to reduce the stress in your life?
9. Do you know the warning signs of a heart attack?
10. Are you trained in CPR?
11. Do you watch your cholesterol level?
12. Are you a "couch potato"?
13. Do you think about your weight in terms of cardiovascular disease?
14. Do you schedule regular physical examinations?

Although the reasons for 90% to 95% of the cases of hypertension are not known, the health risks produced by uncontrolled hypertension are clearly understood. Throughout the body, hypertension makes arteries and arterioles become less elastic and thus incapable of dilating under a heavy workload. Brittle, calcified blood vessels can burst unexpectedly and produce serious strokes (brain accidents), kidney failure (renal accidents), or eye damage (**retinal hemorrhage**). Furthermore, it appears that blood and fat clots are more easily formed and dislodged in a vascular system affected by hypertension. Thus hypertension can be a cause of heart attacks. Clearly, hypertension is a potential killer.

Ironically, despite its deadly nature, hypertension is referred to as "the silent killer" because people with hypertension often are not aware that they have the condition. They cannot feel the sensation of high blood pressure. The condition does not produce dizziness, headaches, or memory loss unless one is experiencing a medical crisis. It is estimated that nearly one-third of the people who have hypertension do not realize they have it.[5] Many who are aware of their hypertension do little to control it. Only a small percentage (27%) of people who have hypertension control it adequately, generally through dietary control, supervised fitness, relaxation training, and drug therapy.

Hypertension is not thought of as a curable disease; rather, it is a controllable disease. Once therapy is stopped, the condition returns. As a responsible adult, use every opportunity you can to measure your blood pressure on a regular basis.

Prevention and treatment

Weight reduction, physical activity, moderation in alcohol use, and sodium restriction are often used to reduce hypertension. For overweight or obese people, a reduction in body weight may produce a significant drop in blood pressure. Physical activity helps lower blood pressure by expending calories (which leads to weight loss) and improving overall circulation. Reducing alcohol consumption to no more than 1–2 drinks daily helps reduce blood pressure in some people.

The restriction of sodium (salt) in the diet also helps some people reduce hypertension. Interestingly, this strategy is effective only for those who are **salt sensitive**—

Key Terms

systolic pressure
Blood pressure against blood vessel walls when the heart contracts.

diastolic pressure
Blood pressure against blood vessel walls when the heart relaxes.

retinal hemorrhage
Uncontrolled bleeding from arteries within the eye's retina.

salt sensitive
Term used to describe people whose bodies overreact to the presence of sodium by retaining fluid and thus experience an increase in blood pressure.

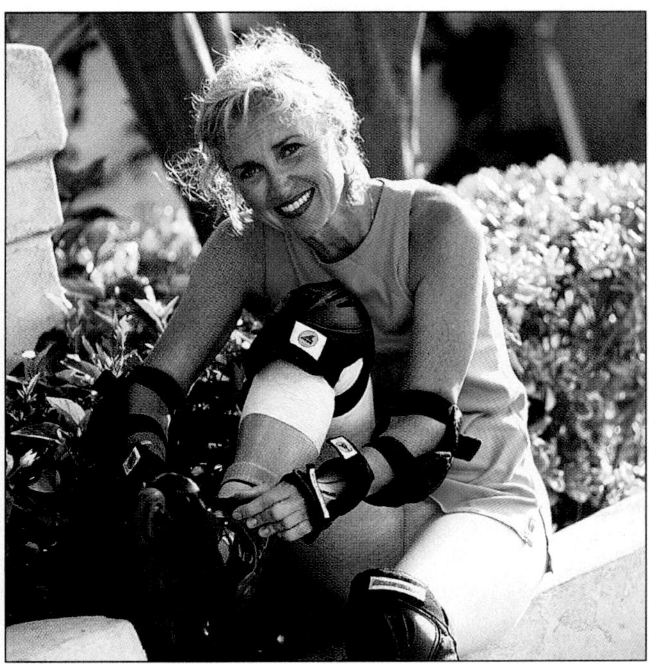

Prevention of hypertension involves weight management and physical activity.

estimated to be about 25% of the population. Reducing salt intake would have little effect on the blood pressure of the rest of the population. Nevertheless, since our daily intake of salt vastly exceeds our need for salt, the general recommendation to curb salt intake still makes good sense.

Many of the stress reduction activities discussed in Chapter 3 are receiving increased attention in the struggle to reduce hypertension. In recent years, behavioral scientists have reported the success of meditation, biofeedback, controlled breathing, and muscle relaxation exercises in reducing hypertension. Look for further research findings in these areas in the years to come.

There are literally dozens of drugs available for use by people with hypertension. Unfortunately, many patients refuse to take their medication on a consistent basis, probably because of the mistaken notion that "you must feel sick to be sick." Nutritional supplements, such as calcium, magnesium, potassium, and fish oil, have not been proven to be effective in lowering blood pressure.

Stroke

Stroke is a general term for a wide variety of crises (sometimes called *cerebrovascular accidents* [CVAs] or brain attacks) that result from blood vessel damage in the brain. African Americans have a much greater risk of stroke than white Americans do, probably because African Americans have a greater likelihood of having hypertension than white Americans. Data for 1998 indicate that 158,448 deaths and half a million new cases of stroke occurred.[2] Just as the heart muscle needs an adequate blood supply, so does the brain. Any disturbance in the proper supply of oxygen and nutrients to the brain can pose a threat.

Perhaps the most common form of stroke results from the blockage of a cerebral (brain) artery. Similar to coronary occlusions, **cerebrovascular occlusions** can be started by a clot that forms within an artery, called a *thrombus,* or by a clot that travels from another part of the body to the brain, called an *embolus* (Figure 10-5, *A* and *B*). The resultant accidents (cerebral thrombosis or cerebral embolism) cause between 80% and 90% of all strokes. The portion of the brain deprived of oxygen and nutrients can literally die.

A third type of stroke can result from an artery that bursts to produce a crisis called *cerebral hemorrhage* (Figure 10-5, *C*). Damaged, brittle arteries can be especially susceptible to bursting when a person has hypertension.

A fourth form of stroke is a *cerebral aneurysm.* An aneurysm is a ballooning or outpouching on a weakened area of an artery (Figure 10-5, *D*). Aneurysms may occur in various locations of the body and are not always life-threatening. The development of aneurysms is not fully understood, although there seems to be a relationship between aneurysms and hypertension. It is quite possible that many aneurysms are congenital defects. In any case, when a cerebral aneurysm bursts, a stroke results. See the Changing for the Better box on p. 243 to learn the warning signs of stroke.

A person who reports any warning signs of stroke or any small stroke, called a **transient ischemic attack (TIA),** will undergo a battery of diagnostic tests, which could include a physical examination, a search for possible brain tumors, tests to identify areas of the brain affected, use of the electroencephalogram, cerebral arteriography, and the use of the **CT** (computed tomography) **scan** or **MRI** (magnetic resonance imaging) **scan.** Many additional tests are also available.

Treatment of stroke patients depends on the nature and extent of the damage. Some patients require surgery (to repair vessels and relieve pressure) and acute care in the hospital. Others undergo drug treatment, especially the use of anticoagulant drugs, including aspirin and TPA (the "clot buster" drug).

The advancements made in the rehabilitation of stroke patients are amazing. Although some severely affected patients have little hope of improvement, our increasing advancements in the application of computer technology to such disciplines as speech and physical therapy offer encouraging signs for stroke patients and their families.

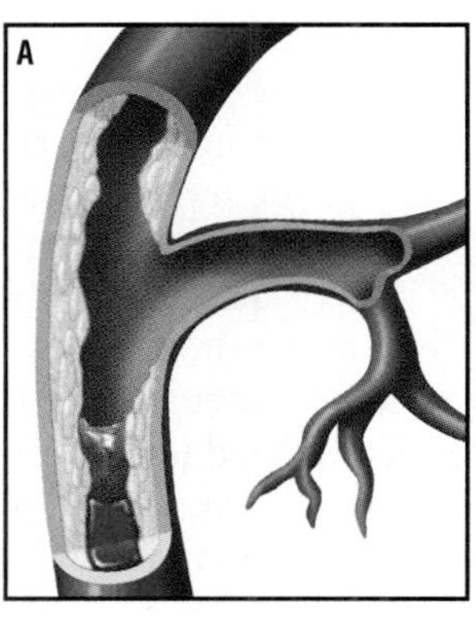

Thrombus
A clot that forms within a narrowed section of a blood vessel and remains at its place of origin.

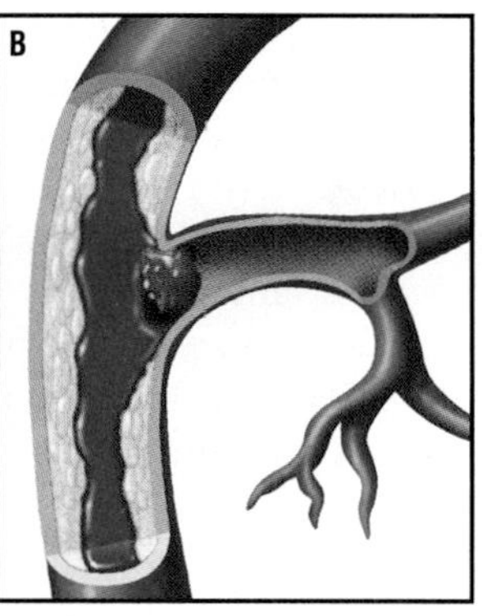

Embolus
A clot that moves through the circulatory system and becomes lodged at a narrowed point within a vessel.

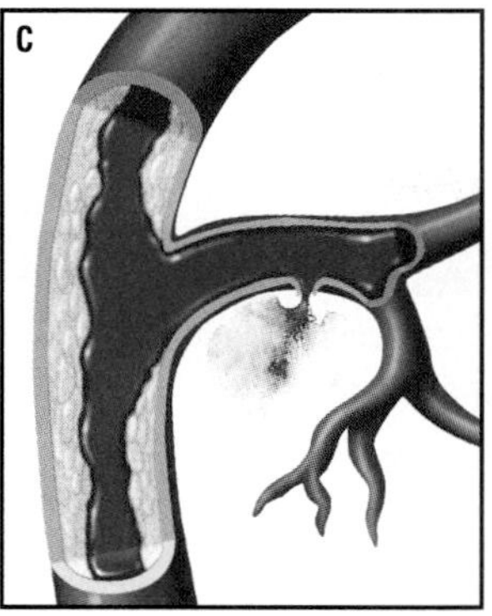

Hemorrhage
The sudden bursting of a blood vessel.

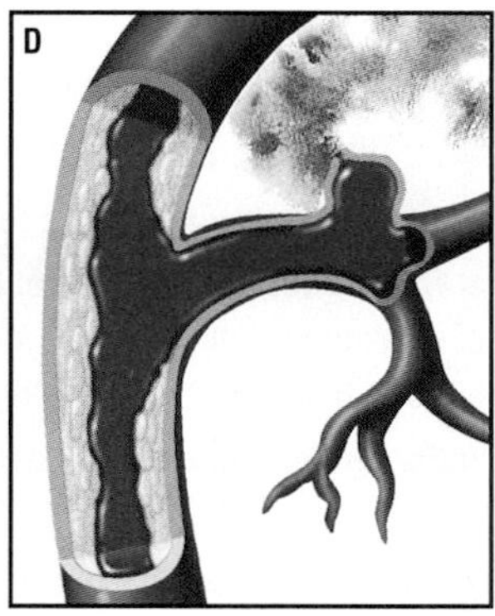

Aneurysm
A sac formed when a section of a blood vessel thins and balloons; the weakened wall of the sac can burst, or rupture, as shown here.

Figure 10-5 Causes of stroke.

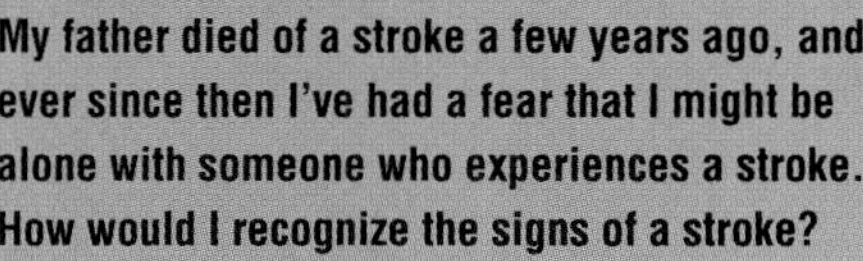

Changing *for the Better*

Recognizing Warning Signs of Stroke

My father died of a stroke a few years ago, and ever since then I've had a fear that I might be alone with someone who experiences a stroke. How would I recognize the signs of a stroke?

Although many stroke victims have little advance warning of an impending crisis, there are some warning signals of stroke that should be recognized. The American Heart Association encourages everyone to be aware of the following signs:

- Sudden, temporary weakness or numbness of the face, arm, and leg on one side of the body
- Temporary loss of speech or trouble in speaking or understanding speech
- Temporary dimness or loss of vision, particularly in one eye
- Unexplained dizziness, unsteadiness, or sudden falls

Many severe strokes are preceded by "little strokes," warning signals like the above, experienced days, weeks, or months before the more severe event. Prompt medical or surgical attention to these symptoms may prevent a fatal or disabling stroke from occurring.

Congenital Heart Disease

A congenital defect is one that is present at birth. The American Heart Association estimates that each year about 40,000 babies are born with a congenital heart defect. In 1998, 4,657 children (mostly infants) died of congenital heart disease.[2]

A variety of abnormalities may be produced by congenital heart disease, including valve damage, holes in the walls of the septum, blood vessel transposition, and an underdevelopment of the left side of the heart. All of

Key Terms

cerebrovascular occlusion
Blockages to arteries supplying blood to the cerebral cortex of the brain; strokes.

transient ischemic attack (TIA)
Strokelike symptoms caused by temporary spasm of cerebral blood vessels.

CT scan
Computed tomography scan; an x-ray procedure that is designed to visualize structures within the body that would not normally be seen through conventional x-ray procedures.

MRI scan
Magnetic resonance imaging scan; an imaging procedure that uses a giant magnet to generate images of body tissues.

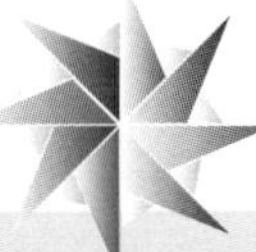

Risk Factors for Congenital and Rheumatic Heart Disease

Risk Factors for Congenital Heart Disease
Fetal exposure to rubella, other viral infections, pollutants, alcohol, or tobacco smoke during pregnancy

Risk Factors for Rheumatic Heart Disease
Streptococcal infection

Common Symptoms of Strep Throat
Sudden onset of sore throat, particularly with pain when swallowing
Fever
Swollen, tender glands under the angle of the jaw
Headache
Nausea and vomiting
Tonsils covered with a yellow or white pus or discharge

these problems ultimately prevent a newborn from adequately oxygenating tissues throughout the body. A bluish skin color (cyanosis) is seen in some infants with such congenital heart defects. These infants are sometimes referred to as *blue babies.*

The cause of congenital heart defects is not clearly understood, although one cause, *rubella,* has been identified. The fetuses of mothers who contract the rubella virus during the first 3 months of pregnancy are at great risk of developing *congenital rubella syndrome (CRS),* a catch-all term for a wide variety of congenital defects, including heart defects, deafness, cataracts, and mental retardation. Other hypotheses about the development of congenital heart disease implicate environmental pollutants; maternal use of drugs, including alcohol, during pregnancy; and unknown genetic factors (see the Star Box above).

Treatment of congenital defects usually requires surgery, although some conditions may respond well to drug therapy. Defective blood vessels and certain malformations of the heart can be surgically repaired. This surgery is so successful that many children respond quite quickly to the increased circulation and oxygenation. Many are able to lead normal, active lives.

Rheumatic Heart Disease

Rheumatic heart disease is the final stage in a series of complications started by a streptococcal infection of the throat (strep throat). The Star Box above lists symptoms of strep throat. This bacterial infection, if untreated, can result in an inflammatory disease called *rheumatic fever* (and a related condition, scarlet fever). Rheumatic fever is a whole-body (systemic) reaction that can produce fever, joint pain, skin rashes, and possible brain and heart damage. A person who has had rheumatic fever is more susceptible to subsequent attacks. Rheumatic fever tends to run in families. Nearly 5000 Americans died from rheumatic fever and rheumatic heart disease in 1998.[2]

Damage from rheumatic fever centers on the heart's valves. For some reason the bacteria tend to proliferate in the heart valves. Defective heart valves may fail either to open fully *(stenosis)* or to close fully *(insufficiency).* Diagnosis of valve damage might initially come when a physician hears a backwashing or backflow of blood (a **murmur**). Further tests—including chest X rays, cardiac catheterization, and echocardiography—can reveal the extent of valve damage. Once identified, a faulty valve can be replaced surgically with a metal or plastic artificial valve or a valve taken from an animal's heart.

Congestive Heart Failure

Congestive heart failure is a condition in which the heart lacks the strength to continue to circulate blood normally throughout the body. In 1998, 46,980 people died from congestive heart failure. During congestive heart failure, the heart continues to work, but it cannot function well enough to maintain appropriate circulation. Venous blood flow starts to "back up." Swelling occurs, especially in the legs and ankles. Fluid can collect in the lungs and cause breathing difficulties and shortness of breath, and kidney function may be damaged.[5]

Congestive heart failure can result from heart damage caused by congenital heart defects, lung disease, rheumatic fever, heart attack, atherosclerosis, or high blood pressure. Generally, congestive heart failure is treatable through a combined program of rest, proper diet, modified daily activities, and the use of appropriate drugs. Without medical care, congestive heart failure can be fatal.

Additional conditions

Besides the cardiovascular diseases already discussed, the heart and blood vessels are also subject to other pathological conditions. Tumors of the heart, although rare, occur. Infectious conditions involving the pericardial sac that surrounds the heart *(pericarditis)* and the innermost layer of the heart *(endocarditis)* are more commonly seen. In addition, inflammation of the veins *(phlebitis)* is troublesome to some people.

Peripheral artery disease. **Peripheral artery disease (PAD),** also called *peripheral vascular disease (PVD),* is a blood vessel disease characterized by pathological changes to the arteries and arterioles in the extremities (primarily the legs and feet but sometimes the hands).

These changes result from years of damage to the peripheral blood vessels. Important causes of PAD are cigarette smoking, a high-fat diet, obesity, and sedentary occupations. In some cases, PAD is aggravated by blood vessel changes resulting from diabetes.

PAD severely restricts blood flow to the extremities. The reduction in blood flow is responsible for leg pain or cramping during exercise, numbness, tingling, coldness, and loss of hair in the affected limb. The most serious consequence of PAD is the increased likelihood of developing ulcerations and tissue death. These conditions can lead to gangrene and may eventually necessitate amputation.

The treatment of PAD consists of multiple approaches and may include efforts to improve blood lipid levels (through diet, exercise, or drug therapy), reduce hypertension, reduce body weight, and eliminate smoking. Blood vessel surgery is also a possible treatment approach.

Key Terms

rheumatic heart disease
Chronic damage to the heart (especially heart valves) resulting from a streptococcal infection within the heart; a complication associated with rheumatic fever.

murmur
An atypical heart sound that suggests a backwashing of blood into a chamber of the heart from which it has just left.

congestive heart failure
Inability of the heart to pump out all the blood that returns to it; can lead to dangerous fluid accumulations in veins, lungs, and kidneys.

peripheral artery disease (PAD)
Damage resulting from restricted blood flow to the extremities, especially the legs and feet.

SUMMARY

- Cardiovascular disorders are responsible for more disabilities and deaths than any other disease.
- The cardiovascular system consists of the heart, blood, and blood vessels. This system performs many functions.
- Our overall health depends on the health of the cardiovascular system.
- A cardiovascular risk factor is an attribute that a person has or is exposed to that increases the likelihood of heart disease.
- The "big six" risk factors are tobacco smoke, physical inactivity, high blood cholesterol level, high blood pressure, diabetes mellitus, and obesity and overweight. These are controllable risk factors.
- Increasing age, male gender, and heredity are risk factors that cannot be controlled.
- Four contributing risk factors to heart disease are individual response to stress, sex hormones, birth control pills, and drinking too much alcohol.
- The major forms of cardiovascular disease include coronary artery disease, hypertension, stroke, congenital heart disease, rheumatic heart disease, and congestive heart failure. Each disease develops in a specific way and may require a highly specialized form of treatment.

REVIEW QUESTIONS

1. Identify the principal components of the cardiovascular system. Trace the path of blood through the heart and cardiovascular system.
2. How much blood does the average adult have? What are some of the important functions of blood?
3. Define cardiovascular risk factor. What relationship do risk factors have to cardiovascular disease?
4. Identify those risk factors for cardiovascular disease that cannot be changed. Identify those risk factors that can be changed. Identify the risk factors that can be contributing factors.
5. What are the six major forms of cardiovascular disease? For each of these diseases, describe what the disease is, its cause (if known), and its treatment.
6. Describe how high-density lipoproteins differ from low-density lipoproteins.
7. What problems does atherosclerosis produce?
8. Why is hypertension referred to as "the silent killer"?
9. What are the warning signals of stroke?
10. What is peripheral artery disease?

THINK ABOUT THIS . . .

- Have you ever considered your potential for developing heart disease?
- In the last week, what have you done to improve your cardiovascular system?
- Do you know your total cholesterol reading? Do you know your levels of LDLs and HDLs?
- When was the last time you had your blood pressure checked? What were the readings?
- What role should men play in reducing the threats of congenital heart disease?
- Are you comfortable talking with your relatives about their possible risk factors?

REFERENCES

1. Kotecki JE, Chamness BE: A valuable tool for evaluating health-related www sites, *Journal of Health Education* 30:1, January/February 1999, 56–58.
2. American Heart Association: *2001 Heart and stroke statistical update,* 2000, The Association.
3. Seeley RR, Stephens TD, Tate P: *Essentials of anatomy and physiology,* ed 3, 1999, McGraw-Hill.
4. Thibodeau GA, Patton KT: *The human body in health and disease,* ed 3, 2001, Mosby.
5. American Heart Association: **www.americanheart.org/Heart_and_Stroke_A_Z_Guide/**, August 29, 2001.
6. American Heart Association: **www.americanheart.org/Heart_and_Stroke_A_Z_Guide/womens/**, September 1, 2001.
7. Hormone replacement therapy: more risk than benefit? *Harvard Health Letter* 25:8, June 2000, 4–5.
8. HDL: the good (but complex) cholesterol, *Harvard Heart Letter* 8:1, September 1997, 1–4.
9. Cholesterol: up with the good, *Harvard Heart Letter* 5:11, July 1995, 3–4.
10. Aspirin for coronary disease: beneficial in women, too, *Harvard Heart Letter* 7:7, March 1997, 8.

SUGGESTED READINGS

American Heart Association: *American Heart Association low-fat, low-cholesterol cookbook: heart-healthy, easy-to-make recipes that taste great,* ed 2, 1998, Times Books.
This revised cookbook was developed by the American Heart Association, the group most dedicated to improving the heart health of the American public. It includes favorite recipes from the earlier edition as well as innovative, tasty new recipes. This cookbook focuses on easy-to-make dishes that will make consumers forget how healthy the food actually is.

Burkman K: *The stroke recovery book: a guide for patients and families,* 1998, Addicus Books.
For the half million people annually who have strokes, this short reference book is a valuable guide for both patients and their families. Written by a physician, this book provides easy-to-understand answers to many of the questions about stroke. The various types of strokes, their causes, and treatments are explained. The author describes how strokes affect both body functioning and mental processes, including emotions and cognitive processes.

Kawalski RE, Kattus AA: *The 8-week cholesterol cure: how to lower your blood cholesterol by up to 40 percent without drugs or deprivation,* 1999, HarperCollins.
This is a revision of an earlier successful book written by Kawalski that features four new chapters. The authors encourage readers to modify their diets to include many more whole grains and other foods and vitamins that help lower blood cholesterol levels. This book also shows readers how to increase the percentages of good cholesterol (HDLs) in the bloodstream.

As we go to Press...

In August 2001, a popular cholesterol-lowering drug was taken off the market after thirty-one deaths in the United States were linked to its use. The deaths were apparently related to an uncommon side effect called rhabdomyolysis, which destroys muscle cells and allows them to enter the bloodstream and threaten kidney and other organ functioning. At the time of the recall, Baycol (cerivastatin), manufactured by Bayer, was being used by 700,000 Americans. Baycol was in a classification of drugs known as statins. As we go to press, patients using Baycol were encouraged to see their physicians and consider switching to one of the five other popular statin drugs (Lescol, Lipitor, Mevacor, Pravachol, and Zocor).

Name ______________________ **Date** __________ **Section** __________

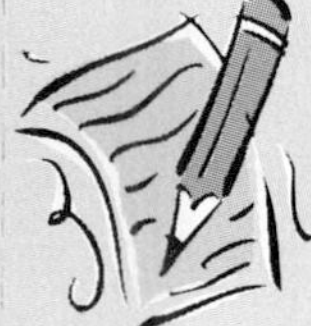

Personal Assessment

What Is Your Risk for Heart Disease?

Cholesterol

Your serum cholesterol level is:

0	190 or below
+ 2	191 to 230
+ 6	231 to 289
+12	290 to 319
+16	Over 320

Your HDL cholesterol is:

− 2	Over 60
0	45 to 60
+ 2	35 to 44
+ 6	29 to 34
+12	23 to 28
+16	Below 23

Smoking

You smoke now or have in the past:

0 Never smoked, or quit more than 5 years ago
+ 1 Quit 2 to 4 years ago
+ 3 Quit about 1 year ago
+ 6 Quit during the past year

You now smoke:

+ 9 ½ to 1 pack a day
+12 1 to 2 packs a day
+15 More than 2 packs a day

The quality of the air you breathe is:

0 Unpolluted by smoke, exhaust, or industry at home and at work
+ 2 Live or work with smokers in unpolluted area
+ 4 Live and work with smokers in unpolluted area
+ 6 Live or work with smokers **and** live or work in air-polluted area
+ 8 Live **and** work with smokers **and** live and work in air-polluted area

Blood Pressure

Your blood pressure is:

0 120/75 or below
+ 2 120/75 to 140/85
+ 6 140/85 to 150/90
+ 8 150/90 to 175/100
+10 175/100 to 190/110
+12 190/110 or above

Exercise

Your exercise habits are:

0 Exercise vigorously 4 or 5 times a week
+ 2 Exercise moderately 4 or 5 times a week
+ 4 Exercise only on weekends
+ 6 Exercise occasionally
+ 8 Little or no exercise

Weight

Your weight is:

0 Always at or near ideal weight
+ 1 Now 10% overweight
+ 2 Now 20% overweight
+ 3 Now 30% or more overweight
+ 4 Now 20% or more overweight and have been since before age 30

Stress

You feel overstressed:

0 Rarely at work or at home
+ 3 Somewhat at home but not at work
+ 5 Somewhat at work but not at home
+ 7 Somewhat at work **and** at home
+ 9 Usually at work **or** at home
+12 Usually at work **and** at home

Diabetes

Your diabetic history is:

0 Blood sugar always normal
+ 2 Blood glucose slightly high (prediabetic) or slightly low (hypoglycemic)
+ 4 Diabetic beginning after age 40 requiring strict dietary or insulin control
+ 5 Diabetic beginning before age 30 requiring strict dietary or insulin control

Alcohol

You drink alcoholic beverages:

0 Never or only socially, about once or twice a month, or only one 5-ounce glass of wine or 12-ounce glass of beer or 1½ ounces of hard liquor about 5 times a week
+ 2 Two to three 5-ounces glasses of wine or 12-ounce glasses of beer or 1½-ounce cocktails about 5 times a week
+ 4 More than three 1½-ounce cocktails or more than three 5-ounce glasses of wine or 12-ounce glasses of beer almost every day

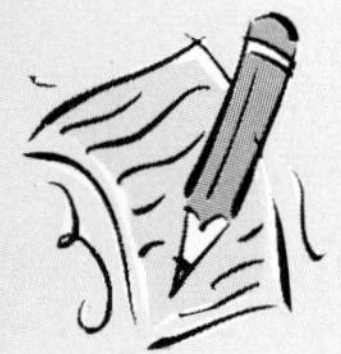

Personal Assessment *continued*

Interpretation

Add all sources and check below

0 to 20: Low risk. Excellent family history and lifestyle habits.

21 to 50: Moderate risk. Family history or lifestyle habits put you at some risk. You might lower your risks and minimize your genetic predisposition if you change any poor habits.

51 to 74: High risk. Habits and family history indicate high risk of heart disease. Change your habits now.

Above 75: Very high risk. Family history and a lifetime of poor habits put you at very high risk of heart disease. Eliminate as many of the risk factors as you can.

To Carry This Further . . .

Were you surprised with your score on this assessment? What were your most significant risk factors? Do you plan to make any changes in your lifestyle to reduce your cardiovascular risks? Why or why not?

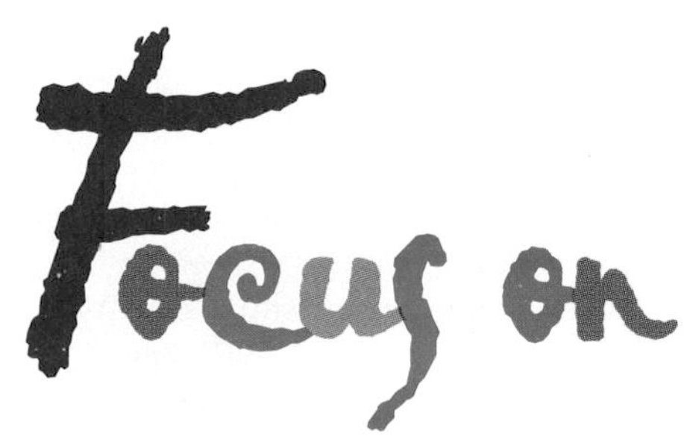

HYPERTENSION IN AFRICAN AMERICANS: TARGETING PREVENTION

Development of disease is an area in which each societal group is disadvantaged in one way or another. Practically every group has a tendency to develop one or more afflictions at a higher rate than the general population. For the African American community, one particular problem is hypertension.

The existing data show that hypertension is more common in African Americans[1,2] and is more aggressive and less well managed in African Americans than in whites. African Americans also have higher rates of morbidity and mortality from diseases related to high blood pressure, such as stroke and renal failure. The natural nocturnal fall in blood pressure is less pronounced in African Americans, and their systolic blood pressure while awake is higher than in people of other races.[1]

The exact causes of these differences have not been pinpointed, but research seems to be focused in two general areas. Some research suggests that certain physical and genetic factors contribute to increased incidence of hypertension in African Americans, whereas other studies have shown that hypertension in African Americans is related to environmental stress. This debate involves not just medical data but socioeconomic factors as well. In short, it is a nature vs. nurture debate, and there are supporting data for both arguments.

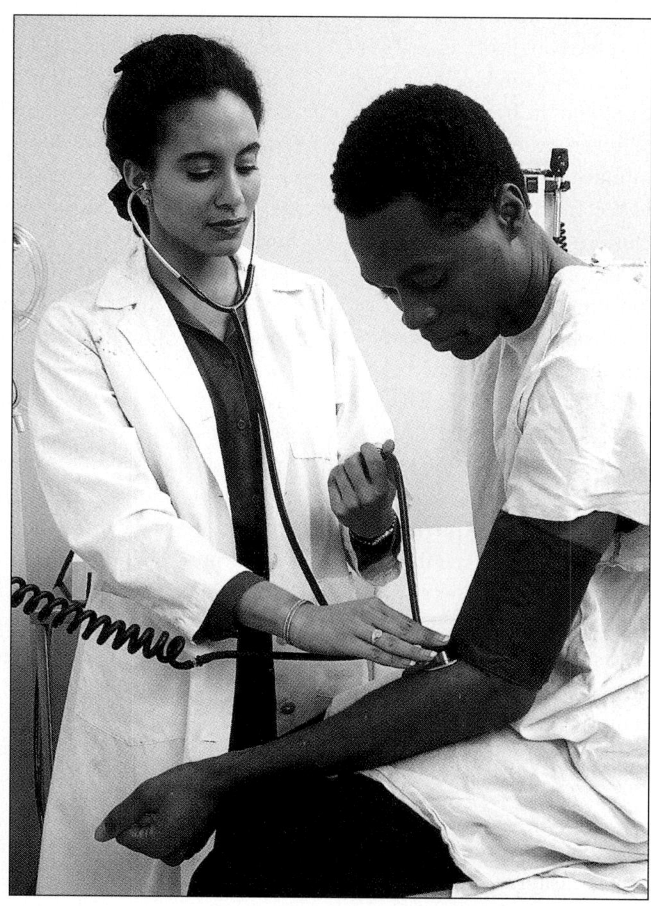

A combination of genetic factors and stress may be responsible for the high incidence of hypertension among African Americans.

Nature vs. Nurture

Studies have shown that environmental stress may contribute to increased hypertension in African Americans. A study conducted by Dr. Norman Anderson of Duke University[3] shows that chronic stress may lead to an increase in the release of the hormone norepinephrine to the bloodstream. Norepinephrine reduces the amount of salt eliminated from the kidneys, and the resulting increase in blood salt content can lead to increased blood pressure. This chain reaction has been shown to occur in animal studies. The high rate of chronic exposure to stress in many African American communities has been well documented.[3] If these studies hold true for humans, it would lend credence to the idea that certain stressful factors found in some African American communities could cause hypertension. Stressors such as poverty, unemployment, the threat of violence, and racial discrimination could be shown to cause kidneys to reduce elimination of salt and thus may also increase the risk of hypertension.[3]

Anger in response to racism may be a significant contributing factor in increased hypertension in African Americans. A study conducted jointly at the University of Tennessee and Saint Louis University showed that blood pressure in African Americans increased significantly when they were shown film clips of racially motivated violence.[4] The responses of African Americans to these scenes of racial discrimination were more pronounced than their responses to viewing scenes that were anger-provoking but had no racial component. The increases in blood pressure were not into the hypertension range, but researchers believe that over time, such continued elevation of blood pressure could become dangerous.

Such conclusions seem to suggest that socioeconomic factors are the main cause of hypertension among African Americans. A study performed on twenty-six African American women on strict low-fat diets seems to support this. The data showed that women of higher socioeconomic status had more excretion of salt than those of lower status.[3] Since proportionately more African Americans are in lower socioeconomic classes than whites, increased stress from lower status could be the main factor behind the inflated rate of hypertension among the African American population.

But is it all due to environment? Perhaps not. Other groups of traditionally lower socioeconomic status, such as Hispanics, Asians, and Native Americans, have been found to have the same incidence of hypertension as whites.[1] African American children have been found to have higher blood pressure in general than white children;[1] it is not known whether stress plays a significant role in affecting the blood pressure of these children so early in life.

There is also evidence that African Americans may be predisposed to hypertension at the cellular level. Microscopic studies of blood vessels in African Americans with severe hypertension revealed that renal arterioles were thickened and had reduced flow. This thickening, not found in the renal arterioles of hypertensive whites, was caused by hypertrophy (excess growth) of smooth muscle cells in the muscle walls of the arterioles. This thickening reduced the size of the lumen (inside opening) of the vessels, and the resulting reduced blood flow may have caused increased blood pressure. The smooth muscle cells were thought to be responding abnormally to growth factors, which caused the hypertrophy to occur.[2] The reason behind this abnormal reaction was not determined, however.

The best explanation of why African Americans are more prone to develop hypertension may not involve environment or genetics alone, but a combination of the two. Stress factors unique to the African American community may serve to aggravate or intensify an existing physical predisposition toward hypertension. It has already been shown that the tendency toward developing hypertension can be passed from parents to their children. Add several unique stress factors to a population already predisposed to high blood pressure, and the potential exists for high numbers of people to develop hypertension. Commenting on the UT-SLU study, Dr. Elijah Saunders agreed that "racism and Black rage are emotional stressors that could worsen a physiological tendency toward hypertension."[4]

Treatment for Hypertension in African Americans

The good news is that African Americans respond to medical treatment in a similar manner to whites. The treatment regimen for African Americans may have to be altered somewhat, however, since they do not respond as well to some hypertension medications as people of other races. For unknown reasons, drugs such as beta-blockers and ACE (angiotensin converting enzyme) inhibitors do not work as well in African Americans and may need to be supplemented by other medications, such as diuretics.[1]

Lifestyle changes may also be needed and may be a more effective tool in lowering blood pressure in African Americans than in people of other races.[1] Effort should be made to exercise and lose weight if needed, since excess weight can be a contributing factor in hypertension. Hypertensive African Americans tend to have lower intakes of potassium and calcium, so diet changes should be made that ensure that these minerals are in adequate supply. A reduction in sodium may also be desirable, since research suggests that African Americans may be more sensitive to the effects of sodium on the cardiovascular system.[1]

Although African Americans are more likely to develop high blood pressure, prevention and treatment can help keep hypertension from becoming a deadly affliction. Proper diagnosis is essential, so people at risk should see their doctors to determine whether they have hypertension or are at risk for developing it. Through recommending lifestyle modifications, prescribing medications, or both, a physician can help manage this condition or help prevent its onset.[5]

For Discussion . . .

Do you feel that people in lower (or higher) socioeconomic groups suffer more from everyday stress? Do you believe physiological or genetic differences may exist between different ethnic or racial groups?

References

1. Kaplan NM: Ethnic aspects of hypertension, *Lancet* 344(8920), 1994.
2. Dustan HP: Growth factors and racial differences in severity of hypertension and renal diseases, *Lancet* 339(8805), 1992.
3. Haywood RL: Why Black Americans suffer with more high blood pressure than Whites, *Jet* Dec 5, 1994, 87(5).
4. Study reveals anger over racism causes high blood pressure in Blacks, *Jet* May 14, 1990, 78(5).
5. Too little attention paid to high blood pressure, *Tufts University Health and Nutrition Letter,* (15:11), January 1998, p. 1.

chapter 11

Living with Cancer and Chronic Conditions

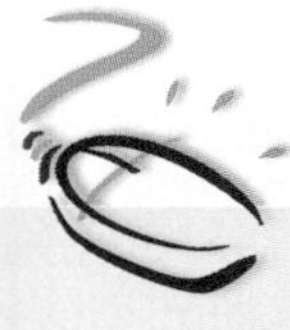

Online Learning Center Resources

www.mhhe.com/hahn6e

Log on to our Online Learning Center (OLC) for access to these additional resources:

- Chapter key terms and definitions
- Learning objectives
- Additional behavior change objectives
- Student interactive question-and-answer sites
- Self-scoring chapter quiz

The OLC also offers web links for study and exploration of health topics. Here are some examples of what you'll find:

- **www.cancer.org** Start your search at the American Cancer Society homepage, which includes ACS fact sheets and other publications.
- **http://cancernet.nci.nih.gov/index.html** Check out this excellent source for researching a broad range of cancer-related topics.
- **www.cansearch.org** This site offers great support resources for cancer patients and their families.

Taking Charge of Your Health

- Stay attuned to media reports about chronic conditions so that you can make informed choices.
- Support agencies devoted to the prevention of chronic health conditions.
- Monitor your work, home, and recreational environments to determine whether they are placing you at risk for cancer.
- Perform regular self-examinations for forms of cancer that can be detected through these techniques.
- Undergo the recommended cancer screening procedures for your age and sex.
- If you have cancer or a chronic condition, participate actively in your own treatment.

Eye on the Media

Support Is Just a Click Away

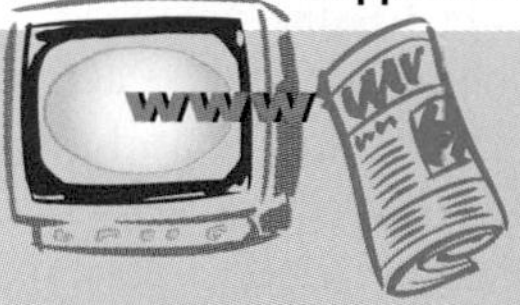

Support groups are composed of people who come together to help each other through the demands of a chronic health condition. These groups have traditionally been organized by institutions in the local health care community, such as hospitals, by the local affiliates of national organizations, such as the American Cancer Society, or by citizens who have the same chronic condition. Increasingly common today, however, are support groups whose members are connected, not by physical proximity, but by the Internet.

Health self-help groups on the Internet develop in one of two ways. The first occurs when a brick-and-mortar organization, such as a national agency or health care institution, develops a support group for its homepage. The second way is for a person with the condition (or a family member of that person) to organize an online group.

You can find a health support group simply by surfing the net. Or you can be referred to a site by a health care professional, friend, family

Eye on the Media *continued*

member, colleague, or someone with a similar condition. You can also go to the homepage of a medical institution or a national agency to find out if it provides a support group link.

For someone with a newly diagnosed chronic condition, the initial contact with a support group may be made to get information about the condition and its treatment. For others, it is a way of connecting with other people who have the condition. Web support groups provide windows to the outside world, particularly for those whose conditions limit their mobility and social contacts. The Internet support group transcends the restrictions of various diseases to make new connections possible.

It's important to realize that the online support group's members are rarely physicians or other highly trained health professionals. So you shouldn't rely on this source for specific technical information. Instead, your main sources of information about medical management of a chronic condition should be your health care providers. Seasoned members of support groups need to remind themselves that newly diagnosed members are inexperienced and vulnerable. It will take them time to adjust to the frankness and clinical sophistication demonstrated by some group members in addressing their health problems.

Some hospitals provide laptop computers to patients so they can maintain contact with their support groups. In this way, health care institutions are encouraging patients to support their efforts and, perhaps, helping them recover more quickly.

Most illnesses are disruptive, affecting your ability to participate in day-to-day activities. When you are ill, school, employment, and leisure activities are replaced by periods of decreased activity and sometimes bed rest or hospitalization. When an illness is **chronic,** the effect may extend over long periods, perhaps an entire lifetime. People with chronic illness must eventually find a balance between day-to-day function and the continuous presence of their condition. Cancer is an illness that is usually chronic in nature.

THE STATUS OF CANCER TODAY AND TOMORROW

It is estimated that 1,268,000 new cases of cancer were diagnosed and 553,400 Americans died of the disease in 2001.[1] In spite of our knowledge about cancer and our ongoing attempts to prevent and cure it, progress in cancer prevention is limited. It could be a combination of factors, including the aging of the population, our failure to curb tobacco use, the high fat content of the typical American diet, the continuing urbanization and pollution of our environment, the presence of millions of people without health insurance to pay for early diagnosis and proper treatment, or, simply, our ability to recognize its true role in deaths once ascribed to other causes. Regardless, cancer needs to be brought under control.

CANCER: A PROBLEM OF CELL REGULATION

Just as a corporation depends on competent individuals to staff its various departments, the body depends on its basic units of function—the cells. Cells band together as tissues, such as muscle tissue, to perform a prescribed function. Tissues in turn join to form organs, such as the heart, and organs are assembled into the body's several organ systems, such as the cardiovascular system. This is the "corporate structure" of the body.

If individuals and cells are the basic units of function for their respective organizations, the failure of either to perform in a prescribed, dependable manner can erode the overall organization to the extent that it might not be able to continue. Cancer, the second leading cause of death among adults, reflects cell dysfunction in its most extreme form.[2] In cancer the normal behavior of cells ceases.

Cell Regulation

Most of the tissues of the body lose cells over time. This continual loss requires that replacement cells be brought forward from areas of young and less specialized cells. The process of *specialization* required to turn the less specialized cells into mature cells is carefully controlled by genes within the cells. Upon becoming specialized, these newest cells copy, or *replicate,* themselves. These two processes are carefully monitored by the cells' **regulatory genes.** Failure to regulate specialization and replication results in abnormal, or cancerous, cells.

Cells also have genes designed to repair mistakes in the copying of genetic material (the basis of replication) and genes to suppress the growth of abnormal cells if they occur. Thus *repair genes* and *suppressor genes,* such as the *p53* gene, join regulatory genes to prevent the development of abnormal cells.[2] If these genes fail to function properly and malignant (cancerous) cells develop, the immune system (see Chapter 12) will, ideally, recognize their presence and remove them before a clinical (diagnosable) case of cancer can develop.

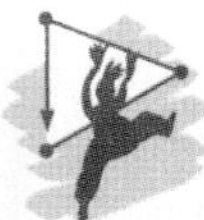

HealthQuest Activities

- The self-assessment activity *Cancer: What's Your Risk?,* found in the Cancer Module, allows you to examine how your family history, personal health history, occupation, environment, and behavior affect your risk of developing cancer. *HealthQuest* will estimate whether you are at decreased, average, or above-average risk of developing several kinds of cancer. Complete the self-assessment and then gather more information about the cancers for which you are at increased risk. Use the "Cancer Info" feature to help you.
- Like other chronic diseases that occur more frequently as people age, cancer may appear to be an unlikely possibility to young adults. Review the *Cancer Info* feature to learn how cancer affects quality of life. Then read the article on social support for people with cancer. Finally, increase your awareness of skin cancer prevention by using the *Skin Cancer Exploration.* List the factors that put a person at highest and at lowest risk for skin cancer. Then determine which factors are modifiable and which are not.

Because specialization, replication, repair, and suppressor genes can become cancer-causing genes, or **oncogenes,** when they do not work properly, these four types of genes can also be referred to as **protooncogenes,** or potential oncogenes.[2] The failure of tumor suppressor genes to regulate the formation of abnormal cells is now thought to be a critical factor in the development of cancer. In addition to the *p53* gene, other specific genes have been associated with certain types of breast cancer, ovarian cancer, colon cancer, and prostate cancer.[2] In the future, scientists may discover that virtually all cancers have genetic predispositions or specific oncogenes associated with their development.

Oncogene Formation

All cells have protooncogenes. But what changes normal cancer-preventing genes so that they become cancer-causing genes? Three mechanisms—genetic mutations, viral infections, and carcinogens—have received much attention.

Genetic mutations develop when dividing cells miscopy genetic information. If the gene that is miscopied is a protooncogene, the oncogene that results will stimulate the formation of cancerous cells. A variety of factors, including aging, free radical formation, radiation, and an array of carcinogens, are associated with the miscopying of the complex genetic information that comprises the genes found within the cell, including those intended to prevent cancer.

In both animals and humans, *cancer-producing viruses,* such as the leukemia virus in cats and the human immunodeficiency (HIV) virus, herpes virus, and human papillomavirus (HPV) in humans (see Chapter 12), have been identified. These viruses seek out cells of a particular type, such as those of the immune system, and alter their genetic material to convert these cells into virus-producing cells. In the process, they change the makeup of one or more of the regulatory genes, converting these protooncogenes into oncogenes. Once converted into oncogenes, the altered genes are passed on through cell division.

A third possible explanation for the conversion of protooncogenes into oncogenes is the presence of environmental agents known as *carcinogens.* Over an extended period, carcinogens, such as chemicals found in tobacco smoke, polluted air and water, toxic wastes, and the high fat content of foods, may convert protooncogenes into oncogenes. These carcinogens may work alone or in combination *(co-carcinogens).* Thus people might develop lung cancer only if they are exposed to the right combination of carcinogens over an extended period.

Our understanding of the role of genes in the development of cancer is expanding rapidly. In conjunction with the **Human Genome Project** and the *Cancer Genome Anatomy Project (CGAP),*[3] the scientific community has now identified over 160 oncogenes, tumor suppressor protooncogenes, and other genetic markers for human cancers.[4] Among the most familiar to the public are the *p16* oncogene for lung cancer, the *BRCA1* and *BRCA2* tumor suppressor genes for breast cancer and ovarian cancer, and the *MSH2* and *MSH1* genes for colon cancer. As geneticists continue to discover additional genetic links to cancer, the possibility of some form of "gene-repair" technology or a "gene chip" to aid screening becomes a possibility in the war against cancer.

Key Terms

chronic
Develops slowly and persists for a long period of time.

regulatory genes
Genes within the cell that control cellular replication, or doubling.

oncogenes
Genes that are believed to activate the development of cancer.

protooncogenes
Normal regulatory genes that may become oncogenes.

Human Genome Project
International quest by geneticists to identify the location and composition of every gene within the human cell.

The Cancerous Cell

In comparison with their noncancerous cousins, cancer cells are both similar and dissimilar in how they function. It is the dissimilar aspects that usually make them unpredictable and more difficult to manage.

One unique aspect of cancerous cells is their infinite life expectancy. It appears that cancerous cells can produce an enzyme, *telomerase,* that blocks the biological clock that tells normal cells that it's time to die.[5] In spite of this ability to live forever, cancer cells do not necessarily divide more quickly than normal cells. In fact, they can divide at the same rate or even at a slower rate.[2]

Because cancerous cells do not possess the *contact inhibition* (a control mechanism that influences the number of cells that can occupy a particular space) of normal cells, they can accumulate and eventually alter the structure of a body organ or break through its wall into neighboring areas (invasion). Also, the absence of *cellular cohesiveness* (a property seen in normal cells that "keeps them at home") allows cancer cells to spread through the circulatory or lymphatic system to distant points via **metastasis** (Figure 11-1). A final unique characteristic of cancerous cells is their ability to command extra blood supply to meet their metabolic needs and provide additional routes for metastasis. This *angiogenesis potential* of cancer cells makes them extremely hardy in comparison with noncancerous cells, although progress against this capability is being made. Today at least ten angiogenesis-inhibiting drugs are under development or in clinical trials.[6] As an example, Thalidomide, a drug once associated with severe birth defects when given as a sedative to women early in their pregnancies, is being used to treat breast, prostate, and brain cancers.

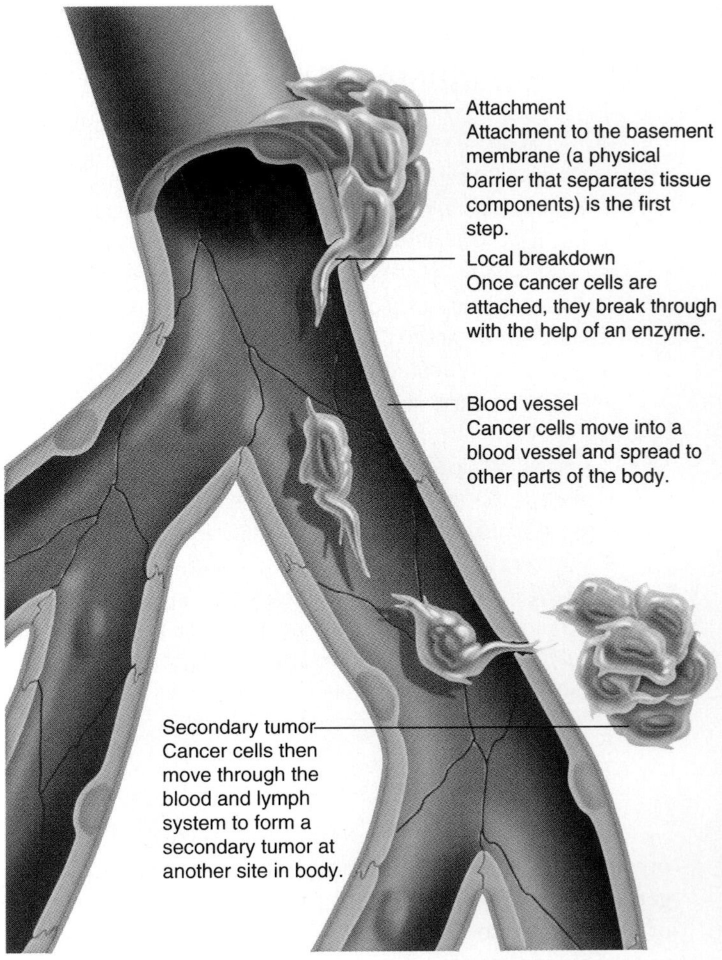
Attachment
Attachment to the basement membrane (a physical barrier that separates tissue components) is the first step.
Local breakdown
Once cancer cells are attached, they break through with the help of an enzyme.
Blood vessel
Cancer cells move into a blood vessel and spread to other parts of the body.
Secondary tumor
Cancer cells then move through the blood and lymph system to form a secondary tumor at another site in body.

Figure 11-1 How cancer spreads. Locomotion is (movement) essential to the process of metastasis (spread of cancer). Scientists have identified a protein that causes cancer cells to grow arms, or pseudopodia, enabling them to move to other parts of the body.

Benign Tumors

Noncancerous, or **benign,** tumors can also form in the body. These tumors are usually enclosed by a fibrous membrane and do not spread from their point of origin as cancerous tumors can. Benign tumors are dangerous, however, when they crowd out normal tissue within a confined space.

Types of Cancer and Their Locations

Cancers are named on the basis of the type of tissues where they occur. The classifications below are used by physicians to describe malignancies to the layperson:

carcinoma Found most frequently in the skin, nose, mouth, throat, stomach, intestinal tract, glands, nerves, breasts, urinary and genital structures, lungs, kidneys, and liver; approximately 85% of all malignant tumors are classified as carcinomas

sarcoma Formed in the connective tissues of the body; bone, cartilage, and tendons are the sites of sarcoma development; only 2% of all malignancies are of this type

melanoma Arises from the melanin-containing cells of skin; found most often in individuals who have had extensive sun exposure, particularly a deep, penetrating sunburn; although once rare, the amount of this cancer has increased markedly in recent years; remains among the most deadly forms of cancer

neuroblastoma Originates in the immature cells found within the central nervous system; neuroblastomas are rare; usually found in children

adenocarcinoma Derived from cells of the endocrine glands

hepatoma Originates in cells of the liver; although not thought to be directly caused by alcohol use, hepatomas are more frequently seen in individuals who have experienced **sclerotic changes** in the liver

Men	Incidence	Deaths
Lung	90,700	90,100
Kidney	18,700	8,900
Stomach	13,400	7,400
Pancreas	14,200	14,100
Colon/rectum	67,300	27,700
Bladder	39,200	8,300
Prostate	198,100	31,500
Leukemia/ lymphoma	52,700	26,500
All sites	643,000	286,100

Women	Incidence	Deaths
Lung	78,800	67,300
Breast	192,200	40,200
Stomach	8,300	5,400
Pancreas	15,000	14,800
Colon/rectum	68,100	29,000
Ovary	23,400	13,900
Uterus	51,200	11,000
Leukemia/ lymphoma	42,400	22,600
All sites	625,000	267,300

Figure 11-2 These 2001 estimates of cancer incidence and deaths reveal some significant similarities between men and women. Note that lung cancer is the leading cause of cancer deaths for both genders.

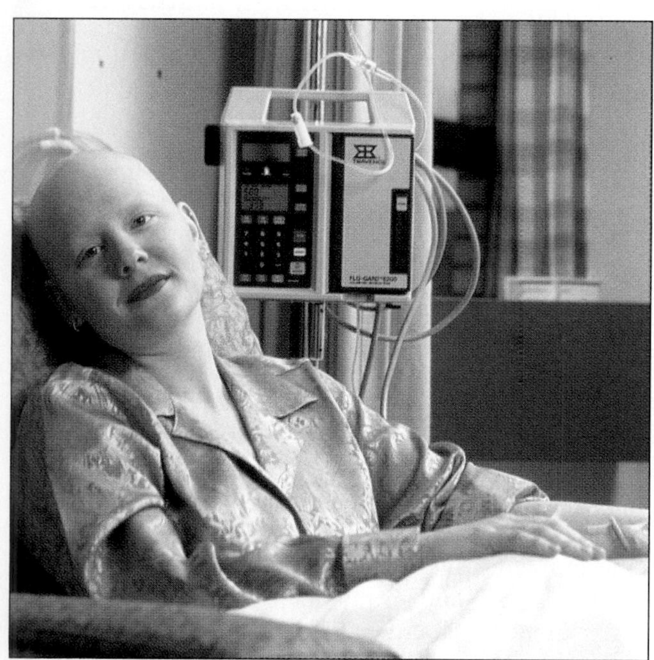

Chemotherapy is a treatment for many types of cancer.

leukemia Found in cells of the blood and blood-forming tissues; characterized by abnormal, immature white blood cell formation; multiple forms found in children and adults

lymphoma Arises in cells of the lymphatic tissues or other immune system tissues; includes lymphosarcomas and Hodgkin's disease, characterized by abnormal white cell production and decreased resistance

Figure 11-2 presents information about the incidence of cancer and the deaths from cancer at various sites in both men and women.[1]

CANCER AT SELECTED SITES IN THE BODY

A second, more familiar way to describe cancer is according to the organ (or tissue) site where it occurs. The following discussion focuses on some of these familiar sites.

Key Terms

metastasis
The spread of cancerous cells from their site of origin to other areas of the body.

benign
Noncancerous; tumors that do not spread.

sclerotic changes
Thickening or hardening of tissues.

Changing *for the Better*

Summary of American Cancer Society Recommendations for the Early Detection of Cancer in Asymptomatic People

Cancer runs in my family—on both sides. What cancer screening tests should each family member get, and when?

Site	Recommendation
Cancer-related checkup	A cancer-related checkup is recommended every 3 years for people age 20–40 and every year for people age 40 and older. This exam should include health counseling and, depending on a person's age, might include examinations for cancers of the thyroid, oral cavity, skin, lymph nodes, testes, and ovaries, as well as for some nonmalignant diseases.
Breast	Women 40 and older should have an annual mammogram, an annual clinical breast exam (CBE) performed by a health care professional, and should perform monthly breast self-examination. The CBE should be conducted close to and preferably before the scheduled mammogram. Women ages 20–39 should have a clinical breast exam performed by a health care professional every three years and should perform monthly breast self-examination.
Colon and rectum	Men and women aged 50 or older should follow *one* of the examination schedules below: • A fecal occult blood test every year and a flexible sigmoidoscopy every five years* • A colonoscopy every 10 years.* • A double-contrast barium enema every five years.* • A digital rectal exam should be done at the same time as sigmoidoscopy, colonoscopy, or double-contrast barium enema. People who are at moderate or high risk for colorectal cancer should talk with a doctor about a different testing schedule.
Prostate	The ACS recommends that both the prostate-specific antigen (PSA) blood test and the digital rectal examination be offered annually, beginning at age 50, to men who have a life expectancy of at least 10 years and to younger men who are at high risk. Men in high-risk groups, such as those with a strong familial predisposition (i.e., two or more affected first-degree relatives), or African Americans may begin at a younger age (i.e., 45 years).
Uterus	**Cervix:** All women who are or have been sexually active or who are 18 and older should have an annual Pap test and pelvic examination. After three or more consecutive satisfactory examinations with normal findings, the Pap test may be performed less frequently. Discuss the matter with your physician. **Endometrium:** Women at high risk for colon cancer should be offered an endometrial biopsy annually when menopause begins.

Source:

Regular screening procedures can lead to early identification of cancer at these sites (see the Changing for the Better box above).

Lung

Lung cancer is one of the most lethal forms of cancer. Primarily because its symptoms first appear when the disease is at an advanced stage, only 14% of all lung cancer victims survive 5 years beyond diagnosis.[1] By the time victims are sufficiently concerned about their persistent cough, blood-streaked sputum, and chest pain, it is often too late for treatment to be effective.

Today it is known that a genetic predisposition exists in the development of lung cancer. As many as 12% of the people who develop this form of cancer may have an inherited "headstart."[7] When people who are genetically at risk also smoke, their level of risk for developing lung cancer is hundreds of times greater than it is for nonsmokers. About 30% of lung cancer cases appear in people who smoke but are not genetically predisposed. Smokers account for 87% of all reported cases of lung cancer, and lung cancer causes 30% of all cancer deaths.[1] Environmental agents, such as passive tobacco smoke, radon, asbestos, and air pollutants, contribute to a lesser degree in the development of lung cancer.

According to the World Health Organization, the incidence of lung cancer has risen 200% for women, paralleling their increased smoking. Currently, lung cancer exceeds breast cancer as the leading cause of cancer deaths in women. The incidence of lung cancer has shown an encouraging decline in men while their use of tobacco is decreasing.

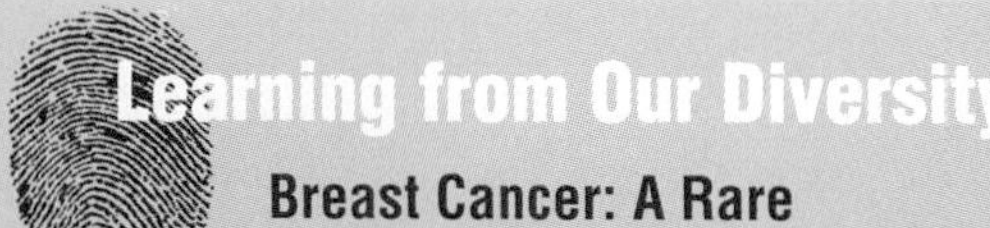

Breast Cancer: A Rare Diagnosis in Men

With all the attention given to breast cancer in women—in the news, by physicians, and by research foundations—you may be surprised to learn that men can also be diagnosed with this condition. For every 100 women who develop breast cancer, however, only one case will be reported among men. Estimates for the year 2001 suggest that no more than 1,500 American men will develop breast cancer. When compared to the 192,200 cases anticipated in women during the same year, the rarity of breast cancer in men becomes apparent.

The typical male breast cancer victim is usually older than 60 and often has a family history of the disease. The *BRCA2* tumor suppressor gene mutation is also found within the victim's genetic linage. In some cases, the male breast cancer victim has the inherited condition of Klinefelter's syndrome, in which a second X (or female) sex chromosome is present. The presence of the extra sex chromosome produces enhanced estrogen within the male body, resulting in adolescent development of prominent breasts and a higher risk of breasts cancer later in life. Other conditions, such as various forms of liver disease, also result in higher levels of estrogen and, eventually, a greater risk of male breast cancer.

In most ways male breast cancer is very similar in type to that seen in women. Infiltrating ductal cancer, ductal carcinoma in situ, and a form of cancer arising from the ducts immediately beneath the nipple (Paget's disease) have been reported. Because of this close similarity to female breast cancer, medical management of male breast cancer closely parallels that seen in women. Surgery (a modified radical mastectomy), chemotherapy, external radiation, and hormonal therapy are used alone or in combination. The latter therapy may include not only drugs to block the influence of estrogen on estrogen-sensitive cancer cells, but removal of testicles as well. As with virtually all forms of cancer, early diagnosis and treatment are of critical importance.

Breast

Surpassed only by lung cancer, breast cancer is the second leading cause of death from cancer in women. Now, nearly 1 in 8 women will develop breast cancer. As they age, women are increasingly at risk for developing breast cancer. Early detection is the key to complete recovery. In fact, 97% of women who discover their breast cancer before it has spread will survive more than 5 years.[1]

Although all women and men are at some risk for developing breast cancer, women whose menstrual periods began when they were young and for whom menopause was late (longer exposure to higher estrogen levels), women who had no children (high risk seen later in life) or had their first child later in life (nursing helps lower risk, however), and women with a family history of breast cancer are at greater risk. Also, women whose diets are high in saturated fats and who have excessive fat in the waist-hip area are more likely to develop breast cancer, although the exact role of dietary fats remains contested. Alcohol consumption, use of an oral contraceptive, and use of estrogen replacement therapy (ERT) still foster controversy regarding their influence in women's risk for developing breast cancer. The influence of breast density and sedentary lifestyle on breast cancer is currently being investigated. Regional influences on the occurrence of breast cancer now appear to be less powerful than once thought.[8]

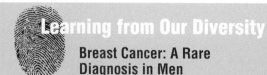

The incidence of breast cancer among men is discussed in the Learning from Our Diversity box above. The Personal Assessment on p. 275 will help you evaluate your own risk for developing breast cancer.

Today it is recommended that women age 40 and older undergo annual mammography, an annual breast examination performed by a physician, and monthly breast self-examinations (see the Changing for the Better box on p. 258. For women between ages 20 and 39, a breast examination should be performed by a physician once every 3 years, as well as breast self-examination on a monthly basis.

Regardless of age, each woman has a unique risk profile. Therefore the recommendation of her physician should be given careful consideration. It is strongly advised that the mammography procedure be performed in a facility that does a large number of mammography studies on a regular basis (with the most recent equipment, more skilled technicians, and more experienced radiologists reading the films).

In addition to breast self-examination and mammography, new techniques for detection are being considered. For example, contrast media-based MRIs can see through dense tissue areas and collected breast fluid more effectively than X rays can.

Women who have the *BRCA1* or *BRCA2* genetic mutation need to be monitored closely;[9] they may elect to undergo a *prophylactic mastectomy.*[10] This inheritance pattern, however, may affect only 5% of all women.

Regardless of the detection method, if a lump is found, a breast biopsy can determine what the lump is. If the lump is cancerous, treatment is highly effective if the cancer is found in an early stage. Since many choices exist about the type of surgery used to remove the cancer, women should seek a second opinion. The least extensive

Changing *for the Better*

Breast Self-Examination

I've never felt confident about doing a breast self-exam. What is the proper technique?

The following explains how to do a breast self-examination:

1. In the shower: Examine your breasts during a bath or shower; hands glide more easily over wet skin. With your fingers flat, move gently over every part of each breast. Use right hand to examine left breast, left hand for right breast. Check for any lump, hard knot, or thickening. This self-examination should be done monthly, preferably a day or two after the end of the menstrual period.
2. Before a mirror: Inspect your breasts with arms at your sides. Next, raise your arms high overhead. Look for any changes in contour of each breast, a swelling, dimpling of skin, changes in the nipple. Then rest palms on hips, and press down firmly to flex your chest muscles. Left and right breast will not exactly match—few women's breasts do.
3. Lying down: To examine your right breast, put a pillow or folded towel under your right shoulder. Place right hand behind your head—this distributes breast tissue more evenly on the chest. With left hand, fingers flat, press gently in small circular motions around an imaginary clock face. Begin at outermost top of your right breast for 12 o'clock, then move to 1 o'clock, and so on around the circle back to 12 o'clock. A ridge of firm tissue in the lower curve of each breast is normal. Then move in an inch toward the nipple; keep circling to examine every part of your breast, including the nipple. This requires at least three more circles. Now slowly repeat the procedure on your left breast with a pillow under your left shoulder and left hand behind head. Notice how your breast structure feels. Finally, squeeze the nipple of each breast gently between thumb and index finger. Any discharge, clear or bloody, should be reported to your doctor immediately.

Breast cancer can occur in men too. Therefore this examination should be performed monthly by men. Regular inspection shows what is normal for you and will give you confidence in your examination.

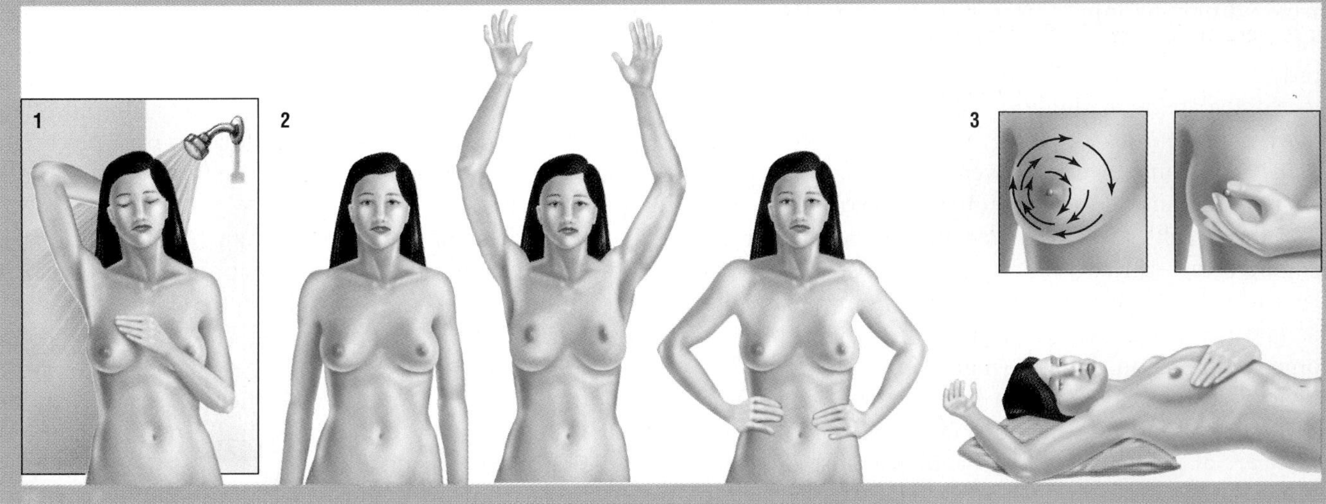

surgery, the lumpectomy, in combination with drug therapy, has proved highly effective. For advanced cancers, chemotherapeutic drugs or radiation therapy may be used in combination with surgery. In addition, experimental therapy involving immune system suppression followed by the infusion of embryonic stem cells to "re-program" the immune system has also been explored. However, for some women, even when their cancer is in an early stage, radical **mastectomy** may be the preferred route of treatment. Breast reconstruction is often possible after more radical surgery.

During much of the last decade, the potential for preventing breast cancer was thought to be at hand—with a family of drugs that block the influence of estrogen on abnormal breast cells. These *selective estrogen-receptor modulators* (SERMs) were given to women who were at high risk for breast cancer. Tamoxifem, the best studied SERM, was joined by Raloxifene as an approved preventive agent. Currently, however, uncertainty exists about the exact role that SERMs should play in breast cancer prevention, particularly in terms of their influence on the development of estrogen receptor-negative tumors.[11]

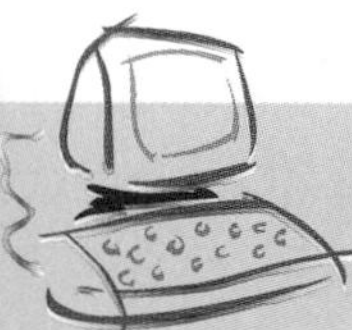

OnSITE/InSIGHT

Learning to Go: Health

Are you concerned about developing cancer? Want to know how to live with a chronic condition? Click on the Motivator icon, and check out the following chapters:

Lesson 30: Guard against breast cancer.
Lesson 31: Protect your skin from the sun.
Lesson 32: Reduce your risk of cancer.
Lesson 34: Learn to live with diabetes.
Lesson 35: Control your chronic pain.
Lesson 36: Learn how to manage your asthma.

STUDENT POLL

Has your life been affected by cancer or another chronic condition? Go to the Online Learning Center at **www.mhhe.com/hahn6e**. Click on Student Resources to access the Student Poll. Answer these questions and then find out what other students said.

1. Have any of your family members or friends been diagnosed with cancer?
2. Are you taking measures to reduce your risk of developing cancer?
3. Do you think you're at risk for a certain type of cancer?
4. Is there a pattern of cancer in your family history?
5. Do you perform self-examinations for cancer (breast or testicular) regularly?
6. Can you name the seven warning signs of cancer?
7. Do any chronic conditions (other than cancer) run in your family?
8. Do you have diabetes?
9. Do you suffer from asthma?

Uterus

In 2001, approximately 51,200 new cases of cancer of the uterus were anticipated in the United States.[1] Included in this figure were 38,300 cases of cancer of the uterine lining (endometrial cancer) and 12,900 cases of cancer of the uterine neck (cervical cancer). The death rate from uterine cancer has dropped greatly since 1950, largely because of the use of the **Pap test.** This test looks for precancerous changes in the cells taken from the cervix.

The importance of women having a Pap test for cervical cancer on a routine basis cannot be overemphasized. Without screening, a 20-year-old of average risk has a 250 in 10,000 chance of getting cervical cancer and a 118 in 10,000 chance of dying from it. With screening, a 20-year-old of average risk has a 35 in 10,000 chance of getting this form of cancer and only an 11 in 10,000 chance of dying from it. The Pap test is not perfect, however; about 7% of the tests will miss finding abnormal changes.[12] Further, not all women whose test results are abnormal receive adequate follow-up care, nor do they have subsequent Pap tests on a regular enough basis. Today more effective computerized tests are available, and as their use increases, the incidence of inaccurate tests should fall.

TALKING POINTS • Three risk factors are associated with HPV-induced cervical cancer: early age of first sexual intercourse, higher-than-average number of partners, and lack of protection against sexually transmitted diseases (e.g., condoms). How would you introduce this topic to a teenage daughter, sister, or niece?

In addition to changes discovered by a Pap test, symptoms suggesting cancer of the uterus include abnormal bleeding between periods. Risk factors associated with this form of cancer include early age of first intercourse, number of sexual partners, history of infertility, HPV infections (see p. 300 in Chapter 12), and excessive fat tissue around the waist. Women who have received ERT (see p. 257) may also have a higher risk. A lower level of risk for uterine cancer is seen in women who have used barrier contraceptives (condoms, diaphragms, and spermicides). The Personal Assessment on p. 275 will help you evaluate your risk of developing cervical cancer.

Vagina

Although rare, cancer of the vagina (the passage leading to the uterus) is of concern to a particular group of women: the daughters of over 3 million mothers who were given the drug DES (diethylstilbestrol) to prevent miscarriages. Because of the effects of DES on the fetal development of the reproductive system, these daughters now face the risk

Key Terms

mastectomy
Removal of breast tissue.

Pap test
A cancer screening procedure in which cells are removed from the cervix and examined for precancerous changes.

of developing a form of vaginal (and cervical) cancer called *clear cell cancer.* Since the risk was identified nearly 50 years ago, the medical community has been following large groups of daughters to better assess their level of risk. To date, 1 in every 1000 exposed daughters has developed this form of cancer, some as early as 15 years of age.

Ovary

In the United States in 2001, it was estimated that 23,400 new cases of ovarian cancer would be identified and 13,900 affected women would die. Most cases develop in women who are older than 40 and who have not had children or began menstruation at an early age. The highest rate is in women over 60. The incidence of ovarian cancer is greatest among women who have had a relatively longer exposure to hormones during their menstrual cycles and, perhaps, in women receiving HRT for more than 10 years.[13] The inheritance of the *BRCA1* tumor suppressor gene mutation and, particularly, the *BRCA2* mutation (see p. 257) increases the risk of developing ovarian cancer.

Because of its vague symptoms, ovarian cancer has been referred to as a *silent* cancer. Digestive disturbances, gas, and stomach distention are often its only symptoms. Today, diagnosis of this highly lethal cancer is made using transvaginal ultrasound and surgery. A three-drug combination, which includes Taxol, has extended average remission by nearly 2 years.

Prostate

The prostate gland is a walnut-size gland located near the base of the penis. It surrounds the neck of the bladder and the urethra. Cancer of the prostate is the most common form of cancer in men and a leading cause of death from cancer in older men. On the basis of current statistics, approximately 1 out of 6 men will develop this form of cancer. Men with a family history of prostate cancer are at greater risk of developing this form of cancer than men without this family history. Additionally, a link between prostate cancer and dietary patterns, such as excessive red meat and dairy product consumption, has been suggested. African American men are also at a higher risk of developing prostate cancer.

The symptoms of prostate disease, including prostate cancer, are listed in the Star Box above. If these symptoms appear, particularly in men 50 years of age and older, it is important to consult a physician. Screening for prostate cancer should begin by age 50. It involves an annual rectal examination and the prostate-specific antigen (PSA) blood test. This test has been joined by a more sensitive version that can identify the "free" antigen most closely associated with prostate cancer, thus cutting down on false positives and the extensive use of biopsies. In addition, an ultrasound rectal examination is used in men whose PSA scores are abnormally high.

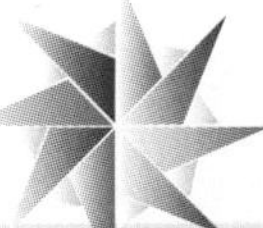

Symptoms of Prostate Disease

- Difficulty in urinating
- Frequent urination, particularly at night
- Continued wetness for a short time after urination
- Blood in the urine
- Low back pain
- Ache in upper thighs

Traditionally, prostate cancer has been treated through surgery or the use of radiation and chemotherapy, with a survival rate of 100% when diagnosed early and 93% overall.[1] Because this type of cancer grows slowly, it is increasingly likely that men whose cancer is very localized and whose life expectancy is less than 10 years at the time of diagnosis will not receive treatment but rather will be closely monitored for any progression in the cancer.[14]

Testicle

Cancer of the testicle is among the least common forms of cancer; however, it represents the most common solid tumor in men between the ages of 20 and 34 years. Testicular cancer has a tendency to run in families and is more common in men whose testicles were undescended during childhood. The incidence of this cancer has been increasing in recent years. However, no single explanation can be given for this increase. Factors such as a difficult pregnancy, elevated temperature in the groin, or mumps may be involved. The incidence of this cancer has increased by 100% since 1930, and a corresponding drop in sperm count has been seen. Agricultural pesticide toxicity may be involved in both of these changes. In 2001, 7,200 new cases were diagnosed and 300 deaths occurred.[1]

Symptoms of cancer of the testicles include a small, painless lump on the side of the testicle, a swollen or enlarged testicle, or heaviness or a dragging sensation in the groin or scrotum. Risk factors include confirmed injury, mumps, and hormonal treatments given to the mother before the child's birth. The importance of testicular self-examination, as well as early diagnosis and prompt treatment, cannot be overemphasized for men in the at-risk age group of 20 to 34 years. The Changing for the Better box on p. 261 explains how to perform a testicular self-examination.

Changing *for the Better*

Testicular Self-Examination

I feel unsure about how to perform a testicular self-exam. What is the correct method?

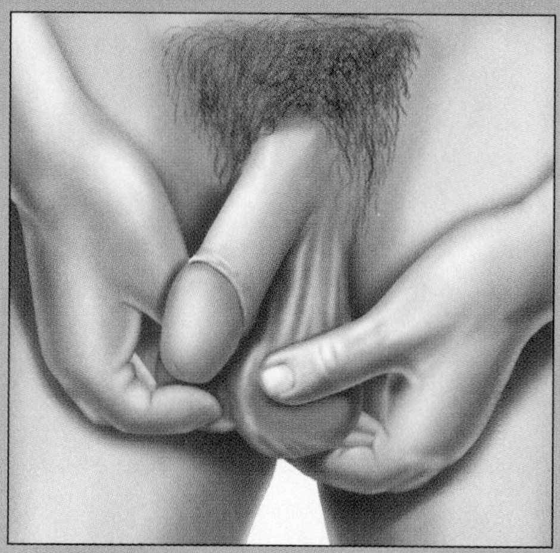

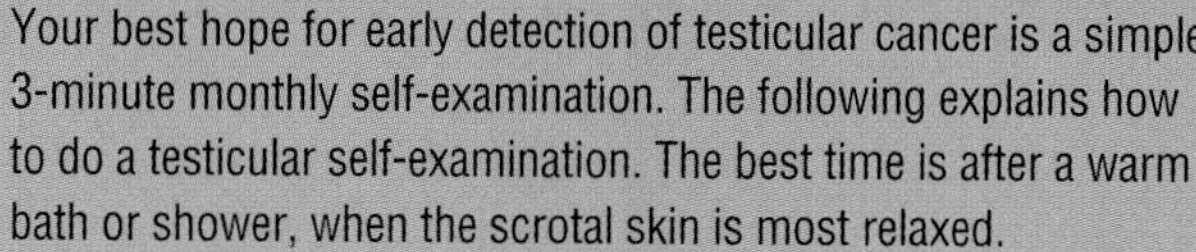

Your best hope for early detection of testicular cancer is a simple 3-minute monthly self-examination. The following explains how to do a testicular self-examination. The best time is after a warm bath or shower, when the scrotal skin is most relaxed.

1. Roll each testicle gently between the thumb and fingers of both hands.
2. If you find any hard lumps or nodules, you should see your doctor promptly. They may not be malignant, but only your doctor can make the diagnosis.

After a thorough physical examination, your doctor may perform certain X ray studies to make the most accurate diagnosis possible.

Monthly testicular self-examinations are as important for men as breast self-examinations are for women.

Colon and Rectum

Cancer of the colon and rectum (colorectal cancer) has a combined incidence and death rate third only to that of breast and lung cancer. Two types of tumors, carcinoma and lymphoma, can be found in both the colon and rectum. Fortunately, when diagnosed in a localized state, colorectal cancer has a relatively high survival rate of 90% through the first 5 years.[1] Genes have recently been discovered that lead to familial colon cancer and familial polyposis (abnormal tissue growth that occurs before formation of cancer) and are believed to be responsible for the tendency for colon and rectal cancer to run in families. These forms of cancer may be higher in people whose diets are both high in saturated fat from red meat and low in fruits and vegetables, which contain antioxidant vitamins and fiber. However, a recent study disputes the influence of dietary fiber in preventing colorectal cancer.[15] An even more recent study supports the role of fiber from fruits and vegetables, but not dietary fiber.[16] An association between colorectal cancer and smoking has also been identified.

Symptoms associated with colorectal cancers include bleeding from the rectum, blood in the stool, or a change in bowel habits. Also, a family history of inflammatory bowel disease, polyp formation, or colorectal cancer. In people over 50, any sudden change in bowel habits that lasts 10 days or longer should be evaluated. The American Cancer Society recommends preventive health care beginning at age 50 that includes digital (manual) rectal examination, a stool blood test every 5 years, and a flexible sigmoidoscopy examination every 5 years, and a colonoscopy every 10 years (see Changing for the Better on page 256). Prompt removal of polyps has been shown to be effective in lowering the risk of developing colorectal cancer. Further, there is evidence that the development of colorectal cancer may be prevented or slowed through regular exercise and through the regular use of aspirin.[17]

The treatment of colorectal cancer involves surgery combined with the use of chemotherapy drugs. A *colostomy* is required in 15% of the cases of colon and rectal cancer.

Pancreas

Pancreatic cancer is one of the most lethal forms of cancer, with a survival rate of only 4% at 5 years after diagnosis.[1] In light of the organ's important roles in both digestion and metabolic processes (see the discussion of diabetes mellitus on p. 268), its destruction leaves the body in a state incompatible with living.

In 2001, 29,200 new cases of pancreatic cancer were diagnosed.[1] The disease is more common in men than women and occurs most frequently in African American men. Early detection of this cancer is difficult because of the absence of symptoms until late in its course. Risk of developing this form of cancer increases with age; with diabetes mellitus, pancreatitis (inflammation of the pancreas), or cirrhosis (see Chapter 8); and with diets high in fat. To date, little success in effective treatment has been achieved.

How to look for melanoma

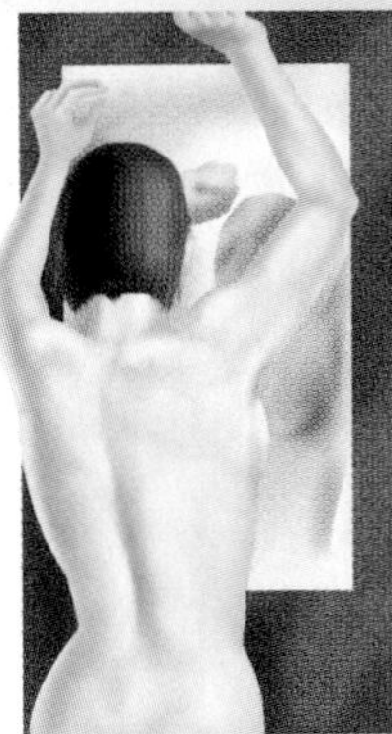

1. Examine your body front and back in the mirror, then right and left sides with arms raised.

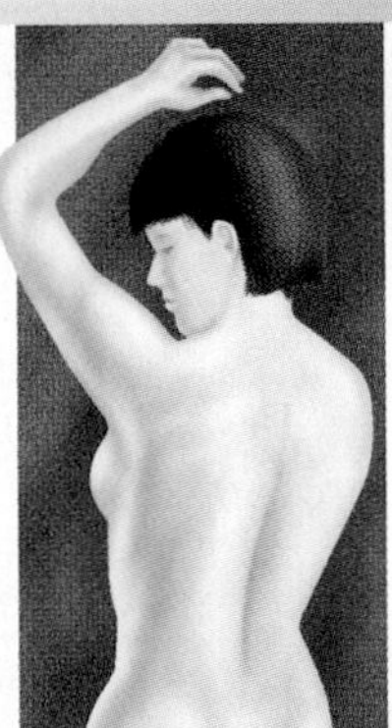

2. Bend your elbows and carefully look at your palms, forearms, and under your upper arms.

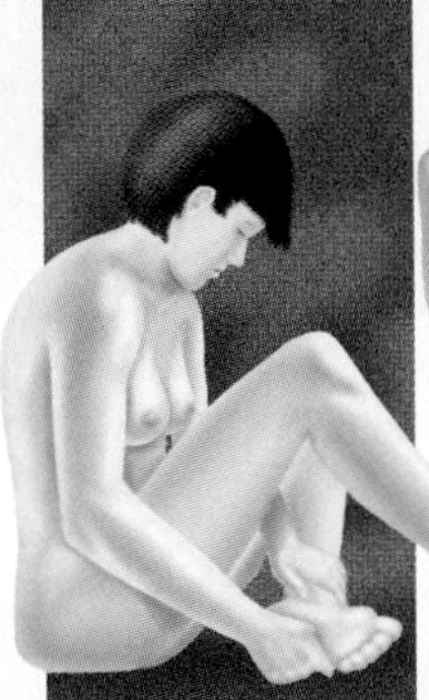

3. Look at the backs of your legs and feet, the spaces between your toes, and the soles of your feet.

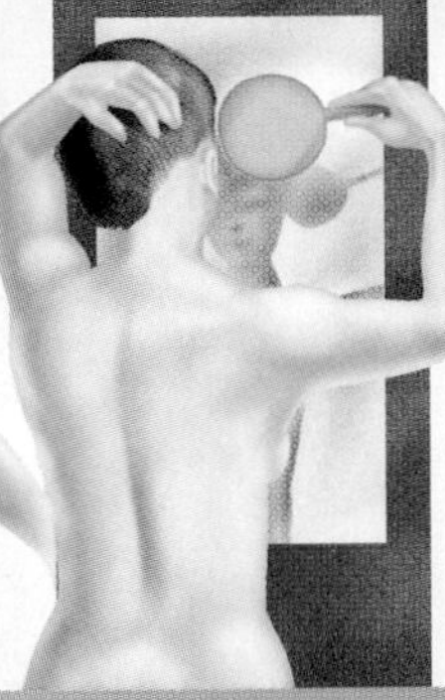

4. Examine the back of your neck and scalp with a hand mirror. Part your hair for a closer look.

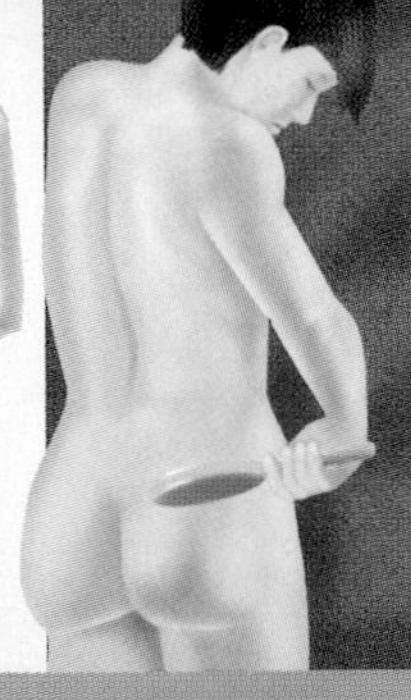

5. Finally, check your back and buttocks with a mirror.

What to look for

Potential signs of malignancy in moles or pigmented spots:

Asymmetry

One half unlike the other half

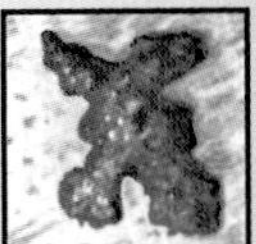

Irregularity

Border irregular or poorly defined

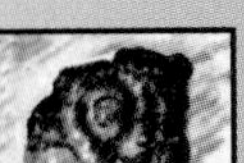

Color

Color varies from one area to another; shades of tan, brown, or black

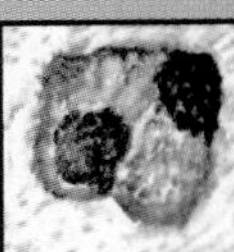

Size

Diameter larger than 6 mm, as a rule (diameter of a pencil eraser)

Skin

Thanks largely to a desire for a fashionable tan, too many teens and adults are spending more time in the sun (and in tanning booths) than their skin can tolerate. As a result, skin cancer, once common only among those people who worked in the sun, is occurring with alarming frequency. In 2001, more than 1 million Americans developed basal or squamous cell skin cancer[1] and 51,400 cases of highly dangerous malignant melanoma were diagnosed.[1] Severe sunburning during childhood and chronic sun exposure during adolescence and younger adulthood are responsible for these increases in skin cancer.

Although many doctors do not emphasize this point enough, the key to the successful treatment of skin cancer lies in early detection. In the case of basal cell or squamous cell cancer, the development of a pale, waxlike, pearly nodule or red, scaly patch may be the first symptom. For others, skin cancer may be noticed as a gradual change in the appearance of an already existing skin mole. If such a change is noted, a physician should be contacted. Melanoma usually begins as a small molelike growth that increases progressively in size, changes color, ulcerates, and bleeds easily. For help in detecting melanoma, the American Cancer Society recommends using the guidelines below:

A is for **a**symmetry
B is for **b**order irregularity
C is for **c**olor (change)
D is for a **d**iameter greater than 6 mm
E is for **e**levation (raised margins)

The photographs show a mole that would be considered harmless and one that clearly demonstrates the ABCD characteristics described above. Again, it is important to be observant and not fail to recognize the changing status of a mole or other skin lesion. The illustration on page 262 depicts the steps to take in making a regular inspection of the skin.

When nonmelanoma skin cancer is found, an almost 100% cure rate can be expected. Treatment of these skin cancers can involve surgical removal, destruction through burning or freezing, or X ray therapy. When the more serious melanomas are found in an early stage, a high cure rate is accomplished using the same techniques. However, when malignant melanomas are more advanced, extensive surgery and chemotherapy become necessary and recovery is rare.

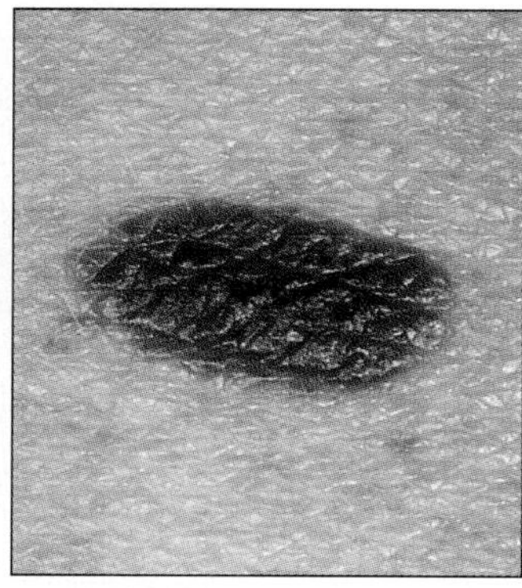

Normal mole. This type of lesion is often seen in large numbers on the skin and may affect any body site. Note its symmetrical shape, regular borders, uniform color, and relatively small size (less than 6 millimeters).

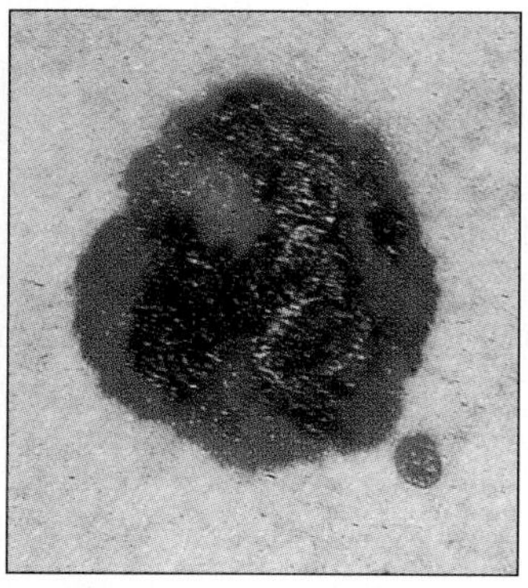

Malignant melanoma. Note its asymmetrical shape, irregular borders, uneven color, and relatively large size (about 2 centimeters).

Prevention of skin cancer should be a high priority for people who enjoy the sun or must work outdoors. The use of sunscreen is of great importance. In addition, parents can help their children prevent skin cancer later in life by restricting their outdoor play from 11:00 AM to 2:00 PM, requiring them to wear hats that shade their faces, and applying a sunscreen with SPF 15 regardless of a child's skin tone.

A relationship between the presence of certain abnormal moles, called *dysplastic nevi,* and the risk of developing malignant melanoma has recently been established. By counting these "indicator moles," physicians can estimate a patient's risk of developing this serious form of skin cancer before it appears.[18] The Personal Assessment on p. 275 will help you determine your own risk of developing this kind of cancer.

THE DIAGNOSIS OF CANCER

Is cancer survivable? The answer is, of course, yes. The chances for survival (defined as living without reoccurrence at least 5 years after diagnosis) depend greatly on the promptness of diagnosis and treatment. Thus the chances for recovery from cancer are best when cancer is detected early. The familiar "cancer's seven warning signals" can serve as a basis for early detection (see the Star Box above). Also, unexplained weight loss can be a signal for the presence of a malignancy. Weight loss, however, is not usually an early indicator of cancer. Persistent headaches and vision changes should be evaluated by a physician.

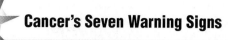

Cancer's Seven Warning Signs

Listed below are the seven warning signs of cancer, which the acronym CAUTION will help you remember:

1. **C**hange in bowel or bladder habits
2. **A** sore that does not heal
3. **U**nusual bleeding or discharge
4. **T**hickening or lump in breast or elsewhere
5. **I**ndigestion or difficulty in swallowing
6. **O**bvious change in a wart or mole
7. **N**agging cough or hoarseness

If you have a warning sign that persists for more than 5 days, see your doctor!

In addition to the recognition of danger signals, undergoing regularly scheduled screening for malignancy-related changes is important. A monthly breast self-examination for all women over the age of 20 is recommended. For men, monthly testicular self-examinations are strongly recommended. Step-by-step procedures for both of these self-examinations are provided in the Changing for the Better boxes on pp. 258 and 261. The remaining screening procedures require the services of a medical practitioner.

Treatment

In today's approach to cancer treatment, proven therapies and promising new experimental approaches are often combined. The traditional therapies are surgery, radiation, and chemotherapy. Used independently or in combination, they form the backbone of our increasingly successful efforts in treating cancer. Newer, more experimental therapies are also being used on a limited basis. One or more experimental approaches may be combined with surgery, radiation, and chemotherapy as a basis for treatment. In the sections that follow, a brief description of each treatment is given.

Surgery

Surgical removal of tissue suspected to contain cancerous cells is the oldest approach to cancer therapy. When undertaken early in the course of the disease, surgery is particularly suited for cancers of the skin, gastrointestinal tract, breast, uterus, cervix, prostate gland, and testicle. Minimal procedures are undertaken whenever possible, and radiation or chemotherapy is often used with surgery to ensure maximum effectiveness.

Radiation

Radiation is capable of killing cancer cells by altering their genetic material during cell division. Since neighboring cells also divide, they are exposed to the damaging effects of radiation as well. However, by carefully planning the length of exposure and time of treatment and by focusing the radiation with precision, damage to noncancerous cells can be held to a minimum.

Chemotherapy

The important advances in successful cancer treatment can be attributed to advances in chemotherapy, including new drugs and the more effective combination of new drugs and familiar chemotherapeutic agents. Most often, these drugs work by destroying cancer cells' ability to use important materials or carry out cell division in a normal manner. Because chemotherapy influences cell division, it will influence noncancerous cells that divide frequently. Among the cells most susceptible to this influence are those that make up bone marrow, the lining of the intestinal tract, and the hair follicles. People who are undergoing chemotherapy often have immune system suppression, diarrhea, and hair loss.

Anti-Cancer Drugs

Although many chemotherapy agents have been in use for decades and new ones are being developed, there is an array of anti-cancer drugs that do not fit into the traditional five classes of chemotherapy agents. More than 402 drugs are now in various stages of development and clinical trials. Perhaps the most familiar to the general public are the **anti-angiogenesis** drugs, which "starve" tumors by restricting their blood supply, and Herceptin, which may prevent the development of breast cancer in some people. Early reports on the effectiveness of the anti-angiogenesis drugs have been somewhat disappointing.

Another newer chemotherapy agent is C225, which blocks receptors on the cancer cell's membrane, which normally recognizes the presence of epidermal growth factor (EGF), a substance that allows cancer cells to grow at a faster than normal pace.[19] This targeted cancer therapy is at the forefront of the pharmacological treatment of cancer.

Immunotherapy

Immunotherapy is the use of a variety of substances to trigger a person's own immune system to attack cancer cells or prevent them from becoming activated. Among these new forms of immunotherapy are the use of interferon, monoclonal antibodies, interleukin-2, tumor necrosis factor (TNF), and certain bone marrow growth regulators. In addition, two cancer vaccines are undergoing early clinical trials. One vaccine has shown some ability to provide a period of disease remission for patients with a particular form of pancreatic cancer, while a second vaccine is been used with some success in patients with metastatic kidney cancer. In both vaccine trials, radiation and other chemotherapy agents were also employed.

Alternative (complementary) cancer therapies

Many Americans have called for the evaluation and greater availability of complementary alternative forms of cancer prevention and treatment. The National Institutes of Health has begun an in-depth study of alternative or nonconventional cancer treatments. Through the use of new and carefully controlled studies and the reassessment of research and records already available, the NIH is trying to better understand the benefits of alternative or complementary therapies.

Among the treatments to be given closer and more careful consideration are chiropractic (the manipulation of the spine), acupressure (finger and thumb pressure to relieve pain), and acupuncture (needles inserted to relieve pain and promote the flow of energy within the body). Additional areas of investigation include ayurveda (a traditional Indian lifestyle that involves the use of herbs and a particular diet), biofeedback (monitoring of body functions to control body processes), homeopathy (use of minuscule doses of toxic substances), and naturopathy (use of natural remedies, including sunshine and vitamins). Further focus will be directed toward oxidizing agents (substances believed to kill viruses), reflexology (the massaging of points on the feet), therapeutic touch (redirecting of "life forces" through touching areas of the body), and visualization (learning to "see" a cure occurring).

Regardless of the efficacy of these therapies, cancer patients frequently turn to alternative approaches. In a recent survey, it was found that 46% of the cancer patients questioned used mega-doses of vitamins, 34% used herbal products, 16% used non-herbal products (such as shark cartilage), and 4% employed various mind-body therapies in their attempt to recover.[20]

RISK REDUCTION

Because cancer will probably continue to be the second most common cause of death among adults, it is important for you to explore ways of reducing your risk of developing cancer. The following factors, which could make you vulnerable to cancer, can be controlled or at least recognized.

- *Know your family history.* You are the recipient of the genetic strengths and weaknesses of your biological parents and your more distant relatives. If cancer is prevalent in your family medical history, you cannot afford to disregard this fact. It may be appropriate for you to be screened for certain types of cancer more often or at a younger age.
- *Select your occupation carefully.* Because of recently discovered relationships between cancer and occupations that bring employees into contact with carcinogenic agents, you must be aware of risks with certain job selections and assignments. Worksites associated with frequent contact with pesticides, strong solvents, volatile hydocarbons, and airborne fibers could pay well but also shorten life.
- *Do not use tobacco products.* You may want to review Chapter 9 on the overwhelming evidence linking all forms of tobacco use (including smokeless tobacco) to the development of cancer. Smoking is so detrimental to health that it is considered the number one preventable cause of death.
- *Follow a sound diet.* The Changing for the Better box above provides general guidelines on eating to reduce your cancer risk. In addition, review Chapter 5 for information regarding dietary practices and the incidence of various diseases, including cancer. That chapter also discusses the role of fruits and vegetables known to be sources of cancer-preventing phytochemicals.
- *Control your body weight.* Particularly for women, obesity is related to a higher incidence of cancer of the uterus, ovary, and breast. Maintaining a desirable body weight could improve overall health and lead to more successful management of cancer if it develops.
- *Exercise regularly.* Chapter 4 discusses in detail the importance of regular moderate exercise to all aspects of health, including reducing the risk of chronic illnesses. Moderate exercise increases the body's ability to deliver oxygen to its tissues and thus to reduce the formation of cancer-enhancing free radicals formed during incomplete oxidation of nutrients. Moderate exercise also stimulates the production of enzymes that remove free radicals. Some concern exists, however, that extensive exercise might actually reduce the body's ability to produce the enzymes previously mentioned and thus contribute to the development of free-radical–based cellular changes, including cancer.
- *Limit your exposure to sun.* It is important to heed this message, even if you enjoy many outdoor activities. Particularly for people with light complexions, the radiation received through chronic exposure to the sun may foster the development of skin cancer.
- *Consume alcohol in moderation—if at all.* Heavier users of alcohol experience an increased prevalence of several types of cancer, including cancer of the oral cavity, larynx, and esophagus. It should be noted, however, that moderate alcohol consumption is now believed to be a positive factor in prevention of cardiovascular disease. Drinking lightly (see Chapter 8) is therefore recommended for persons who already enjoy alcoholic beverages, but abstinence is equally acceptable for those who do not.

Changing *for the Better*

Eat to Lower Your Cancer Risk

I know several people who have developed cancer recently, and I want to decrease my chance of getting this disease. What can I do right now to lower my risk?

The American Cancer Society recommends the following dietary precautions to help reduce the risk of getting cancer:

- Avoid obesity.
- Reduce total fat intake.
- Eat a wide variety of vegetables such as cauliflower, broccoli, and brussels sprouts, which contain *phytochemicals,* known to reduce the risk of cancer, and fruits that are high in vitamin A, vitamin C, and fiber.
- Avoid smoked, salt-cured, and nitrate-cured foods.
- Limit alcohol consumption.

When these suggestions are given careful consideration, it should be obvious that you can do much to prevent or at least minimize the development of cancer. A wellness-oriented lifestyle is the best weapon in your "personal war against cancer." However, in the final analysis, all risk factor reduction is relative. Life cannot be totally structured around the desire to achieve maximum longevity or reduce morbidity at all costs. Most people need a balance between a life that is emotionally, socially, and spiritually satisfying and one that is structured around living a long time and minimizing illness. Regardless of your personal lifestyle, you can, however, educate others, give comfort and support to those who are living with cancer, and aid the funding of continuing and innovative new cancer research. Resources available for people with cancer and their families are listed in the Star Box on p. 266.

Key Term

anti-angiogenesis
Drug-based therapy that prevents cancerous tumors from developing an enriching blood supply.

Resources for People Living with Cancer

For people with cancer and their families, many telephone hot lines have been set up offering information and referrals:

- **American Cancer Society National Hotline:** (800) ACS-2345. Also, ACS recommends calling local ACS chapters for support group information.
- **National Cancer Institute Cancer Information Service:** (800) 4-CANCER.
- **National Coalition for Cancer Survivorship** (umbrella group for cancer survivor units nationwide): (877) 622-7937.
- **Candlelighters Childhood Cancer Foundation:** Information on support groups for children with cancer and their families: (301) 657-8401 and (800) 366-2223.
- **Surviving:** Support group. Publishes newsletter for Hodgkin's disease survivors. Stanford University Medical Center, Radiology Dept, Room C050, 300 Pasteur Dr, Stanford, CA 94305.
- **Vital Options:** Support group for people 17 to 40 who are cancer survivors: (818) 508-5657.
- **The Resource Center:** American College of Obstetricians and Gynecologists, 409 12th St. S.W., Washington, DC 20224-2188. Send a self-addressed, business-size envelope for *Detecting and Treating Breast Problems.*
- **American College of Radiology,** for accredited mammography centers, (800) ACR-LINE (members only) or (703) 648-8900, ask for mammography.

TALKING POINTS • A close friend justifies her high cancer–risk lifestyle by saying that "Everyone will die of something." How would you counter this point?

CHRONIC HEALTH CONDITIONS

In addition to the two most widely recognized chronic health problems of adulthood—cardiovascular disease and cancer—adults can experience an array of other chronic health conditions. What all of these chronic conditions have in common is the ability to cause significant change in the lives of people—both on the part of the affected person and his or her family members and friends (see Exploring Your Spirituality on p. 267).

Some of these conditions are seen in early adulthood, such as lupus and Crohn's disease. Others, such as diabetes mellitus Type II, generally do not appear until nearer middle age. However, some chronic diseases seen during adulthood have their origins in childhood, such as diabetes mellitus Type I.

Systemic Lupus Erythematosus

Systemic lupus erythematosus (SLE), or simply *lupus,* is perhaps the most familiar of a class of chronic conditions know as **autoimmune** disorders, or connective tissue diseases. Collectively, these conditions reflect a concentrated and inappropriate attack by the body's immune system on its own tissues, which then serve as *self-antigens* (see Chapter 12 for a discussion of the immune response).

The name *systemic lupus erythematosus* reflects the widespread (systemic, or system-wide) destruction of fibrous connective tissue and other tissues and the appearance in some patients of a reddish rash (erythematosus) that imparts a characteristic "mask" to the face. Lupus is most often seen in women who developed the condition during young adulthood. The course of the condition is gradual, with intermittent periods of inflammation, stiffness, fatigue, pleurisy (chest pain), and discomfort over wide areas of the body, including muscles, joints, and skin. Similar changes may also occur with tissue of the nervous system, kidneys, and heart.[21] Diagnosis is made on the basis of symptoms and several laboratory tests.

Why the immune system turns on the body in such an aggressive manner is not fully understood. It is likely, however, that a combination of genetic predisposition and an earlier viral infection or environmental exposure may be involved. Episodes (called *flares*) of lupus often follow exposure to the sun, periods of fatigue, or an infectious disease; all these should be avoided to the fullest extent possible. Management of the condition generally may involve long-term (and low-dose) use of prednisone (a corticosteroid) to suppress the adrenal gland's cortisone, or newer medications, such as Plaquenil (hydroxychloroquine), may be employed. In come cases the immune system itself also may be medically suppressed.

Crohn's Disease

A wide array of chronic conditions that involve the gastrointestinal system are collectively referred to as inflammatory bowel disease (IBD). One type of IBD is Crohn's disease, a deterioration of the inner surface and muscular layer of the intestinal wall that affects nearly 500,000 Americans, many of traditional college age. The disease commonly affects the terminal end of the small intestine and the beginning of the large intestine, or colon. When the disease is active (it frequently has long periods of remission), symptoms include abdominal pain, fever, diarrhea, weight loss, and rectal bleeding that leads to anemia.

Although the cause of Crohn's disease is not fully understood, a genetic predisposition and an autoimmune response may be the principal factors. Multiple forms of Crohn's disease are thought to exist, with each reflecting different genetic components.[22]

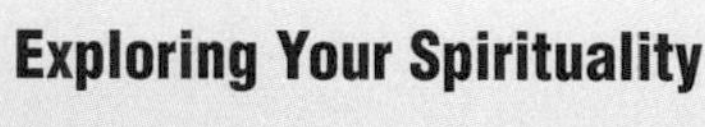

Exploring Your Spirituality

Chronic Illness—The End or a Turning Point?

Most people diagnosed with a chronic illness go through a period of serious adjustment. For college students, the necessary adaptations feel particularly burdensome because so few of their peers are faced with equal demands. Not only must self-care routines be changed, but the help of others may be necessary to carry out that care. The limitations imposed by a chronic illness restrict the activities and behavior of the affected individual and his or her family and friends. Financial matters (including the ability to afford medications), the need to see physicians frequently, and insurance issues add to the person's stress. When young peoples' lives change so profoundly, they can feel isolated and singled out in a negative way.

People respond to the diagnosis of a chronic illness in various ways. Frequently, their first reaction is denial. When this occurs, care may be delayed. At the same time, school and work performance and relationships begin to suffer from the internalized stress. Eventually, though, denial gives way to anger, which is often directed at others. Common targets of this anger are people close to the ill person, such as family and friends. Then the anger broadens to include the world or a God (for "letting these things happen"). Eventually, the demands of the illness, combined with a sense of futility, give way to acceptance. At this stage, the individual's resourcefulness surfaces as he or she looks within for untapped sources of strength. Gradually, the person becomes open to the assistance offered by others, begins to discover new interests and abilities, and realizes that life is not over—just different.

The decision to accept the chronic condition often brings a sense of inner peace and allows for a new approach to living. People who believe that they will not be given a burden too great for them to bear may rise to the challenge and find a level of strength that they—and others—didn't know they had. With acceptance come new learning experiences. The person begins to understand the limitations of the body, to appreciate what true friendships are, and to recognize the importance of emotional resources once taken for granted. Even more significant is the realization that the spiritual dimension of health is bountiful. As the daily challenges of the illness continue, the person realizes that his or her personal beliefs and values have not only survived but are even stronger.

When a person reports the symptoms just described, the physician quickly suspects some form of IBD, such as Crohn's disease. Accordingly, blood tests and a complete series of gastrointestinal (GI) X rays are undertaken. Additional diagnostic procedures could include a CT scan of the of the GI tract, endoscopic examination of the GI tract, and a biopsy of the intestinal wall. Positive results of these tests confirm the existence of Crohn's disease.

Today an array of medications is available or in development for use in management of Crohn's disease. Among the most recently introduced of these medications is infliximab (Remicade), an antibody to tumor necrosis factor (TNF) that has proven effective in managing some forms of the disease.

Although Crohn's disease can be well managed, intestinal obstructions can occur as a result of the progressive thickening of the intestinal wall in the areas of inflammation. Surgery may be necessary to remove the obstruction. People with Crohn's disease many encounter further complications, including gallstones, arthritis, and chronic irritation of the skin.

Multiple Sclerosis

For proper nerve conduction to occur in the brain and spinal cord, an insulating sheath of myelin must surround the neurons. In the progressive disease multiple sclerosis (MS), the cells that produce myelin are destroyed and myelin production ceases. Eventually, the vital functions of the body can no longer be carried out. The cause of MS is not fully understood. Research continues to focus on virus-induced autoimmune mechanisms in which T cells attack viral-infected myelin-producing cells.

Usually, MS first appears during the young adult years. It may take one of three forms, depending on the interplay of periods of stabilization (remitting), renewed deterioration (relapsing), and continuous deterioration (progressive). The initial symptoms are often visual impairment, prickling and burning in the extremities, or an altered **gait.** Deterioration of nervous system function occurs in various forms during the course of MS. In the most advanced stages of MS, movement is greatly impaired, and mental deterioration may be present.

Key Terms

autoimmune
An immune response against the cells of a person's own body.

gait
Pattern of walking.

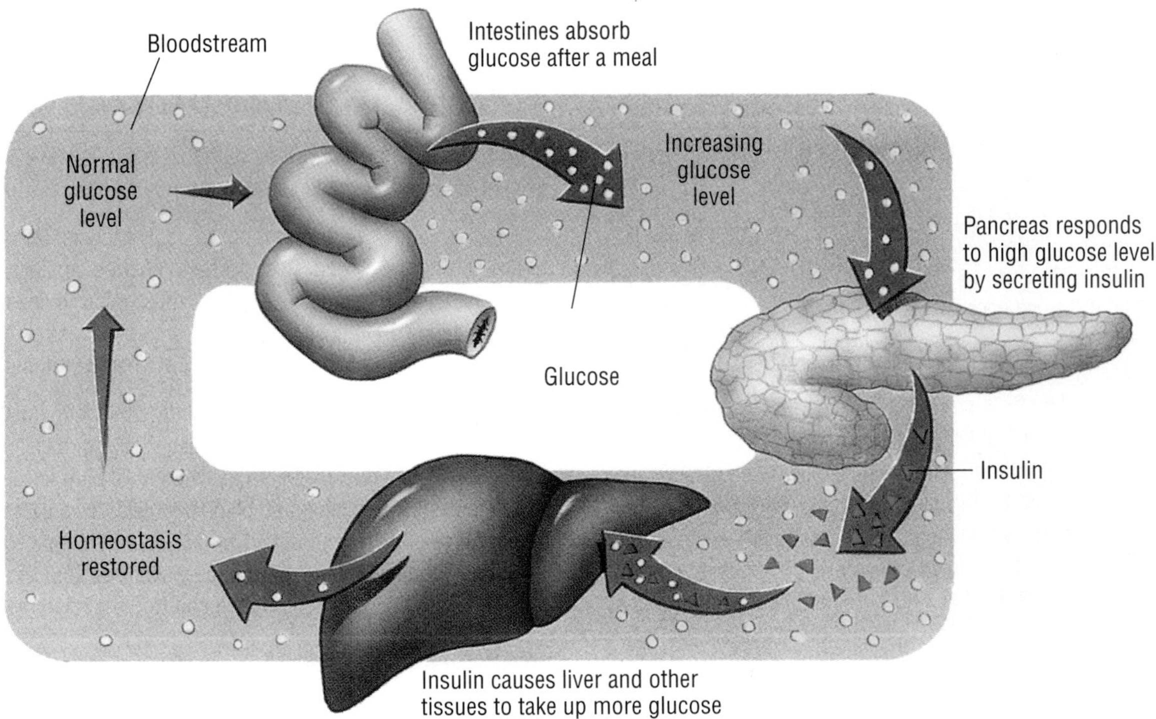
Bloodstream
Intestines absorb glucose after a meal
Normal glucose level
Increasing glucose level
Pancreas responds to high glucose level by secreting insulin
Glucose
Insulin
Homeostasis restored
Insulin causes liver and other tissues to take up more glucose

Figure 11-3 The secretion of insulin is regulated by a mechanism that tends to reverse any deviation from normal. Thus an increase in blood glucose level triggers secretion of insulin. Since insulin promotes glucose uptake by cells, blood glucose level is restored to its lower, normal level.

Treatment of MS involves reducing the severity of the symptoms and extending the periods of remission. Today a variety of therapies are used, including immune-targeted drugs, steroid drugs, drugs that relieve muscle spasms, injection of nerve blockers, and physical therapy.

The development of immune system–related medications is at the center of today's treatment of MS. Interferon beta-1a (Betaseron), a genetically engineered form of interferon, effectively reduces the symptoms of MS but may not slow the progression of the disease. More recently, interferon beta-1a (Avonex) and Glatiramer acetate (Copaxone), drugs that slow the development of the disease and delay periods of relapse, are also available.[23] A newer drug, Zanaflex, intended to reduce the muscle spasticity that accompanies MS, is also available.

In addition to drug therapy, psychotherapy is an important adjunct to the treatment of MS. Profound periods of depression often accompany the initial diagnosis of this condition. Emotional support is helpful in dealing with the progressive impairments associated with most forms of the condition.

Diabetes Mellitus

Diabetes mellitus is not a single condition but rather two metabolic disorders with important similarities and differences.

Non–insulin-dependent diabetes mellitus (Type II)

In people who do not have diabetes mellitus the body's need for energy is met through the "burning" of glucose (blood sugar) within the cells. Glucose is absorbed from the digestive tract and carried to the cells by the blood system. Passage of glucose into the cell is achieved through a transport system that moves the glucose molecule across the cell's membrane. Activation of this glucose transport mechanism requires the presence of the hormone insulin (Figure 11-3). Specific receptor sites for **insulin** can be found on the cell membrane. In addition to its role in the transport of glucose into sensitive cells, insulin is required for the conversion of glucose into glycogen in the liver and the formation of fatty acids in adipose cells. Insulin is produced in the cells of the islets of Langerhans in the pancreas. The release of insulin from the pancreas corresponds to the changing levels of glucose within the blood.[24]

In adults with a **genetic predisposition** for developing non–insulin-dependent diabetes mellitus, a trigger mechanism (most likely obesity) begins a process through which the body cells become increasingly less sensitive to the presence of insulin, although a normal (or slightly greater than normal) amount of insulin is produced by the pancreas. The growing ineffectiveness of

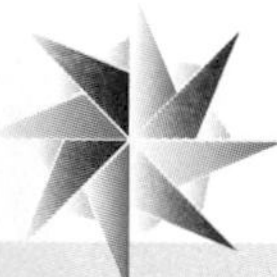

Alzheimer's Disease

Although it affects less than 2% of the elderly, **Alzheimer's disease** is an incapacitating, emotionally painful, and costly affliction. It is the best known of the dementia disorders, affecting an estimated 4 million adults. Today, more than ever before, it is *the* disease associated with aging.

The first signs of Alzheimer's disease are often subtle and may be confused with mild depression. Initially, the person might have difficulty answering questions such as "What is today's date?" Over the next few months, greater memory loss, confusion, and *dementia* (or loss of normal thought processes) occur. In the advanced stages, people with Alzheimer's disease become incontinent, show infantile behavior, and finally become incapacitated as brain tissue is destroyed. With advanced Alzheimer's disease, institutionalization becomes necessary.

Alzheimer's disease is difficult to diagnose because its symptoms are similar to those of other types of dementia. It is only after the person's death, if an autopsy is performed, that the characteristic changes in the brain can be used to make a definitive diagnosis. As a practical matter, a probable diagnosis of Alzheimer's disease is made by the process of elimination. Newer medical imaging technologies, such as MRI scans, have become so refined that it is now almost possible to confirm the diagnosis of Alzheimer's disease before death.

Effective drugs to treat Alzheimer's disease do not exist at this time. However, three currently available drugs (tacrine, donepezil, and rivastigamine) provide temporary improvement in intellectual function during the early stages of the disease by inhibiting the breakdown of acetylcholine, whose diminished availability is the basis of the disease. At least six additional drugs are in various clinical trial phases, including metrifonate and physostigmine.

Several theories have been advanced about the cause of Alzheimer's disease. Increasing evidence indicates that genetic mutations on chromosomes 10, 14, 19 and 21 may encourage the development of the disease. Research into the function of various proteins in fostering the disease's development is also under way. Prevention-oriented trials involving the use of ibuprofen, folic acid, estrogen and vitamin E are also continuing. Research into a method of stopping and reversing the course of the disease through implantation of embryonic stem cells is also under consideration.

Additionally, two vaccines intended to block the development of the disease are under development. One is currently in human trials, while the second, and most likely the least toxic to humans, is nearing clinical trial status.

insulin in getting glucose into cells results in the buildup of glucose in the blood. Elevated levels of glucose lead to *hyperglycemia,* a hallmark symptom of non–insulin-dependent diabetes mellitus.

In response to this buildup, the kidneys begin the process of filtering glucose from the blood. Excess glucose then spills over into the urine. This removal of glucose in the urine demands large amounts of water, a process called *diuresis,* a second important symptom of adult-onset diabetes. Increased thirst, a third symptom of developing diabetes, results in response to the movement of fluid from extracellular spaces into the circulatory system to maintain homeostasis.

For many adults with diabetes, dietary modification (with an emphasis on monitoring total carbohydrate intake, not just sugar) and regular exercise is the only treatment required to maintain an acceptable glucose level. Weight loss will improve the condition by "releasing" more insulin receptors, and exercise increases the actual number of receptor sites. With better insulin recognition, the affected person can better maintain glucose levels.

For people whose condition is more advanced, dietary modification and weight loss are not sufficient, and a hypoglycemia agent must be used. Most recently, Rezulin, a widely used medication that increases the cells' sensitivity to available insulin, was shown to be associated with serious liver damage. However, a similar drug, Avandia, which has fewer harmful effects on the liver, has won FDA approval. For those who require insulin by injection or other delivery methods (e.g., nasal spray or implanted pump), management is much more demanding.

TALKING POINTS • You learn that two young women who are your co-workers have recently been diagnosed with lupus and Crohn's disease, respectively. How can you be supportive of them? What should you say to them about their conditions, particularly on days when it is obvious that they are not feeling well?

Key Terms

insulin
A pancreatic hormone required by the body for the effective metabolism of glucose (blood sugar).

genetic predisposition
An inherited tendency to develop a disease process if necessary environmental factors exist.

Alzheimer's disease
Gradual development of memory loss, confusion, and loss of reasoning; will eventually lead to total intellectual incapacitation, brain degeneration, and death.

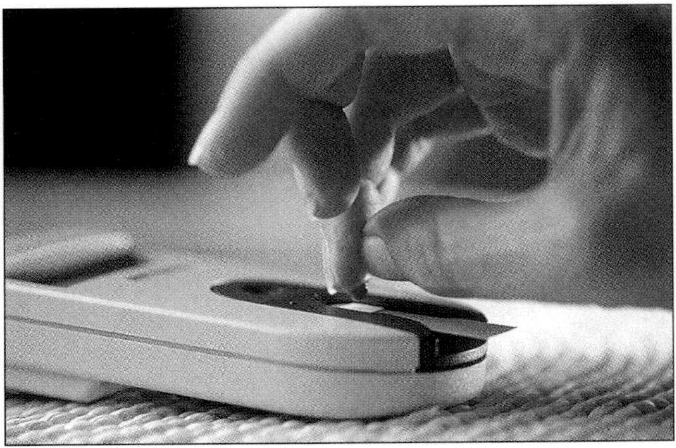

To successfully manage their condition, people with type 1 diabetes mellitus must periodically test their blood glucose level.

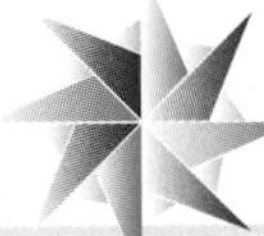

Differences between Types of Diabetes Mellitus

Insulin-Dependent (Type I)
(These symptoms usually develop rapidly.)

- Extreme hunger
- Extreme thirst
- Frequent urination
- Extreme weight loss
- Irritability
- Weakness and fatigue
- Nausea and vomiting

Non–Insulin-Dependent (Type II)
(These symptoms usually develop gradually.)

- Any of the symptoms for insulin-dependent diabetes
- Blurred vision or a change in sight
- Itchy skin
- Tingling or numbness in the limbs

If you notice these symptoms occurring, bring them to the attention of your physician.

In addition to genetic predisposition and obesity, unresolved stress appears to be involved in the development of hyperglycemic states. Although stress alone probably cannot produce a diabetic condition, it is likely that stress can create a series of endocrine changes that can lead to a state of hyperglycemia.

Diabetes can cause serious damage to several important structures within the body. The rate and extent to which people with diabetes develop these changes can be markedly influenced by the nature of their condition and their compliance with its management requirements. For those who already have diabetes, an understanding of the condition and a commitment to its management are important elements in living with diabetes mellitus. However, for the estimated 15 million people who are thought to be "borderline" diabetics and not yet diagnosed, the need to be "discovered" is a growing concern. Accordingly, initial blood glucose testing should ideally begin during young adulthood (by age 25), rather than at middle age, when it typically begins.

Insulin-dependent diabetes mellitus (Type I)

A second type of diabetes mellitus is insulin-dependent diabetes mellitus, or Type I diabetes. The onset of this condition generally occurs before age 35, most often during childhood. In contrast to Type II diabetes, in which insulin is produced but is ineffective because of insensitivity, in Type I diabetes the body does not produce insulin at all. Destruction of the insulin-producing cells of the pancreas by the person's immune system (possibly in combination with a genetic predisposition) accounts for this sudden and irreversible loss of insulin production.[24]

In most ways the two forms of diabetes are similar, with the important exception that insulin-dependent diabetes mellitus requires the use of insulin from an outside source. Today this insulin is obtained either from animals or through genetically engineered bacteria. It is taken by injection (one to four times per day), through the use of an insulin pump that provides a constant supply of insulin to the body, by transdermal patch, or through nasal inhalation. An insulin pill, now under development, will hopefully be available within the next few years.[25] The use of a glucometer, a highly accurate device for measuring the amount of glucose in the blood, allows for sound management of this condition and a life expectancy that is essentially normal. With both forms of diabetes mellitus, sound dietary practice, weight management, planned activity, and control of stress are important for keeping blood glucose levels within normal ranges. Without good management of diabetes mellitus, several serious problems can result, including blindness, gangrene of the extremities, kidney disease, and heart attack. These and other common complications of diabetes are listed in the Star Box on p. 271. People who cannot establish good control are likely to live a shorter life than those who can.

Sickle-Cell Trait and Sickle-Cell Disease

Among the hundreds of human diseases, few are found almost exclusively in a particular racial or ethnic group. Such is the case, however, for the inherited condition *sickle-cell trait/sickle-cell disease.* In the United States, sickle-cell abnormalities are virtually unique to African Americans.

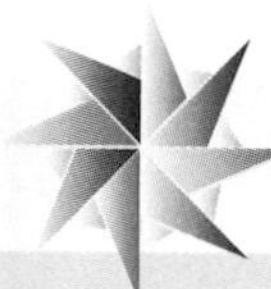

Common Complications of Diabetes

- Cataract formation
- Glaucoma
- Blindness
- Dental caries
- Stillbirths/miscarriages
- Neonatal deaths
- Congenital defects
- Cardiovascular disease
- Kidney disease
- Gangrene
- Impotence

Of all the chemical compounds found in the body, few occur in as many forms as hemoglobin, which helps bind oxygen to red blood cells. Two forms of hemoglobin are associated with sickle-cell trait and sickle-cell disease. African Americans can be the recipients of either form of this abnormal hemoglobin. Those who inherit the trait form do not develop the disease but can transmit the gene for abnormal hemoglobin to their children. In the past, those who inherited the disease form faced a shortened life characterized by periods of pain and impairment. Today, however, with effective screening and new medications, people with sickle-cell disease can reach age 50. Also, bone marrow transplants have extended life expectancy to near-normal ranges. Most recently, an experimental blood transfusion technique was reported to have cured a teenage boy of the sickle-cell disease.

About 8% of all African Americans have the gene for sickle-cell trait; they experience little impairment, but they can transmit the abnormal gene to their children. For about 1.5% of African Americans, sickle-cell disease is a painful, incapacitating, and life-shortening disease.

In the fully expressed disease form, red blood cells are elongated, crescent-shaped (sickled), and unable to pass through the body's minute capillaries. The body responds to the presence of these abnormal red blood cells by removing them very quickly. This sets the stage for anemia. Thus the condition is often called *sickle-cell anemia.* In addition to anemia, the disease form of the condition can cause many serious medical problems, including impaired lung function, congestive heart failure, gallbladder infections, bone changes, and abnormalities of the eye and skin.

If a key exists for preventing sickle-cell trait and disease, it lies in genetic counseling and testing in preparation for reproduction or in the use of in vitro fertilization followed by genetic testing of the embryo before implantation. At present, both of these preventive approaches are very expensive and limited in availability. However, further research and testing could make these methods more affordable and increase their availability to people who are at high risk.

SUMMARY

- The "war on cancer" has made gains in many areas, but it is far from being won, with overall death rates having climbed since 1971.
- Cancer is a condition reflecting the body's inability to control the growth and specialization of cells.
- Genes that control replication, specialization, repair, and suppression of abnormal activity hold the potential of becoming oncogenes and thus can be considered protooncogenes.
- A variety of agents, including genetic mutations, viruses, and carcinogens (and co-carcinogens) stimulate the conversion of regulatory genes (protooncogenes) into oncogenes. The identification of oncogenes continues at a rapid pace in conjunction with the Human Genome Project and the Cancer Genome Anatomy Project.
- Cancer cells demonstrate a variety of interesting characteristics in comparison with normal cells of the same type. Benign tumors, made up of noncancerous cells, can present serious health problems.
- Cancer can be described on the basis of the type of tissue in which it has its origin—carcinoma, sarcoma, melanoma, etc.
- Cancer can be described on the basis of its location within the body—lung, breast, prostate, etc.
- Cigarette smoking and having a genetic predisposition are both related to the development of lung cancer.
- Breast cancer demonstrates clear familial patterns that suggest a genetic predisposition. Mammograms are recommended as an important component of breast cancer identification. Important options should be considered before the treatment of breast cancer.
- Regular use of Pap tests is related to the early detection of uterine (cervical) cancer. A group of middle-aged women who are the daughters of mothers given the drug DES during pregnancy have high levels of vaginal cancer. Ovarian cancer is often "silent" in its presentation of symptoms.
- The PSA test improves the ability to diagnose prostate cancer. A more sensitive PSA test will soon be available.

- Regular self-examination of the testicles leads to early detection of testicular cancer.
- Colon and rectal cancers have strong familial links and is possibly related to diets high in fat and low in fruits and vegetables.
- Pancreatic cancer is very difficult to survive, in part because of the absence of symptoms early in the disease's course.
- Skin cancer prevention requires protection from excessive sun exposure.
- Early detection based on self-examination and screening is the basis for the identification and successful treatment of many cancers. Conventional and alternative treatment methods can be used to treat cancer.
- Adults can display an array of chronic conditions, some of which are expressed for the first time during the traditional college years.
- Chronic conditions, such as lupus, reflect the immune system's failure to recognize the body's own tissue as being "self."
- Crohn's disease, a member of the irritable bowel diseases, causes the deterioration of the inner and muscular layers of the intestinal wall.
- Multiple sclerosis involves the autoimmune destruction of the insulating cover of neurons.
- Diabetes mellitus, in both of its forms, is a chronic condition in which the body is unable to use glucose in the normal manner.

REVIEW QUESTIONS

1. What is the relationship between regulatory genes and tumor suppressor genes in the development of cancer? Why are regulatory genes called both protooncogenes and oncogenes?
2. What are some of the major types of cancer, based on the tissue in which they have their origin?
3. What are the principal factors that contribute to the development of lung cancer? Of breast cancer?
4. When should regular use of mammography begin, and which women should begin using it earliest?
5. How does the PSA test contribute to the early detection of prostate cancer?
6. What signs indicate the possibility that a skin lesion has become cancerous?
7. What important information can be obtained with the use of Pap tests?
8. What are the steps for effective self-examination of the breasts and testicles?
9. Why is ovarian cancer described as a "silent" cancer?
10. What are the conventional and alternative cancer treatments most often used in the treatment of cancer?
11. Which chronic conditions discussed in this chapter are most likely to be first expressed during the traditional college years?
12. What is the role of immune system in the connective tissue disorder known as systemic lupus erythematosus? How does exposure to sun influence the expression of lupus?
13. To what larger family of chronic conditions does Crohn's disease belong. How is it diagnosed and treated?
14. What is thought to be the role of the immune system in the development of MS? What are the ABCs of the fight against MS?
15. How do Type I and Type II diabetes mellitus differ? To what extent are they similar conditions?

THINK ABOUT THIS . . .

- Do you believe you could cope with a significant health problem at this time in your life?
- Do you know anyone who has or has had cancer? How did cancer affect that person's life?
- How regularly do you perform either breast or testicular self-examination?
- If you were diagnosed as having a terminal illness, how willing would you be to serve as a subject in a research project that tested a potentially toxic experimental drug?
- Which conditions in this chapter are you likely to develop, and which are you not likely to develop?

REFERENCES

1. American Cancer Society, *Cancer facts and figures: 2001*, 2001, The Society.
2. Songer J, oncologist: Personal interview, December 1999.
3. A library of hope: the Cancer Genome Anatomy Project, *Cancer Smart* 4(3):6–7, 1998.
4. *CGAP tumor suppressor and oncogene directory*, December 13, 1999.
5. Program cell death: natural cancer suppression, *Cancer Smart* 4(2):6–7, 1998.

6. Starving the tumor—not the patient, *Cancer Smart* 4(4):6–8, 1998.
7. Wood ME et al: The inherited nature of lung cancer: a pilot study, *Lung Cancer* 30(2):135–144, 2000.
8. Laden F et al: Geographic variation in breast cancer incidence rates in a cohort of U.S. women, *J Natl Cancer Inst* 89(18):1373–1378, 1997.
9. Struewing JP, Hartge P, Wacholder S: The risk of cancer associated with specific mutations of *BRCA1* and *BRCA2* among Ashkenazi Jews, *N Engl J Med* 336(20):1401–1408, 1997.
10. Eisen A, Weber BL: Prophylactic mastectomy—the price of fear, *N Engl J Med* 340(2):137–138, 1999.
11. Tamoxifen unsuitable for primary prevention of breast cancer, uncertain efficacy, clear risk (panel consensus), *Prescrire Int* 9(46):56–58, 2000.
12. Janerich DT et al: The screening histories of women with invasive cervical cancer, Connecticut, *Am J Public Health* 85(6):791–794, 1995.
13. Rodriguez C et al: Estrogen replacement therapy and ovarian cancer mortality in large prospective study of U.S. women, *JAMA* 285(11):1460–1465, 2001.
14. Albertsen PC et al: Competing risk analysis of men aged 55 to 74 years at diagnosis managed conservatively for clinically localized prostate cancer, *JAMA* 280(11):975–980, 1998.
15. Potter JD: Fiber and colorectal cancer—where to now? *N Engl J Med* 340(3):223–224, 1999.
16. Terry P et al: Fruit, vegetables, dietary fiber, and the risk of colorectal cancer, *J Natl Cancer Inst* 93(7):525–533, 2001.
17. Giocannucci E et al: Aspirin and the risk of colorectal cancer in women, *N Engl J Med* 332(14):609–614, 1995.
18. Kanzler MH, Mraz-Gernhard S: Primary cutaneous malignant melanoma and its precursor lesions: diagnostic and therapeutic overview, *J Am Acad Dermatol* 45(2):260–276, 2001.
19. Stephenson J: Researchers describe findings for targeted cancer therapies, *JAMA* 284(3):293–295, 2000.
20. Metz JM et al: Cancer patients use unconventional medical therapies far more frequently than standard history and physical examination suggest, *Cancer* 7(2):149–154, 2001.
21. Price SA, Wilson L (editors): *Pathophysiology: clinical concepts of disease processes,* ed 5, Mosby, 1996.
22. Sartor RB: IBD researchers are breaking new ground, *Under the Microscope* (research news bulletin from the Crohn's & Colitis Foundation of America) 5:2, 1998.
23. King M: Avonex, Betaseron, and Copaxone: the new ABC of multiple sclerosis, *Inside MS* 17(4):20–26, 1999.
24. Saladin KS: *Anatomy and physiology: the unity of form and function,* 1998, McGraw-Hill.
25. Gura T: New lead found to a possible "insulin pill," *Science* 284(5416):866, 1999.

SUGGESTED READINGS

Arnot RB: *The breast cancer prevention diet: the powerful foods supplements, and drugs that can save your life,* 1998, Little, Brown.

The author, a physician and NBC's chief medical correspondent, advances a diet-based approach to the prevention of breast cancer that has failed to impress many of his peers. Respected nutritionists applaud the book's emphasis on better nutrition, but they also remind readers that many of the author's contentions about the role of specific nutrients and supplements in preventing cancer are not supported by research. This book will appeal to people who wish to be proactive in preventing cancer and other chronic conditions.

Link J: *The breast cancer survival manual: a step-by-step guide for the woman with newly diagnosed breast cancer,* 1998, Owl Books.

This book, written by an experienced oncologist, is highly informative. Dr. Link provides practical advice about topics such as mastectomy versus breast conservation with radiation, the criteria necessary to justify chemotherapy, how to interpret the staging system used by pathologists, and when a second opinion is appropriate. The author also explores decisions regarding adjuncts to medical therapies—such as structuring proper nutrition, the use of dietary supplements, and the role of exercise—in a very understandable way. Readers are cautioned, though, about the author's tendency to be overly supportive of his own institution in comparison to most others.

Meyer B, Davidson AI, Zorda R (editors): *Diabetes mellitus: diagnosis and treatment,* ed 4, 1998, W.B. Saunders.

Although directed primarily at health care professionals, this highly regarded book, in its fourth edition, has also been well received by lay people. Using the latest scientific research as the book's technical core, the authors provide additional information for patient management of both Type I and Type II diabetes. Topics include fasting before special diagnostic procedures, foot care management, and criteria for making subtle insulin adjustments. In addition to clinicians and persons with diabetes mellitus, this is an excellent book for caregivers.

Piver MS, Wilder G, Bull J: *Gilda's disease: sharing personal experiences and a medical perspective on ovarian cancer,* 1998, Bantam Doubleday Dell Publishing.

For those who remember Gilda Radner's death from ovarian cancer in 1989, a moving new dimension, her husband's deeply personal relationship with his wife and her disease, is added to the story. The addition of medical perspectives by Steven Piver, MD, regarding ovarian cancer and the various treatment options makes this book an important resource for persons interested in the "silent killer."

Name ______________________ **Date** __________ **Section** __________

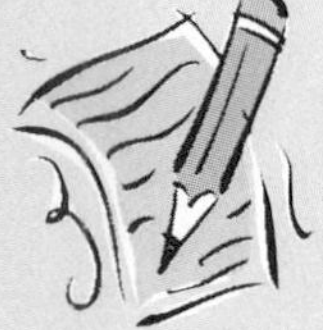

Personal Assessment

Are You at Risk for Skin, Breast, or Cervical Cancer?

Some people may have more than an average risk of developing particular types of cancer. These people can be identified by certain risk factors.

This simple self-testing method is designed by the American Cancer Society to help you assess your risk factors for three common types of cancer. These are the major risk factors but by no means represent the only ones that might be involved.

Check your response to each risk factor. Add the numbers in the parentheses to arrive at a total score for each cancer type. Find out what your score means by reading the information in the "Interpretation" section. You are advised to discuss the information with your physician if you are at a higher risk.

Skin Cancer

1. Frequent work or play in the sun
   a. Yes (10)
   b. No (1)
2. Work in mines, around coal tars, or around radio activity
   a. Yes (10)
   b. No (1)
3. Complexion—fair skin or light skin
   a. Yes (10)
   b. No (1)

Your total points __________

Explanation

1. Excessive ultraviolet light causes skin cancer. Protect yourself with a sunscreen.
2. These materials can cause skin cancer.
3. Light complexions need more protection than others.

Interpretation

Numerical risks for skin cancer are difficult to state. For instance, a person with a dark complexion can work longer in the sun and be less likely to develop cancer than a light-complected person. Furthermore, a person wearing a long-sleeved shirt and a wide-brimmed hat may work in the sun and be less at risk than a person who wears a bathing suit and stays in the sun for only a short period. The risk increases greatly with age.

The key here is if you answered "yes" to any question, you need to realize that you have above-average risk.

Breast Cancer

1. Age group
   a. 20–34 (10)
   b. 35–49 (40)
   c. 50 and over (90)
2. Race/nationality
   a. Asian American (5)
   b. African American (20)
   c. White (25)
   d. Mexican American (10)
3. Family history of breast cancer
   a. Mother, sister, or grandmother (30)
   b. None (10)
4. Your history
   a. No breast disease (10)
   b. Previous noncancerous lumps or cysts (25)
   c. Previous breast cancer (100)
5. Maternity
   a. First pregnancy before age 25 (10)
   b. First pregnancy after age 25 (15)
   c. No pregnancies (20)

Your total points __________

Interpretation

Under 100	Low-risk women should practice monthly breast self-examination (BSE) and have their breasts examined by a doctor as part of a cancer-related checkup.
100–199	Moderate-risk women should practice monthly BSE and have their breasts examined by a doctor as part of a cancer-related checkup. Periodic mammograms should be included as your doctor may advise.
200 or more	High-risk women should practice monthly BSE and have the examinations and mammograms described earlier.

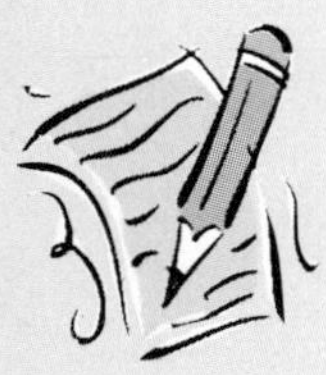

Personal Assessment *continued*

Cervical Cancer*

1. Age group
   a. Less than 25 (10)
   b. 25–39 (20)
   c. 40–54 (30)
   d. 55 and over (30)

2. Race/nationality
   a. Asian American (10)
   b. Puerto Rican (20)
   c. African American (20)
   d. White (10)
   e. Mexican American (20)

3. Number of pregnancies
   a. 0 (10)
   b. 1 to 3 (20)
   c. 4 and over (30)

4. Viral infections
   a. Herpes and other viral infections or ulcer formations on the vagina (10)
   b. Never (1)

5. Age at first intercourse
   a. Before 15 (40)
   b. 15–19 (30)
   c. 20–24 (20)
   d. 25 and over (10)

6. Bleeding between periods or after intercourse
   a. Yes (40)
   b. No (1)

YOUR TOTAL POINTS ___________

Explanations

1. The highest occurrence is in the 40-and-over age group. The numbers represent the relative rates of cancer for different age groups. A 45-year-old woman has a risk three times higher than a 20 year old.
2. Puerto Ricans, African Americans, and Mexican Americans have higher rates of cervical cancer.
3. Women who have delivered more children have a higher occurrence.
4. Viral infections of the cervix and vagina are associated with cervical cancer.
5. Women with earlier intercourse and with more sexual partners are at a higher risk.
6. Irregular bleeding may be a sign of uterine cancer.

Interpretation/To Carry This Further . . .

40–69 — This is a low-risk group. Ask your doctor for a Pap test. You will be advised how often you should be tested after your first test.

70–99 — In this moderate-risk group, more frequent Pap tests may be required.

100 or higher — You are in a high-risk group and should have a Pap test (and pelvic examination) as advised by your doctor.

*Lower portion of uterus. These questions would not apply to a woman who has had a complete hysterectomy.

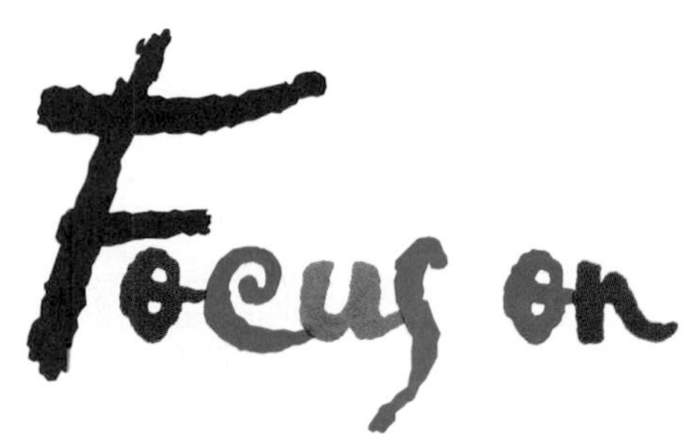

MANAGING CHRONIC PAIN

Carlotta loved to spend her spare time puttering around in her flower garden. Every weekend, she would work outside for hours—tilling soil, putting in new plants, pruning, and landscaping. One Saturday afternoon as she was lifting some railroad ties to create a new border for her plants, she heard a loud popping noise and felt a sharp pain in her lower back. She tried aspirin, bed rest, massage, and heat, but the pain was still excruciating after 2 weeks. She went to see her doctor, who prescribed pain medication and a brief course of physical therapy, but the pain persisted. Finally, after nearly a year passed with no relief, her doctor recommended back surgery. Carlotta spent almost 3 months recovering from the surgery, after which she hoped to lead a normal, pain-free life.

Unfortunately, Carlotta's pain persists today, almost 2 years since her initial injury. Carlotta suffers from chronic pain, a type of pain that persists beyond the expected healing time. Chronic pain differs from most other kinds of pain, such as pain resulting from a headache, a fall, or surgery. According to the American Pain Society, chronic pain is difficult to treat because it doesn't respond to normal pain treatments. Also, some of the usual signs that accompany acute pain, such as sweating, increased heart rate, and dilated pupils, are not present in individuals with chronic pain.[1]

Causes of Chronic Pain

Chronic pain occurs as the result of one of three primary causes. In some patients, it is linked to injuries to the central or peripheral nervous systems, according to John D. Loeser, M.D., director of the Multidisciplinary Pain Center at the University of Washington School of Medicine.[1] In these patients, no tissue damage ever occurred in the part of their body that hurts. Whenever the nervous system heals itself, the functions of the nerve cells lost in the injury are not restored. As a result, the patient's neurological functions are impaired. This type of pain can occur as a result of limb amputation, shingles, diabetes, or surgery.

A second cause of chronic pain is linked to degenerative changes in joints. In these cases, tissue damage has not healed properly. Patients have both inflammation of the joints and chronic degenerative problems.[1] This cause of pain is often involved in diseases such as arthritis and lupus.

The third "cause" of pain is the catch-all category: "no known pathological mechanism."[1] Doctors are unsure why these patients are having pain. The one criterion used to place a patient in this category is whether the patient's pain complaints exceed the physician's expectations based on the illness or injury the patient has suffered.

Conditions Associated with Chronic Pain

Several types of conditions are commonly associated with sufferers of chronic pain, but the most common one is the headache. Up to 57% of men and 76% of women in the adolescent and young adult age-groups experience recurrent headaches. The National Headache Foundation estimates that 45 million Americans suffer from chronic headaches. The four most common types of headaches associated with chronic pain are tension headaches, migraines, cluster headaches, and sinus headaches.[2]

Four out of five Americans experience back pain at some point in their lives. The problem usually resolves itself. However, it is estimated that more than 11 million Americans have back pain that is severe enough to cause impairment. This cause of chronic pain is particularly troublesome because of its economic impact on society. Based on all analyses of possible cost factors, back pain costs society anywhere from $75 billion to $100 billion annually.[1]

Another debilitating condition commonly associated with chronic pain is arthritis. More than 35 million Americans have a form of this disease. Two principal types of arthritis exist. *Osteoarthritis* is the breaking down of the cartilage found at the ends of the long bones. Weight-bearing and frequently used joints are the areas most commonly affected. *Rheumatoid arthritis* is an autoimmune disorder in which the patient's own immune system produces antibodies that attack the tissues in the joints of the body. Symptoms of both types include stiffness and swelling of the joints.

Cancer and Chronic Pain

Although cancer is often associated with chronic pain, pain experts put it in a class by itself. Chronic cancer pain is complex because the pain can occur as a result of bone invasion, tumors compressing nerves, tumors affecting internal organs, obstruction of blood vessels, surgery, chemotherapy, or radiation treatment.[1]

Effects of Chronic Pain

Because chronic pain is such a disruptive, ongoing phenomenon, it can affect most aspects of an individual's life. For example, because of chronic pain many people find it difficult to continue their usual recreational pursuits, such as running, bicycling, and gardening. Also, tasks of daily living, such as dressing oneself and preparing meals, can become difficult or impossible to do without assistance.

The devastation of losing a job is another potential effect of suffering with chronic pain. Because the pain is so invasive and persistent, it affects a person's ability to concentrate, perform essential job duties, or even go to work. The time spent away from work to attend therapy sessions or to visit a physician can become an issue in performance evaluations and may affect a person's ability to keep his or her job.

Sleep disorders are a third potential effect of chronic pain. Sleep disorders can come about in two ways. Either a patient is unable to sleep because of the pain, or the individual becomes dependent on a pain or sleep medication that disrupts the sleep cycle. As sleep deprivation increases, the person's emotional outlook becomes increasingly fragile, interpersonal relationships may begin to show signs of strain, and the probability of accidents increases.

Serious psychological problems can also result from chronic pain. Depression is one of the most common problems. As the individual becomes increasingly impaired by the chronic pain, a lack of motivation sets in. As the level of depression deepens, job performance deteriorates, contact with other people is lessened, and, eventually, a sense of isolation takes over. Fortunately, the depressive aspects of chronic pain can be controlled through a combination of antidepressive medication and psychological intervention.

The final significant side effect of chronic pain is potential damage to the immune system. This effect can be particularly troublesome in patients whose chronic pain is the result of cancer. Studies have shown that pain can suppress the immune system, causing cancer patients to have difficulty recovering.[3] Since this problem can have fatal results, it is especially important for cancer patients to have prompt and effective treatment of their pain.

Methods of Managing Chronic Pain

Although chronic pain has several negative side effects, many of them can be controlled. Most pain specialists recommend a multidisciplinary management approach that involves a combination of methods to achieve the most relief.

One of the most common and effective methods of achieving relief of chronic pain is the use of opioid drugs, also known as *Schedule II* drugs. These drugs have been proven to provide quick relief of pain, particularly among cancer patients and headache sufferers. However, physicians are often reluctant to prescribe these drugs for several reasons. First, doctors are afraid that if they are perceived as prescribing too many opioids, they could be reported to the medical board and ultimately lose their licenses. Second, American society in general disapproves of prescribing narcotics because of the fear of addiction and the idea that all narcotics are "bad," despite their potential for pain relief. Finally, medical personnel tend to underestimate the amount of pain that patients suffer. Most people who suffer severe pain and request narcotics will not become addicts. Yet some medical personnel who work with pain sufferers have the mindset that people with chronic pain do not hurt as badly as they claim to.

For chronic headache sufferers, several other types of drugs also offer hope. For example, the antidepressant Deseryl has been found effective in persons who have trouble falling sleeping for any of several reasons, including the chronic pain of headaches.[4]

Other drugs that provide relief include beta-blockers, calcium channel blockers, and anticonvulsants. Doctors may try several combinations of these drugs to see which one will most effectively relieve headache symptoms, with the eventual goal of removing as many medications as possible from the patient's daily regimen.[5]

For patients with arthritis, two classes of drugs appear to offer the most relief. The first type is known as *nonsteroidal antiinflammatory drugs,* or *NSAIDs.* The most well-known of these drugs are Advil, Nuprin, Naprosyn, and Anaprox. New to this class of NSAIDSs are two highly effective medications that provide pain relief with greatly reduced gastric irritation. These medications, Vioxx and Celebrex, block pain from the joints without affecting the enzymes that protect the sensitive linings of the stomach and intestinal tract.[4] Recently, however, some researchers have questioned this protective capacity.[6] One advantage is that these drugs provide relief within 2 hours. A second type of antiarthritic medicine is known as *slow-acting antirheumatic drugs,* or *SAARDs.* These drugs provide time-released, long-lasting relief.

Surgery is another option for managing chronic pain. This method is most effective in helping patients with cancer. Surgery may also become necessary for the arthritis pain sufferer. Replacement of cartilage or an affected joint will often help a sufferer lead a more normal, less painful life. Surprisingly, however, surgery is generally not an effective option for back pain sufferers.

Because the mind is such a powerful instrument of healing, pain specialists often recommend that patients undertake psychological methods of pain relief in conjunction with traditional methods. For example, many headache specialists recommend biofeedback techniques so that patients can learn to control their responses to pain. Pain specialists also recommended deep-breathing exercises and meditation techniques to promote relaxation.

Physical methods of managing pain can add another dimension to chronic pain management. One time-tested method of relief is massage. Other helpful treatments include nerve blocks to the affected area, physical therapy, and exercises as prescribed by a physical therapist or physician. Finally, a patient can make some lifestyle changes to lessen the pain. Eating regularly, getting plenty of rest, and reducing caffeine intake have all been found to be particularly helpful to headache sufferers. This approach may also help others afflicted with chronic pain.

Although there is still no cure for chronic pain, it can be managed successfully with the help of trained personnel from a variety of fields. However, chronic pain sufferers must be vocal and persistent to get the help they desperately need. Doctors and patients alike must realize that chronic pain is not "all in the patient's head" but a real, treatable condition.

For Discussion . . .

Have you ever known someone who suffered (or still suffers) from chronic pain? What were your feelings about this person and his or her pain? If you suffered from chronic pain, what treatments do you think would be the best for you? Would you be willing to try nonconventional therapies like the ones described in this article, or would you be more comfortable with traditional methods of therapy? Why?

References

1. Cowles J: *Pain relief!—how to say "no" to acute, chronic, and cancer pain,* 1993, Master Media.
2. Marcus NJ, Arbeiter JS (contributor): *Freedom from pain: the breakthrough method of pain relief based on the New York Pain Treatment Program at Lenox Hill Hospital,* 1995, Fireside.
3. Buterbaugh L: Breaking through cancer pain barriers, *Medical World,* Oct 15, p 10, 1993.
4. *Physicians' desk reference 2000,* 1999, Medical Economics Data.
5. Brooks PM: Clinical management of rheumatoid arthritis, *Lancet* (341): 8840, 1993.
6. Josefson D: COX 2 inhibitors can affect the stomach lining, *BMJ* 391: 1518, 1999.

chapter **12**

Preventing Infectious Diseases

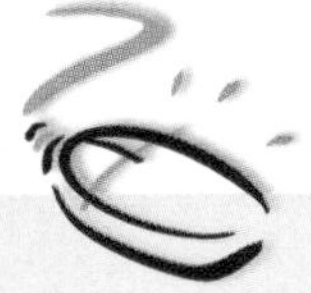

Online Learning Center Resources

www.mhhe.com/hahn6e

Log on to our Online Learning Center (OLC) for access to these additional resources:

- Chapter key terms and definitions
- Learning objectives
- Additional behavior change objectives
- Student interactive question-and-answer sites
- Self-scoring chapter quiz

The OLC also offers web links for study and exploration of health topics. Here are some examples of what you'll find:

- **www.cdc.gov/ncidod/id_links.htm** Visit this CDC website for the single best group of links covering infectious diseases.
- **www.hsph.harvard.edu/Organizations/hai/home_pg.html** Look here for highly specialized scientific and medical information on HIV/AIDS.
- **www.ashastd.org** Find answers to frequently asked questions about sexually transmitted diseases (STDs).

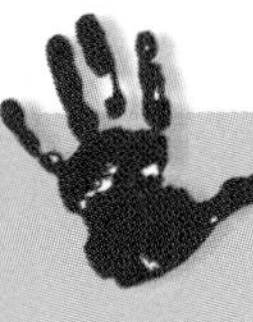

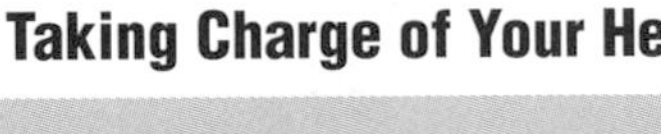

Taking Charge of Your Health

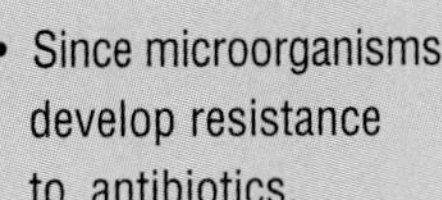

- Since microorganisms develop resistance to antibiotics, continue taking all such medications until gone, even when the symptoms of the infection have subsided.
- Check your current immunization status to make sure you are protected against preventable infectious diseases.
- If you are a parent, take your children to receive their recommended immunizations as necessary (see p. 286).
- Because of the possibility of contracting HIV/AIDS and sexually transmitted diseases, incorporate disease prevention into all your sexual activities.
- Use the Personal Assessment on p. 307 to determine your risk of contracting a sexually transmitted disease.
- If you have ever engaged in high-risk sexual behavior, get tested for HIV.

Eye on the Media

From Fear to Hope—AIDS in the News

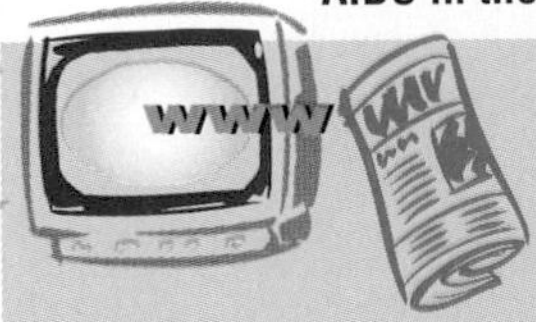

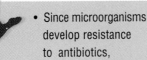

In the early days of news coverage about AIDS, magazines like *Time* and *Newsweek* ran articles called: "The AIDS Epidemic," "Epidemic of Fear," "Plague Mentality," "Fear of Sex," "The Growing Threat," "A Spreading Scourge," "The New Untouchables," "AIDS Spreading Panic Worldwide," "A Grim Race Against the Clock," and "The Lost Generation." The titles reflected fear of the unknown, a new killer disease.

When the case of Kimberley Bergalis broke into the news in 1991, a routine visit to the dentist was suddenly fraught with risk. Bergalis was the first American to die of AIDS after being infected by her dentist, Dr. David Acer. Four of Acer's other patients became infected with AIDS—all traced back to Acer. The public's reaction was near-hysteria. *Time* ran an article called "Should You Worry About Getting AIDS from Your Dentist?" People started asking their dentists (and other doctors) about their use of sterile precautions and even whether they had been tested for HIV.

Eye on the Media *continued*

By 1996, when the "cocktail" approach to AIDS treatment started showing remarkably good results, Magic Johnson was on the cover of both *Time* and *Newsweek* the same week. After more than 4 years of retirement from pro basketball—and the announcement that he had tested positive for HIV—he was back in the game. The secret to his survival? New drug treatments, a healthy diet, regular exercise, support from family and friends, and a positive attitude.

Recently, many news articles reflect a more hopeful tone: "Living Longer with AIDS," "Hope with an Asterisk," "Are Some People Immune?" and "What—I'm Gonna Live?" Doctors, too, are feeling more positive about the disease. As one AIDS specialist said: "I go to work feeling like there's something I can do for my patients."

For people with HIV/AIDS, the future holds different things. For some, who can't afford or tolerate the new drugs, it's still a matter of waiting to die. Others feel that they've been given a second chance. They can think about having relationships again—something many put on hold when they learned they were HIV positive. They can make plans for what they want to do with the rest of their lives—however long that may be.

Most people with HIV/AIDS are buying time—hoping for the big breakthrough, the cure for AIDS. They're trying new drug treatments, hoping that one treatment won't disqualify them from the next one. They're watching TV news, reading the newspapers, and using the Internet with greater attention. Will protease-inhibiting drugs be the answer? Or will the next new drug be the one? Will they live to try it?

Both medical experts and patients agree that it's time for cautious optimism. As one AIDS survivor said: "Everything is still phrased in the conditional for me. It's just that the conditions are more positive." Another voiced the mixed feelings of uncertainty, change, hope, and joy experienced by many who are living longer than they expected: "For a while . . . I didn't have to worry about the future. I didn't have to worry about retirement, getting older. . . . Now it's all come back. But it's great."

INFECTIOUS DISEASES IN THE 2000s

In the 1900s, infectious diseases were the leading cause of death. These deaths resulted from exposure to organisms that produced diseases such as smallpox, tuberculosis (TB), influenza, whooping cough (pertussis), typhoid, diphtheria, and tetanus. However, by midcentury, improvements in public sanitation, the widespread use of antibiotic drugs as a treatment method, and vaccinations as preventive therapy had considerably reduced the number of people who died from infectious diseases.

Today, we have a new respect for infectious diseases. AIDS continues to threaten millions of people in many areas of the world. We are witnessing the resurgence of TB. We recognize the role of pelvic infections in infertility. We also know that failure to fully immunize children, particularly in developing countries, has laid the groundwork for a return of whooping cough, polio, and other serious childhood diseases.

New dimensions of infectious disease have recently come to our attention. These include the appearance of extremely virulent viruses, such as the Ebola virus in Zaire, which is fatal to 75% of the people who contract it and for which there is no immunization or understanding of its transmission; the increasing resistance of bacteria such as *Staphylococcus aureus, Enterococcus,* and *Mycobacterium* (which causes TB) to antibiotics because of overuse, improper use, and biological "redesign" of the organisms themselves; the role of a bacterium *(Helicobacter pylori)* in the development of gastric ulcers; and, finally, the growing concern over transmission of infectious organisms through contaminated food, improper preparation of food, and contamination of water. The development of new antibiotics and more cautious use of current ones represent an encouraging trend.

INFECTIOUS DISEASE TRANSMISSION

Infectious diseases can generally be transferred from person to person, although that transfer is not always direct. These diseases can be especially dangerous because of their ability to spread to large numbers of people, producing *epidemics,* in which a large number of people are infected within a specific geographical area, such as a region of the country, or *pandemics,* in which an infectious disease crosses national borders and infects millions of people worldwide.

The sections that follow explain the process of disease transmission and the stages of infection. For a discussion of preventing infectious disease transmission, turn to the Focus on article on p. 309.

Pathogens

For a disease to be transferred, a person must come into contact with the disease-producing agent, or **pathogen,**

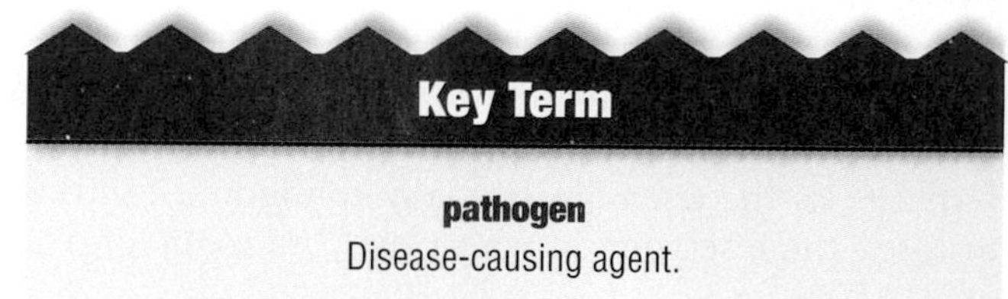

pathogen
Disease-causing agent.

Table 12-1 Pathogens and Common Infectious Diseases

Pathogen	Description	Representative Disease Processes
Viruses	Smallest common pathogens; nonliving particles of genetic material (DNA) surrounded by a protein coat	Rubeola, mumps, chicken pox, rubella, influenza, warts, colds, oral and genital herpes, shingles, AIDS, genital warts
Prion	A protein particle that lacks DNA and is believed to be infectious to animals, including humans	Creutzfeldt-Jakob disease, scrapie, mad cow disease
Bacteria	One-celled microorganisms with sturdy, well-defined cell walls; three distinctive forms: spherical (cocci), rod shaped (bacilli), and spiral shaped (spirilla)	Tetanus, strep throat, scarlet fever, gonorrhea, syphilis, chlamydia, toxic shock syndrome, Legionnaires' disease, bacterial pneumonia, meningitis, diphtheria, food poisoning, Lyme disease
Fungi	Plantlike microorganisms; molds and yeasts	Athlete's foot, ringworm, histoplasmosis, San Joaquin Valley fever, candidiasis
Protozoa	Simplest animal form, generally one-celled organisms	Malaria, amebic dysentery, trichomoniasis, vaginitis
Rickettsia	Viruslike organisms that require a host's living cells for growth and replication	Typhus, Rocky Mountain spotted fever, rickettsialpox
Parasitic worms	Many-celled organisms; represented by tape-worms, leeches, and roundworms	Dirofilariasis (dog heartworm), elephantiasis, onchocerciasis

such as a virus, bacterium, or fungus. When pathogens enter our bodies, they are sometimes able to resist body defense systems, flourish, and produce an illness. This is commonly called an *infection.* Because of their small size, pathogens are sometimes referred to as *microorganisms, microbes,* or *germs.* Table 12-1 describes the more familiar infectious disease agents and some of the illnesses they produce.

Chain of Infection

The transmission of a pathogenic agent through the various links in the chain of infection (Figure 12-1) forms the basis for an understanding of how diseases spread. However, not every pathogenic agent will move all the way through the chain of infection because various links in the chain can be broken. Therefore the presence of a pathogen creates only the potential for a disease.

Agent

The first link in the chain of infection is the disease-causing **agent.** Although some agents are very **virulent** and cause serious infectious illnesses such as HIV, which causes AIDS, others produce far less serious infections, such as the common cold. Through mutation (change), some pathogenic agents, particularly viruses, become more virulent than they once were.

Reservoir

Infectious agents must have the support and protection of a favorable environment to survive. This environment forms the second link in the chain of infection and is referred to as the *reservoir.* In many common infectious diseases, the reservoirs in which the pathogenic organisms live are the bodies of already infected people. Here the agents thrive before being spread to others. These infected people are the **hosts** for particular disease agents.

For other infectious diseases, the reservoirs in which the agents are maintained are the bodies of animals. Rabies is among the most familiar of the animal-reservoir diseases. Affected animals will not always be sick or show symptoms similar to those of an infected person.

The third type of reservoir in which disease-causing agents can reside is a nonliving environment, such as the soil. (The spores of the tetanus bacterium can survive in soil for up to 50 years, entering the human body in a puncture wound.) Warm and moist locker room floors are another example of this environment because the fungi that cause ringworm and jock itch can survive there.

Portal of exit

For pathogenic agents to cause diseases and illnesses in others, they must leave their reservoirs. The third link in the chain of infection is the portal of exit, or the point where agents leave their reservoirs.

In infectious diseases that involve human reservoirs, the principal portals of exit are familiar—the digestive system, the urinary system, the respiratory system, the reproductive system, and the blood.

Mode of transmission

The fourth link in the chain of infection is the mode of transmission, or the way that pathogens are passed from reservoirs to susceptible hosts. Two principal methods are *direct transmission* and *indirect transmission.*

Three types of direct transmission are observed in human-to-human transmission. These include *contact*

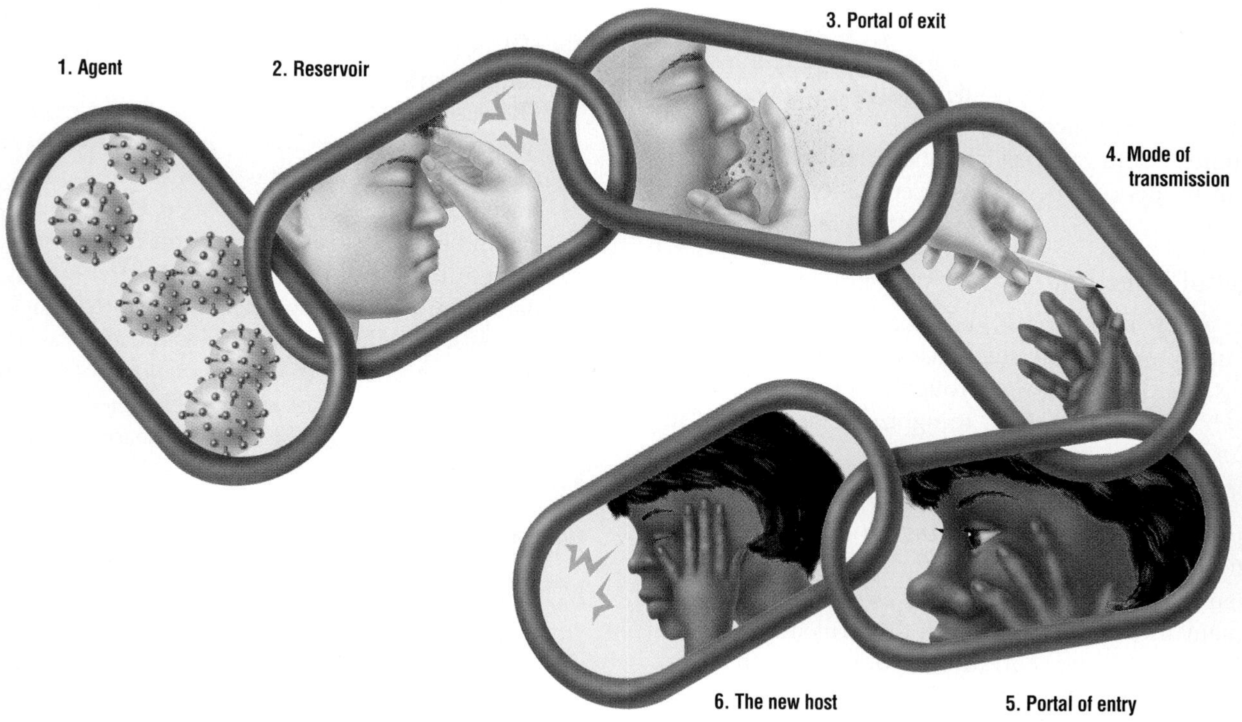

Figure 12-1 The six links in the chain of infection. The example above shows a rhinovirus, which causes the common cold, being passed from one person to another. I, The *agent* (pathogen) is a rhinovirus; 2, The *reservoir* is the infected person; 3, The *portal of exit* is the respiratory system (coughing); 4, The *mode of transmission* is indirect hand contact; 5, The *portal of entry* is the mucous membranes of the uninfected person's eye; 6, The virus now has a *new host.*

between body surfaces (such as kissing, touching, and sexual intercourse), *droplet spread* (inhalation of contaminated air droplets), and *fecal-oral spread* (feces on the hands are brought into contact with the mouth).

Indirect transmission occurs between infected and uninfected people when infectious agents travel by means of nonhuman materials. Vehicles of transmission include *inanimate objects,* such as water, food items, soil, towels, clothing, and eating utensils.

A second method of indirect transmission of infectious agents occurs in conjunction with vectors. The term *vector* is related to living things, such as insects, birds, and other animals that carry diseases from human to human. An example of a vector is the deer tick that transmits Lyme disease.

Airborne indirect transmission involves the *inhalation* (breathing in) of infected particles that have been suspended in an air source for an extended period. Unlike droplet transmission, in which both infected and uninfected people must be in close physical proximity, noninfected people can become infected through airborne transmission by sharing air with infected people who were in the same room hours earlier. Viral infections such as German measles may be spread in this manner.

Portal of entry

The fifth link in the chain of infection is the portal of entry. As with the portals of exit, there are three primary portals of entry for pathogenic agents to enter the bodies of uninfected people. These are the digestive system, the respiratory system, and the reproductive system. In addition, a break in the skin provides another portal of entry. In most infectious conditions the portals of entry are within the same system as the portals of exit. In the case of HIV, however, cross-system transmission occurs. Oral and anal sex allow for infectious agents to pass between the warm, moist tissues of the reproductive system and those of the digestive system.

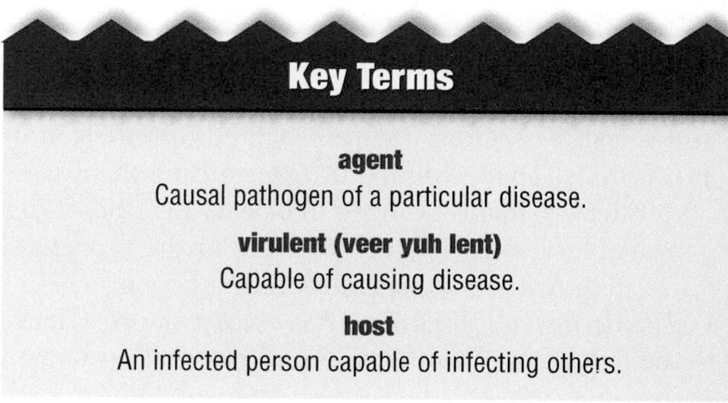

Key Terms

agent
Causal pathogen of a particular disease.

virulent (veer yuh lent)
Capable of causing disease.

host
An infected person capable of infecting others.

The new host

In theory, all people are at risk for contracting infectious diseases and so can be considered as susceptible hosts. In practice, however, factors such as overall health, acquired immunity, health care services, and health-related behavior can influence a person's susceptibility to infectious diseases.

Stages of Infection

When a new host is assaulted by a pathogenic agent, a reasonably predictable sequence of events takes place. That is, the disease moves through five rather distinctive stages.[1] You may be able to recognize these stages of infection each time you catch a cold.

1. *The incubation stage.* This stage lasts from the time a pathogen enters your body until it multiplies enough to produce signs and symptoms of the disease. The length of this stage can vary from a few hours to many months, depending on the virulence of the organisms, the concentration of organisms, the host's (your) level of immune responsiveness, and other health problems you may have. This stage has been called a *silent stage.* Transmission of the pathogen to a new host is possible but not probable during this stage: a host may be infected during this stage but not infectious. HIV infection is an exception to this rule.
2. *The prodromal stage.* The incubation stage is followed by a short period during which you may experience a variety of general signs and symptoms, including watery eyes, runny nose, slight fever, and overall tiredness. These symptoms are nonspecific and may not be strong enough to force you to rest. During this stage the pathogenic agent continues to multiply. Now you (the host) can transfer pathogens to a new host. In fact, because the activity level of the host is generally not restricted and you may still feel well, some believe that this stage is as infective as is the clinical or acute stage. Self-imposed isolation should be practiced during this stage to protect others. Again, HIV infection is different in regard to this stage.
3. *The clinical stage.* This stage, also called the *acme* or *acute stage,* is often the most unpleasant stage for you, the host. At this time the disease reaches its highest point of development. All of the clinical (observable) signs and symptoms for the particular disease can be seen or analyzed by appropriate laboratory tests. The likelihood of transmitting the disease to others is highest during this peak stage; all of our available defense mechanisms are in the process of resisting further damage from the pathogen.
4. *The decline stage.* During this stage, you experience the first signs of recovery. The infection is ending or, in some cases, being reduced to a subclinical level. Relapse may occur if you overextend yourself. In HIV and AIDS, this is almost always the last stage before death.
5. *The recovery stage.* Also called the *convalescence stage,* this stage is characterized by apparent recovery from the invading agent. Disease transmission during this stage is possible but not probable. Until your overall health has been strengthened, you may be especially susceptible to another (perhaps different) disease pathogen. Fortunately, after the recovery stage, further susceptibility to the pathogenic agent should be reduced because of the body's buildup of immunity. Such immunity is not always permanent; for example, many sexually transmitted diseases can be contracted repeatedly.

BODY DEFENSES: MECHANICAL AND CELLULAR IMMUNE SYSTEMS

Much as a military installation is protected by a series of defensive alignments, so too is the body. These defenses can be classified as mechanical or cellular (Figure 12-2). *Mechanical defenses* are first-line defenses. They physically separate the internal body from the external environment. Examples are the skin, the mucous membranes that line the respiratory and gastrointestinal tracts, earwax, the tiny hairs and cilia that filter incoming air, and even tears. These defenses serve primarily as a shield against foreign materials that may contain pathogenic agents. They can, however, be disarmed, as happens when tobacco smoke kills the cilia that protect the airway, resulting in chronic bronchitis, or when contact lenses decrease tearing, leading to irritation and eye infection.

The second component of the body's protective defenses is the *cellular* system or, more commonly, the **immune system.** In comparison with the mechanical defenses, this cell-based component is far more specific. Its primary purpose is to eliminate microorganisms, foreign proteins, and cells foreign to the body. A wellness-oriented lifestyle, including sound nutrition, effective stress management, and regular exercise, strengthens this important division of the immune system. The microorganism, foreign proteins, or abnormal cells whose presence activates this cellular component are identified collectively as *antigens.*[2]

Divisions of the Immune System

Closer examination of the immune system, or cellular defenses, reveals two separate but highly cooperative groups of cells. One group of cells has its origins in the fetal thymus gland. It produces *T cell–mediated immunity,* or simply cell-mediated immunity. The second group of cells consists of the B cells (bursa of Fabricius),

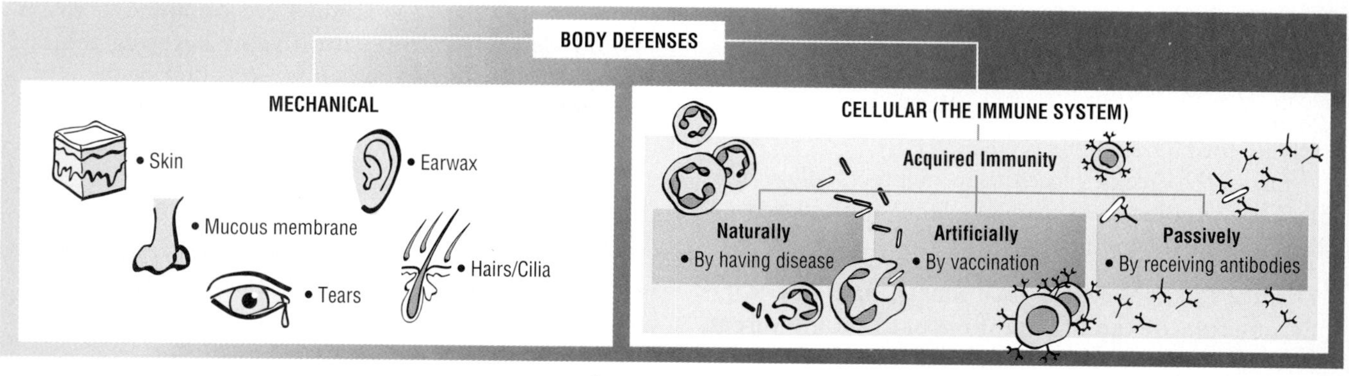

Figure 12-2 The body has a variety of defenses against invading organisms. Mechanical defenses are the first means of protection, since they separate the internal body from the external environment. Cellular defenses include chemicals and specialized cells that provide immunity to subsequent infections.

which are the working units of *humoral immunity.*[2] Cellular elements of both cell-mediated and humoral immunity are found in the bloodstream, the lymphatic tissues of the body, and the fluid that surrounds body cells.

Although you were born with the structural elements of both cell-mediated and humoral immunity, for you to develop an immune response, the components of these cellular systems had to encounter and successfully defend against specific antigens. Once this occurred, your immune system was primed to respond quickly and effectively if the same antigens were encountered again. This confrontation resulted in the development of a state of **acquired immunity (AI).** As seen in Figure 12-2, the development of AI can occur in different ways.

- **Naturally acquired immunity (NAI)** occurs when the body is exposed to infectious agents. When you catch an infectious disease, you fight the infection and in the process become immune (protected) from developing that illness again.
- **Artificially acquired immunity (AAI)** occurs when your body is exposed to weakened or killed infectious agents introduced through vaccination or immunization. As in NAI, the body engages the infectious agents and remembers how to fight the same battle again. A Recommended Childhood Immunization Schedule for children birth through 16 years is available from the American Academy of Pediatrics (AAP) **www.aap.org/family/parents/immunize.htm.**[3,4] Adults with questions about their immunization status or required immunizations for travel abroad should consult their primary care physicians.
- **Passively acquired immunity (PAI)** results when antibodies are introduced into the body. These antibodies, for a variety of specific infections, are produced outside the body (either in animals or by the genetic manipulation of microorganisms). When introduced into the human body, they provide immediate protection until a more natural form of immunity can be developed.

Collectively, these three forms of immunity can provide important protection against infectious disease.

IMMUNIZATIONS

Although the incidence of several childhood communicable diseases is at or near the lowest level ever, the risk of a resurgence of diseases such as measles, polio, diphtheria, and rubella is very real. This possible upturn in childhood infectious diseases could be prevented if parents ensured

Key Terms

immune system
System of cellular elements that protects the body from invading pathogens and foreign materials.

acquired immunity (AI)
The "arming" of the immune system through its intial exposure to an antigen.

naturally acquired immunity (NAI)
Type of acquired immunity resulting from the body's response to naturally occurring pathogens.

artificially acquired immunity (AAI)
Type of acquired immunity resulting from the body's response to pathogens introduced into the body through immunizations.

passively acquired immunity (PAI)
Temporary immunity achieved by providing antibodies to a person exposed to a particular pathogen.

that their children were fully immunized. Overall, about 90% of children receive all necessary immunizations. There are regional variations in the level of immunization, and some racial/ethnic groups are below this overall level (see the Focus on box on p. 309).

Currently, vaccines against several potentially serious infectious conditions are available and should be given. These include the following:

- *Diphtheria:* a potentially fatal illness that leads to inflammation of the membranes that line the throat, swollen lymph nodes, and heart and kidney failure
- *Whooping cough:* a bacterial infection of the airways and lungs that results in deep, noisy breathing and coughing
- *Hepatitis B:* a viral infection that can be transmitted sexually or through the exchange of blood or body fluids and causes serious liver damage
- *Haemophilus influenzae type B:* a bacterial infection that can damage the heart and brain, resulting in meningitis, and can also produce profound hearing loss
- *Tetanus:* a fatal infection caused by bacteria found in the soil that damages the central nervous system
- *Rubella (German measles):* a viral infection of the upper respiratory tract that can cause damage to a developing fetus when the mother contracts the infection during the first trimester of pregnancy
- *Measles (red measles):* a highly contagious viral infection leading to a rash, high fever, and other upper respiratory tract symptoms
- *Polio:* a viral infection capable of causing paralysis of the large muscles of the extremities
- *Mumps:* a viral infection of the salivary glands
- *Chicken pox:* a varicella zoster virus spread by airborne droplets leading to a sore throat, rash, and fluid-filled blisters

Parents of a newborn should take their infant to their family care physician, pediatrician, or well-baby clinic (operated by county health departments) to begin the immunization schedule. The development of new vaccines and the evaluation of currently used vaccines are ongoing processes for preventing infectious diseases in this country. Even the immunization schedule now being used is likely to undergo slight modification. For example, in December of 1999, the American Academy of Pediatrics recommended that the use of oral polio vaccine (OPV), which is made with weakened or attenuated virus, no long be administered. Also, a vaccine against the rotavirus associated with serious childhood diarrhea, only recently approved, has been withdrawn because of safety concerns. On a more positive note, a new vaccine against the bacterium that causes pneumococcal pneumonia in children has received a supportive recommendation from an advisory panel of the FDA. This newly recommended vaccine could also prove to be effective in lowering the incidence of otitis media, a painful infection of the middle ear that commonly develops in infants and younger children.

TALKING POINTS • Through community service work, you meet a couple who say they have not had their children immunized. Would you try to change their minds or notify your local health department?

THE IMMUNE RESPONSE

To fully understand the function of the immune system, a substantial knowledge of human biology is required, and this is beyond the scope of this text. Figure 12-3 provides a simplified view of the immune response.

When antigens—microorganisms, foreign substances, or abnormal cells—are discovered within the body, some antigens are confronted by various types of white blood cells and their number is initially reduced by the destructive action of these blood cells. At the same time, macrophages (a very large white blood cell) encounter other antigens and signal components of cell-mediated immunity called *helper T cells* to assist in the immune response.

Once activated by the presence of the macrophage/antigens complex, helper T cells notify a second component of cellular immunity, the *killer T cells,* and a component of humoral immunity, *B cells.* Killer T cells produce powerful chemical messengers that activate specific white blood cells that are capable of destroying antigens. At the same time, B cells, with the assistance of helper T-cells, are transformed into plasma cells capable of producing **antibodies** and into memory cells, which record information pertaining to the antigen and the appropriate immune system response.

While the helper T cells and killer T cells are engaged in destroying invading antigens, two additional components of cellular immunity are formed: memory T cells and suppressor T cells. As the name suggests, the memory T cells remember additional aspects of the immune system's responses so that reinfections can be encountered even more quickly and decisively. Suppressor T cells are specialized T cells that moderate B cell activity by offsetting the action of helper T cells. Their action allows the production of antibodies to be reduced once it is apparent that the immune system has won its battle.

Clearly, without a normal immune system involving both cellular and humoral elements, we would quickly become the victims of serious and life-shortening infections and malignancies. As you will see later, this is exactly what occurs in virtually all people infected with HIV.

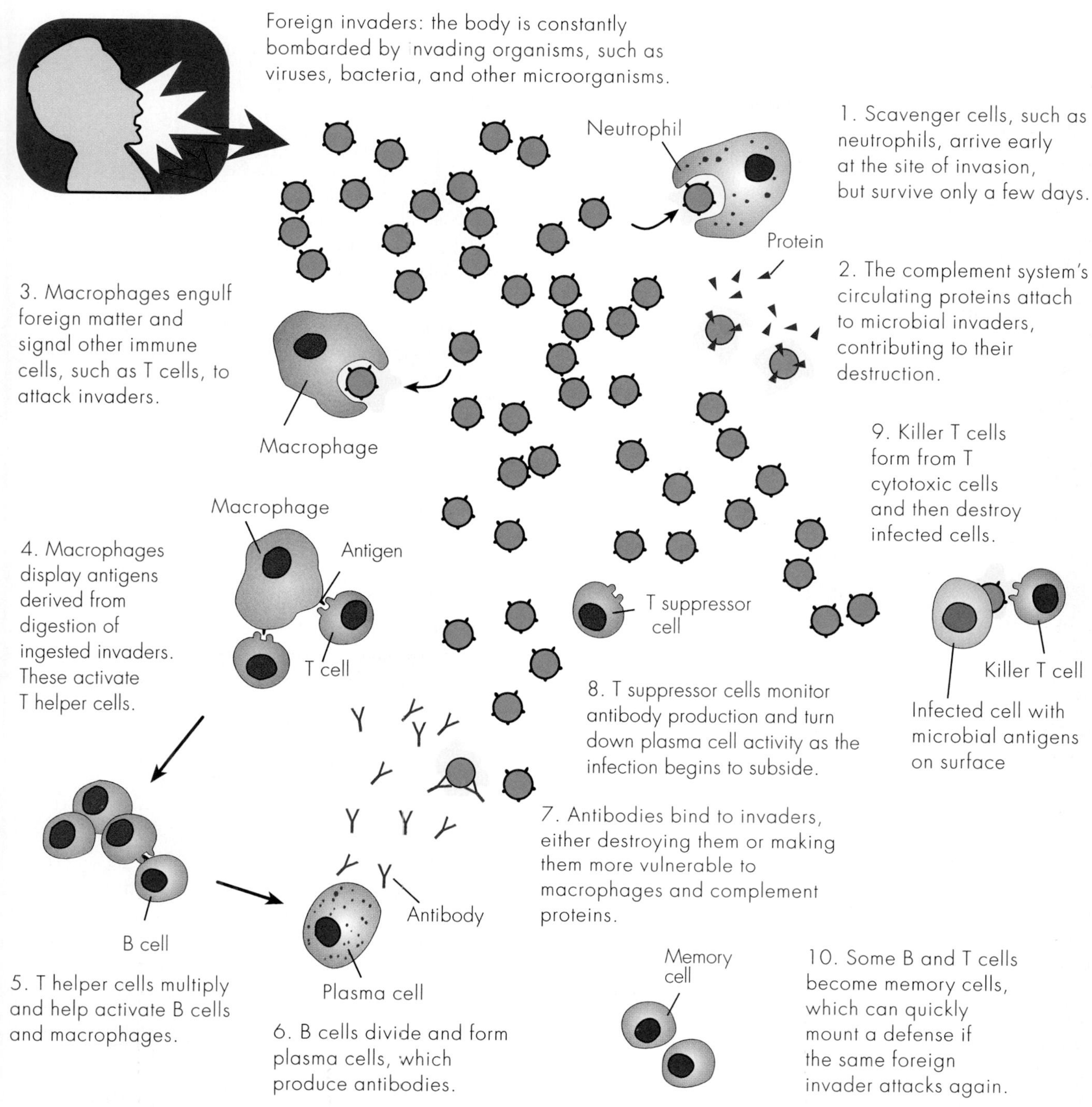

Foreign invaders: the body is constantly bombarded by invading organisms, such as viruses, bacteria, and other microorganisms.
Neutrophil
1. Scavenger cells, such as neutrophils, arrive early at the site of invasion, but survive only a few days.
Protein
2. The complement system's circulating proteins attach to microbial invaders, contributing to their destruction.
3. Macrophages engulf foreign matter and signal other immune cells, such as T cells, to attack invaders.
Macrophage
9. Killer T cells form from T cytotoxic cells and then destroy infected cells.
Macrophage
Antigen
4. Macrophages display antigens derived from digestion of ingested invaders. These activate T helper cells.
T cell
T suppressor cell
Killer T cell
Infected cell with microbial antigens on surface
8. T suppressor cells monitor antibody production and turn down plasma cell activity as the infection begins to subside.
7. Antibodies bind to invaders, either destroying them or making them more vulnerable to macrophages and complement proteins.
Antibody
B cell
Plasma cell
Memory cell
5. T helper cells multiply and help activate B cells and macrophages.
6. B cells divide and form plasma cells, which produce antibodies.
10. Some B and T cells become memory cells, which can quickly mount a defense if the same foreign invader attacks again.

Figure 12-3 Biological warfare. The body commands an army of defenders to reduce the danger of infection and guard against repeat infections. Antigens are the ultimate targets of all immune responses.

CAUSES AND MANAGEMENT OF SELECTED INFECTIOUS DISEASES

This section focuses on some of the common infectious diseases and some that, although less common, are serious. This information provides reference points you can use to judge your own disease susceptibility.

Key Term

antibodies
Chemical compounds produced by the body's immune system to destroy antigens and their toxins.

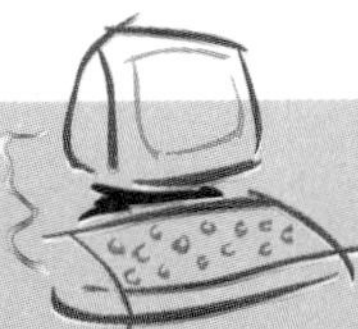

OnSITE/InSIGHT

Learning to Go: Health

What's your best defense against infectious disease? Click on the Motivator icon to find these lessons, which will show you how to protect yourself:

Lesson 36: Protect yourself from infections.
Lesson 37: Practice safe sex.

STUDENT POLL

Are you up to date on infectious diseases? Visit the Online Learning Center at **www.mhhe.com/hahn6e**. Click on Student Resources to find the Student Poll. There you can answer the following questions. When you're finished, see how others responded.

1. Are you more concerned about infectious diseases since starting college?
2. Do you practice safe sex?
3. Have you ever had a sexually transmitted disease?
4. Are you concerned about contracting HIV or AIDS?
5. Do you often get colds?
6. Do you have at least one bout with the flu every year?
7. Do you wash your hands frequently?
8. Have you ever had chickenpox?
9. Does it concern you that meningitis is common among college-age people?
10. Have you ever suffered from mononucleosis ("mono")?
11. Are you tested for TB on a regular basis?
12. Have you been immunized against hepatitis B?
13. Have you ever had pneumonia?
14. If you're often tired, do you think you might have chronic fatigue syndrome?
15. Do you think that your immune system is strong?

The Common Cold

The common cold, an acute upper respiratory tract infection, is humankind's supreme infectious disease. Also known as **acute rhinitis,** this highly contagious viral infection can be caused by any of the nearly 200 known rhinoviruses. Colds are particularly common during periods when people spend time in crowded indoor environments, such as classrooms.

The signs and symptoms of a cold are fairly predictable. Runny nose, watery eyes, general aches and pains, a listless feeling, and a slight fever may all accompany a cold in its early stages. Eventually the nasal passages swell, and the inflammation may spread to the throat. Stuffy nose, sore throat, and coughing may follow. The senses of taste and smell are blocked, and the appetite declines.

With the onset of symptoms, management of a cold should begin promptly. After a few days, most of the cold's symptoms subside. In the meantime, you should isolate yourself from others, drink plenty of fluids, eat moderately, and rest. Keep in mind that antibiotics are effective only against bacterial infections—not viral infections such as colds.

Management of a cold can be aided by using some of the many OTC cold remedies. These remedies will not cure your cold but may lessen the discomfort associated with it. Nasal decongestants, expectorants, cough syrups, and aspirin or acetaminophen can all provide some temporary relief. Use of some of these products for more than a few days is not recommended, however, since a rebound effect may occur.

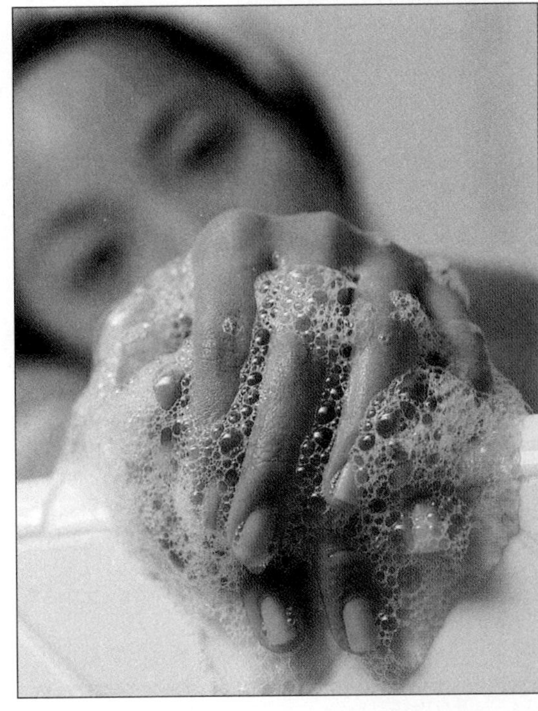

Washing your hands often is the best way to prevent the common cold.

If a cold appears to become more persistent—as evidenced by prolonged chills, noticeable fever above 103° F, chest heaviness or aches, shortness of breath, coughing up rust-colored mucus, or persistent sore throat or hoarseness—contact a physician. Also, it is now recognized that a certain virus associated with the common cold can result in a rare form of potentially serious heart dysfunction. Therefore, if you are not feeling back to normal after having had a cold for 2 to 4 weeks, you should contact a physician.[5]

Preventing colds is almost impossible. Since colds are now thought to be transmitted most readily by hand contact, frequent handwashing and the use of tissues are recommended.

Influenza

Influenza is also an acute, contagious disease caused by viruses. Some influenza outbreaks have produced widespread death, as seen in the influenza pandemics of 1889 to 1890, 1918 to 1919, and 1957. The viral strains that produce this infectious disease have the potential for more severe complications than the viral strains that produce the common cold. The viral strain for a particular form of influenza enters the body through the respiratory tract. After brief incubation and prodromal stages, the host develops signs and symptoms not just in the upper respiratory tract but throughout the entire body. These symptoms include fever, chills, cough, sore throat, headache, gastrointestinal disturbances, and muscular pain. Physicians may recommend only aspirin, fluids, and rest. Parents are reminded not to give aspirin to children.

In recent years, several antiviral medications have been developed to reduce the duration of flu symptoms. Vaccines against various strains of the flu have also been in development. A newly developed oral medication (Tamiflu) has shown the ability to reduce the degree of viral activity within the body and reduce associated symptoms of the flu when administered immediately before and immediately after exposure to a particular flu virus.[6] Another recently developed medication, (Relenza) delivered by nasal inhalation, has shown a protective effect during the course of a single flu season in much the same way that the injectable flu vaccines do.[7] All flu vaccines must be accurately formulated to match the viruses expected to be prevalent during an upcoming flu season. Both the oral medication and the inhalation medication described are now available. (See Table 12-2 for a comparison of influenza with the common cold.)

Most young adults can cope with the milder strains of influenza that are prevalent each winter or spring. However, pregnant women and older people—especially older people with additional health complications—are not so capable of handling this viral attack. They may quickly develop secondary bacterial complications, especially pneumonia, which can prove fatal. Flu vaccinations are routinely recommended for older people, but they have also proved effective for younger adults.

Table 12-2 Is It a Cold or the Flu?

	Cold	Flu
Symptoms		
Fever	Rare	Characteristic, high (102°–104° + F); lasts 3–4 days
Headache	Rare	Prominent
General aches, pains	Slight	Usual; often severe
Fatigue, weakness	Quite mild	Can last up to 2–3 weeks
Extreme exhaustion	Never	Early and prominent
Stuffy nose	Common	Sometimes
Sneezing	Usual	Sometimes
Sore throat	Common	Sometimes
Chest discomfort, cough	Mild to moderate; hacking cough	Common; can become severe
Complications	Sinus congestion, earache	Pneumonia, bronchitis; can be life threatening
Prevention	Avoidance of infected people	Annual vaccination; amantadine or rimantadine (antiviral drugs)
Treatment	Temporary relief	Amantadine or rimantadine within 24–48 hours after onset of symptoms

Tuberculosis

Until the mid-1980s, TB, a bacterial infection of the lungs resulting in chronic coughing, weight loss, and even death, was considered to be under control in the United States. Then, however, an upsurge in cases occurred, with a peak of 26,283 cases in 1992. Since that time, a decline has been noted, with 7% fewer cases between 1995 (22,860) and 1996 (21,327).[8] Another decline was noted for 1997, the most recent year for which data are available. However, immigration of people from areas of the world in which TB is more prevalent and the emergence of drug-resistant strains of the bacterium require that greater attention be paid to this infectious disease. Today, for example, the epidemic spread of TB in Russia is being watched closely. The 2 million new cases reported in Russia during 1999, many involving drug-resistant bacterial strains, will make Europe and North America vulnerable in a very short time.

Key Term

acute rhinitis
The common cold; the sudden onset of nasal inflammation.

Because TB is spread through coughing, the disease thrives in crowded places, where infected people are in constant contact with others. Prisons, hospitals, public housing units, and college residence halls are places where close day-to-day contact occurs. In such settings a single infected person can spread the TB agents to many others.

When healthy people are exposed to TB agents, their immune systems generally are able to contain the bacteria to prevent the development of symptoms and to reduce the likelihood of infecting others. However, when the immune system is damaged, such as in the elderly, the malnourished, and those who are infected with HIV, the disease can become established and may eventually be transmitted to other people at risk.

Multiple drug–resistant (MDR) TB has been reported as 2% of all TB cases. Increasingly prevalent in this country, MDR TB is the result of patients' inability to follow their physicians' instructions (for various reasons) when initially treated, inadequate treatment by physicians, and increased exposure of HIV-infected people to TB. Only 50% of people with this form of TB can be cured.

Health officials are again requesting that TB testing programs be implemented. They are also recommending that those infected, once identified, be isolated and closely supervised during the entire 6 to 8 months of treatment required for complete recovery. New diagnostic tests have been developed and should result in more prompt treatment and effective control of the transmission of the disease.

Pneumonia

Pneumonia is a general term used for a variety of infectious respiratory conditions. Bacterial, viral, fungal, rickettsial, mycoplasmal, and parasitic forms of pneumonia exist.[9] However, bacterial pneumonia is the most common form. It is often seen in conjunction with other illnesses that weaken the body's immune system. This is why even healthy young people should consider colds and flu as potentially serious and treat them properly. In fact, pneumonia is so common in the frail elderly that it is often the specific condition causing death. *Pneumocystis carinii* pneumonia, a parasitic form, is of great importance today, since it is a principal opportunistic infection associated with the diagnosis of AIDS in HIV-infected people.

Among older adults with a history of chronic obstructive lung disease, cardiovascular disease, diabetes, or alcoholism, a midwinter form of pneumonia known as *acute community-acquired pneumonia* is often a serious health problem.[9] The sudden onset of chills, chest pain, and a cough producing sputum are characteristics of this condition. Additionally, a symptom-free form of pneumonia known as *walking pneumonia* is also commonly seen in adults and can become serious without warning. Individuals with any of these illnesses should be watched carefully during the high-risk season of the year and provided with effective treatment if symptoms develop.

Mononucleosis

Of all the common infectious diseases that a college student can contract, **mononucleosis ("mono")** can force a lengthy period of bed rest during a semester or quarter when it can least be afforded. Other common diseases that are likely to affect you can be managed with minimal amounts of disruption. However, the overall weakness and fatigue seen in many people with mono sometimes require 1 or 2 months of rest and recuperation.

Mono is a viral infection in which the body produces an excessive number of mononuclear leukocytes (a type of white blood cell). After uncertain, perhaps lengthy, incubation and prodromal stages, the acute symptoms of mono can appear, including weakness, headache, low-grade fever, swollen lymph glands (especially in the neck), and sore throat. Mental fatigue and depression are sometimes reported as side effects of mononucleosis. Usually after the acute symptoms disappear, the weakness and fatigue remain—perhaps for a few months. Mono is diagnosed on the basis of characteristic symptoms. Also, the Monospot blood smear can be used to determine the prevalence of abnormal white blood cells. In addition, an antibody test can detect activity of the immune system that is characteristic of the illness.

Since mononucleosis is caused by a virus (Epstein-Barr virus), antibiotic therapy is not recommended. Treatment most often includes bed rest and the use of OTC remedies for fever (aspirin or acetaminophen) and sore throat (lozenges). In extreme cases, corticosteroid drugs can be used. Appropriate fluid intake and a well-balanced diet are also important in the recovery stages of mono. Fortunately, the body tends to develop NAI to the mono virus, so subsequent infections of mono are unusual.

For years, mono has been labeled the "kissing disease"; however, mono is not highly contagious and is known to be spread by direct transmission in ways other than kissing. No vaccine has been developed to confer AAI for mononucleosis. The best preventive measures include the steps that you can take to increase your resistance to most infectious diseases: (1) eat a well-balanced diet, (2) exercise regularly, (3) sleep sufficiently, (4) use health care services appropriately, (5) live in a reasonably healthful environment, and (6) avoid direct contact with infected people.

Chronic Fatigue Syndrome

Perhaps the most perplexing "infectious" condition seen by physicians is **chronic fatigue syndrome (CFS).** First identified in 1985, this mononucleosis-like condition is most commonly seen in women in their thirties and forties. People with CFS, many of whom are busy professional people, report flu-like symptoms, including severe exhaustion, fatigue, headaches, muscle aches, fever, inability to concentrate, allergies, intolerance to exercise, and depression. Examinations done on the first people with CFS revealed antibodies to the Epstein-Barr virus. Thus it was assumed to be an infectious viral disease (and initially called *chronic Epstein-Barr syndrome*).

Since its first appearance, the condition has received a great deal of attention regarding its exact nature. Today, opinions vary widely as to whether the condition is a specific viral infection, a condition involving both viral infections and nonviral components, or some other disorder.[10]

In recent years it has been noted that another chronic condition, fibromyalgia, appears in a manner similar to CFS. As in CFS, the person with fibromyalgia demonstrates fatigue, inefficient sleep patterns, localized areas of tenderness and pain, morning stiffness, and headaches. The onset of this condition, like that of CFS, can follow periods of stress, infectious disease, physical trauma such as falls, thyroid dysfunction, or in conjunction with a connective tissue disorder.[11] Therefore some clinicians believe that the two conditions might be very closely related,[12] drawing on an explanation based on immune system involvement.

Regardless of its cause or causes, CFS is extremely unpleasant for its victims. Certainly, those experiencing the symptoms over an extended time need to be seen by a physician experienced in dealing with CFS.

Measles

Previously thought to be only a childhood disease, *red measles* (also called **rubeola** or *common measles*) has recently been seen in large numbers on some American college campuses. Red measles is the highly contagious type of measles characterized by a short-lived, relatively high fever (103° to 104° F) and a whole-body red spotty rash that lasts about a week. The other type of measles, German measles (**rubella,** or 3-day measles), is a much milder form that has serious implications for newborn babies of mothers who contracted this disease during pregnancy. Highly successful vaccines are now available for both varieties of measles and are usually given in the same injection. Women should receive these vaccinations before they become pregnant.

The outbreak of red measles among college students during the early 1990s points to the fact that our society mistakenly believes that most infectious diseases have now been eliminated. Public health experts now realize that those who contracted the disease either had never been vaccinated or had been vaccinated with a killed variety vaccine used before 1969. Only students who had already had red measles as children or who had been vaccinated with a live virus were guaranteed full immunity against the red measles virus. Nontraditional college students in particular should attempt to determine whether their immunization status is based on use of the older, less effective vaccine.

Today, most public school systems are requiring documented proof of immunization from a physician or clinic before children can attend classes. As an educated parent, you should be conscientious about adhering to immunization schedules for your children. In fact, measles immunization efforts have increased so effectively because of school and public health department involvement that the number of measles cases fell from 55,000 cases between 1989 and 1991 to 488 cases in 1996. Most recently (1998), only 100 cases of measles were reported, and many of these cases were among visitors to the United States.[13]

Bacterial Meningitis

Over the last few years, a formerly infrequently seen, but potentially fatal infectious disease, meningococcal meningitis, has appeared on college campuses suggesting that college students are currently at greater risk of contracting the disease than their noncollege peers.[14] Particularly interesting is the fact that among college students, the risk of contracting this infection on campus appears to be highest for those students living in residence halls, suggesting that close living quarters, as well as smoking and alcohol consumption, favors transmission of the bacteria.

Meningococcal meningitis is a bacterial infection of the thin membranous coverings of the brain. In its earliest stages, this disease can easily be confused with the flu. Symptoms usually include a high fever, severe headache, stiff neck, nausea with vomiting, extreme tiredness, and the formation of a progressive rash. For about 10% of people who develop this condition, the infection is fatal, often within 24 hours. Therefore the mere presence of the symptoms described above signals the need for immediate medical evaluation. If done promptly, treatment is

Key Terms

mononucleosis ("mono")
Viral infection characterized by weakness, fatigue, swollen glands, sore throat, and low-grade fever.

chronic fatigue syndrome (CFS)
Illness that causes severe exhaustion, fatigue, aches, and depression; mostly affects women in their thirties and forties.

rubeola (roo BE oh luh)
Red or common measles.

rubella
German or 3-day measles.

highly effective. In response to the increasing incidence of this infection on college campuses, impetus is growing for the immunization of incoming college students, although immunization does not provide complete protection.[15]

Lyme Disease

An infectious disease that is becoming increasingly common in Eastern, Southeastern, upper Midwestern, and West Coast states is **Lyme disease,** with 16,273 cases reported in 1999. This bacterial disease results when infected deer ticks, usually in the nymph (immature) state, attach to the skin and inject the infectious agent as they feed on the host's blood. Deer ticks become infected by feeding on infected white-tailed deer or white-footed mice.

The symptoms of Lyme disease are variable, but they generally first appear within 30 days as small red bumps surrounded by a circular red rash at the site of bites. During this phase I stage, flu-like symptoms may appear, including chills, headaches, muscle and joint aches, and low-grade fever. For approximately 20% of infected people, a phase II stage develops in which nervous system or heart disorders may occur. For affected people who still remain untreated, a phase III stage can develop in which chronic arthritis, lasting up to 2 years, can occur. Fortunately, Lyme disease can be treated with antibiotics. However, no immunity develops, so subsequent infections can occur. The ability to diagnose the presence of Lyme disease in children may be more difficult than for adults. For adults who are at high risk for tick bites, a three-step immunization (LYMErix) should be considered (although it is not effective for everyone). Most recently, progress has been made in improving the accuracy and speed of the diagnostic test for Lyme disease so that treatment can be started as quickly as possible.[16]

For people living in high-risk areas, outdoor activities can expose them to the nearly invisible tick nymphs that have fallen from deer into the grass. So people who are active outdoors should check themselves frequently to be sure that they are tick-free. Shirts should be tucked into pants, pants tucked into socks, and gloves and hats worn when possible. It is also helpful to shower after coming in from outdoors and to check clothing for evidence of ticks. Pets can also carry infected ticks into the house. If ticks are found, they should be carefully removed from the skin with tweezers and the affected area washed. A physician should be consulted if you notice symptoms or if you are concerned that you might have been exposed.

The tick that carries Lyme disease has also been responsible for a potentially fatal bacterial infection, *human granulocytic ehrlichiosis* (HGE). This disease is associated with high fever, headache, muscle aches, and chills. HGE is successfully treated with doxycycline, an antibiotic that can also be used in the treatment of Lyme disease. People with these symptoms, particularly "outdoor people" and those living in areas of the country where Lyme disease is reported, should make certain that HGE is also considered in the diagnosis and treatment of their symptoms.

TALKING POINTS • You suspect that you have Lyme disease, but your doctor thinks that this is highly unlikely and is not investigating this possibility. How would you go about convincing her to test you?

Hantavirus Pulmonary Syndrome

Since 1993, a small but rapidly growing number of people have died of extreme pulmonary distress caused by the leakage of plasma into the lungs. In all of the initial cases, the people living in the Southwest, had been well until they began developing flu-like symptoms over 1 or 2 days, then quickly experienced difficulty breathing, and died only hours later. Epidemiologists quickly suspected a viral agent such as the hantavirus known to exist in Asia and, to a lesser degree, in Europe. Exhaustive laboratory work led to the culturing of the virus and confirmed that all of the victims had been infected with an American version of the hantavirus. The latest infectious condition, *hantavirus pulmonary syndrome,* was identified.[17]

Today, this hantavirus disease has been reported in areas beyond the Southwest, including most of the Western states and some of the Eastern states. The common denominator in all areas in which the hantavirus infection has occurred is the presence of deer mice. It is now known that this common rodent serves as the reservoir for the virus.

The mode of transmission of the virus from deer mice to humans involves the inhalation of dust contaminated with dried virus-rich rodent urine or saliva-contaminated materials, such as nests. In areas with deer mouse populations (most of the United States), health experts are now warning people to be extremely careful when cleaning houses and barns in which deer mouse droppings are likely to be found. If it is necessary to remove rodent nests, wear rubber gloves, pour Lysol or bleach on the nests and soak them thoroughly, pick up nests with shovels, and then burn them or bury them several feet deep in the ground. The first case of human-to-human transmission of hantavirus was reported in Argentina. Eighteen people were infected, including physicians who were caring for patients, and nine of them died.

There is no vaccine for hantavirus pulmonary syndrome, but the illness is currently recognized more quickly. Since the importance of early evaluation of flu-like symptoms is now understood, the death rate has begun to fall. In 1998, sixteen new cases of hantavirus were investigated in the Four Corners area of the American Southwest.[18]

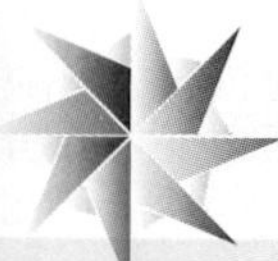

Signs and Symptoms of Toxic Shock Syndrome

- Fever (102° F or above)
- Headache
- Vomiting
- Sore throat
- Diarrhea
- Muscle aches
- Sunburnlike rash
- Low blood pressure
- Bloodshot eyes
- Disorientation
- Reduced urination
- Peeling of skin on the palms and soles of the feet

Toxic Shock Syndrome

Toxic shock syndrome (TSS), first reported in 1978, made front-page headlines in 1980, when it was reported by the CDC that there was a connection between TSS and the presence of a specific bacterial agent (*Staphylococcus aureus*) in the vagina and the use of tampons.

TSS is characterized by the signs and symptoms listed in the Star Box above. Superabsorbent varieties of tampons apparently can irritate the vaginal lining three times more quickly than regular tampons. This vaginal irritation is enhanced when the tampons remain in the vagina for a long time (over 5 hours). Once this irritation has begun, the staphylococcal bacteria (which are commonly present in the vagina) have relatively easy access to the bloodstream. Proliferation of these bacteria in the circulatory system and their resultant toxins produce TSS. Left untreated, the victim can die—usually as a result of cardiovascular failure. Currently, only about 5% of women diagnosed as having TSS die from the condition.

Although the extent of this disease is still quite limited (only about 3 to 6 cases per 100,000 women per year) and the mortality figures are low (comparable with those in women who use oral contraceptives), each woman should show reasonable caution in using tampons. Recommendations are that (1) tampons should not be the sole form of sanitary protection used, and (2) tampons should not be in place for too long. Women should change tampons every few hours and intermittently use sanitary napkins. Tampons should not be used during sleep.

The incidence of TSS has dropped significantly since the early 1980s. Possible reasons for this decrease are the removal of some superabsorbent tampons from the market and the standardization of the labels for junior, super, and super-plus tampons that began in 1990. However, the CDC still reports about 1,300 cases of TSS per year and suggests that this number may be substanially underreported.

Hepatitis

Hepatitis is an inflammatory process of the liver that can be caused by several viruses. Types A, B (once called non-A), C (once called non-B), D, and E have been recognized. Hepatitis can also be caused indirectly from abuse of alcohol and other drugs. General symptoms of hepatitis include fever, nausea, loss of appetite, abdominal pain, and jaundice (yellowing of the skin and eyes).

Type A hepatitis is often associated with consuming fecal-contaminated water or food, such as raw shellfish. Poor sanitation, particularly in the handling of food and diaper-changing activities has produced outbreaks in child-care centers. Experts estimate that up to 200,000 people per year are infected. In 1995, the FDA approved a vaccine for hepatitis type A.

TALKING POINTS • You've noticed that one of your restaurant coworkers doesn't wash her hands after using the restroom. Would you say something to her about this or notify the manager?

Type B hepatitis (HBV) is spread in various ways, including sexual contact, intravenous drug use, tattooing, and medical and dental procedures. Chronic HBV infection has been associated with liver cirrhosis and liver cancer. An effective immunization for hepatitis B is now available. Although usually given during childhood, it should be seriously considered for a wide array of people, including all health care professionals (physicians, dentists, nurses, laboratory technicians, dental assistants, athletic trainers, etc.), food service workers, day care center staff, social workers, police officers, teachers, and college students. An AIDS drug, 3TC (lamivudine), was recently approved for the treatment of hepatitis B.

Type C hepatitis is contracted in ways similar to type B (sexual contact, tainted blood, and shared needles). The pool of infected people is in excess of 4 million, and the death rate is expected to climb. Of particular concern is the high incidence of the disease within the prison

Key Terms

Lyme disease
Bacterial infection transmitted by deer ticks.

toxic shock syndrome (TSS)
Potentially fatal condition resulting from the proliferation of certain bacteria in the vagina that enter the general blood circulation.

population. In 1998, the FDA approved a dual-drug therapy for HCV, but there is no vaccine for the disease.

The newly identified *type D* (delta) hepatitis is very difficult to treat. It is found almost exclusively in people already suffering from type B hepatitis. This virus, like type B hepatitis and HIV, makes unprotected sexual contact, including oral and anal sex, very risky. *Type E* hepatitis, associated with water contamination, is rarely seen in this country, except in people returning from affected areas of the world.

AIDS

AIDS is rapidly becoming the most devastating infectious disease of modern times. On the basis of current data, since the initial reporting of the disease in 1981 through December 2000, 774,467 Americans have been diagnosed with AIDS and 448,060 (58% of all cases) have died from the disease.[19] The monetary cost of caring for people with HIV/AIDS is also considerable. During the mid-1990s, the yearly cost to care for an HIV/AIDS patient was estimated to be between $36,000 and 50,700. Recently, principally because of the new drugs that have improved the quality of health and reduced the need for hospitalization, the annual cost has been reduced to approximately $20,000.[20]

Cause of AIDS

AIDS is caused by HIV, a virus that attacks the helper T cells of the immune system (see p. 286). When HIV attacks helper T cells, people lose the ability to fight off a variety of infections that normally would be easily controlled. Because these infections develop when people are vulnerable, they are collectively called *opportunistic infections.* HIV-infected people become vulnerable to infection by bacteria, protozoa, fungi, and a number of viruses. Although not infections, a variety of malignancies (see Chapter 11) also develop during this period of immune system vulnerability.

During the initial years of the HIV/AIDS epidemic, specific diagnosable conditions formed the basis for applying the clinical label of *HIV with AIDS.* Among these were *Pneumocystis carinii* pneumonia and Kaposi's sarcoma, a rare but deadly form of skin cancer. Gradually, additional conditions were recognized as being associated with advancing deterioration of the immune system, and these were added to the list of AIDS conditions. Eventually, this list contained nearly thirty (see page 296) definitive conditions, with more being added as they become apparent. Among the conditions included in the current version of the list are toxoplasmosis within the brain, cytomegalovirus retinitis with loss of vision, lymphoma involving the brain, recurrent *Salmonella* septicemia, and a wasting syndrome that includes invasive cervical cancer in women, recurrent pneumonia, and recurrent tuberculosis. Today, however, there is a growing tendency to assign the label of *HIV with AIDS* to HIV-infected people when their level of helper T cells drops below 200 cells per cubic millimeter, regardless of whether specific conditions are present.

Spread of HIV

HIV cannot be contracted easily. The chance of contracting HIV through casual contact with HIV-infected people at work, school, or home is extremely rare. HIV is known to be spread only by direct sexual contact involving the exchange of body fluids (including blood, semen, and vaginal secretions), sharing of hypodermic needles, transfusion of infected blood or blood products, and perinatal transmission (from an infected mother to a fetus or newborn baby). HIV can also be transmitted during the early days of breastfeeding, if the infected mother is untreated. Drug treatment of the mother before delivery and of the infant immediately following birth appears to reduce the risk of breast feeding-induced transmission considerably.[21] On a more positive note, HIV is not transmitted by sweat, saliva (unless blood-contaminated), or tears, although the virus may be found in very low concentrations in these fluids. Oral transmission of HIV, however, should also be considered a possibility because of gingivitis and bleeding gums. However, the presence of enzymes in the digestive tract makes transmission via ingestion impossible. Women are at much greater risk (12 times higher) than men for the heterosexual transmission of HIV because of the higher concentration of HIV in semen than in vaginal secretions.

Signs and symptoms of HIV infection

Most people infected with HIV initially feel well and have no symptoms (that is, they are asymptomatic). The incubation period for HIV infection is generally considered to range from 6 months to 10 years or more, with the average being approximately 6 years. Despite the lengthy period between infection and the first clinical signs of damage to the immune system, antibodies to HIV may appear within several weeks to 3 months of contracting the virus. Relatively few people are tested for HIV infection *at any time* during the incubation period. Therefore infected people may remain in the asymptomatic state (currently referred to as *HIV+ without symptoms*) and be carriers of HIV for years before they would notice signs of illness sufficient to warrant a physical examination.

Because of the delay between the appearance of antibodies and the accuracy of early screening for HIV, a very small "window of opportunity" has existed to protect our blood supply. However, the use of carefully constructed screening profiles for selecting donors and immediate testing of blood virtually closed that window. Today, the use of two tests, one very sensitive to HIV an-

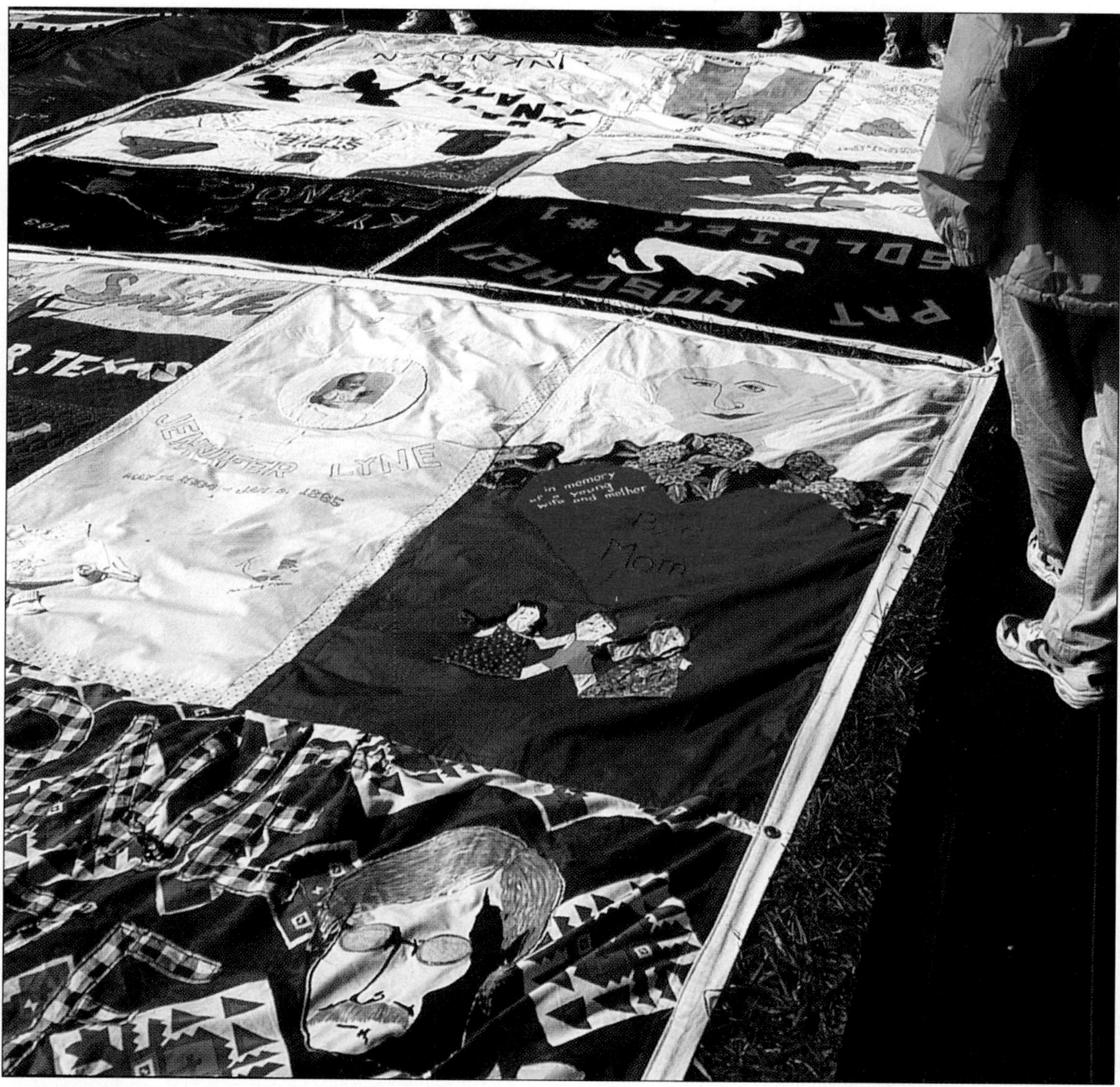

Each panel of the AIDS quilt is crafted by loved ones in memory of a family member or friend who has died. People with HIV/AIDS are living longer, and researchers are working hard to find a cure.

tibodies, followed by a second less sensitive test, has closed the window even further; no more than one person in 10,000 may be infected yet capable of being a blood donor.[22]

In the absence of symptoms of immune system deterioration and HIV testing results, sexually active people need to redefine the meaning of *monogamous*. Today, it is possible that two people in the absence of both having been tested and retested, need to account for the HIV status of all the sexual partners they have had, in addition to the HIV status of the sexual partners that those sexually partners have had, over a 10-year period before it is safe to assume that their sexual relationship is HIV-free. Since this strict approach is uncommon, some are labeling today's late adolescents and young adults as "a generation in jeopardy."

TALKING POINTS • You're dating someone you like very much, and you think you might become sexually involved with her soon. How would you ask her about her HIV status?

Virtually all people infected with HIV eventually develop signs and symptoms of a more advanced stage of the disease. These include tiredness, fever, loss of appetite and weight, diarrhea, night sweats, and swollen glands (usually in the neck, armpits, and groin). At this point, they are said to have HIV+ with symptoms. Table 12-3 indicates that these people are infectious and have damage to the immune system.

It is estimated that given sufficient time, possibly as long as 15 years, the vast majority (95%) of infected people will move beyond HIV with symptoms to develop

Table 12-3 The Spectrum of HIV Infection

	HIV+ Without Symptoms (Asymptomatic)	HIV+ With Symptoms	HIV+ With AIDS
External signs	No symptoms Looks well	Fever Night sweats Swollen lymph glands Weight loss Diarrhea Minor infections Fatigue	Kaposi's sarcoma *Pneumocystis carinii* pneumonia and/or other predetermined illnesses Neurological disorders One or more of an additional 25 + diagnosable conditions or a T4 helper cell count below 200 per cubic milliliter
Incubation	Invasion of virus to 10 years	Several months to 10 or more years	Several months to 10–12 or more years
Internal level of infection	Antibodies are produced Immune system remains intact Positive antibody test	Antibodies are produced Immune system weakened Positive antibody test	Immune system deficient Positive antibody test
Infectious?	Yes	Yes	Yes

one or more of the nearly thirty conditions whose presence leads to the label *HIV with AIDS* or *AIDS* being applied. Although this situation is not fully understood, a small percentage of infected people (5%) possess an ability to hold the infection in check and have survived for two decades without developing AIDS.

In addition to the use of the label *AIDS* for individuals who are HIV positive and have one or more of the conditions specified, the label is applied to those people whose helper T cell count falls below 200 per cubic millimeter. A normal helper T cell range is 800 to 1000.

Diagnosis of HIV infection

The CDC has established specific criteria that physicians and researchers use to define HIV infection. In addition to a clinical examination and laboratory tests for accompanying infections, HIV infection is diagnosed by the use of an initial screening test, the enzyme-linked immunosorbent assay (ELISA). If antibodies to HIV are identified, a confirming test, the Western blot, can be performed. Once clinical services are begun, more specific tests can be used to determine the drug-resistant status of a patient's specific form of HIV. Of course, if initial testing is done to soon after exposure, a false negative screening test will result due to the absence of antibodies to the virus at that early stage.

These two basic screening tests can be undertaken anonymously, in which the individual being tested is unknown to the testing laboratory other than on the basis of an assigned number, or confidentially, in which the identity of the person being tested is known, but neither the identity of that person nor the results of the test is released to anyone other than the person tested. Home tests, such as Home Access and Confide, provide accurate, anonymous results within 24 hours through a blood droplet sample that is mailed to the company for analysis. The Learning from Our Diversity box on p. 297 explores the challenges facing older adults who have a chronic condition, such as HIV/AIDS.

Treatment of HIV and AIDS

There is no cure for HIV and AIDS. The most effective treatment seems to be a "drug cocktail" in which a *protease inhibitor* is combined with two reverse transcriptase inhibitors. The protease inhibitor blocks the action of an enzyme that the virus needs to uncouple polypeptides into smaller fragments for use in reproducing itself within the host's cells. The reverse transcriptase inhibitors block the copying of RNA into a form that can enter a host cell's nucleus, a process known as *reverse transcription.* The combined effect of the protease inhibitors and reverse transcriptase inhibitors is to inhibit the ability of HIV to reproduce. These agents can reduce the viral load to a level at which the virus can no longer be detected in the blood.

The introduction of the protease inhibitors has revolutionized HIV/AIDS care. The number of deaths from AIDS fell in 1996 for the first time since the virus was identified. That decline continued until very recently, when it began to level off, perhaps because of the demand of undergoing the drug therapy. It should also be noted that protease inhibitors can have serious side effects and can cause viral resistance. In addition, these agents have no effect on viral particles that have taken shelter (sequestered) in other immune cells, within neurons, and within cells of the testes. In fact,

Learning from Our Diversity

Infectious Disease: A Challenge for Older Adults

It's not always easy for young adults in excellent health to recover quickly and completely from some infectious diseases. Later in life the recovery often becomes much more difficult and in some cases impossible. For a variety of reasons older adults do not respond to infectious conditions with the same resiliency as they once did.

Central to this issue is the gradual degradation of the immune system over time. For reasons not fully understood, the immune system loses both its ability to recognize the presence of pathogens that have entered the body and its ability to mount an effective response against them. Particularly important in this regard are the decreased prevalence of active immune system cells and the inability of existing immune cells to respond effectively. Whether this reduced level of immune protections is a "programmed" aspect of aging (all human life does end at some point in time) or whether it reflects a process that is preventable (perhaps through lifestyle modifications) remains hotly debated. Perhaps no group of older adults is at greater risk because of a compromised immune system than are those with AIDS. The nearly eighty thousand persons over age 50 with this immune system–destroying disease have a decreased ability to resist all infectious conditions, even when their HIV levels are suppressed through drug therapy.

In addition to the normal aging of their immune systems, older adults are generally afflicted with a variety of chronic conditions. The presence of multiple chronic illnesses (known as comorbidity) places the body under great stress, which also undermines the immune system. The combined effects of these conditions result in damage to different organ systems of the body—most importantly, the cardiovascular system, the respiratory system, and the renal system. Any time these systems are compromised by the effects of illness, either chronic or acute, the body becomes particularly vulnerable to infectious agents that routinely exist in our environment.

Compounding this situation is the inability of many older adults to understand the potential seriousness of infections at this stage of their lives. They may even have a false sense of confidence that their bodies are just as "good" at warding off infections as they once were. In addition, a lack of social support, isolation from health care facilities, and the inability to afford expensive prescription medication together make important medical care less available at a time when it could be effective.

When these factors are combined, as they are for many older adults, serious and even fatal infectious conditions become a reality. Therefore, anyone who is responsible for the health and well-being of older persons needs to understand their susceptibility to infectious conditions and recognize the fact that timely and competent care is of critical importance.

---

when drug treatment is stopped, for even a short time, previously sequestered viral particles rapidly begin reappearing in body fluids. Thus a cure for HIV/AIDS remains elusive.

A vaccine effective in the prevention of HIV infection does not yet exist. In the United States alone, over twenty different experimental vaccines are in the early stages of research and at least one vaccine, AIDSVAX, has entered large-scale phase III human trials. Internationally, an additional twenty experimental vaccines are in the research and development stage. Encouraging results have been achieved in animal trials,[23] and numerous small-scale human trials have demonstrated acceptable levels of safety for various vaccines. The failure to develop a vaccine most likely reflects the ability of HIV to change its appearance so often that dozens of strains of HIV exist at all times in the United States. So there may even be more than one strain of HIV within a single individual at any given time.

Reports stemming from the AIDS Vaccine 2001 Conferences held in Philadelphia suggest a high level of optimism. Of course, HIV infection remains largely preventable through the application of safer sex practices, the careful selection of sexual partners, and the discontinuation of needle sharing.

Prevention of HIV infection

Can HIV infection be prevented? The answer is a definite yes. Although HIV infection rates on college campuses are thought to be low (approximately 0.2%), students can be at risk. There are a number of steps you can take to reduce your risk of contracting and transmitting HIV. All of these steps involve understanding your behavior and the methods by which HIV can be transmitted. Particularly applicable for college-aged people are *abstinence, safer sex, sobriety,* and *communication* with potential sexual partners. Abstaining from sexual activity offers the highest level of protection from HIV. However, many people do not want to make that choice. The Changing for the Better box on p. 299 lists specific points that relate to safer sex, sobriety, and the exchange of honest, accurate information regarding sexual histories—all of which are practical approaches to minimizing your risk of contracting HIV.

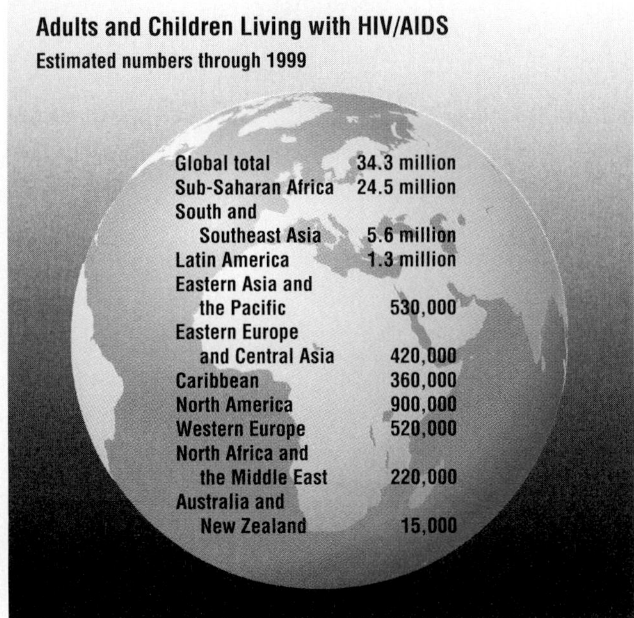

Adults and Children Living with HIV/AIDS
Estimated numbers through 1999
Global total 34.3 million
Sub-Saharan Africa 24.5 million
South and Southeast Asia 5.6 million
Latin America 1.3 million
Eastern Asia and the Pacific 530,000
Eastern Europe and Central Asia 420,000
Caribbean 360,000
North America 900,000
Western Europe 520,000
North Africa and the Middle East 220,000
Australia and New Zealand 15,000

Figure 12-4 For every person counted in these statistics, there is a face and a story. What are you doing to protect yourself from HIV?

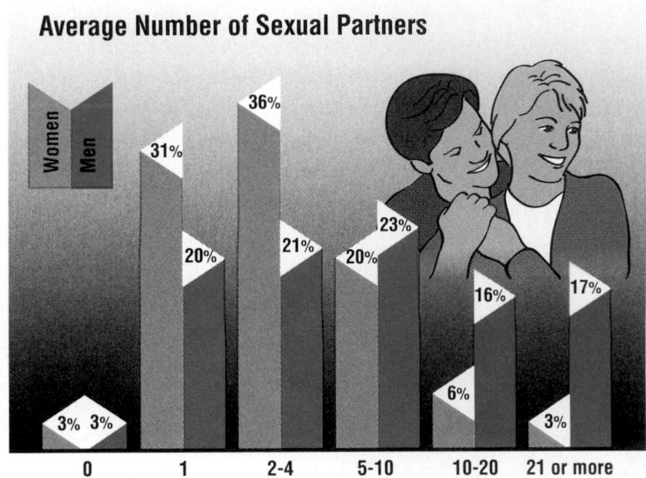

Figure 12-5 Average number of sexual partners men and women have had since age 18. The fewer the number of partners you've had, the lower your risk of contracting HIV or an STD.

To carry protection further, the U.S. Public Health Service has provided recommendations for the following groups: (1) the general public, (2) people at increased risk of infection (including health-care workers), and (3) people with a positive HIV antibody test. The Public Health Service has a toll-free AIDS hot line (1-800-342-AIDS), and local or state hot lines are also available. It is vital for you to keep informed about HIV infection and AIDS. Exploring Your Spirituality on p. 300 offers some suggestions on coping with the demands of a chronic illness such as HIV.

SEXUALLY TRANSMITTED DISEASES

Sexually transmitted diseases (STDs) were once referred to as venereal diseases (for Venus, the Roman goddess of love). Today the term *venereal disease* has been replaced by the broader term *sexually transmitted disease.* The current emphasis is on the successful prevention and treatment of STDs rather than on the ethics of sexuality (Figure 12-5). The following points about STDs should be remembered: (1) more than one STD can exist in a person at a given point in time; (2) the symptoms of STDs can vary over time and from person to person; (3) little immunity is developed for STDs; and (4) STDs can predispose people to additional health problems, including infertility, birth defects in their children, cancer, and long-term disability. Additionally, the risk of HIV infection is higher when sexual partners are also infected with STDs.

This section focuses on the STDs most frequently diagnosed among college students (chlamydia, gonorrhea, human papillomavirus infection, herpes simplex, syphilis, and pubic lice). A short section follows, covering common vaginal infections, some of which may occur without sexual contact. Completing the Personal Assessment on p. 307 will help you determine your own risk of contracting an STD. Also, refer to the Changing for the Better box on p. 299 for safer sex practices.

Chlamydia (Nonspecific Urethritis)

Chlamydia is considered the most prevalent STD in the United States today. Chlamydia infections occur an estimated 5 times more frequently than gonorrhea and up to 10 times more frequently than syphilis. In 1999, 656,721 cases of chlamydia were reported to the CDC, with approximately 18% of the cases occurring in men and 82% in women.

Chlamydia trachomatis is the bacterial agent that causes the chlamydia infection. Chlamydia is the most common cause of nonspecific urethritis (NSU). NSU refers to infections of the **urethra** and surrounding tissues that are not caused by the bacterium responsible for gonorrhea. Only when a culture for suspected gonorrhea proves negative do clinicians diagnose NSU, usually by calling it *chlamydia.* Although not as accurate as a culture, new diagnostic tests, such as Test Pack, should allow a diagnosis to be made more quickly. About 80% of men with chlamydia describe gonorrhea-like signs and symptoms, including painful urination and a whitish pus discharge

Changing *for the Better*

Reducing Your Risk of Contracting HIV

I've had only one partner in the past, but now I'm starting to date others with whom I may become sexually active. What should I do to protect myself from HIV and sexually transmitted diseases?

It is important to keep in mind that sexual partners may not reveal their true sexual history or drug habits. If you are sexually active, you can lower your risk of infection with HIV and STDs by adopting the following safer sex practices.

- Learn the sexual history and HIV status of your sex partner.
- Limit your sexual partners by practicing abstinence or by maintaining long-term monogamous relationships.
- Always use condoms correctly and consistently.
- Avoid contact with body fluids, feces, and semen.
- Curtail use of drugs that impair good judgment.
- Never share hypodermic needles.
- Refrain from sex with known injectable drug abusers.*
- Avoid sex with HIV-infected patients, those with signs and symptoms of AIDS, and the partners of high-risk individuals.*
- Get regular tests for STD infections.
- Do not engage in unprotected anal intercourse.

How easy will it be to adopt these behaviors? How real is your risk of becoming HIV-positive?

*Current studies indicate that the elimination of high-risk people as sexual partners is the single most effective safer sex practice that can be implemented.

from the penis. As in gonorrheal infections and many other STDs, most women report no overt signs or symptoms. A few women might exhibit a mild urethral discharge, painful urination, and swelling of vulval tissues. Whereas oral forms of penicillin are used in the treatment of gonococcal infections, oral tetracycline or doxycycline is prescribed for chlamydia and other NSUs.

As with all STDs, both sexual partners should receive treatment to avoid the ping-pong effect: the back-and-forth reinfection that occurs among couples when only one partner receives treatment. Furthermore, as with other STDs, having chlamydia does not effectively confer immunity.

Unresolved chlamydia can lead to the same negative health consequences that result from untreated gonorrheal infections. In men the pathogens can invade and damage the deeper reproductive structures (prostate gland, seminal vesicles, and Cowper's glands). Sterility can result. The pathogens can spread further and produce joint problems (arthritis) and heart complications (damaged heart valves, blood vessels, and heart muscle tissue).

In women the pathogens enter the body through the urethra or the cervical area. If not properly treated, the invasion can reach the deeper pelvic structures, producing a syndrome called **pelvic inflammatory disease (PID).** The inner uterine wall (endometrium), the fallopian tubes, and any surrounding structures may be attacked to produce this painful syndrome. A variety of further complications can result, including sterility and **peritonitis.** Infected women can transmit a chlamydia infection to the eyes and lungs of newborns during a vaginal birth. For both men and women the early detection of chlamydia and other NSUs is of paramount concern.

Human Papillomavirus

Human papillomavirus (HPV) infections are generally asymptomatic, and so the exact extent of the disease is unknown. A study of a group of sexually active college women found HPV infection in approximately 20% of the women. HPV-related changes to the cells of the cervix are found in nearly 5% of the Pap smears taken from women under age 30. It is currently believed that for women, risk factors for HPV infection include: (1) sexual activity before age 20, (2) intercourse with three or more partners before age 35, and (3) intercourse with a partner who has had three or more partners.[24] The extent of HPV infection in men is even less clearly known, but it is likely widespread.

The concern about HPV infections is centered on the ability of some of the more than fifty forms of the virus

Key Terms

sexually transmitted diseases (STDs)
Infectious diseases that are spread primarily through intimate sexual contact.

chlamydia
The most prevalent sexually transmitted disease. Caused by a nongonococcal bacterium.

urethra (yoo REE thra)
Passageway through which urine leaves the urinary bladder.

pelvic inflammatory disease (PID)
Acute or chronic infection of the peritoneum or lining of the abdominopelvic cavity; associated with a variety of symptoms and a potential cause of sterility.

peritonitis (pare it ton EYE tis)
Inflammation of the peritoneum or lining of the abdominopelvic cavity.

human papillomavirus (HPV)
Sexually transmitted virus capable of causing precancerous changes in the cervix; causative agent for genital warts.

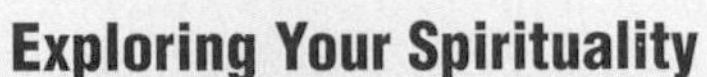

Exploring Your Spirituality

Living with an Infectious Disease—Life Is Not Over, Just Different

A chronic infectious disease can wear down your body and your spirit. First, you've got to deal with the pain, fatigue, and medicinal side effects associated with the condition. But you also need to learn to adapt everything—your routine, your relationships, and your work—to the illness. As the quality of your life changes dramatically, you may feel depressed, frustrated, and alone. What is the best way to handle the different aspects of your life as you learn to cope with a long-term illness such as chronic fatigue syndrome, hepatitis, or HIV? Will it ever be possible to enjoy a full life again?

Your workplace may present the first big challenge. Since your energy level will be decreased by your illness, you may have trouble completing tasks on time and handling your normal workload. Your allotted sick time and vacation days may be used up quickly for doctor's appointments, hospitalizations, and those days when you are simply too exhausted to go to work. Your coworkers and your supervisor may discriminate against you in subtle ways, making you feel that you're not doing your fair share. The best way to handle these challenges is to maintain a positive and friendly attitude, carefully manage your time off, promote open communication with your employer, and do your best to produce quality work even when you're not feeling well.

Your intimate relationships may also be strained. Your partner may not understand the new limits your illness places on your activities, especially if you were very active before. The best approach is open and honest communication. Try to dispel (or come to terms with) any fears your partner may have about your illness. Take all necessary precautions to avoid infecting your partner if the disease is transmissible. Also, reassure your partner that you're taking these precautions so that he or she won't become ill. Make a point of including your partner in your daily routines. Keep him or her informed of all doctor's appointments, procedures you must undergo, and any news of progress or setbacks. Share your feelings as a way of reducing anxiety for both of you. Create adaptations so that you can still enjoy a romantic relationship. Make the most of your time together, and find new ways to enjoy each other's company.

If you have children, they will also be affected by your illness. Young children may not understand why you can't take them for a sled ride when you feel sick or why you can't go to a school play because of a doctor's appointment. It's best to let children know that their fears and anxieties are valid and that you want them to share them with you. Tell them about your prognosis, taking care not to make any false promises of recovery if that is not expected. Spend time with each child—helping with homework, reading a story, or doing light chores around the house. Always allow the child to ask questions.

From your home to your workplace, your life will change along with your chronic condition. As you adapt to your new situation, it is important to:

- *Be your own best friend.* Eat well, exercise as much as you can, rest when you need to, and follow the treatments prescribed by your physician.
- *Know and understand your limits.* Don't feel guilty about not doing things you used to do before you got sick. Instead, set goals and handle responsibilities as your condition allows.
- *Find new things to do for fun.* This is a good time to start a new hobby that's relaxing. You can also make adaptations so that you can continue activities you've always enjoyed. Maybe you can't run 3 miles a day, but an after-dinner walk might be a pleasant substitute.
- *Communicate openly with others.* Share your feelings respectfully, and allow others around you to share theirs. Together, you can calm your fears, instill hope in each other, and foster a sense of belonging.
- *Remain positive.* Remember, life is not over—just different. Look forward to the good days, when you feel well, and take advantage of them. Create new ways to fulfill your needs and desires. Remain positive about the future and your treatment. New discoveries do occur, and treatments are always evolving. However, be realistic about your situation. Joining a support group may be one of the best things you can do for yourself.

What you learn about yourself throughout your illness may surprise you. You may discover a strength of spirit you never knew you had. Some days may be very hard, but somehow you get through them. You may see life in a new way—slowing down and taking pleasure in a job well done, enjoying friendships more, listening to your inner voice, spending time with your children, taking a second look at nature, and being thankful for today and tomorrow.

to foster precancerous changes in the cervix. In addition, HPV is associated with the development of genital warts (condyloma acuminata). These pinkish-white lesions may be found in raised clusters that resemble tiny heads of cauliflower (see the photograph on p. 301). Found most commonly on the penis, scrotum, labia, cervix, and around the anus, genital warts are the most common symptomatic viral STD in this country. Although most genital wart colonies are small, they may become very large and block the anus or birth canal during pregnancy.

Treatment for HPV, including genital warts, may include burning, freezing, removal with a CO_2 laser, or the use of various medications. Regardless of treatment, however, return of the viral colonies will most likely occur. Condom use should be encouraged in an attempt to prevent transmission of HPV.

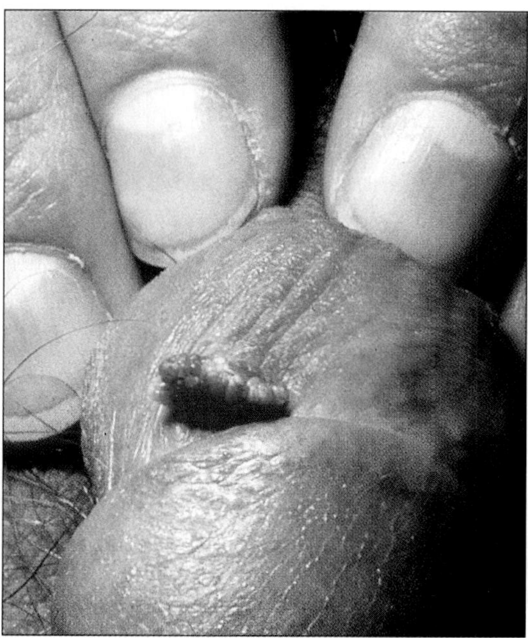

A human papillomavirus infection (genital warts).

Gonorrhea

Another extremely common STD, gonorrhea is caused by a bacterium (*Neisseria gonorrhoeae*). In men this bacterial agent can produce a milky-white discharge from the penis, accompanied by painful urination. About 80% of men who contract gonorrhea report varying degrees of these symptoms. This figure is approximately reversed for women: only about 20% of women are symptomatic and thus report varying degrees of frequent, painful urination, with a slimy yellow-green discharge from the vagina or urethra. Oral sex with an infected partner can produce a gonorrheal infection of the throat (pharyngeal gonorrhea). Gonorrhea can also be transmitted to the rectal areas of both men and women. In 1998, 322,286 cases of gonorrhea, about equally divided between men and women, were reported to the CDC. In light of the asymptomatic (showing no symptoms) nature of the disease in women, the equal number of reported cases for men and women suggests a high level of self-referral by women, regular preventive reproductive health care by women, and cooperative case finding on the part of both men and women.

Diagnosis of gonorrhea is made by culturing the bacteria. Antibiotic treatment regimens include use of penicillin, tetracycline, ampicillin, or other drugs. Some strains of gonorrhea (penicillin-resistant strains) are much more difficult to treat than others.

Testing for gonorrhea is included as a part of prenatal care so that infections in mothers can be treated before birth. If the birth canal is infected, newborns could easily contract the infection in the mucous membranes of the eye. Most states still require that drops be placed in the eyes of all newborns to prevent this infection.

Changing *for the Better*

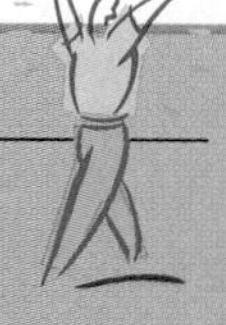

Talking with Your Partner about Herpes

My girlfriend told me she has herpes and said she's "taking care of everything." What can I do to get things out in the open?

Although herpes rarely has serious consequences, the lesions are infectious and tend to reappear. It is important to talk openly with your partner about this sexually transmitted disease. Here are some tips to make things easier:

- *Educate yourself.*
  Be aware that herpes is rarely dangerous.
  Learn when the disease is most contagious (during the eruption and blister stage), and that herpes can be spread even during the non-eruption, non-blister periods—traditionally defined as safe periods.
- *Choose the right time to talk.*
  Discuss herpes with your partner only after you have gotten to know each other.
- *Listen to your partner.*
  Be prepared to answer any questions that he or she may have.
- *Together, put things in perspective.*
  Keep a positive outlook.
  Remember that you are not alone.
  Be aware that using a condom and abstaining from coitus during the most infectious period can prevent transmission of the disease.
  Although there is no known cure, research continues on an antiviral drug.
  Join a local support group together.

Herpes Simplex

Public health officials think that the sexually transmitted genital herpes virus infection rivals chlamydia as the most prevalent STD. Recent studies show that about 20% of the adult population (about 45 million people) is infected with genital herpes virus, although most people are asymptomatic for genital herpes.[25] Herpes is really a family of over fifty viruses, some of which produce recognized diseases in humans (chicken pox, **shingles,**

Key Term

shingles
Viral infection affecting the nerve endings of the skin.

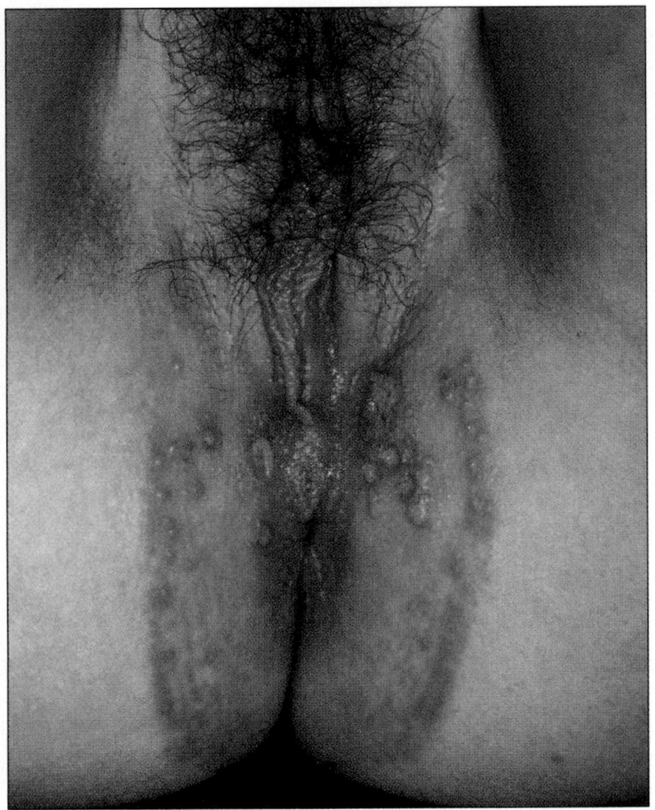

A severe herpes infection.

mononucleosis, and others). One subgroup called *herpes simplex 1 virus* (HSV-1) produces an infection called *labial herpes* (oral or lip herpes). Labial herpes produces common fever blisters or cold sores seen around the lips and oral cavity. Herpes *simplex 2 virus* (HSV-2) is a different strain that produces similar clumps of blisterlike lesions in the genital region. Laypeople have referred to this second type of herpes as the STD type, although both types produce identical clinical pictures. Both forms can exist at either site. Oral-genital sexual practices have resulted in genital herpes cases now being caused by HSV-1.

Herpes appears as a single sore or as a small cluster of blisterlike sores (see the photograph above). These sores burn, itch, and (for some) become quite painful. The infected person might also report swollen lymph glands, muscular aches and pains, and fever. Some patients feel weak and sleepy when blisters are present. The lesions may last from a few days to a few weeks. A week is the average time for active viral shedding; then the blisters begin scabbing, and new skin is formed.

Herpes is an interesting virus for several reasons. It can lie dormant for extended periods. However, for reasons not well understood but perhaps related to stress, diet, or overall health, the viral particles can be stimulated to travel along the nerve pathways to the skin and then create an active infection. Thus herpes can be considered a recurrent infection. Fortunately for most people, recurrent infections are less severe than the initial episode and do not last as long. Herpes is also interesting because, unlike most STDs, no treatment method has been successful at killing the virus. Recommended treatment for an initial outbreak of herpes calls for the use of one of three medications. These medications are taken orally, multiple times each day, for 7 to 10 days. Since these medications only temporarily suppress the infectious process, some clinicians choose to treat each recurrence, but others prefer to use medications on a continuing basis in an attempt to suppress recurrences.[26] There are also some medications that may provide symptomatic relief. Diagnosis of genital herpes is almost always made by a clinical examination.

The best prevention against ever getting a herpes infection is to avoid all direct contact with a person who has an active infection. Do not kiss someone with a fever blister—or let them kiss you (or your children) if they have an active lesion. Do not share drinking glasses or eating utensils. Check your partner's genitals. Do not have intimate sexual contact with someone who displays the blisterlike clusters or rash. (Condoms are only marginally helpful and cannot protect against lesions on the female vulva or the lower abdominal area of men). Be careful not to infect yourself by touching a blister and then touching any other part of your body. The Changing for the Better box on p. 301 provides helpful advice for talking to your partner if you have genital herpes.

Newborn babies are especially susceptible to the virus if they come into contact with an active lesion during the birth process. Newborns have not developed the defense capabilities to resist the invasion. They can quickly develop a systemic general infection (neonatal herpes) that is often fatal or local infections that produce permanent brain damage or blindness. Most of these possible problems can be prevented through proper prenatal care. If there is any chance that the viral particles may be present at birth, a cesarean delivery can be performed, although this is less commonly done today than in the past.

Syphilis

Like gonorrhea, syphilis is caused by a bacterium (*Treponema pallidum*) and is transmitted almost exclusively by sexual intercourse. The incidence of syphilis, a CDC-reportable disease, is far lower than that of gonorrhea. In 1950 a record 217,558 cases of syphilis were reported in this country. The number of cases then fell steadily to less than 80,000 cases in 1980. From 1980 through 1990 the incidence climbed, reaching nearly 140,000 cases in 1990. A subsequent decline then began, and in 1994 the number of cases dropped to 81,695 and continued to decline, reaching 35,628 in 1999.[27] In spite of a downward trend, an alarming number of today's cases have also been associated with HIV infections. Additionally, an alarming increase in infant syphilis has been noted in children born to mothers who use drugs and support their habit through sexual activity.

Unlike other STDs, syphilis is characterized by a progression through a series of stages that unfold over several decades. Following an incubation period of 10 to 90 days, the *primary stage* of syphilis is characterized by the formation of a small, raised, painless sore called a *chancre.* In 90% of women and 50% of men, this highly infectious lesion is not easily identified, and so treatment is generally not received. Even in the absence of treatment, however, the chancre will heal in 4 to 5 weeks, marking the end of this stage.

Following an asymptomatic period of several weeks, the *secondary stage* of the disease appears. In this extremely contagious stage, the bacteria have become systemically distributed and may result in a variety of symptoms, including a generalized body rash, a sore throat, bone and joint soreness, or a patchy loss of hair. A blood test (VDRL) will be positive, and treatment can be effectively administered. If the disease is untreated, this stage will subside within 2 to 6 weeks. It is during this stage that syphilis is easily transmitted by a pregnant woman to her fetus. Congenital syphilis often results in a stillbirth or an infant born with a variety of life-threatening complications. Early treatment of a pregnant women can prevent this.

After the secondary stage has subsided, an extended *latency period* develops, lasting from many months to many years. During this stage there are no visible signs of the illness, and infected persons are noninfectious because the bacteria have become sequestered, only to reappear many years later.

The *late stage* of syphilis generally occurs two or more decades following the initial infection. In this terminal stage of the disease, soft rubbery tumors can be found on the body, either in ulcerated or partially healed states. In addition to this skin damage, extensive damage to the brain, heart and circulatory system, and eyes has also occurred. At this stage, treatment is at best only partially effective and death generally ensues.

In all stages of the disease, including the latency period, treatment involves the use of antibiotics. When treatment is begun during the later stages of syphilis, damage being done to the body can be stopped, but any damage that has already occurred is unlikely to be reversed.

Pubic Lice

Three types of lice infect humans: the head louse, the body louse, and the pubic louse all feed on the blood of the host. Except for the relatively uncommon body louse, these tiny insects do not carry diseases. They are, however, quite annoying.

Pubic lice, also called *crabs,* attach themselves to the base of the pubic hairs, where they live and attach their eggs (nits). These eggs move into a larval stage after 1 week; after 2 more weeks, they develop into mature adult crab lice.

People usually notice they have a pubic lice infestation when they are confronted with intense itching in the genital region. Both prescription and OTC creams, lotions, and shampoos are extremely effective in killing both the lice and their eggs.

Lice are not transmitted exclusively through sexual contact, but also by contact with bedsheets and clothes that may be contaminated. If you develop a pubic lice infestation, you will have to treat yourself, your clothes, your sheets, and your furniture.

Vaginal Infections

Two common pathogens produce uncomfortable vaginal infections in women. The first is the yeast or fungus *Candida (Monilia) albicans.* This organism, commonly found in the vagina, seems to multiply rapidly when some unusual stressor (pregnancy, use of the birth control pill or antibiotics, diabetes) affects a woman's body. This infection, now called *vulvovaginal candidiasis (VVC),* is signaled by a white or cream-colored vaginal discharge that resembles cottage cheese. Vaginal itching and vulvar swelling are also commonly reported. Current treatment is based on the use of one of several prescription and OTC drugs.

Nonprescription products offer effective home treatment. You should consult a physician before using these products for the first time. (Men rarely report this infection, although some may report mildly painful urination or a barely noticeable discharge at the urethral opening or beneath the foreskin of the penis.)

The protozoan *Trichomonas vaginalis* also produces a vaginal infection. This parasite can be transmitted through sexual intercourse or by contact with contaminated (often damp) objects, such as towels, or toilet seats, that may contain some vaginal discharge. In women, this infection, called *trichomoniasis,* or "trich," produces a foamy, yellow-green, foul-smelling discharge that may be accompanied by itching, swelling, and painful urination. Although topically applied treatments with limited effectiveness are available, more highly effective oral medications are also available. Men infrequently contract trichomoniasis but may harbor the organisms without realizing it. They also should be treated to minimize reinfection of partners.

The vagina is warm, dark, and moist, an ideal breeding environment for a variety of organisms. Unfortunately, some commercial products seem to increase the incidence of vaginal infections. Among these are tight panty hose (without cotton panels), which tend to increase the vaginal temperature, and commercial vaginal douches, which can alter the acidity of the vagina. Both of these products might promote infections. Women are also advised to wipe from front to back after every bowel movement to reduce the opportunity of direct transmission of pathogenic agents from the rectum to the vagina. Although difficult to do in many cases, avoiding public restrooms is also a good practice. If you notice any unusual discharge from the vagina, you should report this to your physician.

Cystitis and Urethritis

Cystitis, an infection of the urinary bladder, and *urethritis,* an infection of the urethra, occasionally can be caused by a sexually transmitted organism. Such infections can also be traced to the organisms that cause vaginitis and organisms found in the intestinal tract. A culture is required to identify the specific pathogen associated with a particular case of cystitis or urethritis. The symptoms are pain when urinating, the need to urinate frequently, a dull aching pain above the pubic bone, and the passing of blood-streaked urine.

Physicians can easily treat cystitis and urethritis with antibiotics when the specific organism has been identified. In fact, newer medications can be effective in a single dose.

If cystitis or urethritis is left untreated, the infectious agent could move upward in the urinary system and infect the ureters and kidneys. These upper urinary tract infections are more serious and require more extensive evaluation and aggressive treatment. Therefore you should obtain medical care immediately if symptoms are noticed.

Preventing cystitis and urethritis depends partly on the source of the infectious agent. You can generally reduce the incidence of infection by urinating completely (to fully empty the bladder) and by drinking ample fluids to flush the urinary tract. It has also been recognized that compounds found in cranberry juice may be helpful in reducing urinary tract infections.[28]

SUMMARY

- Progress has been made in reducing the incidence of some forms of infectious disease, but other infectious conditions are becoming more prevalent.
- A variety of pathogenic agents are responsible for infectious conditions.
- A chain of infection with six links characterizes every infectious condition.
- Infectious conditions progress through five distinct stages.
- Immunity can be acquired through both natural and artificial means. Immunization should be received on a regularly scheduled basis.
- The immune system's response to infection relies on cellular and humoral elements.
- The common cold and influenza display many similar symptoms but differ in terms of infectious agents, incubation period, prevention, and treatment.
- Tuberculosis and pneumonia are potentially fatal infections of the respiratory system.
- Mononucleosis and chronic fatigue syndrome are infections that result in chronic tiredness.
- Fibromyalgia is a chronic condition that may be similar in some ways to chronic fatigue syndrome.
- Measles is a childhood infection that can be harmful when contracted during adulthood.
- Bacterial meningitis is of growing concern on college campuses.
- Lyme disease is a bacterial infection contracted in conjunction with outdoor activities.
- Hantavirus pulmonary syndrome is caused by a virus carried by deer mice.
- Hepatitis B (serum hepatitis) is a bloodborne infectious condition that can lead to serious liver damage. Hepatitis A, C, D, and E also exist.
- HIV/AIDS is a widespread, incurable viral disease transmitted through sexual activity, intravenous drug use, the use of infected blood products, across the placenta during pregnancy, and in breast milk
- The definitive definition of AIDS can be based on the presence of specific conditions or the diminished number of helper T cells.
- Effective treatment of HIV and AIDS is considerably improved but still not capable of resulting in a cure, and prevention through the use of an effective vaccine is nonexistent.
- A variety of sexually transmitted conditions exists, many of which do not produce symptoms in most infected women and many infected men.
- Safer sex practices can reduce the risk of contracting STDs.

REVIEW QUESTIONS

1. What are the agents responsible for the most familiar infectious conditions?
2. What are the six links that form the chain of infection?
3. What are the five stages that characterize the progression of infectious conditions?
4. What are the two principal components of the immune system, and how do they cooperate to protect the body from infectious agents and abnormal cells?
5. How are the common cold and influenza similar? How do they differ in terms of causative agents, incubation period, prevention, and treatment?
6. What symptoms make mononucleosis, chronic fatigue syndrome, and fibromyalgia similar? What aspects of each are different?
7. Why is measles a more serious condition when it develops in adults?
8. What is the relationship between bacterial meningitis and living patterns on the college campus?
9. Why is outdoor activity a risk factor in contracting Lyme disease?
10. How is hepatitis B transmitted, and which occupational group is at greatest risk of contracting this infection? How do forms A, C, D, and E compare with hepatitis B?
11. How is HIV transmitted? To what extent is the treatment of HIV/AIDS effective? What is meant by the term *safer sex?*
12. What specific infectious diseases could be classified as being STDs?
13. Why are women more often asymptomatic for STDs than men?
14. To what extent and in what manner can STD transmission be prevented?

THINK ABOUT THIS . . .

- How do you feel when a classmate or coworker comes to class or work ill? Is it fair to expose you to his or her illness?
- Which infectious disease have you had in the recent past? What impact did this infection have on your day-to-day activities?
- What diseases have you been immunized against?
- How do you feel about parents who do not have their children immunized?
- What would your initial reaction be if you found out that someone close to you had a sexually transmitted disease?

REFERENCES

1. Hamann B: *Disease: identification, prevention and control,* ed 2, 2001, McGraw-Hill.
2. Saladin KS: *Anatomy and physiology: unit of form and function,* ed 2, 2001, McGraw-Hill.
3. Recommended Childhood Immunization Schedule, United States, January–December 1999. American Academy of Pediatrics, December 1999. **www.aap.org/family/parents/immunize.htm**
4. AAP updates policy on recommended use of inactivated polio vaccine (IPV) for routine immunization. Press Release, December 6, 1999. **www.aap.org/advocacy/release/decipv.htm**
5. Pauschinger M, et al: Detection of adenoviral genome in the myocardium of adult patients with idiopathic left ventricular dysfunction. *JAMA* 99(10):1348–1354, 1999.
6. Hayden FG, et al: Use of the oral neuraminidase inhibitor oseltamivir in experimental human influenza: randomized controlled trials for prevention and treatment. *JAMA* 282(13):1240–1246, 1999.
7. Nichol KL, et al: Effectiveness of live, attenuated intranasal influenza virus vaccine in healthy, working adults: a randomized controlled trial. *JAMA* 282(2):137–144, 1999.
8. Centers for Disease Control: Tuberculosis—United States, *MMWR* 46(30):695–699, 1996.
9. Mandell GL, Bennett JE, Dolin R: *Principles and practice of infectious disease,* ed 5, 1999, Churchill Livingstone.
10. National Institute of Allergy and Infectious Diseases (NIAID): *Chronic fatigue syndrome—etiological theories,* 1999. **www.niaid.nih.gov/publication/cfs/etio.htm**
11. *Fibromyalgia basics: symptoms, treatments and research,* 1999, **www.fmnetnews.com/pages/basic.html**
12. *Diagnostic criteria for fibromyalgia and CFS,* 1999. **www.fmnetnews.com/pages/criteria.html**
13. Centers for Disease Control and Prevention: Summary of notifiable diseases, United States, 1998, *MMWR* 47(53), Dec 31, 1999.
14. Harrison LH, et al: Risk of meningococcal meningitis in college students. *JAMA* 281(20):1906–1910, 1999.
15. Centers for Disease Control and Prevention: Meningococcal disease among college students, Press Release, October 20, 1999. **www.cdc.gov/ncidod/dbmd/diseaseinfo/meningococcal_college.htm**
16. Schutzer SE, et al: *Borrelia burgdorferi*—specific immune complexes in acute Lyme disease. *JAMA* 282(20):1942–1946, 1999.

17. Hart CA, Bennett M: Hantavirus infections: epidemiology and pathogenesis. *Microbes Infect* 1(14):1229–1237, 1999.
18. Rodriquez-Moran P, Kelly C, Hjelle B: Hantavirus infection in the Four Corners region of USA in 1998. *Lancet* 352(9137):1353, 1998.
19. Centers for Disease Control and Prevention: *U.S. HIV and AIDS cases reported through December 2000. Year-End edition,* 12(2):3–48, 2001.
20. Bozzette SA et al: The care of HIV-infected adults in the United States, HIV Cost and Services Utilization Study Consortium, *N Engl J Med,* 229(26):1897–1904, 1998.
21. Musoke P, et al: A phase I/II study of the safety and pharmacokinetics of nevirapine in HIV-1 infected pregnant Ugandan women and their neonates (HIVNET 006). *AIDS* 13(4):479–486, 1999.
22. Jafee H (presentation): Sixth Conference on Retroviruses and Opportunistic Infections, Chicago, February 2, 1999.
23. Crooty S et al: Protection against simian immunodeficiency virus vaginal challenge by using Sabin poliovirus vectors *J Virol.* 75(16):7435–7452, 2001.
24. Hatcher R, et al: *Contraceptive technology: 1998,* ed 17, 1998, Irvington.
25. Flemming DT, et al: Herpes simplex virus type 2 in the United States, 1976–1994, *N Engl J Med* 337(16):1105–1111, 1997.
26. 1998 Guidelines for treatment of sexually transmitted diseases. *MMWR* (suppl) 1997 Jan; 47(RR-1):1–16.
27. Summary of notifiable diseases, United States, *MMWR* 48(53):1–101, 2001.
28. Howell AB, et al: Inhibition of the adherence of P-fimbriated *Escherichia coli* to uroepithelial-cell surfaces by proanthocyanidin extracts from cranberries. *N Engl J Med* 339(15):1085–1086, 1998.

SUGGESTED READINGS

Homes F, et al: *Sexually transmitted diseases,* ed 3, 1999, McGraw-Hill.

This book is a valuable resource for people who need to know about STDs from the widest range of perspectives, including microbiological, clinical, legal, and social. It is intended for professionals who work in the fields of STD care and prevention, although it would be an equally good resource for students majoring in public health.

Farrell J: *Invisible enemies: stories of infectious disease,* 1998, Farrar, Straus & Giroux.

The book's author, Jeanette Farrell, literally tells the story of seven of the most important and interesting infectious diseases, including leprosy, the plague, cholera, and smallpox. Her narrative style carries the younger reader through the epidemiological backroads that lead to a fuller understanding of how these diseases were discovered, how they are treated, what is currently being learned about each one, and what the outcome of treatment is most likely to be. This book would be an excellent addition to the science education major's professional library.

Marr L: *Sexually transmitted disease: a physician tells you what you need to know,* 1998, The Johns Hopkins University Press.

Here is a simple, understandable, and helpful source of information about the cause, treatment, and prevention of subsequent infections. It is presented by a physician who is experienced in the treatment of infectious conditions. The author addresses the many myths about STD transmission and treatment.

Turkington C: *Hepatitis C: the silent killer.* 1998, Contemporary Books.

The intended audience for this book is people who have recently been diagnosed with hepatitis C and their loved ones. In a very understandable way, the author presents current information about the cause, treatment, and management of this viral infection of the liver.

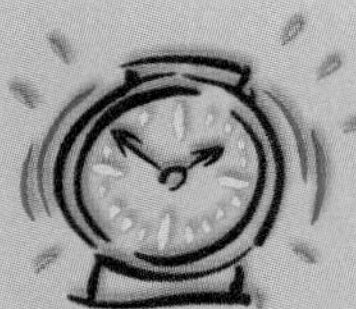

As we go to Press...

First detected in New York City in 1999, the West Nile virus had been isolated in thirteen states to date, principally in the eastern half of the United States, from Florida to Canada. This infectious virus is transmitted from a vector, most often birds, by mosquitoes. The mosquitoes in turn introduce the virus into humans while taking a blood meal. Thousands of birds, most commonly the American crow, have died from the West Nile virus. In 2000, twenty-one people in the United States were reported as having illnesses directly related to the West Nile virus, compared to sixty-two in 1999.

Health authorities predict a continuing movement of the virus westward, due to bird migration, and eventual isolation in every area of the country. Although treatable, West Nile virus infection can result in severe neurological illnesses and, sometimes, death.

Name ______________________ **Date** __________ **Section** __________

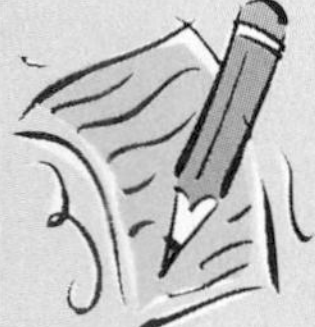

Personal Assessment

What Is Your Risk of Contracting a Sexually Transmitted Disease?

A variety of factors interact to determine your risk of contracting a sexually transmitted disease (STD). This inventory is intended to provide you with an estimate of your level of risk.

Circle the number of each row that best characterizes you. Enter that number on the line at the end of the row (points). After assigning yourself a number in each row, total the number appearing in the points column. Your total points will allow you to interpret your risk for contracting an STD.

						Points
Age						
1	3	4	5	3	2	_____
0–9	10–14	15–19	20–29	30–34	35+	
Sexual Practices						
0	1	2	4	6	8	_____
Never engage in sex	One sex partner	More than one sex partner but never more than one at a time	Two to five sex partners	Five to ten sex partners	Ten or more sex partners	
Sexual Attitudes						
0	1	8	1	7	8	_____
Will not engage in nonmarital sex	Premarital sex is okay if it is with future spouse	Any kind of premarital sex is okay	Extramarital sex is not for me	Extramarital sex is okay	Believe in complete sexual freedom	
Attitudes toward Contraception						
1	1	6	5	4	8	_____
Would use condom to prevent pregnancy	Would use condom to prevent STDs	Would never use a condom	Would use the birth control pill	Would use other contraceptive measure	Would not use anything	
Attitudes toward STD						
3	3	4	6	6	6	_____
Am not sexually active so I do not worry	Would be able to talk about STD with my partner	Would check an infection to be sure	Would be afraid to check out an infection	Can't even talk about an infection	STDs are no problem—easily cured	

YOUR TOTAL POINTS _____

Interpretation

5–8	Your risk is well below average
9–13	Your risk is below average
14–17	Your risk is at or near average
18–21	Your risk is moderately high
22+	Your risk is high

To Carry This Further . . .

Having taken this Personal Assessment, were you surprised at your level of risk? What is the primary reason for this level? How concerned are you and your classmates and friends about contracting an STD?

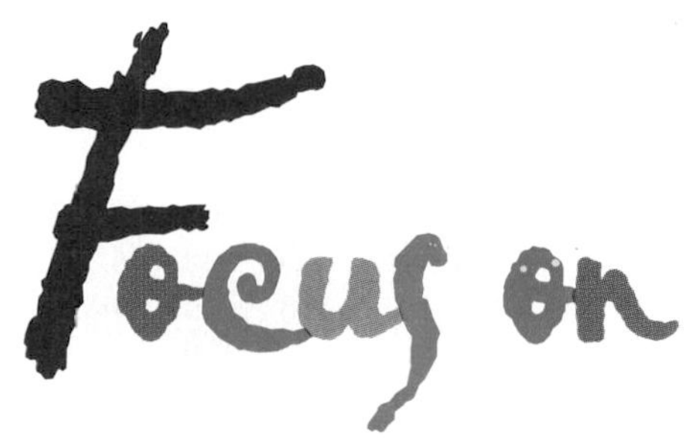

CHILDHOOD IMMUNIZATIONS—PROGRESS AND CHALLENGES

Although the American population is becoming increasingly heterogeneous, the level of childhood immunization in this country is considerably higher than it was 20 years ago. This level is substantially higher than that of many other nations. In fact, it approaches the level seen in the most homogeneously populated developed countries. This high level of immunization demonstrates our understanding that familiar infectious diseases exist and that new infectious agents are being identified each year.

In the 1980s, just over one-half of American 2-year-olds had received all of the recommended immunizations. Today, three-quarters of all American 2-year-olds have received all of the recommended immunizations, and well over 90% have received all immunizations for measles, mumps, rubella, polio, and *Haemophilus influenzae* type b (Hib). Two immunizations—a vintage form for diphtheria, tetanus, and pertussis (DPT) and a relatively recent one for hepatitis B—are only slightly below the 90% level.[1] The newer vaccination for varicella (chicken pox) will require additional time to reach the acceptable 90% level.

Much of the credit for this progress can be given to the President's Childhood Immunization Initiative.[2] This federal initiative increased funding for immunization coverage among disadvantaged groups, encouraged the development of new methods of monitoring compliance levels, and promoted educational programs to underscore the importance of full protection from preventable infectious diseases. Most recently, the Bill and Melinda Gates Foundation pledged $750 million to improve immunization rates throughout the world, including this country.[3] Programs funded by this grant are likely to be directed toward specific groups of children who remain underserved by our health care system.

Why do approximately 10% of our nation's children remain less than fully immunized against the eleven infectious conditions that can be prevented through immunization? The reasons vary widely.[4] For many, the principal reasons are poverty and isolation from health care services. However, other reasons help to explain the small segment of our children who have less than full protection or no protection. These include parental concerns over the small but always present risk of injury and illness resulting from the immunization process or the vaccines used. Religious and philosophical considerations are also involved in the decisions that some parents make about immunization for their children. Additionally, some health care providers fail to monitor the compliance of their patients, and so partially protected children (or not yet protected infants) go undetected. Finally, apathy on the part of some parents and caregivers causes them to neglect the need to protect vulnerable children from preventable infectious diseases.

Despite these deficiencies, the advances toward complete immunization coverage made in the last decade are impressive. However, this progress can be eroded in the course of one generation if future parents do not continue this practice of having their children immunized and if governmental support and private initiatives are not continued. Children are dependent on parental and community awareness, concern, and initiative for their protection from infectious diseases.

What Parents Need to Know

The American Academy of Pediatrics recommends the following immunization schedule (released January 2000):

Birth to 2 months: hepatitis B
1 to 4 months: hepatitis B
2 months: diphtheria/tetanus/pertussis, *H. influenzae* type B, polio
4 months: diphtheria/tetanus/pertussis, *H. influenzae* type B, polio
6 to 18 months: hepatitis B, polio
6 months: diphtheria/tetanus/pertussis, hepatitis B
12 to 15 months: hepatitis B, measles/mumps/rubella
12 to 18 months: varicella
15 to 18 months: diphtheria/tetanus/pertussis
24 months: hepatitis A (in selected areas)
4 to 6 years: diphtheria/tetanus/pertussis, polio, measles/mumps/rubella
11 to 12 years: hepatitis B, measles/mumps/rubella, varicella
11 to 16 years: tetanus/diphtheria.

Note: The AAP advises that you check with your pediatrician or health clinic at each visit to find out if your child needs any booster shots or if any new vaccines have been recommended since this schedule was prepared.

References

1. Teitelbaum MA, Edmunds M: Immunization and vaccine preventable illness, United States, 1992 to 1997. *Stat Bull Metrop Insur Co* 80(2):13–20, April–June, 1999.
2. The National Vaccine Advisory Committee: Strategies to sustain success in childhood immunizations. *JAMA* 282(4):363–370, 1999.
3. The Bill and Melinda Gates Foundation: A $750 Million Gift to the Global Alliance for Vaccines and Immunization (GAVI), November 11, 1999. **www.gatesfoundation.org/pressRelease/991123Health.html**
4. Orenstein W: National Immunization Program, Centers for Disease Control and Prevention, 33rd National Immunization Conference, Dallas, June 1999.

part 5

Sexuality and Reproduction

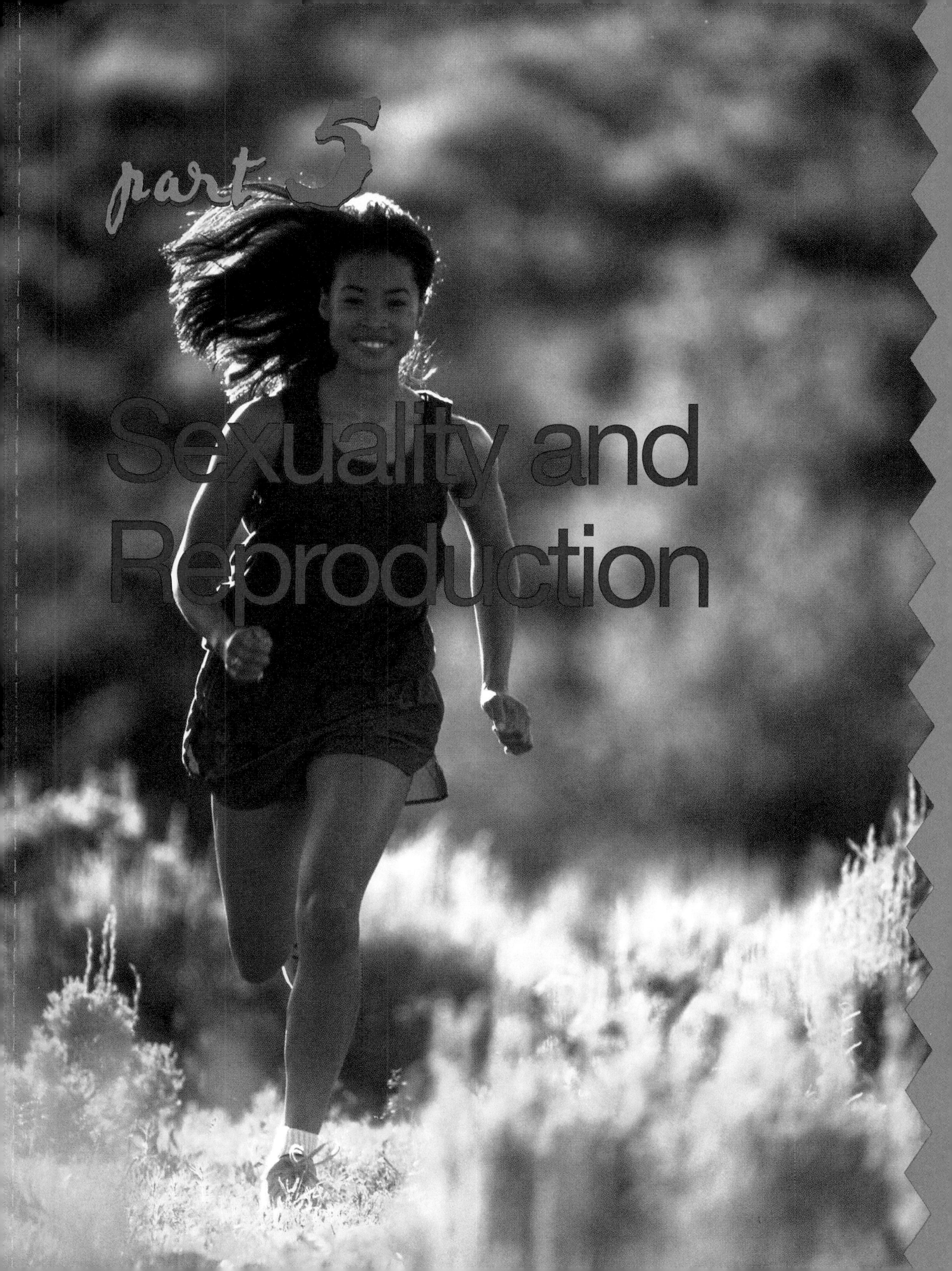

chapter **13**

Understanding Sexuality

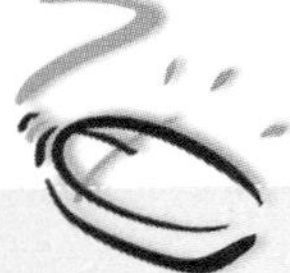

Online Learning Center Resources

www.mhhe.com/hahn6e

Log on to our Online Learning Center (OLC) for access to these additional resources:

- Chapter key terms and definitions
- Learning objectives
- Additional behavior change objectives
- Student interactive question-and-answer sites
- Self-scoring chapter quiz

The OLC also offers web links for study and exploration of health topics. Here are some examples of what you'll find:

- **www.indiana.edu/~kinsey** Study the findings of the Kinsey Institute for Research in Sex, Gender, and Reproduction.
- **www.positive.org/JustSayYes/contents.html** Take an online tour here, through the most important topics for teens who are sexually active or just thinking about it.
- **www.sexualitydata.com** Click on *Index of Topics* to browse, or use the search function to find specific information.

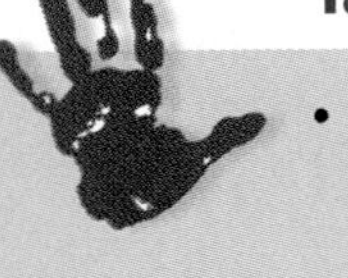

Taking Charge of Your Health

- Take the Personal Assessment on p. 339 to understand your sexual attitudes better.
- Use the Personal Assessment on p. 341 to find out how sexually compatible you and your partner are.
- If being around someone whose sexual orientation is different from yours makes you feel uncomfortable, focus on getting to know that person better as an individual.
- If you are in an unhealthy relationship, take the first step toward getting out of it through professional counseling or group support.
- If you are in a sexual relationship, communicate your sexual needs to your partner clearly. Encourage him or her to do the same so that you will both have a satisfying sex life.
- Consider whether your lifetime plan will involve marriage, singlehood, or cohabitation. Evaluate your current situation in relation to that plan.

Eye on the Media

MTV's *Loveline:* The Relationship Clinic

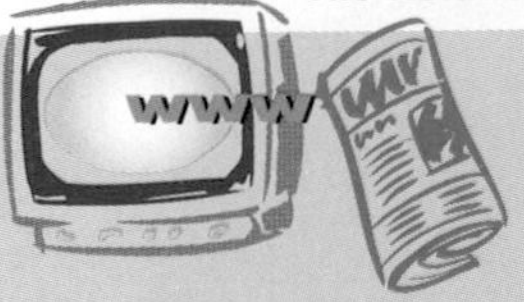

Where have many of today's young adults gone for information about relationships and sex? Since 1996, millions of young viewers have been captivated by the one-hour MTV show called *Loveline.* This is a studio-based, call-in program hosted by comedian Adam Carolla and Dr. Drew Pinsky, a board-certified physician who is the medical director of the chemical dependency services at a Pasadena, California, hospital. "Dr. Drew" has the medical credibility, and Adam has the funny, sarcastic wit that connects well with young people. In 2001, the *Loveline* television show ended, but reruns occasionally appear.

Carolla and Pinsky have continued their brand of relationship and sex advice through their co-hosting of the radio version of *Loveline.* This syndicated call-in radio show originates from Los Angeles's KROQ radio and is heard on more than fifty radio stations across the country. The hosts take listeners' calls that involve any issue related to sex and relationships: sexual performance, sexually transmitted diseases, sexual orientation, sexual abuse, drugs and sex, dating intimacy, starting and ending relationships, and sexual identity. Many of the questions might

Eye on the Media *continued*

be considered kinky by conservative adults. It's not uncommon for the hosts to identify a caller who has fabricated a completely outrageous story. The hosts frequently ask follow-up questions to understand the caller's concerns better. Celebrity guests, often rock musicians or actors, frequently make appearances on the show.

Part of the fun is that the show is so unpredictable. Although Dr. Drew tries to provide factual information in a clear, concise way to help the caller and the listeners, Carolla cannot resist using his comic wit to lighten any frank discussion. Although *Loveline* provides generally excellent information, the show is not for everyone. To learn more about *Loveline,* Dr. Drew, or Carolla, check out the following websites: **www.kroq.com/loveline**, **www.drdrew.com**, and **www.geocities.com/tomsters**.

Currently, we have reached an understanding of both the biological and psychosocial factors that contribute to the complex expression of our **sexuality.** As a society, we are now inclined to view human behavior in terms of a complex script written on the basis of both biology and conditioning. Reflecting this understanding is how we use the words "male" or "female" to refer to the biological roots of our sexuality and the words "man" or "woman" to refer to the psychosocial roots of our sexuality. This chapter explores human sexuality as it relates to the dynamic interplay of the biological and psychosocial bases that form your **masculinity** or **femininity.**

BIOLOGICAL BASES OF HUMAN SEXUALITY

Within a few seconds after the birth of a baby, someone—a doctor, nurse, or parent—emphatically labels the child: "It's a boy," or "It's a girl." For the parents and society as a whole, the child's **biological sexuality** is being displayed and identified. Another female or male enters the world.

Genetic Basis

At the moment of conception, a Y-bearing or an X-bearing sperm cell joins with the X-bearing ovum to establish the true basis of biological sexuality.[1] A fertilized ovum with sex chromosomes XX is biologically female, and a fertilized ovum bearing the XY sex chromosomes is biologically male. Genetics forms the most basic level of an individual's biological sexuality.

Gonadal Basis

The gonadal basis for biological sexuality refers to the growing embryo's development of **gonads.** Male embryos develop testes about the seventh week after conception, and female embryos develop ovaries about the twelfth week after conception.

Structural Development

The development of male or female reproductive structures is initially determined by the presence or absence of hormones produced by the developing testes—androgens and the müllerian inhibiting substance (MIS). With these hormones present, the male embryo starts to develop male reproductive structures (penis, scrotum, vas deferens, seminal vesicles, prostate gland, and Cowper's glands).

Because the female embryo is not exposed to these male hormones, it develops the characteristic female reproductive structures: the uterus, fallopian tubes, vagina, labia, and clitoris.

Biological Sexuality and the Childhood Years

The growth and development of the child in terms of reproductive organs and physiological processes have traditionally been thought to be "latent" during the childhood years. However, a gradual degree of growth occurs in both girls and boys. The reproductive organs, however, will undergo more greatly accelerated growth at the onset of **puberty** and will achieve their adult size and capabilities shortly.

Key Terms

sexuality
The quality of being sexual; can be viewed from many biological and psychosocial perspectives.

masculinity
Behavioral expressions traditionally observed in males.

femininity
Behavioral expressions traditionally observed in females.

biological sexuality
Male and female aspects of sexuality.

gonads
Male or female sex glands; testes produce sperm and ovaries produce eggs.

puberty
Achievement of reproductive ability.

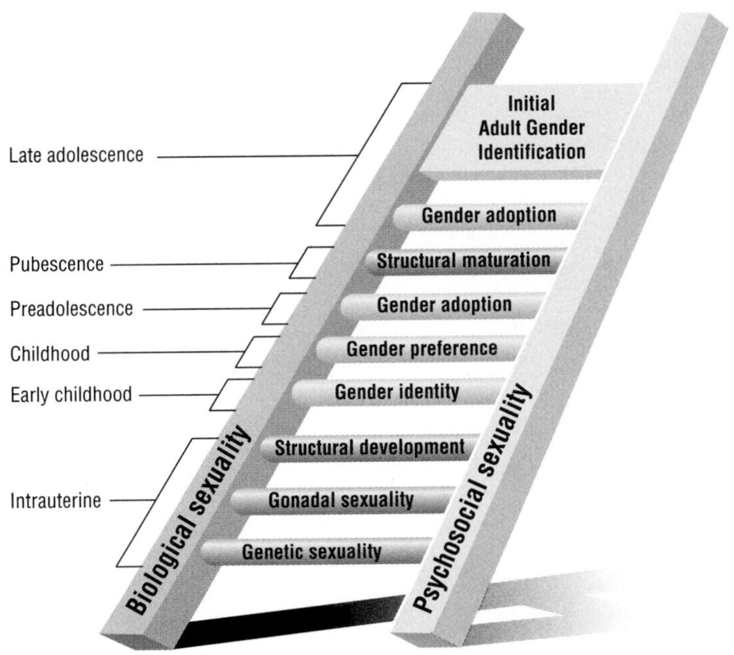

Figure 13-1 Our sexuality develops through biological and psychosocial stages.

Puberty

The entry into puberty is a gradual maturing process for young girls and boys. For young girls, the onset of menstruation, called **menarche,** usually occurs around age 13 but may come somewhat earlier or later.[2] Early menstrual cycles tend to be **anovulatory.** Menarche is usually preceded by a growth spurt that includes the budding of breasts and the growth of pubic and underarm hair.

Young males follow a similar pattern of maturation, including a growth spurt followed by a gradual sexual maturity. However, this process takes place about 2 years later than in young females. Genital enlargement, underarm and pubic hair growth, and a lowering of the voice commonly occur. The male's first ejaculation is generally experienced by the age of 14, most commonly through **nocturnal emission** or masturbation. For many young boys, fully mature sperm do not develop until about age 15.

Reproductive capability only gradually declines over the course of the adult years. In the woman, however, the onset of **menopause** signals a more definite turning off of the reproductive system than is the case for the male adult. By the early to mid-fifties, virtually all women have entered a postmenopausal period, but for men, relatively high-level **spermatogenesis** may continue for a decade or two.

The story of sexual maturation and reproductive maturity cannot, however, be solely focused on the changes that take place in the body. The psychosocial processes that accompany the biological changes are also important.

PSYCHOSOCIAL BASES OF HUMAN SEXUALITY

If growth and development of our sexuality were to be visualized as a stepladder (Figure 13-1), one vertical rail of the ladder would represent our biological sexuality. The rungs would represent the sequential unfolding of the genetic, gonadal, and structural components.

Because humans, more than any other life form, can rise above a life centered on reproduction, a second dimension (or rail) to our sexuality exists—our **psychosocial sexuality.** The reason we possess the ability to be more than reproductive beings is a question for the theologian or philosopher. We are considerably more complex than the functions determined by biology. The process that transforms a male into a man and a female into a woman begins at birth and continues to influence us through the course of our lives.

Gender Identity

Although expectant parents may prefer to have a child of one **gender** over the other, they know that this matter is determined when the child is conceived. External genitals "cast the die," and femininity or masculinity is traditionally reinforced by the parents and society in general. By age 18 months, typical children have both the language and the insight to correctly identify their gender. They have established a **gender identity.**[3] The first rung rising from the psychosocial rail of the ladder has been climbed.

Gender Preference

During the preschool years, children receive the second component of the *scripting* required for the full development of psychosocial sexuality—the preference for the gender to which they have been assigned. The process through which **gender preference** is transmitted to the child is a less subtle form of the practices observed during the gender identity period (the first 18 months). Many parents begin to control the child's exposure to experiences traditionally reserved for children of the opposite gender. This is particularly true for boys; parents will stop play activities they perceive as being too feminine.

With the increasing importance of competitive sports for women, many of the skills and experiences once reserved for boys are now being fostered in young girls. What effect, if any, this movement will have on the speed at which gender preference is reached is a topic for further research.*

Gender Adoption

The process of reaching an initial adult gender identification requires a considerable period of time. The specific knowledge, attitudes, and behavior characteristic of adults must be observed, analyzed, and practiced. The process of acquiring and personalizing these "insights" about how men and women think, feel, and act is reflected by the term **gender adoption,** the first and third rungs below the initial adult gender identification rail of the ladder in Figure 13-1.

In addition to developing a personalized version of an adult sexual identity, it is important that the child—and particularly the adolescent—construct a *gender schema* for a member of the opposite gender. Clearly, the world of adulthood, involving intimacy, parenting, and employment, will require that men know women and women know men. Gender adoption provides an opportunity to begin to assemble this equally valuable "picture" of what the other gender is like.

Initial Adult Gender Identification

By the time young people have climbed all of the rungs of the sexuality ladder, they have arrived at the chronological point in the life cycle when they need to construct an initial adult **gender identification.** You might notice that this label seems remarkably similar to the terminology used to describe one of the developmental tasks being used in this textbook. In fact, the task of forming an initial adult identity is closely related to developing an initial adult image of oneself as a man or a woman. Although most of us currently support the concept of "person" in many gender-neutral contexts (for some very valid reasons), we still must identify ourselves as either a man or a woman.

Transsexualism

Students are often intrigued by a sexual variance that is first noticed during one or two of the psychosocial stages just discussed. Transsexualism is a sexual variance of the most profound nature because it represents a complete rejection by an individual of his or her biological sexuality. The male transsexual believes that he is female and thus desires to be the woman that he knows he is. The female transsexual believes that she is male and wants to become the man that she knows she should be. Psychiatrists, sex therapists, and transexuals do not view transexualism as a homosexual orientation.

For transsexuals, the periods of gender preference and gender adoption are perplexing as they attempt, with limited success, to resolve the conflict between

Key Terms

menarche (muh NAR key)
Time of a female's first menstrual cycle.

anovulatory (an OH vyu luh tory)
Not ovulating.

nocturnal emission
Ejaculation that occurs during sleep; "wet dream."

menopause
Decline and eventual cessation of hormone production by the female reproductive system.

spermatogenesis (sper mat oh JEN uh sis)
Process of sperm production.

psychosocial sexuality
Masculine and feminine aspects of sexuality.

gender
General term reflecting a biological basis of sexuality; the male gender or the female gender.

gender identity
Recognition of one's gender.

gender preference
Emotional and intellectual acceptance of one's own gender.

gender adoption
Lengthy process of learning the behavior that is traditional for one's gender.

gender identification
Achievement of a personally satisfying interpretation of one's masculinity or femininity.

*If you want to test the existence of gender preference, ask a group of first- or second-grade boys or girls if they would be happier being a member of the opposite gender. Be prepared for some frank replies.

what their mind tells them is true and what their body displays. Adolescent and young adult transsexuals often cross-dress, undertake homosexual relationships (which they view as being heterosexual relationships), experiment with hormone replacement therapy, and sometimes actively pursue a **sex reassignment operation.** Several thousand of these operations have been performed at some of the leading medical centers in the United States.

ANDROGYNY: SHARING THE PLUSES

Over the last 25 years our society has increasingly accepted an image of a person who possesses both masculine and feminine qualities. This accepted image has taken years to develop because our society traditionally has reinforced rigid masculine roles for men and rigid feminine roles for women.

In the past, from the time a child was born, we assigned and reinforced only those roles and traits that were thought to be directly related to his or her biological gender. Boys were not allowed to cry, play with dolls, or help in the kitchen. Girls were not encouraged to become involved in sports; they were told to learn to sew, cook, and baby-sit. Men were encouraged to be strong, expressive, dominant, aggressive, and career oriented, and women were encouraged to be weak, shy, submissive, passive, and home oriented.

These traditional biases have resulted in some interesting phenomena related to career opportunities. Women were denied jobs requiring above-average physical strength, admittance into professional schools requiring high intellectual capacities, such as law, medicine, and business, and entry into most levels of military participation. Likewise, men were not encouraged to enter traditionally feminine careers, such as nursing, clerical work, and elementary school teaching.

For a variety of reasons, the traditional picture has changed. **Androgyny,** or the blending of both feminine and masculine qualities, is more clearly evident in our society now than ever before. Today it is more acceptable to see men involved in raising children (including changing diapers) and doing routine housework. It is also more acceptable to see women entering the workplace in jobs traditionally managed by men and participating in sports traditionally played by men. Men are not scoffed at when they are seen crying after a touching movie. Women are not laughed at when they choose to assert themselves. The disposal of numerous sexual stereotypes has probably benefited our society immensely by relieving people of the pressure to be 100% "womanly" or 100% "macho."

Research data suggest that androgynous people are more flexible, have greater self-esteem, and show more social skills and motivation to achieve.[3] This should encourage you to be unafraid to break the gender role stereotype.

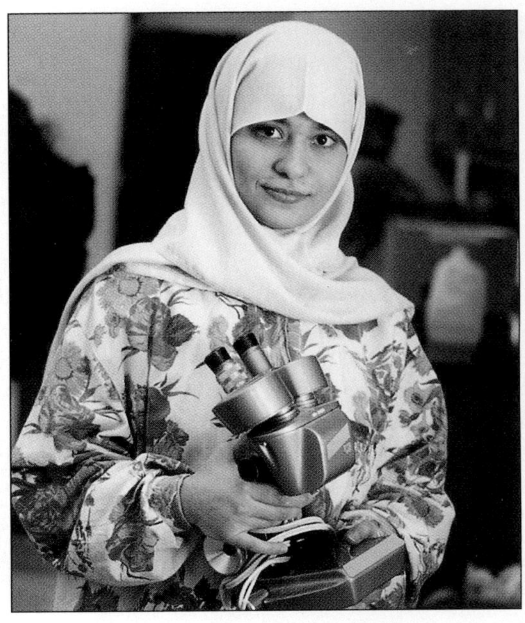

The number of women choosing professions that were once considered "male," such as law and medicine, is continually increasing.

TALKING POINTS • How could you demonstrate to your grandmother that the blending of gender roles is a positive development?

REPRODUCTIVE SYSTEMS

The most familiar aspects of biological sexuality are the structures that compose the reproductive systems. Each structure contributes to the reproductive process in unique ways. Thus, with these structures, males have the ability to impregnate. Females have the ability to become pregnant, give birth, and nourish infants through breastfeeding. Many of these structures are also associated with nonreproductive sexual behavior.

Male Reproductive System

The male reproductive system consists of external structures of genitals (the penis and scrotum) and internal structures (the testes, various passageways or ducts, seminal vesicles, the prostate gland, and the Cowper's glands) (Figure 13-2, *A*). The *testes* (also called *gonads* or *testicles*) are two egg-shaped bodies that lie within a saclike structure called the *scrotum.* During most of fetal development, the testes lie within the abdominal cavity. They descend into the scrotum during the last 2 months of fetal life. The testes are housed in the scrotum because a temperature lower than the body core temperature is re-

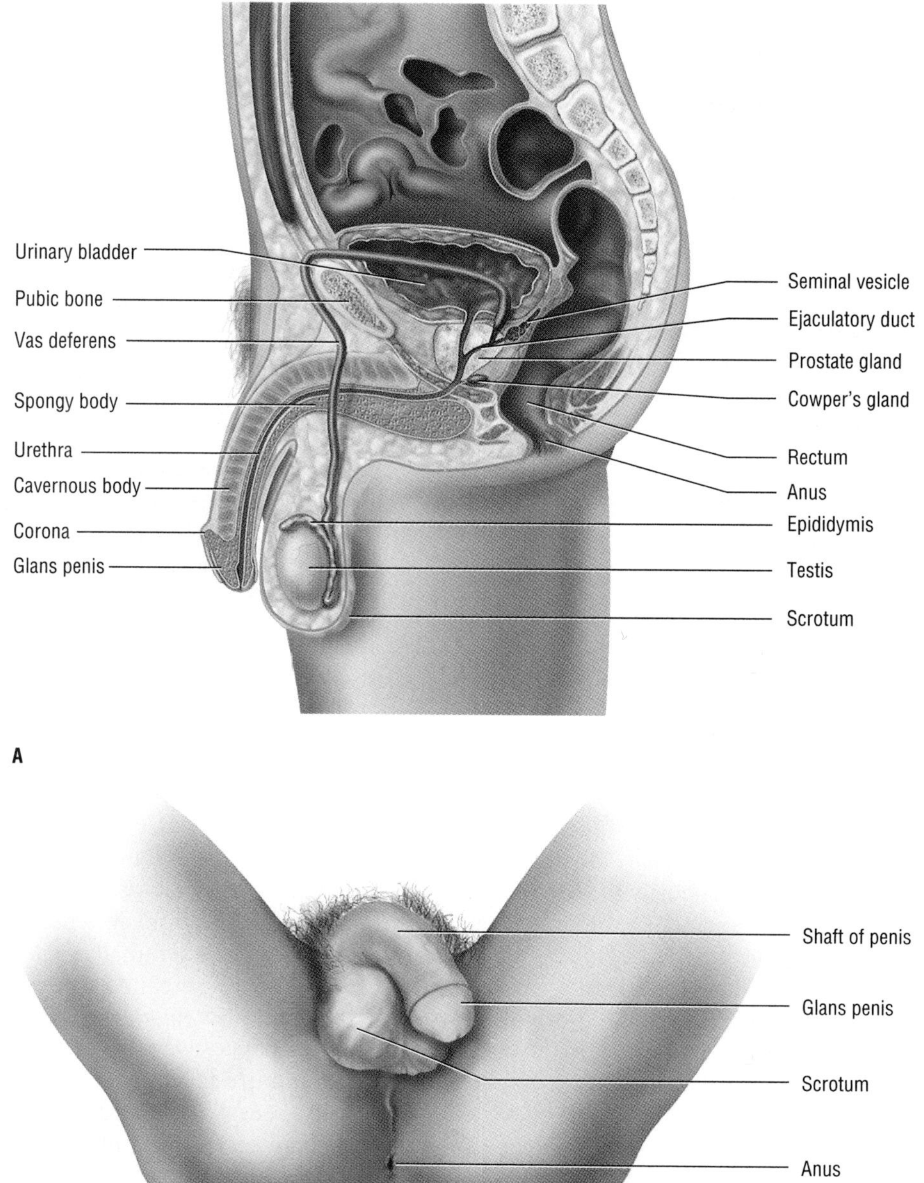

Figure 13-2 The male reproductive system. **A,** Side view, **B,** Front view.

quired for adequate sperm development. The walls of the scrotum are composed of contractile tissue and can draw the testes closer to the body during cold temperatures (and sexual arousal) and relax during warm temperatures. Scrotal contraction and relaxation allow a constant, productive temperature to be maintained in the testes.

Each testis contains an intricate network of structures called *seminiferous tubules* (Figure 13-2, *B*). Within these 300 or so seminiferous tubules, the process of sperm production (spermatogenesis) takes place. Sperm

Key Terms

sex reassignment operation
Surgical procedure designed to remove the external genitalia and replace them with genitalia appropriate to the opposite gender.

androgyny (an droj en ee)
The blending of both masculine and feminine qualities.

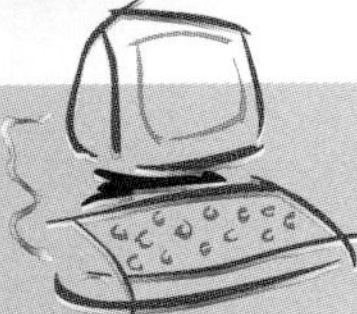

OnSITE/InSIGHT

Learning to Go: Health

Do you think of sexuality as a part of your health? Click on the Motivator icon to find the following lessons related to sexuality:

Lesson 38: Practice safe sex.
Lesson 39: Understand your sexual orientation.
Lesson 40: Enhance your personal relationships.

STUDENT POLL

Is your sexuality important to you? Go to the Online Learning Center at **www.mhhe.com/hahn6e**. Click on Student Resources to find the Student Poll. Answer the following questions and then find out how other students responded.

1. Do you have close friendships?
2. Is it important to you to have one close sexual relationship?
3. Do you believe the way people treat you is directly related to your gender?
4. Do you think you can be intimate with someone without having a sexual relationship with that person?
5. Have you repeatedly found yourself in bad relationships?
6. Is it important to you to always be in a romantic relationship?
7. Do you have a strong desire to love and be loved?
8. Do you feel pressured to always be in a romantic relationship?
9. Are you married, or do you see marriage in your future?
10. Is it important to you to find a partner to spend the rest of your life with?
11. Have you considered remaining single for life?
12. Do you look at single parenthood as a choice?
13. Do you respect people who have a sexual orientation that's different from yours?
14. Do you believe that sexual orientation is a choice?
15. Are different sexual orientations considered acceptable on your college campus?

cell development starts at about age 11 in boys and is influenced by the release of the hormone **ICSH (interstitial cell-stimulating hormone)** from the pituitary gland. ICSH does primarily what its name suggests: it stimulates specific cells (called *interstitial cells*) within the testes to begin producing the male sex hormone *testosterone.* Testosterone in turn is primarily responsible for the gradual development of the male secondary sex characteristics at the onset of puberty. By the time a boy is approximately 15 years old, sufficient levels of testosterone exist so that the testes become capable of full spermatogenesis.

Before the age of about 15, most of the sperm cells produced in the testes are incapable of fertilization. The production of fully mature sperm *(spermatozoa)* is triggered by another hormone secreted by the brain's pituitary gland—**FSH (follicle-stimulating hormone).** FSH influences the seminiferous tubules to begin producing spermatozoa that are capable of fertilization.

Spermatogenesis takes place around the clock, with hundreds of millions of sperm cells produced daily. The sperm cells do not stay in the seminiferous tubules but rather are transferred through a system of ducts that lead into the *epididymis.* The epididymis is a tubular coil that attaches to the back side of each testicle. These collecting structures house the maturing sperm cells for 2 to 3 weeks. During this period the sperm finally become capable of motion, but they remain inactive until they mix with the secretions from the accessory glands (the seminal vesicles, prostate gland, and Cowper's glands).

Each epididymis leads into an 18-inch passageway known as the *vas deferens.* Sperm, moved along by the action of hairlike projections called *cilia,* can also remain in the vas deferens for an extended time without losing their ability to fertilize an egg.

The two vasa deferens extend into the abdominal cavity, where each meets with a *seminal vesicle*—the first of the three accessory structures or glands. Each seminal vesicle contributes a clear, alkaline fluid that nourishes the sperm cells with fructose and permits the sperm cells to be suspended in a movable medium. The fusion of a vas deferens with the seminal vesicle results in the formation of a passageway called the *ejaculatory duct.* Each ejaculatory duct is only about 1 inch long and empties into the final passageway for the sperm—the urethra.

This juncture takes place in an area surrounded by the second accessory gland—the *prostate gland.* The prostate gland secretes a milky fluid containing a variety of substances, including proteins, cholesterol, citric acid, calcium, buffering salts, and various enzymes. The prostate secretions further nourish the sperm cells and also raise the pH level, making the mixture quite alkaline. This alkalinity permits the sperm to have greater longevity as they are transported during ejaculation through the urethra, out of the penis, and into the highly acidic vagina.

The third accessory glands, the Cowper's glands, serve primarily to lubricate the urethra with a clear, viscous mucus. These paired glands empty their small amounts of preejaculatory fluid during the plateau stage of the sexual response cycle. Alkaline in nature, this fluid also neutralizes the acidic level of the urethra. It is hypothesized that viable sperm cells can be suspended in this fluid and can enter the female reproductive tract before full ejaculation by the male.[3] This may account for many of the failures of the "withdrawal" method of contraception.

The sperm cells, when combined with secretions from the seminal vesicles and the prostate gland, form a sticky substance called **semen.** Interestingly, the microscopic sperm actually makes up less than 5% of the seminal fluid discharged at ejaculation. Contrary to popular belief, the paired seminal vesicles contribute about 60% of the semen volume, and the prostate gland adds about 30%.[4] Thus the fear of some men that a **vasectomy** will destroy their ability to ejaculate is completely unfounded (see Chapter 14).

During *emission* (the gathering of semen in the upper part of the urethra), a sphincter muscle at the base of the bladder contracts and inhibits semen from being pushed into the bladder and urine from being deposited into the urethra.[5] Thus semen and urine rarely intermingle, even though they leave the body through the same passageway.

Ejaculation takes place when the semen is forced out of the penis through the urethral opening. The involuntary, rhythmic muscle contractions that control ejaculation result in a series of pleasurable sensations known as *orgasm.*

The urethra lies on the underside of the penis and extends through one of three cylindrical chambers of erectile tissue (two cavernous bodies and one spongy body). Each of these three chambers provides the vascular space required for sufficient erection of the penis. When a male becomes sexually aroused, these areas become congested with blood (*vasocongestion*). After ejaculation or when a male is no longer sexually stimulated, these chambers release the blood into the general circulation and the penis returns to a **flaccid** state.

The *shaft* of the penis is covered by a thin layer of skin that is an extension of the skin that covers the scrotum. This loose layer of skin is sensitive to sexual stimulation and extends over the head of the penis, except in males who have been circumcised. The *glans* (or head) of the penis is the most sexually sensitive (to tactile stimulation) part of the male body. Nerve receptor sites are especially prominent along the *corona* (the ridge of the glans) and the *frenulum* (the thin tissue at the base of the glans).

Female Reproductive System

The external structures (genitals) of the female reproductive system consist of the mons pubis, labia majora, labia minora, clitoris, and vestibule (Figure 13-3). Collectively these structures form the *vulva* or vulval area. The *mons pubis* is the fatty covering over the pubic bone. The mons pubis (or mons veneris, "mound of Venus") is covered by pubic hair and is quite sensitive to sexual stimulation. The *labia majora* are large longitudinal folds of skin that cover the entrance to the vagina, whereas the *labia minora* are the smaller longitudinal skin folds that lie within the labia majora. These hairless skin folds of the labia minora join at the top to form the *prepuce.* The prepuce covers the glans of the *clitoris,* which is the most sexually sensitive part of the female body.

A rather direct analogy can be made between the penis and the clitoris. In terms of the tactile sensitivity, both structures are the most sensitive parts of the male and female genitals. Both contain a glans and a shaft (although the clitoral shaft is beneath the skin surface). Both organs are composed of erectile tissue that can become engorged with blood. Both are covered by skin folds (the clitoral prepuce of the female and the foreskin of the male), and both structures can collect **smegma** beneath these tissue folds.[3]

The *vestibule* is the region enclosed by the labia minora. Evident here are the urethral opening and the entrance to the vagina (or vaginal orifice). Also located at the vaginal opening are the *Bartholin's glands,* which secrete a minute amount of lubricating fluid during sexual excitement.

The *hymen* is a thin layer of tissue that stretches across the opening of the vagina. Once thought to be the only indication of virginity, the intact hymen rarely covers the vaginal opening entirely. Openings in the hymen are necessary for the discharge of menstrual fluid and vaginal secretions. Many hymens are stretched or torn to full opening by adolescent physical activity or by the

Key Terms

ICSH (interstitial cell-stimulating hormone) (in ter STISH ul)
A gonadotropic hormone of the male required for the production of testosterone.

FSH (follicle-stimulating hormone)
A gonadotropic hormone required for initial development of ova (in the female) and sperm (in the male).

semen
Secretion containing sperm and nutrients discharged from the urethra at ejaculation.

vasectomy
Surgical procedure in which the vasa deferens are cut to prevent the passage of sperm from the testicles; the most common form of male sterilization.

flaccid (fla sid)
Nonerect; the state of erectile tissue when vasocongestion is not occurring.

smegma
Cellular discharge that can accumulate beneath the clitoral hood and the foreskin of an uncircumcised penis.

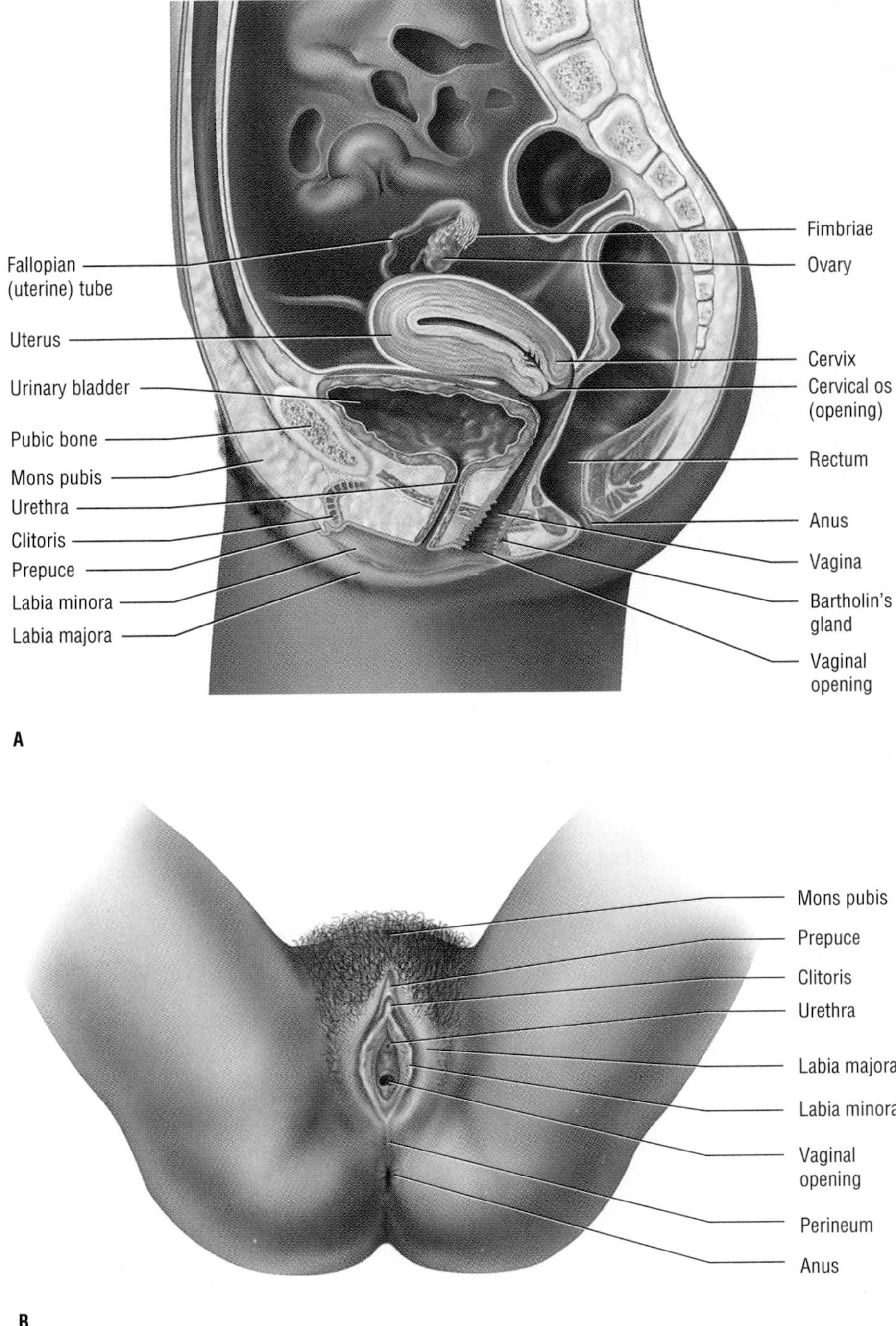

Figure 13-3 The female reproductive system. **A,** Side view, **B,** Front view.

insertion of tampons. In women whose hymens are not fully ruptured, the first act of sexual intercourse will generally accomplish this. Pain may accompany first intercourse in females with relatively intact hymens.

The internal reproductive structures of the female include the vagina, uterus, fallopian tubes, and ovaries. The *vagina* is the structure that accepts the penis during sexual intercourse. Normally the walls of the vagina are collapsed, except during sexual stimulation, when the vaginal walls widen and elongate to accommodate the erect penis. Only the outer third of the vagina is especially sensitive to sexual stimulation. In this location, vaginal tissues swell considerably to form the **orgasmic platform.** This platform constricts the vaginal opening and in effect "grips" the penis (or other inserted object)—regardless of its size.[3] So the belief that a woman receives considerably more sexual pleasure from men with large penises is not supported from an anatomical standpoint.

The *uterus* (or *womb*) is approximately the size and shape of a small pear. This highly muscular organ is capable of undergoing a wide range of physical changes, as evidenced by its enlargement during pregnancy, its contraction during menstruation and labor, and its movement during the orgasmic phase of the female sexual response cycle. The primary function of the uterus is to provide a suitable environment for the possible implantation of a fertilized ovum, or egg. This implantation, should it occur, will take place in the innermost lining of the uterus—the *endometrium*. In the mature female, the endometrium undergoes cyclic changes as it prepares a new lining on a near-monthly basis.

The lower third of the uterus is called the *cervix*. The cervix extends slightly into the vagina. Sperm can enter the uterus through the cervical opening, or *cervical os*. Mucous glands in the cervix secrete a fluid that is thin and watery near the time of ovulation. Mucus of this consistency apparently facilitates sperm passage into the uterus and deeper structures. However, cervical mucus is much thicker during certain points in the menstrual cycle (when pregnancy is improbable) and during pregnancy (to protect against bacterial agents and other substances that are especially dangerous to the developing fetus).

The upper two thirds of the uterus is called the *corpus*, or *body*. This is where implantation of the fertilized ovum generally takes place. The upper portion of the uterus opens into two *fallopian tubes*, or *oviducts*, each about 4 inches long. The fallopian tubes are each directed toward an *ovary*. They serve as a passageway for the ovum in its week-long voyage toward the uterus. Usually, conception takes place in the upper third of the fallopian tubes.

The ovaries are analogous to the testes in the male. Their function is to produce the ovum, or egg. Usually, one ovary produces and releases just one egg each month. Approximately the size and shape of an unshelled almond, an ovary produces viable ova in the process known as *oogenesis*. The ovaries also produce the female sex hormones through the efforts of specific structures within the ovaries. These hormones play multiple roles in the development of female secondary sex characteristics, but their primary function is to prepare the endometrium of the uterus for possible implantation of a fertilized ovum. In the average healthy female, this preparation takes place about 13 times a year for a period of about 35 years. At menopause, the ovaries shrink considerably and stop nearly all hormonal production.

Menstrual cycle

Each month or so, the inner wall of the uterus prepares for a possible pregnancy. When a pregnancy does not occur (as is the case throughout most months of a woman's fertile years), this lining must be released and a new one prepared. The breakdown of this endometrial wall and the resultant discharge of blood and endometrial tissue is known as *menstruation* (or *menses*) (Figure 13-4). The cyclic timing of menstruation is governed by hormones released from two sources: the pituitary gland and the ovaries.

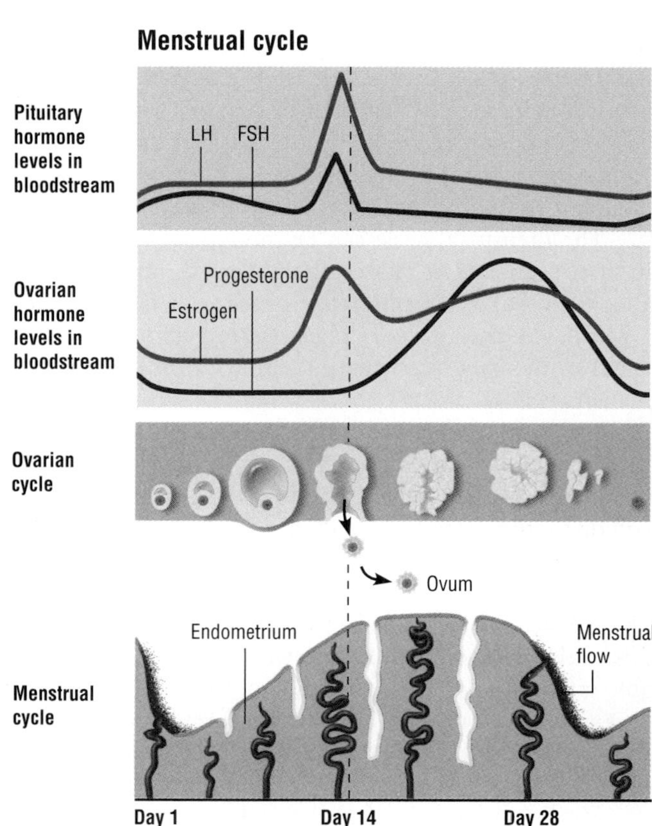

Figure 13-4 The menstrual cycle involves the development and release of an ovum, supported by hormones from the pituitary, and the buildup of the endometrium, supported by hormones from the ovary, for the purpose of establishing a pregnancy.

Key Term

orgasmic platform
Expanded outer third of the vagina that grips the penis during the plateau phase of the sexual response pattern.

Girls generally have their first menstrual cycle, the onset of which is called *menarche,* sometime between 12 and 14 years of age. Body weight, nutrition, heredity, and overall health are factors related to menarche. After a girl first menstruates, she may be anovulatory for a year or longer before a viable ovum is released during her cycle. This cyclic activity will continue until about age 45 to 55.

This text refers to a menstrual cycle that lasts 28 days. However, few women display perfect 28-day cycles. Most women fluctuate by a few days to a week around this 28-day pattern, and some women vary greatly from this cycle.

Your knowledge about the menstrual cycle is critical for your understanding of pregnancy, contraception, menopause, and issues related to the overall health and comfort of women (see the Star Box on this page for a discussion of endometriosis). Although at first this cycle may sound like a complicated process, each segment of the cycle can be studied separately for better understanding.

The menstrual cycle can be thought of as occurring in three segments or phases: the menstrual phase (lasting about 1 week), the proliferative phase (also lasting about 1 week), and the secretory phase (lasting about 2 weeks). Day 1 of this cycle starts with the first day of bleeding, or menstrual flow.

The *menstrual phase* signals the woman that a pregnancy has not taken place and that her uterine lining is being sloughed off. During a 5- to 7-day period, a woman will discharge about ¼ to ½ cup of blood and tissue. (Only about 1 ounce of the menstrual flow is actual blood.) The menstrual flow is heaviest during the first days of this phase. Since the muscular uterus must contract to accomplish this tissue removal, some women have uncomfortable cramping during menstruation. Most women, however, report more pain and discomfort during the few days before the first day of bleeding. (See the discussion of premenstrual syndrome [PMS] on page 323.)

Modern methods of absorbing menstrual flow include the use of internal tampons and external pads. Caution must be exercised by the users of tampons to prevent the possibility of toxic shock syndrome (TSS) (see Chapter 12). Since menstrual flow is a positive sign of good health, women are encouraged to be normally active during menstruation.

The *proliferative phase* of the menstrual cycle starts about the time menstruation stops. Lasting about 1 week, this phase is first influenced by the release of FSH from the pituitary gland. FSH circulates in the bloodstream and directs the ovaries to start the process of maturing approximately 20 primary ovarian *follicles.* Thousands of primary egg follicles are present in each ovary at birth. These follicles resemble shells that house immature ova. As these follicles ripen under FSH influence, they release the hormone estrogen. Estrogen's primary function is to direct the endometrium to start the development of a thick, highly vascular wall. As the estrogen levels increase, the pituitary gland's secretion of FSH is reduced. Now the pituitary gland prepares for the surge of the **luteinizing hormone (LH)** required to accomplish ovulation.[6]

In the days immediately preceding ovulation, one of the primary follicles (called the *graafian follicle*) matures fully. The other primary follicles degenerate and are absorbed by the body. The graafian follicle moves toward the surface of the ovary. When LH is released in massive quantities on about day 14, the graafian follicle bursts to release the fully mature ovum. The release of the ovum is **ovulation.** Regardless of the overall length of a woman's cycle, ovulation occurs 14 days before her first day of menstrual flow.

The ovum is quickly captured by the fingerlike projections (*fimbriae*) of the fallopian tubes. In the upper third of the fallopian tubes, the ovum is capable of being fertilized in a 24- to 36-hour period. If the ovum is not fertilized by a sperm cell, it will begin to degenerate and eventually will be absorbed by the body.

After ovulation, the *secretory phase* of the menstrual cycle starts when the remnants of the graafian follicle restructure themselves into a **corpus luteum.** The corpus luteum remains inside the ovary, secreting estrogen and a fourth hormone called *progesterone.* Progesterone, which literally means "for pregnancy," continues to direct the endometrial buildup. If pregnancy occurs, the corpus lu-

Endometriosis

Endometriosis is a condition in which endometrial tissue that normally lines the uterus is found growing within the pelvic cavity. Because the tissue remains sensitive to circulating hormones, it is the source of pain and discomfort during the latter half of the menstrual cycle. Endometriosis is most commonly found in younger women and is frequently related to infertility.

In addition to discomfort before menstruation, the symptoms of endometriosis include low back pain, pain during intercourse, and a variety of lower digestive tract symptoms, such as diarrhea and constipation. As with the general pain and discomfort of endometriosis, these symptoms are also more noticeable during the latter weeks of the cycle.

Treatment of endometriosis largely depends on its extent. Drugs to suppress ovulation, including birth control pills, may be helpful in mild cases. For more severe cases, surgical removal of the tissue or a hysterectomy may be necessary. For some women, endometriosis is suppressed during pregnancy and does not return after pregnancy.

teum monitors progesterone and estrogen levels throughout the pregnancy. If pregnancy does not occur, high levels of progesterone signal the pituitary gland to stop the release of LH and the corpus luteum starts to degenerate on about day 24. When estrogen and progesterone levels diminish significantly by day 28, the endometrium is discharged from the uterus and out the vagina. The secretory phase ends, and the menstrual phase begins. The cycle is then complete.

PMS. PMS is characterized by psychological symptoms, such as depression, lethargy, irritability, and aggressiveness, or somatic symptoms, such as headache, backache, asthma, and acne, that recur in the same phase of each menstrual cycle, followed by a symptom-free phase in each cycle. Some of the more frequently reported symptoms of PMS include tension, tender breasts, fainting, fatigue, abdominal cramps, and weight gain.

The cause of PMS appears to be hormonal. Perhaps a woman's body is insensitive to a normal level of progesterone, or her ovaries fail to produce a normal amount of progesterone. These reasons seem plausible because PMS types of symptoms do not occur during pregnancy, during which natural progesterone levels are very high, and because women with PMS seem to feel much better after receiving high doses of natural progesterone in suppository form. When using oral contraceptives that supply synthetic progesterone at normal levels, many women report relief from some symptoms of PMS. However, the effectiveness of the most frequently used form of treatment, progesterone suppositories, is now being questioned.

Until the effectiveness of progesterone has been fully researched, it is unlikely that the medical community will deal with PMS through any approach other than a relatively conservative treatment of symptoms through the use of *analgesic drugs* (including *prostaglandin inhibitors*), diuretic drugs, dietary modifications (including restriction of caffeine and salt), vitamin B_6 therapy, exercise, and stress-reduction exercises. The exact nature of PMS has been further complicated by the classification of severe PMS as a mental disturbance by some segments of the American Psychiatric Association.

Fibrocystic breast condition. In some women, particularly those who have never been pregnant, stimulation of the breast tissues by estrogen and progesterone during the menstrual cycle results in an unusually high degree of secretory activity by the cells lining the ducts. The fluid released by the secretory lining finds its way into the fibrous connective tissue areas in the lower half of the breast, where in pocketlike cysts the fluid presses against neighboring tissues. In many women, excessive secretory activity produces a fibrocystic breast condition characterized by swollen, firm or hardened, tender breast tissue before menstruation.

Women who experience a more extensive fibrocystic condition can be treated with drugs that have a "calming" effect on progesterone production. In addition, occasional draining of the fluid-filled cysts can bring relief.

Menopause

For the vast majority of women in their late forties through their mid-fifties, a gradual decline in reproductive system function, called *menopause,* occurs. Menopause is a normal physiological process, not a disease process. It can, however, become a health concern for some middle-aged women who have unpleasant side effects resulting from this natural stoppage of ovum production and menstruation.

As ovarian function and hormone production diminish, a period of adjustment must be made by the hypothalamus, ovaries, uterus, and other estrogen-sensitive tissues. The extent of menopause as a health problem is determined by the degree to which **hot flashes,** vaginal wall dryness, depression and melancholy, breast changes, and the uncertainty of fertility are seen as problems.

In comparison with past generations, today's midlife women are much less likely to find menopause to be a negative experience. The end of fertility, combined with children leaving the home, makes the middle years a period of personal rediscovery for many women.

For women who are troubled by the changes brought about by menopause, physicians may prescribe **hormone replacement therapy (HRT).** This can relieve many symptoms and offer benefits to help reduce the incidence of osteoporosis (see Chapter 4) and coronary artery disease (see Chapter 10).

Key Terms

luteinizing hormone (LH) (LOO ten eye zing)
A gonadotropic hormone of the female required for fullest development and release of ova; ovulating hormone.

ovulation
The release of a mature egg from the ovary.

corpus luteum (kore pus loo tee um)
Cellular remnant of the graafian follicle after the release of an ovum.

hot flashes
Temporary feelings of warmth experienced by women during and after menopause, caused by blood vessel dilation.

hormone replacement therapy (HRT)
Medically administered estrogen and progestin to replace hormones lost as the result of menopause.

HUMAN SEXUAL RESPONSE PATTERN

Although history has many written and visual accounts of the human's ability to be sexually aroused, it was not until the pioneering work of Masters and Johnson[7] that the events associated with arousal were clinically documented. Five questions posed by these researchers gave direction to a series of studies involving the scientific evaluation of human sexual response:

Is There a Predictable Pattern Associated with the Sexual Responses of Males and Females?

The answer to the first question posed by the researchers was an emphatic yes. A predictable sexual response pattern was identified;[7] it consists of an initial **excitement stage,** a **plateau stage,** an **orgasmic stage,** and a **resolution stage.** Each stage involves predictable changes in the structural characteristics and physiological function of reproductive and nonreproductive organs in both the male and the female. These changes are shown in Figure 13-5.

Is the Sexual Response Pattern Stimuli-Specific?

The research of Masters and Johnson[7] clearly established a no answer to the second question concerning stimuli specificity. Their findings demonstrated that numerous senses can supply the stimuli necessary for initiating the sexual response pattern. Although touching activities might initiate arousal in most people and maximize it for the vast majority of people, in both males and females, sight, smell, sound, and *vicariously formed stimuli* can also stimulate the same sexual arousal patterns.

What Differences Occur in the Sexual Response Pattern?

Differences between males and females

Several differences are observable when the sexual response patterns of males and females are compared:

- With the exception of some later adolescent males, the vast majority of males are not multiorgasmic. The **refractory phase** of the resolution stage prevents most males from experiencing more than one orgasm in a short period, even when sufficient stimulation is available.
- Females possess a **multiorgasmic capacity.** Masters and Johnson[7] found that as many as 10% to 30% of all female adults routinely experience multiple orgasms.
- Although they possess multiorgasmic potential, about 10% of all female adults are *anorgasmic*—that is, they never experience an orgasm.[7] For many anorgasmic females, orgasms can be experienced when masturbation, rather than **coitus,** provides the stimulation.
- When measured during coitus, males reach orgasm far more quickly than do females. However, when masturbation is the source of stimulation, females reach orgasm as quickly as do males.[7]

More important than any of the differences pointed out is the finding that the sexual response patterns of males and females are far more alike than they are different. Not only do males and females experience the four basic stages of the response pattern, but they also have similar responses in specific areas, including the **erection** and *tumescence* of sexual structures; the appearance of a **sex flush;** the increase in cardiac output, blood pressure, and respiratory rate; and the occurrence of *rhythmic pelvic thrusting.*[7]

Differences among subjects within a same-gender group

When a group of subjects of the same gender was studied in an attempt to answer questions about similarities and

Key Terms

excitement stage
Initial arousal stage of the sexual response pattern.

plateau stage
Second stage of the sexual response pattern; a leveling off of arousal immediately before orgasm.

orgasmic stage
Third stage of the sexual response pattern; the stage during which neuromuscular tension is released.

resolution stage
Fourth stage of the sexual response pattern; the return of the body to a preexcitement state.

refractory phase
That portion of the male's resolution stage during which sexual arousal cannot occur.

multiorgasmic capacity
Potential to have several orgasms within a single period of sexual arousal.

coitus (CO ih tus)
Penile-vaginal intercourse.

erection
The engorgement of erectile tissue with blood; characteristic of the penis, clitoris, nipples, labia minora, and scrotum.

sex flush
The reddish skin response that results from increasing sexual arousal.

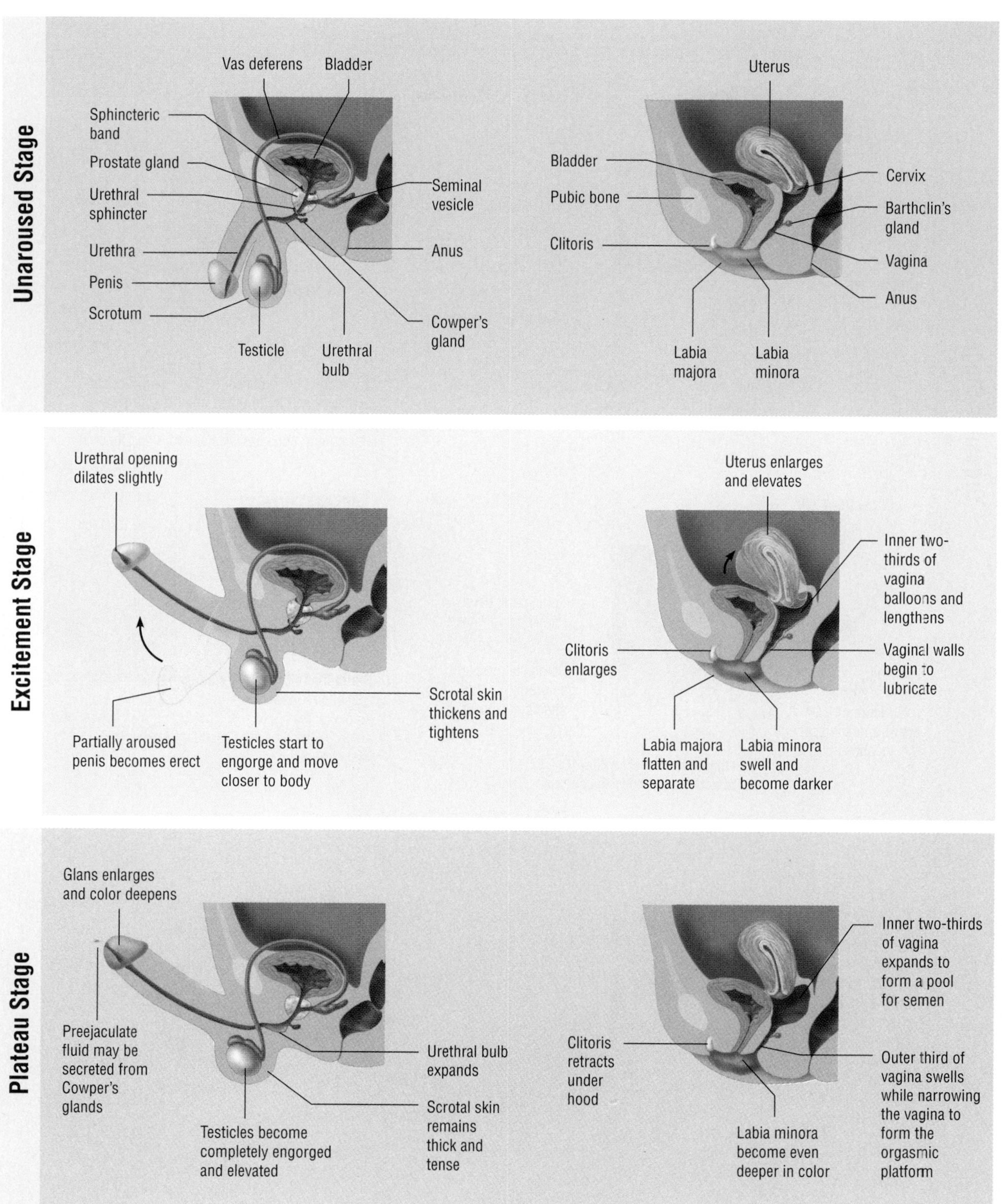

Figure 13-5 The sexual response pattern in men and women. *Continued.*

Orgasmic Stage

SENSATION OF ORGASM

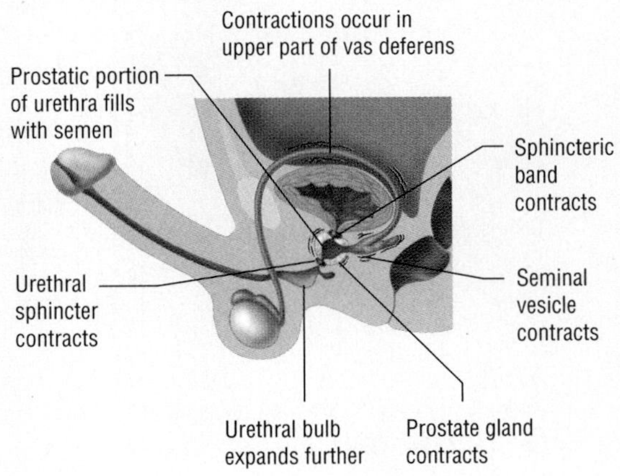
Contractions occur in upper part of vas deferens
Prostatic portion of urethra fills with semen
Sphincteric band contracts
Urethral sphincter contracts
Seminal vesicle contracts
Urethral bulb expands further
Prostate gland contracts

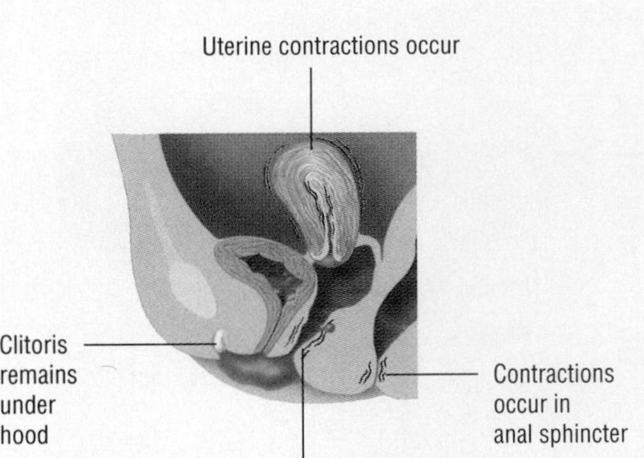
Uterine contractions occur
Clitoris remains under hood
Contractions occur in anal sphincter
Contractions in outer third of the vagina occur rhythmically 3 to 15 times; the first of these contractions are spaced at 0.8-second intervals; later contractions are weaker and occur more slowly

EJACULATION

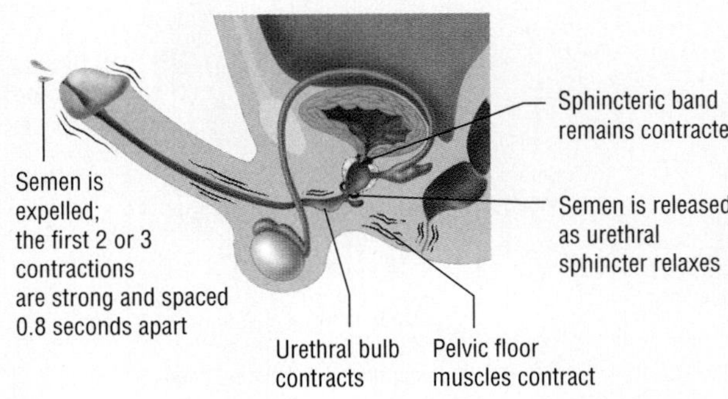
Sphincteric band remains contracted
Semen is expelled; the first 2 or 3 contractions are strong and spaced 0.8 seconds apart
Semen is released as urethral sphincter relaxes
Urethral bulb contracts
Pelvic floor muscles contract

BREAST CHANGES

① **Unaroused stage**

② **Excitement stage**
Breast size increases; nipples become erect; veins become more visible

③ **Plateau and orgasmic stages**
Breast size increases more; areola increases in size (making nipples appear less erect); skin color may become flushed from vasocongestion

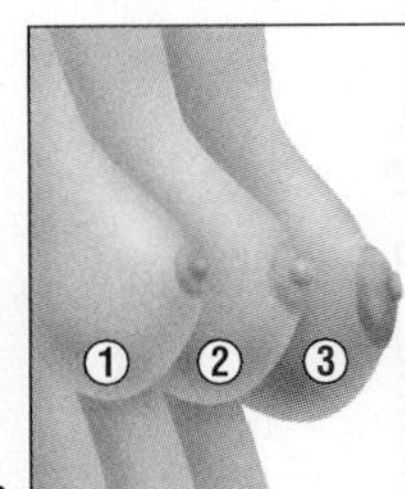
①
②
③

Resolution Stage

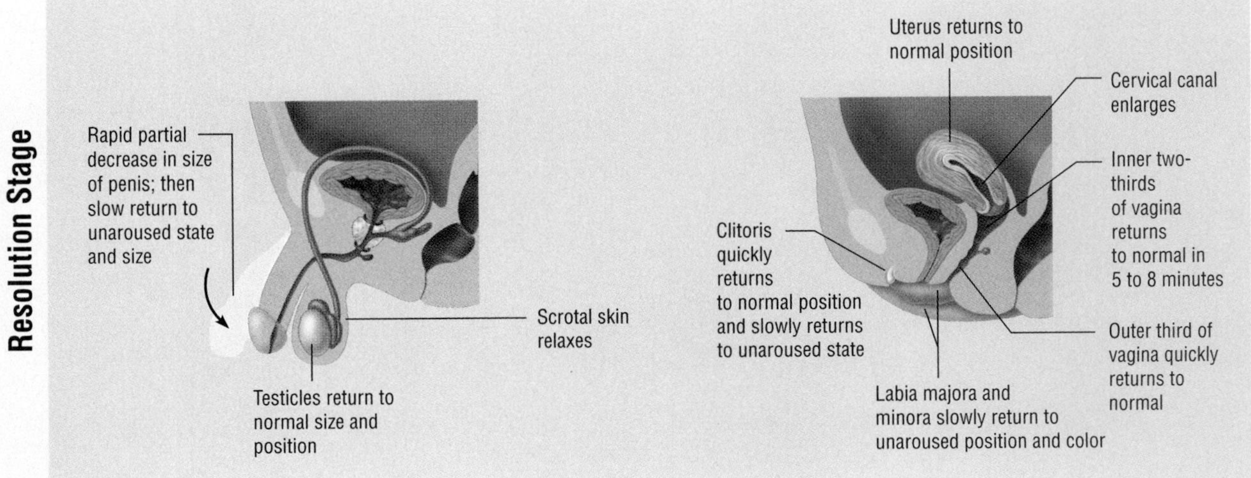
Rapid partial decrease in size of penis; then slow return to unaroused state and size
Scrotal skin relaxes
Testicles return to normal size and position
Uterus returns to normal position
Cervical canal enlarges
Inner two-thirds of vagina returns to normal in 5 to 8 minutes
Clitoris quickly returns to normal position and slowly returns to unaroused state
Outer third of vagina quickly returns to normal
Labia majora and minora slowly return to unaroused position and color

Figure 13-5

differences in the sexual response pattern, Masters and Johnson noted considerable variation. Even when variables such as age, race, education, and general health were held constant, the extent and duration of virtually every stage of the response pattern varied.

Differences within the same individual

For a given person the nature of the sexual response pattern does not remain constant, even when observed over a relatively short period. A variety of internal and external factors can alter this pattern. The aging process, changes in general health status, levels of stress, altered environmental settings, use of alcohol and other drugs, and behavioral changes in a sexual partner can cause one's own sexual response pattern to change from one sexual experience to another. Sexual performance difficulties and therapies are briefly discussed in the Star Box on this page.

What Are the Basic Physiological Mechanisms Underlying the Sexual Response Pattern?

The basic mechanisms in the fourth question posed by Masters and Johnson are now well recognized. One factor, *vasocongestion,* or the retention of blood or fluid within a particular tissue, is critically important in the development of physiological changes that promote the sexual response pattern.[7] The presence of erectile tissue underlies the changes that can be noted in the penis, breasts, and scrotum of the male and the clitoris, breasts, and labia minora of the female.

A second mechanism now recognized as necessary for the development of the sexual response pattern is that of *myotonia,* or the buildup of *neuromuscular tonus* within a variety of body structures.[7] At the end of the plateau stage of the response pattern, a sudden release of the accumulated neuromuscular tension gives rise to the rhythmic muscular contractions and pleasurable muscular spasms that constitute orgasm, as well as ejaculation in the male.

What Role Is Played by Specific Organs and Organ Systems within the Sexual Response Pattern?

The fifth question posed by Masters and Johnson, which concerns the role played by specific organs and organ systems during each stage of the response pattern, can be readily answered by referring to the material presented in Figure 13–5. As you study this figure, remember that direct stimulation of the penis and either direct or indirect stimulation of the clitoris are the principal avenues toward orgasm. Also, intercourse represents only one activity that can lead to orgasmic pleasure.[2]

Sexual Performance Difficulties and Therapies

Despite the predictability of the human sexual response pattern, many people find that at some point in their lives, they are no longer capable of responding sexually. The inability of a person to perform adequately is identified as a sexual difficulty or dysfunction. Sexual difficulties can have a negative influence on a person's sense of sexual satisfaction and on a partner's satisfaction. Fortunately, most sexual difficulties can be resolved through strategies that use individual, couple, or group counseling. Many sexual performance difficulties stem from psychogenic (originating in the mind) factors.

PATTERNS OF SEXUAL BEHAVIOR

Although sex researchers may see sexual behavior in terms of the human sexual response pattern just described, most people are more interested in the observable dimensions of sexual behavior. Complete the Personal Assessment on p. 341 to determine whether your own attitudes toward sexuality are traditional or nontraditional.

Celibacy

Celibacy can be defined as the self-imposed avoidance of sexual intimacy. It is synonymous with sexual abstinence. There are many reasons people could choose not to have a sexually intimate relationship. For some, celibacy is part of a religious doctrine. Others might be afraid of sexually transmitted diseases. For most, however, celibacy is preferred simply because it seems appropriate for them. Celibate people can certainly have deep, intimate relationships with other people—just not sexual relationships. Celibacy may be short-term or last a lifetime, and no identified physical or psychological complications appear to result from a celibate lifestyle.

Key Terms

masturbation
Self-stimulation of the genitals.

sexual fantasies
Fantasies with sexual themes; sexual daydreams or imaginary events.

TALKING POINTS • You have decided to remain celibate until you're ready to make a lifetime commitment to someone. How would you explain this to the person you are now dating?

Masturbation

Throughout recorded history, **masturbation** has been a primary method of achieving sexual pleasure. Through masturbation, people can explore their sexual response patterns. Traditionally, some societies and religious groups have condemned this behavior based on the belief that intercourse is the only "right" sexual behavior. With sufficient lubrication, masturbation cannot do physical harm. Today masturbation is considered by most sex therapists and researchers to be a normal source of self-pleasure.

Fantasy and Erotic Dreams

The brain is the most sensual organ in the body. In fact, many sexuality experts classify **sexual fantasies** and **erotic dreams** as forms of sexual behavior. Particularly for people whose verbal ability is highly developed, the ability to create imaginary scenes enriches other forms of sexual behavior.

Sexual fantasies are generally found in association with some second type of sexual behavior. When occurring before intercourse or masturbation, fantasies prepare a person for the behavior that will follow. As an example, fantasies experienced while reading a book may focus your attention on sexual activity that will occur later in the day.

When fantasies occur in conjunction with another form of sexual behavior, the second behavior may be greatly enhanced by the supportive fantasy. Both women and men fantasize during foreplay and intercourse. Masturbation and fantasizing are inseparable activities.

Erotic dreams occur during sleep in both men and women. The association between these dreams and ejaculation resulting in a nocturnal emission (wet dream) is readily recognized in males. In females, erotic dreams can lead not only to vaginal lubrication but to orgasm as well.

Shared Touching

Virtually the entire body can be an erogenous (sexually sensitive) zone when shared touching is involved. A soft, light touch, a slight application of pressure, the brushing back of a partner's hair, and gentle massage are all forms of communication that heighten sexual arousal.

Genital Contact

Two important uses can be identified for the practice of stimulating a partner's genitals. The first is that of being the tactile component of **foreplay.** Genital contact, in the form of holding, rubbing, stroking, or caressing, heightens arousal to a level that allows for progression to intercourse.

The second role of genital contact is that of *mutual masturbation to orgasm*. Stimulation of the genitals so that both partners have orgasm is a form of sexual behavior practiced by many people, as well as couples during the late stage of a pregnancy. For couples not desiring pregnancy, the risk of conception is virtually eliminated when this becomes the form of sexual intimacy practiced.

As is the case of other aspects of intimacy, genital stimulation is best enhanced when partners can talk about their needs, expectations, and reservations. Practice and communication can shape this form of contact into a pleasure-giving approach to sexual intimacy.

Oral-Genital Stimulation

Oral-genital stimulation brings together two of the body's most erogenous areas: the genitalia and the mouth. Couples who engage in oral sex consistently report that this form of intimacy is highly satisfactory. Some people have experimented with oral sex and found it unacceptable, and some have never experienced this form of sexual intimacy. Some couples prefer not to participate in oral sex because they consider it immoral (according to religious doctrine), illegal (which it is in some states), or unhygienic (because of a partner's unclean genitals). Some couples may refrain because of the mistaken belief that oral sex is a homosexual practice. Regardless of the reason, a person who does not consider oral sex to be pleasurable should not be coerced into this behavior.

Because oral-genital stimulation can involve an exchange of body fluids, the risk of disease transmission is real. Small tears of mouth or genital tissue may allow transmission of disease-causing pathogens. Only couples who are absolutely certain that they are free from all sexually transmitted diseases (including HIV infection) can practice unprotected oral sex. Couples in doubt should refrain from oral-genital sex or carefully use a condom (on the male) or a latex square to cover the female's vulval area. Increasingly, latex squares (dental dams) can be obtained from drug stores or pharmacies. (Dentists may also provide you with dental dams, or you can make your own latex square by cutting a condom into an appropriate shape, or you can use plastic kitchen wrap.)

Three basic forms of oral-genital stimulation are practiced by both heterosexual and homosexual couples.[5] **Fellatio,** in which the penis is sucked, licked, or kissed by the partner, is the most common of the three. **Cunnilingus,** in which the vulva of the female is kissed, licked, or penetrated by the partner's tongue, is only slightly less frequently practiced.

Mutual oral-genital stimulation, the third form of oral-genital stimulation, combines both fellatio and cunnilingus. When practiced by a heterosexual couple, the female partner performs fellatio on her partner while her male partner performs cunnilingus on her. Homosexual couples can practice mutual fellatio or cunnilingus.

Intercourse

Sexual intercourse (coitus) refers to the act of inserting the penis into the vagina. Intercourse is the sexual behavior that is most directly associated with **procreation.** For some, intercourse is the only natural and appropriate form of sexual intimacy.

The incidence and frequency of sexual intercourse is a much-studied topic. Information concerning the percentages of people who have engaged in intercourse is readily available in textbooks used in sexuality courses. Data concerning sexual intercourse among college students may be changing somewhat because of concerns about HIV infection and other STDs, but a reasonable estimate of the percentage of college students reporting sexual intercourse is between 60% and 75%.

These percentages reflect two important concepts about the sexual activity of college students. The first is that a large majority of college students is having intercourse. The second concept is that a sizeable percentage (25% to 40%) of students is choosing to refrain from intercourse. Indeed, the belief that "everyone is doing it" may be a bit shortsighted. From a public health standpoint, we believe it is important to provide accurate health information to protect those who choose to have intercourse and to actively support a person's right to choose not to have intercourse.

Couples need to share their expectations concerning sexual techniques and frequency of intercourse. Even the "performance" factors, such as depth of penetration, nature of body movements, tempo of activity, and timing of orgasm are of increasing importance to many couples. Issues concerning sexually transmitted diseases (including HIV infection) are also critically important for couples who are contemplating intercourse. These factors also need to be explored through open communication.

There are a variety of books (including textbooks) that provide written and visually explicit information on intercourse positions. Four basic positions for intercourse—male above, female above, side by side, and rear entry—each offer relative advantages and disadvantages.

SEXUALITY AND AGING

Students are often curious about how aging affects sexuality. This is understandable because we live in a society that idolizes youth and demands performance. Many younger people become anxious about growing older because of what they think will happen to their ability to express their sexuality. Interestingly, young adults are willing to accept other physical changes of aging (such as the slowing down of basal metabolism, reduced lung capacity, and even wrinkles) but not those changes related to sexuality.

Most of the research in this area suggests that older people are quite capable of performing sexually. As with other aspects of aging, certain anatomical and physiological changes will be evident, but these changes do not necessarily reduce the ability to enjoy sexual activity.[3] Most experts in sexuality report that many older people remain interested in sexual activity. Furthermore, those who are exposed to regular sexual activity throughout a lifetime report being most satisfied with their sex lives as older adults.

As people age, the likelihood of alterations in the male and female sexual response cycles increases. In the postmenopausal women, vaginal lubrication commonly begins more slowly, and the amount of lubrication usually diminishes. However, clitoral sensitivity and nipple erection remain the same as in earlier years. The female capacity for multiple orgasms remains the same, although the number of contractions that occur at orgasm typically is reduced.

In the older man, physical changes are also evident. This is thought to be caused by the decrease in the production of testosterone between the ages of 20 and 60 years. After age 60 or so, testosterone levels remain relatively steady. Thus many men, despite a decrease in sperm production, remain fertile into their eighties. Older men typically take longer to achieve an erection (however, they are able to maintain their erection longer before ejaculation), have fewer muscular contractions at orgasm, and ejaculate less forcefully than they once did. The volume of seminal fluid ejaculated is typically less than in earlier years, and its consistency is somewhat thinner. The resolution phase is usually longer in older men. In spite of these gradual changes, some elderly men engage in sexual intercourse with the same frequency as do much younger men.

Key Terms

erotic dreams
Dreams whose content elicits a sexual response.

foreplay
Activities, often involving touching and caressing, that prepare individuals for sexual intercourse.

fellatio (feh LAY she oh)
Oral stimulation of the penis.

cunnilingus (cun uh LING gus)
Oral stimulation of the vulva or clitoris.

procreation
Reproduction.

LOVE

Love may be one of the most elusive yet widely recognized concepts that describe some level of emotional attachment to another. Various forms of love include friendship, erotic, devotional, parental, and altruistic love. Two types of love are most closely associated with dating and mate selection: *passionate love* and *companionate love.*

Passionate love, also described as romantic love or **infatuation,** is a state of extreme absorption in another person. It is characterized by intense feelings of tenderness, elation, anxiety, sexual desire, and ecstasy. Often appearing early in a relationship, passionate love typically does not last very long. Passionate love is driven by the excitement of being closely involved with a person whose character is not fully known.

If a relationship progresses, passionate love is gradually replaced by companionate love. This type of love is less emotionally intense than passionate love. It is characterized by friendly affection and a deep attachment that is based on extensive familiarity with the partner. This love is enduring and capable of sustaining long-term, mutual growth. Central to companionate love are feelings of empathy for, support of, and tolerance of the partner. Complete the Personal Assessment on p. 341 to determine whether you and your partner are truly compatible.

RECOGNIZING UNHEALTHY RELATIONSHIPS

Clearly, not all dating relationships will continue. Many couples recognize when a partnership is nearing an end, and they reach a mutual decision to break off the relationship. This is a traditional, natural way for people to learn about their interactions with others. They simply decide to split up and move on.

However, sometimes people do not recognize or heed the warning signs of an unstable relationship, so they stay involved long after the risks outweigh the benefits. These warning signs include abusive behavior, including both emotional and physical abuse (see Chapter 16). Another red flag is excessive jealousy about a partner's interactions with others. Sometimes excessive jealousy evolves into controlling behavior, and one partner attempts to manage the daily activities of the other partner. By definition, controlling behavior limits your creativity and freedom.

Other warning signs are dishonesty, irresponsibility, lack of patience, and any kind of drug abuse. We certainly do not want to see these qualities in those we have initially judged to be "nice people," even though these unappealing characteristics may be obvious to others. If you suspect that any of these problems may be undermining your relationship, talk about your concerns with one or two trusted friends, and seek the advice of a professional counselor at your college or university. Try to realize that ending your relationship might be the best thing you could do for yourself.

TALKING POINTS • Your sister is in an unhealthy relationship but doesn't seem to see the warning signs. How could you alert her to the potential dangers?

FRIENDSHIP

One of the exciting aspects of college life is that you will probably meet many new people. Some of these people will become your best friends. Because of your common experiences, it is likely that you will keep in contact with a few of these friends for a lifetime. Close attachments to other people can have an important influence on all of the dimensions of your health.

What is it that draws friends together? With the exception of physical intimacy, many of the same growth experiences seen in dating and mate selection are also seen in the development of friendships. Think about how you and your best friend developed the relationship you now have. You probably became friends when you shared similar interests and experiences. Your friendship progressed (and even faltered at times) through personal gains or losses. In all likelihood, you cared about each other and learned to share your deepest beliefs and feelings. Then, you cemented your friendship by transferring your beliefs into behavior.

Throughout the development of a deep friendship, the qualities of trust, tolerance, empathy, and support must be demonstrated. Otherwise the friendship can fall apart. You may have noticed that the qualities seen in a friendship are very similar to the qualities noted in the description of companionate love. In both cases, people develop deep attachments through extensive familiarity and understanding.

INTIMACY

When most people hear the word **intimacy,** they immediately think about physical intimacy. They think about shared touching, kissing, and even intercourse. However, sexuality experts and family therapists prefer to view intimacy more broadly, as any close, mutual, verbal or nonverbal behavior within a relationship. In this sense, intimate behavior can range from sharing deep feelings and experiences with a partner to sharing profound physical pleasures with a partner.

Intimacy is present in both love and friendship. You have likely shared intimate feelings with your closest friends, as well as with those you love. Intimacy helps us feel connected to others and allows us to feel the full measure of our own self-worth.

TALKING POINTS • **Your teenage son equates intimacy with sex. How would you explain the emotional intimacy involved in marriage?**

MARRIAGE

Just as there is no single best way for two people to move through dating and mate selection, marriage is also a variable undertaking. In marriage, two people join their lives in a way that affirms each as an individual and both as a legal pair. Some are able to resolve conflicts constructively (see the Changing for the Better box below). However, for a large percentage of couples, the demands of marriage are too rigorous, confining, and demanding. They will find resolution for their dissatisfaction through divorce or extramarital affairs. For most, though, marriage will be an experience that alternates periods of happiness, productivity, and admiration with periods of frustration, unhappiness, and disillusionment with the partner. Each of you who marries will find the experience unique in every regard. The Changing for the Better box on p. 332 presents some advice for improving marriage.

Currently, certain trends regarding marriage are evident. The most obvious of these is the age at first marriage. Today men are waiting longer than ever to marry. The average age at first marriage for men is 27 years.[8] In addition, these new husbands are better educated than in the past and are more likely to be established in their careers. Women are also waiting longer to get married and tend to be more educated and career oriented than they were in the past. Recent statistics indicate that the median age at first marriage for women is 25 years.[8]

Marriage still appeals to most adults. Currently, 76% of adults age 18 and older are either married, widowed, or divorced.[9] Thus only about one-fifth of today's adults have not married. Within the last decade, the percentage of adults who have decided not to marry has nearly doubled. Singlehood and other alternatives to marriage are discussed later in this chapter. See the Learning from Our Diversity box on p. 332 for a discussion of same-sex marriage.

Changing *for the Better*

Resolving Conflict

Whenever I have a disagreement with my girlfriend, both of us say hurtful things and end up feeling bad. How can we resolve our conflicts in a positive way?

Here are some successful ways to manage conflict:

- Show mutual respect.
- Identify and resolve the real issue.
- Seek areas of agreement.
- Mutually participate in decision making.
- Be cooperative and specific.
- Focus on the present and future—not the past.
- Don't try to assign blame.
- Say what you are thinking and feeling.
- When talking, use sentences that begin with "I."
- Avoid using sentences that start with "you" or "why."
- Set a time limit for discussing problems.
- Accept responsibility.
- Schedule time together.

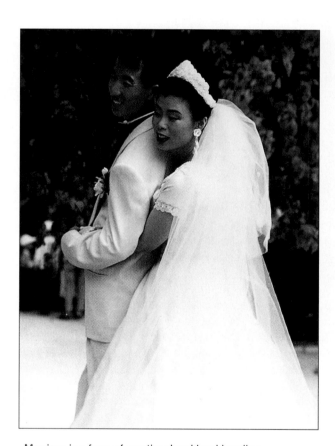

Marriage is a form of emotional and legal bonding.

Key Terms

infatuation
A relatively temporary, intensely romantic attraction to another person.

intimacy
Any close, mutual, verbal or nonverbal behavior within a relationship.

Changing *for the Better*

Can You Improve Your Marriage?

Between working and taking classes, my wife and I both have heavy schedules. One thing that's not getting any attention is our relationship. What can we do to make our marriage better?

Few marital relationships are "perfect." All marriages are faced with occasional periods of strain or turmoil. Even marriages that do not exhibit major signs of distress can be improved, mostly through better communication. Marriage experts suggest that implementing some of these patterns can strengthen marriages:

- Problems that exist within the marriage should be brought into the open so that both partners are aware of the difficulties.
- Balance should exist between the needs and expectations of each partner. Decisions should be made jointly. Partners should support each other as best they can. When a partner's goals cannot be actively supported, he or she should at least receive moral support and encouragement.
- Realistic expectations should be established. Partners should negotiate areas in which disagreement exists. They should work together to determine the manner in which resources should be shared.
- Participating in marriage counseling and marriage encounter groups can be helpful.

A sense of permanence helps sustain a marriage over the course of time. If the partners are convinced that their relationship can withstand difficult times, then they are more likely to take the time to make needed changes. Couples can develop a sense of permanence by implementing some of the patterns described above.

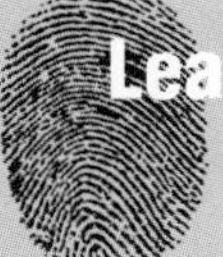

Learning from Our Diversity

The Debate Over Same-Sex Marriage

What is the definition of marriage? Must the marriage partners be a man and woman? Would same-sex marriages weaken our society?

Same-sex marriage would grant gays an array of legal and economic rights, including joint parental custody, insurance and health benefits, joint tax returns, alimony and child support, inheritance of property, hospital visitation rights, family leave, and a spouse's Social Security and retirement benefits.

Same-sex unions actually have been debated for many years. Some U.S. clergy were presiding over gay "marriages" in the 1980s, and several hundred companies now offer benefits to same-sex partners of employees. Gay publications debated the subject in the 1950s. In *Same-Sex Unions in Premodern Europe,* the late John Boswell, a Yale University historian, suggested that ancient marriage ceremonies provide evidence that Greeks and medieval Christians celebrated same-sex relationships.

Some observers predict that this will be the greatest gay rights debate in history. Where do you stand on this issue? Should gay partners be granted the same legal right to marriage as heterosexual couples? Or do you believe legal marriage should be limited to its traditional definition of a union between opposite-sex partners?

DIVORCE

Marriages, like many other kinds of interpersonal relationships, can end. Today, marriages—relationships begun with the intent of permanence "until death do us part"—end through divorce nearly as frequently as they continue.

Why should approximately half of marital relationships be so likely to end? Unfortunately, marriage experts cannot provide one clear answer. Rather, they suggest that divorce is a reflection of unfulfilled expectations for marriage on the part of one or both partners, including the following:

- The belief that marriage will ease your need to deal with your own faults and that your failures can be shared by your partner
- The belief that marriage will change faults that you know exist in your partner
- The belief that the high level of romance of your dating and courtship period will be continued through marriage
- The belief that marriage can provide you with an arena for the development of your personal power, and that

Changing *for the Better*

Coping With a Breakup

My husband and I have been married for 10 years. Recently, he announced that he wants to be "free." There's no one else, he says. He just wants to leave. I'm angry, hurt, and sad. How can I get through this crisis?

The following tips suggest both alternatives to breakup and ways to cope with it.

- *Talk first.* Try to deal effectively and directly with the conflicts. The old theory said that it was good for a couple to fight. However, anger can cause more anger and even lead to violence. Freely venting anger is as likely to damage a relationship as to improve it. So, cool off first, then discuss issues fully and freely.
- *Obtain help.* The services of a *qualified* counselor, psychologist, or psychiatrist may help a couple resolve their problems. Notice the emphasis on the word *qualified.* Some people who have little training or competence represent themselves as counselors. For this reason a couple should insist on verifying the counselor's training and licensing.
- *Trial separation.* Sometimes only a few weeks apart can convince a couple that it is far better to work together than to go it totally alone. It is generally better to establish the rules of such a trial quite firmly. Will the individuals see others? What are the responsibilities if children are involved? There should also be a time limit, perhaps a month or two, after which the partners reunite and discuss their situation again.
- *Allow time for grief and healing.* When a relationship ends, people are often tempted to immediately become as socially and sexually active as possible. This can be a way to express anger and relieve pain. But it can also cause frustration and despair. A better solution for many is to acknowledge the grief the breakup has caused and allow time for healing. Up to a year of continuing one's life and solidifying friendships typically helps the rejected partner establish a new equilibrium.

once married, you will not need to compromise with your partner

- The belief that your marital partner will be successful in meeting all of your needs

If these expectations seem to be ones you anticipate through marriage, then you may find that disappointments will abound. To varying degrees, marriage is a partnership that requires much cooperation and compromise. Marriage can be complicated. Because of the high expectations that many people hold for marriage, the termination of marriage can be an emotionally difficult process to undertake (see the Changing for the Better box above).

Concern is frequently voiced over the well-being of children whose parents divorce. Different factors, however, influence the extent to which divorce affects children. Included among these factors are the gender and age of the children, custody arrangements, financial support, and the remarriage of one or both parents. For many children, adjustments must be made to accept their new status as a member of a blended family.

TALKING POINTS • A couple you know well is going through a divorce. How could you show support for each person without taking sides?

ALTERNATIVES TO MARRIAGE

Although the great majority of you have experienced or will experience marriage, alternatives to marriage certainly exist. This section briefly explores singlehood, cohabitation, and single parenthood.

Singlehood

An alternative to marriage for adults is *singlehood.* For many people, being single is a lifestyle that affords the potential for pursuing intimacy, if desired, and provides an uncluttered path for independence and self-directedness. Other people, however, are single because of divorce, separation, death, or the absence of an opportunity to establish a partnership. The U.S. Bureau of the Census indicates that 42% of women and 39% of men over the age of 18 are currently single.[9]

Many different living arrangements are seen among singles. Some single people live alone and choose not to share a household. Other arrangements for singles include cohabitation, periodic cohabitation, singlehood during the week and cohabitation on the weekends or during vacations, or the *platonic* sharing of a household with others. For young adults, large percentages of single men and women live with their parents.

Like habitation arrangements, the sexual intimacy patterns of singles are individually tailored. Some singles practice celibacy, others pursue heterosexual or homosexual intimate relationships in a **monogamous** pattern, and others may have multiple partners. As in all interpersonal relationships, including marriage, the levels of commitment are as variable as the people involved.

Cohabitation

Cohabitation, or the sharing of living quarters by unmarried people, represents another alternative to marriage. According to the U.S. Bureau of the Census, the number of unmarried, opposite-gender couples living together nearly tripled between 1980 and 1999, from 1.6 million couples to over 4.5 million couples.[9]

Although cohabitation may seem to imply a vision of sexual intimacy between male and female roommates, several forms of shared living arrangements can be viewed as cohabitation. For some couples, cohabitation is only a part-time arrangement for weekends, during summer vacation, or on a variable schedule. In addition, **platonic** cohabitation can exist when a couple shares living quarters but does so without establishing an intimate relationship. Close friends and people of retirement age might be included in a group called *cohabitants.*

Single Parenthood

Unmarried young women becoming pregnant and then becoming single parents is a continuing reality in the United States. A new and significantly different form of single parenthood is, however, also a reality in this country: the planned entry into a single parenthood by older, better educated people, the vast majority of whom are women.

In contrast to the teenaged girl who becomes a single parent through an unwed pregnancy, the more mature woman who desires single parenting has usually planned carefully for the experience. She has explored several important concerns, including questions about how she will become pregnant (with or without the knowledge of a male partner or through artificial insemination), the need for a father figure for the child, the effect of single parenting on her social life, and its effect on her career development. Once these questions have been resolved, no legal barriers stand in the way of her becoming a single parent.

A very large number of women and a growing number of men are actively participating in single parenthood in conjunction with a divorce settlement or separation agreement involving sole or joint custody of children. In 1999, single women headed up 7.8 million households with children under age 18. In contrast, single men headed up 1.7 million households in 1999 with children under age 18.[9]

A few single parents have been awarded children through adoption. The likelihood of a single person's receiving a child this way is small, but more people have been successful recently in single-parent adoptions.

SEXUAL ORIENTATION

Sexual orientation refers to the direction in which people focus their sexual interests. People can focus their attention on opposite-gender partners, same-gender partners, or partners of both genders.

Heterosexuality

Heterosexuality (or heterosexual orientation) refers to an attraction to opposite-gender partners. (*Heteros* is a Greek word that means "the other.") Throughout the world, this is the most common sexual orientation. For reasons related to species survival, heterosexuality has its most basic roots in the biological dimension of human sexuality. Beyond its biological roots, heterosexuality has significant cultural and religious support in virtually every country in the world. Most societies expect men to be attracted to women and women to be attracted to men. Worldwide, laws related to marriage, living arrangements, health benefits, child rearing, financial matters, sexual behavior, and inheritance generally support relationships that are heterosexual in nature.

Homosexuality

Homosexuality (or homosexual orientation) refers to an attraction to same-gender partners. The term *homosexuality* comes from the Greek word *homos,* meaning "same." The word *homosexuality* may be used with regard to males or females. Thus we use the terms *homosexual males* and *homosexual females.* Frequently the word *gay* is used to refer to homosexual orientation in both males and females. *Lesbianism* is also used to refer to the sexual attraction between females.

The distinctions among the three categories of sexual orientation are much less clear than their definitions might suggest. Most people probably fall somewhere along a continuum between exclusive heterosexuality and exclusive homosexuality. In 1948, Kinsey presented just such a continuum.[10]

Why does a given individual have a particular orientation? There is no simple answer to this question. (College human sexuality textbooks devote entire chapters to this topic.) In the mid-1990s, some research pointed to differences in the sizes of certain brain structures as a possible biological basis for homosexuality. However, for sexual orientation in general, no one theory has emerged that fully explains this developmental process. Regardless of the cause, however, reversal to heterosexuality generally does not occur. Furthermore, most homosexuals report that no single event "triggered" their homosexuality. Many homosexuals also indicate that they knew their orientations were "different" from other children as far back as their prepuberty years. See Exploring Your Spirituality for insight into some of the issues that homosexuals often need to face.

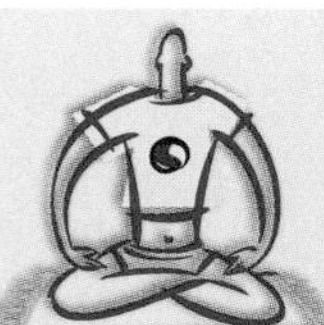

Exploring Your Spirituality

Coming Out—Then What?

If you are openly gay, when you finally told your family and friends about your sexual orientation, a lot of things changed. But one thing probably stayed the same—you still feel like an outsider. Most of the couples holding hands on campus are young men and women. TV sitcoms are centered on heterosexual couples. They may include a gay character, but usually in a minor role. Popular magazines—through their ads, their features, their entire focus—are telling you how to be attractive to the opposite sex.

Being openly gay has probably made you wonder about some of the mixed messages you receive. The person who says it's OK that you're gay also seems to feel sorry for you—because you can't have a "normal" life and enjoy some of the things she does. Your mother makes remarks that suggest she still has hopes that someday you'll marry her best friend's son.

Feeling good about being gay in a straight world doesn't come easily. You've got to work at it. Start by finding support among your gay friends. Knowing that you're not alone is important—especially right after coming out. Realizing that other good, whole people are gay helps to reinforce your self-esteem. Joining a campus gay organization is good for ongoing support, but don't limit yourself to that group. To grow as an individual, you also need to interact with and be part of heterosexual society.

Focus on what you value about yourself. Are you creative? Someone who gets things accomplished? A dependable friend? Think about the contributions you make—to your family, school, friends, church, and community. Remind yourself that you're a worthy person.

What do your friends appreciate about you? Do they value your advice? Like your sense of humor? Admire your courage? Think you're a strong leader?

Reinforcing the fact that you're a whole, worthy person is up to you. Listen to the "tapes" that are constantly playing in your head—both positive and negative. Edit out the negative thoughts, and turn up the volume on the positive ones. Take charge of what you think about yourself, rather than accepting what others think you are or should be.

TALKING POINTS • How would you react if a close family member told you that he or she was gay? How could you be supportive or at least communicate your feelings without anger or criticism?

The extent of homosexuality in our society is a debatable issue. Clearly, gathering valid information of this kind is difficult. The extent of homosexual orientation is probably much greater than many heterosexuals realize. Furthermore, many people refuse to reveal their homosexuality and thus prefer to remain "in the closet."

Although operational definitions of homosexuality may vary from researcher to researcher, Kinsey estimated that about 2% of American females and 4% of American males were exclusively homosexual.[10,11] More recent estimates place the overall combined figure of homosexuals at about 10% of the population. Clearly the expression of same-gender attraction is not uncommon. See the Exploring Your Spirituality box above.

Bisexuality

People whose preference for sexual partners includes both genders are referred to as *bisexuals.* Bisexuals may fall into one of three groups: those who are (1) genuinely attracted to both genders, (2) homosexual but also feel the need to behave heterosexually, or (3) aroused physically by the same gender but attracted emotionally to the opposite gender. Some people participate in a bisexual lifestyle for extended periods. Others move quickly to a more exclusive orientation. The size of the bisexual population is not accurately known.

A particularly pressing reason for learning more about the bisexual lifestyle is its relationship to the transmission of HIV infection. Except for intravenous drug users, bisexuals may hold the greatest potential for extending HIV infection into the heterosexual population. Since the prevalence of bisexuality is unknown, the consistent use of safer sex practices becomes more important than ever.

Key Terms

monogamous (mo NOG a mus)
Paired relationship with one partner.

cohabitation
Sharing of a residence by two unrelated, unmarried people; living together.

platonic (pluh TON ick)
Close association between two people that does not include a sexual relationship.

SUMMARY

- Biological and psychosocial factors contribute to the complex expression of our sexuality.
- The structural basis of sexuality begins as the male and female reproductive structures develop in the growing embryo and fetus. Structural sexuality changes as one moves through adolescence and later life.
- The psychosocial processes of gender identity, gender preference, and gender adoption form the basis for an initial adult gender identification.
- The male and female reproductive structures are external and internal. The complex functioning of these structures is controlled by hormones.
- The menstrual cycle's primary functions are to produce mature ova and to develop a supportive environment for the fetus in the uterus.
- The sexual response pattern consists of four stages: excitement, plateau, orgasm, and resolution.
- Many older people remain interested and active in sexual activities. Physiological changes may alter the way in which some older people perform sexually.
- Although most individuals marry at some time in their lives, alternatives to marriage exist, including singlehood, cohabitation, and single parenthood.
- Three sexual orientations are heterosexuality, homosexuality, and bisexuality.

REVIEW QUESTIONS

1. Describe the following foundations of our biological sexuality: the genetic basis, the gonadal basis, and structural development.
2. Define and explain the following terms: gender identity, gender preference, gender adoption, initial adult gender identification, and transsexualism.
3. Identify the major components of the male and female reproductive systems. Trace the passageways for sperm and ova.
4. Explain the menstrual cycle. Identify and describe the four main hormones that control the menstrual cycle.
5. What similarities and differences exist between the sexual response patterns of males and females?
6. Approximately what percentage of today's college students report having had sexual intercourse?
7. Explain the differences between heterosexuality, homosexuality, and bisexuality. How common are each of these sexual orientations in our society?

THINK ABOUT THIS . . .

- How would you summarize your feelings about the changes in your body that took place during puberty?
- To what extent do you think that knowledge about the menstrual cycle will be pertinent to you as you move through adulthood? (This question is for BOTH men and women.)
- Do you think a celibate lifestyle is possible or practical in this new millennium? Why or why not?
- What are your estimates of the percentages of men and women at your college or university who have had sexual intercourse?
- In comparison with a decade ago, are heterosexuals generally more comfortable or less comfortable with homosexuals in our society? Support your answer with specific examples.

REFERENCES

1. Thibodeau GA: *The human body in health and disease,* ed 2, 1999, Mosby.
2. Hyde JS, DeLamater J: *Understanding human sexuality,* ed 7, 1999, McGraw-Hill.
3. Crooks R, Baur K: *Our sexuality,* ed 7, 1998, Brooks/Cole Publishing Co.
4. Thibodeau GA: *Structure and function of the body,* ed 10, 1999, Mosby.
5. Allgeier ER, Allgeier AR: *Sexual interactions,* ed 5, 2000, Houghton Mifflin.
6. Hatcher RA et al: *Contraceptive technology,* ed 17, 1998, Ardent Media, Inc.
7. Masters W, Johnson V: *Human sexual response,* 1966, Lippincott, Williams & Wilkins.
8. Fields J, Casper LM: America's families and living arrangements: March 2000. *Current Population Reports,* (U.S. Census Bureau) P20–537, p. 9, 2001.
9. U.S. Bureau of the Census: *Statistical abstract of the United States: 2000,* ed 120, 2000, U.S. Government Printing Office.
10. Kinsey AC, Pomeroy WB, Martin CE: *Sexual behavior in the human male,* reprint edition, 1998, Indiana University Press.
11. Kinsey AC et al: *Sexual behavior in the human female,* reprint edition, 1998, Indiana University Press.

SUGGESTED READINGS

Byington J, Bly RW, Eliaz I: *Natural alternatives to Viagra: how to recharge your sexual performance without surgery or prescription drugs,* 1999, Birch Lane Press.

The anti-impotence drug Viagra is not a wonder drug for all men. In fact, it can produce some uncomfortable, even dangerous, side effects for certain men. This book offers a variety of natural methods for coping with erectile problems. It is written in a manner that is easily understandable to both men and women.

Dalton K, Holton W, Dalton K: *Once a month: understanding and treating PMS,* ed 6, 1999, Hunter House.

Researchers estimate that about 75% of women experience some conditions related to premenstrual syndrome. This book describes the most common symptoms of PMS, strategies for coping with these symptoms, and the effect of PMS on the development of osteoporosis.

Gittleman AL, Wright JV: *Before the change: taking charge of your perimenopause,* 1999, Harper.

Perimenopause, roughly the 10 years before menopause, can be a difficult time—emotionally and physically—for some women. This book is a do-it-yourself guide to coping with the symptoms of perimenopause without resorting to hormonal treatments. The symptoms of perimenopause are clearly identified, and a self-diagnosis quiz is included. A perimenopause diet is presented, as well as recommendations for the use of herbs, natural hormones, and vitamin and mineral supplementation.

Gottman JM, Silver N: *The seven principles for making marriage work,* 1999, Crown Publishing.

This book is written by a psychology professor who is the director of the Seattle Marital and Family Institute. Dr. Gottman combines his research findings with his experience as a marital therapist to help couples discover what really matters in a relationship. This book is helpful to married couples as well as to those contemplating marriage.

As we go to Press...

The August 2001 issue of the *American Journal of Public Health* published a study by Stephen Russell and Kara Joyner that found a strong link between same-sex sexual orientation and adolescent suicidal thoughts and suicide attempts. Although this link has been reported in other studies, this research was the first to use nationally representative data coming from the ongoing National Longitudinal Study of Adolescent Health. The researchers found that 15% of the 458 teens who reported having attempted suicide had a same-sex orientation. This percentage was twice the proportional representation of this group in the sample. The authors called for improved suicide intervention and prevention measures for gay and lesbian youth.

Name ______________________ Date __________ Section __________

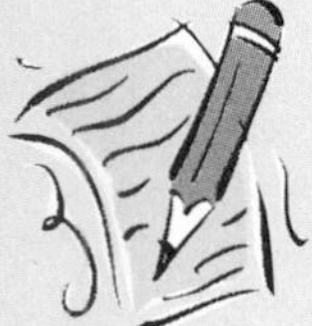

Personal Assessment

Sexual Attitudes: A Matter of Feelings

Respond to each of the following statements by selecting a numbered response (1–5) that most accurately reflects your feelings. Circle the number of your selection. At the end of the questionnaire, total these numbers for use in interpreting your responses.

1 Agree strongly
2 Agree moderately
3 Uncertain
4 Disagree moderately
5 Disagree strongly

Men and women have greater differences than they have similarities.	1	2	3	4	5
Homosexuality and bisexuality are immoral and unnatural.	1	2	3	4	5
Our society is too sexually oriented.	1	2	3	4	5
Pornography encourages sexual promiscuity.	1	2	3	4	5
Children know far too much about sex.	1	2	3	4	5
Education about sexuality is solely the responsibility of the family.	1	2	3	4	5
Dating begins far too early in our society.	1	2	3	4	5
Sexual intimacy before marriage leads to emotional stress and damage to one's reputation.	1	2	3	4	5
Sexual availability is far too frequently the reason that people marry.	1	2	3	4	5
Reproduction is the most important reason for sexual intimacy during marriage.	1	2	3	4	5
Modern families are too small.	1	2	3	4	5
Family planning clinics should not receive public funds.	1	2	3	4	5
Contraception is the woman's responsibility.	1	2	3	4	5
Abortion is the murder of an innocent child.	1	2	3	4	5
Marriage has been weakened by the changing role of women in society.	1	2	3	4	5
Divorce is an unacceptable means of resolving marital difficulties.	1	2	3	4	5
Extramarital sexual intimacy will destroy a marriage.	1	2	3	4	5
Sexual abuse of a child does not generally occur unless the child encourages the adult.	1	2	3	4	5
Provocative behavior by the woman is a factor in almost every case of rape.	1	2	3	4	5
Reproduction is not a right but a privilege.	1	2	3	4	5

YOUR TOTAL POINTS __________

Interpretation

20–34 points	A very traditional attitude toward sexuality
35–54 points	A moderately traditional attitude toward sexuality
55–65 points	A rather ambivalent attitude toward sexuality
66–85 points	A moderately nontraditional attitude toward sexuality
86–100 points	A very nontraditional attitude toward sexuality

To Carry This Further . . .

Were you surprised at your results? Compare your results with those of a roommate or close friend. How do you think your parents would score on this assessment?

Name ______________________ **Date** __________ **Section** __________

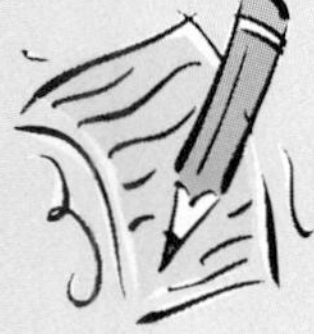

Personal Assessment

How Compatible Are You?

This quiz will help test how compatible you and your partner's personalities are. You should each rate the truth of these twenty statements based on the following scale. Circle the number that reflects your feelings. Total your scores and check the interpretation following the quiz.

1 Never true
2 Sometimes true
3 Frequently true
4 Always true

We can communicate our innermost thoughts effectively.	1	2	3	4
We trust each other.	1	2	3	4
We agree on whose needs come first.	1	2	3	4
We have realistic expectations of each other and of ourselves.	1	2	3	4
Individual growth is important within our relationship.	1	2	3	4
We will go on as a couple even if our partner doesn't change.	1	2	3	4
Our personal problems are discussed with each other first.	1	2	3	4
We both do our best to compromise.	1	2	3	4
We usually fight fairly.	1	2	3	4
We try not to be rigid or unyielding.	1	2	3	4
We keep any needs to be "perfect" in proper perspective.	1	2	3	4
We can balance desires to be sociable and the need to be alone.	1	2	3	4
We both make friends and keep them.	1	2	3	4
Neither of us stays down or up for long periods.	1	2	3	4
We can tolerate the other's mood without being affected by it.	1	2	3	4
We can deal with disappointment and disillusionment.	1	2	3	4
Both of us can tolerate failure.	1	2	3	4
We can both express anger appropriately.	1	2	3	4
We are both assertive when necessary.	1	2	3	4
We agree on how our personal surroundings are kept.	1	2	3	4

YOUR TOTAL POINTS __________

Interpretation

20–35 points	You and your partner seem quite incompatible. Professional help may open your lines of communication.
36–55 points	You probably need more awareness and compromise.
56–70 points	You are highly compatible. However, be aware of the areas where you can improve.
71–80 points	Your relationship is very fulfilling.

To Carry This Further . . .

Ask your partner to take this test too. You may have a one-sided view of a "perfect" relationship. Even if you scored high on this assessment, be aware of areas where you can still improve.

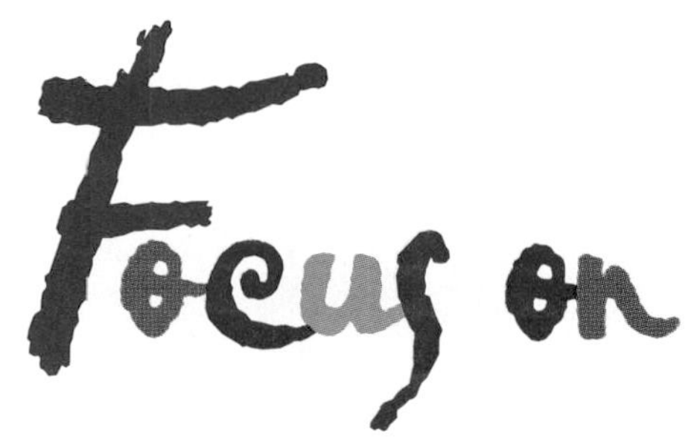

SEX ON THE WEB

It's like a singles bar without the loud music. If you have a computer and a modem, you can gain access to the world's largest "meet market." From the comfort of your home, you can browse the Internet and meet people for conversation, friendship, romance, and even "sex" (such as it is in cyberspace). There is a cover charge, but you won't have to buy drinks to start up a conversation or get your toes smashed on the dance floor. You won't even have to worry about getting diseases (except for the occasional computer virus).

However, there are drawbacks when you enter this hangout. Can you be sure the person you're chatting with is all he or she seems to be? How can you be certain of a person's personality, age, or even his or her gender? And is there a safe way to meet a "cyberfriend" face-to-face? The Internet way of meeting people has its own built-in set of advantages—but inviting the world into your home has its dangers as well.

Today's Internet user can find a variety of potential conversation topics using a web browser and typing in various keywords. As the Internet grows, so do its various websites and USENET discussion groups. Some people see this expansion as a source of entertainment. They think that the Internet is a fun and interesting way to meet people who share their interests. Others think that the Internet allows pornographers, pedophiles, and other deviants to perpetuate their behavior and prey on innocent children. Both groups are attempting to use the law either to keep the Internet as a haven for free speech or to clean it up and make it safer for children. This clash of ideals is creating a continual battle over the nature and character of the Internet.

Fun and Games on the Web

The world wide web is a large group of computer networks, both public and private, that connect millions of computer users in an estimated 150 countries. Over 70,000 private computer bulletin boards exist in the United States alone, and private commercial networks such as Prodigy, America Online, and CompuServe provide nearly 6 million subscribers worldwide with access to the Internet.[1] Although the Internet contains information about all facets of life, the sexually oriented sites are proving to be the most popular areas among the general public. For example, alt.sex, a USENET discussion group where people can chat in real time with other users, is the most often visited site on the Internet.[2] Brian Reid, director of the Network Systems Laboratory at Digital Equipment Corporation, reports that between 180,000 and 500,000 users drop into this discussion group on a monthly basis.[3]

At websites, computer bulletin boards that usually include photographs, interested parties can find almost anything that conforms to their sexual desires. Many pictures of nude men and women that can be found at most adult-oriented video stores and booksellers can be downloaded (placed on a user's computer disk or printed on his or her own printer).[1] However, other types of less common sexual images are also available at websites, including explicit images that many people find objectionable.

The Positive Side of the Web

Despite the potentially offensive graphic images available on-line, the Internet does have several good points. One positive aspect is that people who are interested in meeting others can use the Internet as a sort of virtual pick-up bar without many of the unpleasant consequences. It gives people the freedom either to be themselves without fear of repercussions or to adopt a totally new persona. Best of all, cybersex participants don't have to worry about looking their best during a virtual date.[4] Who you are (or who you pretend to be) becomes more important than what you look like in cyberspace chat rooms.

Sexually oriented Internet sites can also be positive in the sense that they sometimes inspire creative impulses and prevent people from engaging in destructive behavior. Some sites house participatory novels in which users can immerse themselves and create new realities for themselves and other participants.[5] In this respect, these sites are similar to fantasy game pages that house activities such as Dungeons & Dragons. People are able to cast off their old identities and create exciting new personas that are able to engage in sexual practices that the users themselves would never attempt in real life. Thus the Internet becomes a harmless outlet for sexual fantasies: the ultimate safe sex.

A third plus to using the Internet to meet people is that occasionally, people who use it do fall in "virtual love," choose to meet face to face, and end up developing a relationship or even getting married.[4] Although this is a rare occurrence, the chance that it could happen is enough to keep some people involved with on-line romances in the hope of finding a perfect cybermate who will be as good in person.

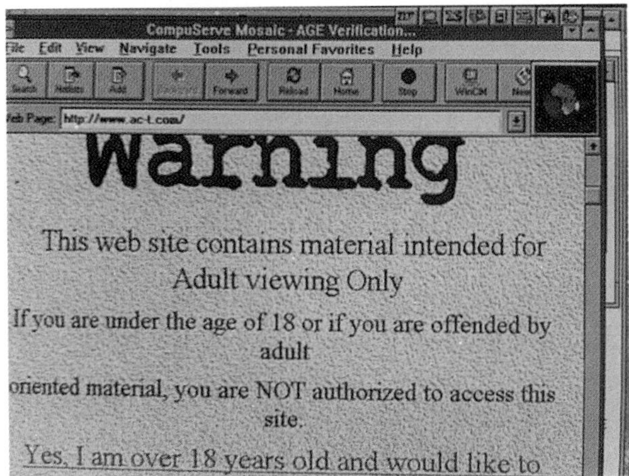

Pitfalls of On-Line Sex

Although virtual sex has many good points in its favor, there are also several negative aspects. One of the worst possible scenarios of on-line sex is discovering that the person with whom you have been pursuing a virtual relationship is not who he or she claims to be. This pitfall is particularly dangerous when one of the parties in the relationship is a minor. In response to a recent on-line query, 130 female teenagers stated that they had posted erotic stories on a sexually oriented bulletin board and corresponded with adult men. In the stories, the teenagers pretended to be adults. Several of the teenagers also admitted that they had scheduled face-to-face meetings with these adult men without telling anyone.[6] Although none of the teenagers reported any negative consequences as a result of these meetings, the potential for danger was most certainly present. A recent case in which a 13-year-old female from Kentucky ended up in Los Angeles after being lured there by her adult male Internet correspondent provides evidence to prove this point.[3] Additionally, several cases exist in which pedophiles have used computer bulletin boards to contact children, learned their names and addresses, and set up meetings with them. Several rapes have occurred as a result of this.[7]

A second drawback to on-line sex is the considerable cost. Although chat rooms are sometimes free and websites have "visitor's passes" that allow sneak previews, most of the hard-core sexual activity can be very expensive. Some chat rooms charge as much as $12 an hour for a conversation.[4] To get to the more explicit photographs and participatory novels on the Internet, a member's fee is required, which ranges anywhere from $19.95 for 6 months to $129.95 for a year. These fees are generally paid by credit card on-line. A digital video camera, which is necessary to create real-time pictures to transmit through a personal computer, costs at least $100.[8] Upgrades to computer memory and equipment to handle more technologically advanced transmissions such as video clips can also be costly, running into the thousands of dollars.

A third potential problem is cybersex addiction. Some people become so involved with virtual reality that they find themselves uninterested in the real world. A librarian at a large college recently reported that many college students have to be asked to log off the library's computers that have Internet connections. These students ignore library policy that limits their Internet use to 30 minutes. One student had to be threatened by campus police; he was logged onto a sexually oriented chat room for almost 4 hours. In another case at the same college a library employee was disciplined after he was caught downloading sexually explicit material.[9] As a result of these incidents the college now blocks many sexually explicit sites and has disabled its computers' ability to download any material.

Avoiding Sex on the Internet

With all the publicity and notoriety surrounding sexually oriented Internet sites, many concerned parents want to ensure that their children do not have access to sexual material through their personal computers. Other people are offended by cybersex and do not want it coming into their homes for religious or moral reasons. For these people, several options exist. Parents can subscribe to an on-line service that blocks potentially offensive sites. CompuServe, one of the largest on-line providers, recently suspended 200 sex discussion groups in response to German authorities' contention that the groups violated German obscenity laws.[10] Also, America Online and Prodigy have mechanisms available on their services to block access to areas that most parents would consider inappropriate for their children.[3] These mechanisms are available free of charge with subscription to the services.

A second option is to purchase a program that will block out undesirable material. One such program, Surf-watch, will automatically block access to 1000 sites and will let you screen all user groups, websites, and other electronic avenues. The cost of this program is $49.95 plus a $5.95 monthly service fee. Other types of blocker programs include NetNanny, which lets parents monitor everything that passes through their computer, and Time's Up, which lets parents set up time limits and appropriate times for their children to use the computer.[8]

A third, decidedly low-tech option is the most obvious and also the most overlooked. Parents should watch what their children are doing while they are on-line and monitor all activities, perhaps by making computer use a family activity.[3] As columnist Michael J. Miller points out, much of the fear that children will accidentally stumble onto a sexually oriented site is unfounded. Unlike broadcast media, on the Internet, you must enter a specific address or follow a specific link to reach a sexually oriented site. Parents who watch their kids will know exactly where the kids go during an on-line jaunt. Additionally, parents should teach their children some basic safety information such as never to give out their real name, address, or telephone number to people they meet on-line. Children should understand that even though they may have on-line friends, these people are really strangers that they know little about.[3–8]

The Telecommunications Competition and Deregulation Act

In February 1996, President Clinton signed into law the Telecommunications Competition and Deregulation Act, a law that contains a provision called the Telecommunications Decency Act to block indecency on-line. Anyone caught transmitting obscene, lewd, or indecent communications by any electronic means could be fined as much as $100,000 and sent to prison for as long as 2 years.[1,10,11] Civil libertarians and users of sexually oriented Internet sites oppose this law, stating that the First Amendment guarantees freedom of speech and that this freedom should include the Internet. They also believe that the law as written is too broad and confusing; it could be interpreted as banning any use of profanity or nudity on-line, including news reports, legal documents, literature, and even the Bible.[11]

Some parents and religious groups, on the other hand, are applauding this new act. They feel it gives them more control over what kinds of materials are coming into their homes. They believe that this legislation is necessary to protect children from being exposed to pornography on-line. They also believe the law is good because it specifically targets material that is patently offensive and depicts graphic sexual activity.[11]

A line has been drawn in the sand regarding sex on the Internet. Supporters of the new law are joining organizations such as Enough is Enough, the National Coalition against Pornography, and the American Family Association Law Center.[7] These groups work to defend traditional values and fight against increased pornography. Meanwhile, web search engines such as Yahoo protested the legislation by turning their web pages to black with white lettering for 48 hours to demonstrate "virtual mourning," and the American Civil Liberties Union filed a federal court complaint to block enforcement of the law.[11]

Using the Internet for sexual purposes can have both positive and negative consequences; therefore people who do so should weigh all factors involved before they decide to enter the world of cybersex. Parents should be especially careful about what they allow to come into their homes via the personal computer. Although blocking methods and the new federal laws provide some protection from sexually oriented material, it is ultimately the individual's responsibility to choose and to monitor what types of information come up while surfing the Internet.

For Discussion . . .

Have you or someone you know ever explored sexually oriented websites on the Internet? If so, was it a positive or a negative experience? Would you be willing to meet a virtual friend face to face? Why or why not? Do you support the new Telecommunications Indecency Act? Why or why not?

REFERENCES

1. Lewis PH: Despite a new plan for cooling it off, cybersex stays hot, *New York Times,* p A1, March 26, 1995.
2. Nashawatz C: Where the wild things are: anonymous sex is back, *Entertainment Weekly,* Sept 23, 1994.
3. Levy S, Stone B: No place for kids: a parents' guide to sex on the Net, *Newsweek,* July 3, 1995.
4. Van der Leur G: Twilight zone of the id, *Time,* 145(12), p 36, Special Issue, Spring 1995.
5. Machure B: MUDs and MUSHes and MOOs, *PC Magazine,* p 10, April 30, 1995.
6. Bennahan DS: Lolitas on-line, *Harper's Bazaar,* p 3406, Sept 1995.
7. Zipperer J: The naked city, *Christianity Today,* Sept 12, 1994.
8. Miller MJ: Cybersex shock, *PC Magazine,* Oct 10, 1995.
9. Anonymous: Personal communication, March 23, 1996.
10. Mezer M: A bad dream comes true in cyberspace, *Newsweek,* p 2, Jan 8, 1996.
11. Wagner M: Tempers flare over web censorship, *Computerworld,* Feb 12, 1996.

chapter **14**

Managing Your Fertility

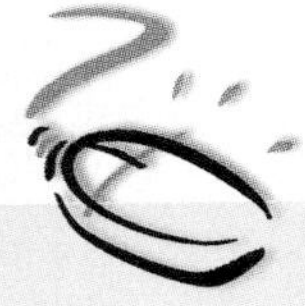

Online Learning Center Resources

www.mhhe.com/hahn6e

Log on to our Online Learning Center (OLC) for access to these additional resources:

- Chapter key terms and definitions
- Learning objectives
- Additional behavior change objectives
- Student interactive question-and-answer sites
- Self-scoring chapter quiz

The OLC also offers web links for study and exploration of health topics. Here are some examples of what you'll find:

- **www.plannedparenthood.org** Check here for family planning, contraception, abortion, and counseling services information.
- **www.naral.org** Visit this site for a pro-choice point of view about abortion.
- **www.nrlc.org** Look here for a different point of view—includes information on alternatives to abortion and the politics of the pro-life movement.

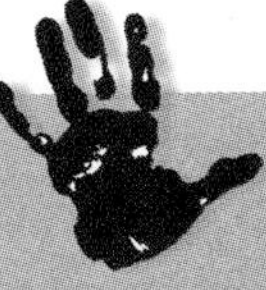

Taking Charge of Your Health

- Use the Personal Assessment on p. 373 to help you determine which birth control method is best for you.
- Talk to your doctor about the health aspects of different types of birth control before making your decision.
- If the method of birth control you are currently using is unsatisfactory to you or your partner, explore other options.
- Reduce your risk of infertility by choosing a birth control method carefully, protecting yourself from infections of the reproductive organs, and maintaining good overall health.
- If you plan to have children, set a time frame that takes into account decreased fertility with advancing age.

Eye on the Media

Information Online—Birth Control and Sexuality

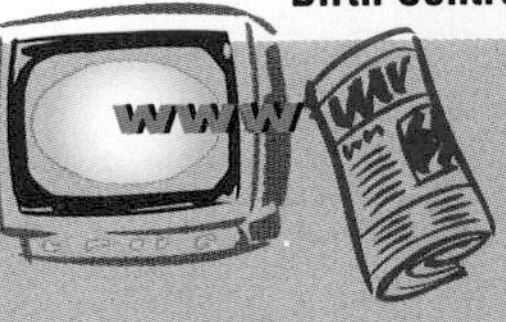

The Internet offers a number of resources for locating information about contraception, birth control, and related topics. Planned Parenthood Federation of America provides one of the most comprehensive sites at **www.plannedparenthood.org**. Here you can find a wide selection of pamphlets, books, newsletters, and videotapes, as well as links to other websites.

If you're looking for birth control information, click on Planned Parenthood's "Frequently Asked Questions," "Fact Sheets," "Sexual Health Glossary," and "Links." Some of the frequently asked questions are:

- Am I pregnant?
- What can I do if I am pregnant?
- Do I have a sexually transmitted disease?
- What are the laws in my state about teens' access to abortion services and birth control?
- How can I get access to birth control?

Of course, answers follow each of these questions. Planned Parenthood

Eye on the Media *continued*

believes that when people are empowered with knowledge, they are better able to make sound decisions about their health and sexuality.

The "Fact Sheets" option at Planned Parenthood's website provides various reports on specific topics, such as abortion, birth control, family planning, sexually transmitted diseases, and teen pregnancy and abortion. The "Sexual Health Glossary" is a listing of hundreds of terms related to sexuality. The "Links" option lists twenty-four topical categories, each one displaying links to related websites.

Three additional online sites offer reliable information about sexuality and reproductive choices. The first is the Alan Guttmacher Institute website at **www.agi-usa.org.** This institute is dedicated to protecting the reproductive choices of women and men throughout the world. It fulfills its mission by disseminating information and the results of scientific research on the subject. The Guttmacher Institute's menu of options includes abortion, law and public policy, pregnancy and birth, prevention and contraception, sexual behavior, and sexually transmitted diseases and youth.

The American Social Health Association's website is **www.ashastd.org.** This organization is dedicated to stopping the spread of sexually transmitted diseases. ASHA operates a network of national hotlines that answers over 2 million calls each year. The website's menu offers selections on sexually transmitted diseases, frequently asked questions, a sexual health glossary, and support groups.

The Sex Information and Education Council of the United States is a nonprofit organization dedicated to developing, collecting, and disseminating information about sexuality. SIECUS has its website at **www.siecus.org.** This organization promotes comprehensive sexuality education and advocates the right of individuals to make responsible sexual choices. SIECUS publishes and distributes thousands of pamphlets, booklets, and bibliographies each year to professionals and the general public.

If you wish to search for information about certain sexuality topics from a pro-life perspective, you might wish to examine the website for The Ultimate Pro-life Resource List at **www.prolifeinfo.org.** This site is supported by the non-profit Women and Children First organization. The Ultimate Pro-life Resource List provides links to information related to abortion alternatives, Roe vs. Wade, euthanasia and assisted suicide, pregnancy help, pro-life news and pro-life organizations.

How you decide to control your **fertility** will have an important effect on your future. Your understanding of information and issues related to fertility control will help you make responsible decisions in this complex area.

For traditional-age students, these decisions may be fast approaching (see Exploring Your Spirituality on p. 348 for a discussion of decision making about sex and the spiritual dimension of sexuality). Frequently, nontraditional students are parents who have had experiences that make them useful resources for other students in the class.

BIRTH CONTROL VS. CONTRACEPTION

Any discussion about the control of your fertility should start with an explanation of the subtle differences between the terms **birth control** and **contraception.** Although many people use the words interchangeably, they reflect different perspectives about fertility control. *Birth control* is an umbrella term that refers to all of the procedures you might use to prevent the birth of a child. Birth control includes all available contraceptive measures, as well as sterilization, abortion procedures, and perhaps the use of the intrauterine device (IUD).

Contraception is a much more specific term for any procedure used to prevent the fertilization of an ovum. Contraceptive measures vary widely in the mechanisms they use to accomplish this task. They also vary considerably in their method of use and their rate of success in preventing conception. A few examples of contraceptive methods are the use of condoms, oral contraceptives, spermicides, diaphragms, and perhaps IUDs.

Beyond the numerous methods mentioned, certain forms of sexual behavior not involving intercourse could be considered forms of contraception. For example, mutual masturbation by couples virtually eliminates the possibility of pregnancy. This practice, as well as additional forms of sexual expression other than intercourse (such as kissing, touching, and massage), has been given the generic term **outercourse.** Not only does outercourse

Key Terms

fertility
The ability to reproduce.

birth control
All of the methods and procedures that can prevent the birth of a child.

contraception
Any method or procedure that prevents fertilization.

outercourse
Sexual activity that does not involve intercourse.

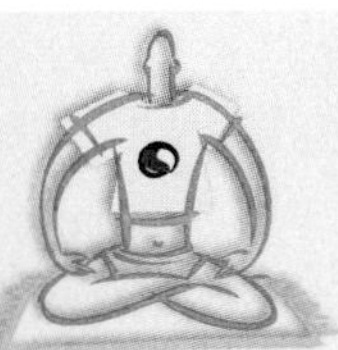

Exploring Your Spirituality

There's More to Sex than You Thought . . .

Are you ready for sex? If you're not sure, take time to think it over. If you start having sex before you're ready, you might feel guilty. You might feel bad because you realize this step isn't right for you now. Or your religious upbringing may make you feel as though you're doing something wrong. You also may not be ready for the emotional aspects of a sexual relationship. Most important, you will probably have difficulty handling the complexities of an unplanned pregnancy or a sexually transmitted disease.

If you do feel ready for sex, you still have a choice. Sex may be OK for you now. It may be personally fulfilling, something that enhances your self-esteem. Alternatively, you can choose to abstain from sex until later—another way of enhancing your self-esteem. You'll feel empowered by making the decision for yourself, rather than doing what is expected. Being strong enough to say "no" can also make you feel good about yourself. For some, making this decision may reflect a renewed commitment to spiritual or religious concerns.

If you're married, sex is a good way of connecting as a couple. It's something that the two of you alone share. It's a time to give special attention to each other—taking a break from the kids, your jobs, and your other responsibilities. It's a way of saying: "This relationship is important—it's something I value."

Going through a pregnancy together is another opportunity for closeness. From the moment you know that you're going to be parents, you're connected in a new way. Your focus becomes the expected child. You'll watch the fetus grow on ultrasound, go to parenting and Lamaze classes together, visit the doctor together, mark the various milestones, and share new emotions. When your child is born, you'll be connected as never before.

Whether you're thinking about starting to have sex, making the decision to wait, or examining the sexual life you have now, you can't ignore the possibilities and the consequences. Is the time right for you? Are you doing this for yourself or for someone else? What do you think you will gain from waiting? Do you expect your future partner to also have made the decision to wait? What do you expect to get from a sexual relationship—pleasure, intimacy, love? What do you expect to give? Do you want an emotional commitment? Do you view sex and love as inseparable? Do you understand how sex can enhance your spirituality? Taking time to consider these questions can make you feel good about yourself—no matter what you decide.

protect against unplanned pregnancy, it may also significantly reduce the transmission of sexually transmitted diseases (STDs), including HIV infection.

THEORETICAL EFFECTIVENESS VS. USE EFFECTIVENESS

People considering the use of a contraceptive method need to understand the difference between the two effectiveness rates given for each form of contraception. *Theoretical effectiveness* is a measure of a contraceptive method's ability to prevent a pregnancy when the method is used precisely as directed during every act of intercourse. *Use effectiveness,* however, refers to the effectiveness of a method in preventing conception when used by the general public. Use effectiveness rates take into account factors that lower effectiveness below that based on "perfect" use. Failure to follow proper instructions, illness of the user, forgetfulness, physician (or pharmacist) error, and a subconscious desire to experience risk or even pregnancy are a few of the factors that can lower the effectiveness of even the most theoretically effective contraceptive technique.

Effectiveness rates are often expressed in terms of the percentage of women users of childbearing age who do not become pregnant while using the method for 1 year. For some methods the theoretical- and use-effectiveness rates are vastly different; the theoretical rate is always higher than the use rate. Table 14-1 presents data concerning effectiveness rates, advantages, and disadvantages of many birth control methods.

SELECTING YOUR CONTRACEPTIVE METHOD

In this section, we discuss some of the many factors that should be important to you as you consider selecting a contraceptive method. Remember that no method possesses equally high marks in all of the following areas. It is important that you and your partner select a contraceptive method that is both acceptable and effective, as determined by your unique needs and expectations. Completing the Personal Assessment on p. 373 will help you make this decision.

For a contraceptive method to be acceptable to those who wish to exercise a large measure of control over their fertility, the following should be given careful consideration:

- *It should be safe.* The contraceptive approach you select should not pose a significant health risk for you or your partner.
- *It should be effective.* Your approach must have a high success rate in preventing pregnancy.

Table 14-1 Effectiveness Rates of Birth Control for 100 Women during 1 Year of Use

Method	Estimated Effectiveness: Theoretical	Estimated Effectiveness: Use	Advantages	Disadvantages
No method (chance)	15%	15%	Inexpensive	Totally ineffective
Withdrawal	96%	81%	No supplies or advance preparation needed; no side effects; men share responsibility for family planning	Interferes with coitus; very difficult to use effectively; women must trust men to withdraw as orgasm approaches
Periodic abstinence Calendar Basal body temperature Cervical mucus method Symptothermal	91%–99%	75%	No supplies needed; no side effects; men share responsibility for family planning; women learn about their bodies	Difficult to use, especially if menstrual cycles are irregular, as is common in young women; abstinence may be necessary for long periods; lengthy instruction and ongoing counseling may be needed
Cervical cap (no prior births)	91%	80%	No health risks; helps protect against some STDs and cervical cancer	Limited availability
Spermicide (gel, foam, suppository, film)	94%	74%	No health risks; helps protect against some STDs; can be used with condoms to increase effectiveness considerably	Must be inserted 5 to 30 minutes before coitus; effective for only 30 to 60 minutes; some women may find them awkward or embarrassing to use
Diaphragm with spermicide	94%	80%	No health risks; helps protect against some STDs and cervical cancer	Must be inserted with jelly or foam before every act of coitus and left in place for at least 6 hours after coitus; must be fitted by health care personnel; some women may find it awkward or embarrassing to use; may be inconvenient to clean, store, and carry
Male condom Male condom with spermicide	97% 99%	86% 95%	Easy to use; inexpensive and easy to obtain; no health risks; very effective protection against some STDs; men share responsibility for family planning	Must be put on just before coitus; some men and women complain of decreased sensation
Female condom	95%	79%	Relatively easy to use; no prescription required; polyurethane is stronger than latex; provides some STD protection; silicone-based lubrication provided; useful when male will not use a condom	Contraceptive effectiveness and STD protection not as high as with male condom; couples may be unfamiliar with a device that extends outside the vagina; more expensive than male condoms
IUD Copper Progestin	 99%+ 98%	 99%+ 98%	Easy to use; highly effective in preventing pregnancy; does not interfere with coitus; repeated action not needed; depending on the device, can be effective for up to 10 years	May increase risk of pelvic inflammatory disease (PID) and infertility in women with more than one sexual partner; not usually recommended for women who have never had a child; must be inserted by health care personnel; may cause heavy bleeding and pain in some women
Combined pill Minipill	99%+ 99%+	95% 95%	Easy to use; highly effective in preventing pregnancy; does not interfere with coitus; regulates menstrual cycle; reduces heavy bleeding and menstrual pain; helps protect against ovarian and endometrial cancer	Must be taken every day; requires medical examination and prescription; minor side effects such as nausea or menstrual spotting; possibility of circulatory problems, such as blood clotting, strokes, and hypertension, in a small percentage of users
Depo-Provera (3 month) Lunelle (1 month)	99%+	99%+	Easy to use; highly effective for an extended period; continued use prevents menstruation	Requires supervision by a physician; administered by injection; some women experience irregular menstrual spotting and weight gain in early months of use
Subdermal implants	99%+	99%+	Highly effective for 5-year period; helps prevent anemia and regulates menstrual cycle	Requires minor surgery; some women experience irregular menstrual spotting and difficult removal
Tubal ligation	99%+	99%+	Permanent; removes fear of pregnancy	Surgery-related risks; generally considered irreversible
Vasectomy	99%+	99%+	Permanent; removes fear of pregnancy	Generally considered irreversible

Adapted from Hatcher RA et al: *Contraceptive Technology*, 17th rev. ed, 1998, Ardent Media, Inc.

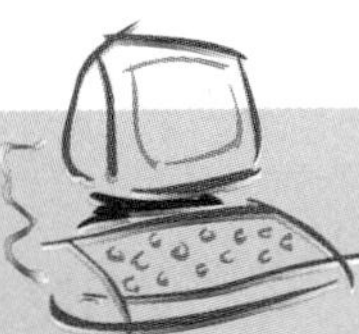

OnSITE/InSIGHT

Learning to Go: Health

Do you have questions about fertility? Click on the Motivator icon to explore these lessons on the topic:

Lesson 41: Choose a contraceptive that fits your lifestyle.
Lesson 42: Deal with an unintended pregnancy.
Lesson 43: Raise healthy, happy children.
Lesson 44: Unlock the mysteries of pregnancy and childbirth.

STUDENT POLL

Ever been concerned about accidental pregnancy? Go to the Online Learning Center at **www.mhhe.com/hahn6e**. Click on Student Resources. Then go to the Student Poll to answer these questions and find out how other students responded.

1. Are you sexually active?
2. Do you believe in contraception?
3. Do you, or does your partner, currently use some form of birth control?
4. Is it important to you to use a contraceptive?
5. Have you ever used emergency contraception?
6. Do you feel well informed about the various forms of contraceptives?
7. Have you ever been faced with an unplanned pregnancy?
8. Would you consider abortion if you (or your partner) had an unplanned pregnancy?
9. Are your fertility choices affected by your moral values?
10. Do you plan to have children some day?
11. Have you, or has your partner, ever had a miscarriage?
12. Has infertility ever been a concern of yours?
13. Have you ever considered in vitro fertilization?
14. Is adoption something you would consider?
15. Do you support the practice of surrogate parenting?

- *It should be reliable.* The form you select must be able to be used over and over again with consistent success.
- *It should be reversible.* Couples who eventually want to have a family should select a method that can be reversed.
- *It should be affordable.* The cost of a particular method must fit comfortably into a couple's budget.
- *It should be easy to use.* Complicated instructions or procedures can make a method difficult to use effectively.
- *It should not interfere with sexual expression.* An ideal contraceptive fits in comfortably with a couple's intimate sexual behavior.

TALKING POINTS • The method of birth control your partner prefers doesn't allow for spontaneous sex. How would you explain that this decreases your enjoyment?

CURRENT BIRTH CONTROL METHODS

Withdrawal

Withdrawal, or **coitus interruptus,** is the contraceptive practice in which the erect penis is removed from the vagina just before ejaculation of semen. Theoretically this procedure prevents sperm from entering the deeper structures of the female reproductive system. The use effectiveness of this method, however, reflects how unsuccessful this method is in practice (see Table 14-1).

There is strong evidence to suggest that the clear preejaculate fluid that helps neutralize and lubricate the male urethra can contain *viable* (capable of fertilization) sperm.[1] This sperm can be deposited near the cervical opening before withdrawal of the penis. This phenomenon may in part explain the relatively low effectiveness of this method. Furthermore, withdrawal does not protect users from the transmission of STDs.

Periodic Abstinence

There are four approaches included in the birth control strategy called **periodic abstinence:** (1) the calendar method, (2) the basal body temperature (BBT) method, (3) the Billings cervical mucus method, and (4) the symptothermal method.[2] All four methods attempt to determine the time a woman ovulates. Figure 14-1 shows a day-to-day fertility calendar used to estimate fertile periods. Most research indicates that an ovum is viable for only about 24 to 36 hours after its release from the ovary. (Once inside the female reproductive tract, some sperm can survive up to a week.)

When a woman can accurately determine when she ovulates, she must refrain from intercourse long enough for the ovum to begin to disintegrate. Of course, some couples are trying to become pregnant, and their goal will be to find the most fertile days that unprotected intercourse could produce a pregnancy.

Fertility awareness, rhythm, natural birth control, and *natural family planning* are terms interchangeable with periodic abstinence. Remember that periodic abstinence

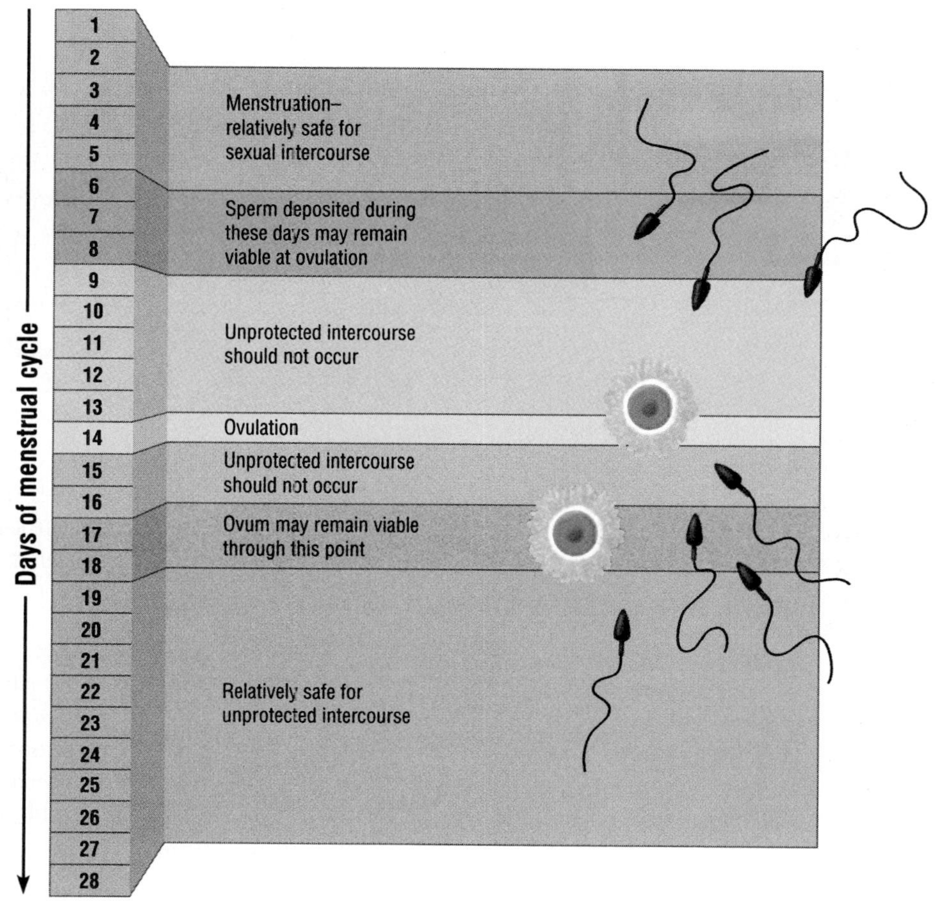

Figure 14-1 Periodic abstinence (fertility awareness or natural family planning) can combine use of the calendar, basal body temperature measurements, and Billings mucus techniques to identify the fertile period. Remember that most women's cycles are not consistently perfect 28-day cycles, as shown in most illustrations.

methods *do not* provide protection against the spread of STDs and HIV infection.

Periodic abstinence is the only acceptable method endorsed by the Roman Catholic Church. For some people who have deep concerns for the spiritual dimensions of their health, the selection of a contraceptive method other than periodic abstinence may indicate a serious compromise of beliefs.

The **calendar method** requires close examination of a woman's menstrual cycle for at least eight cycles. Records are kept of the length (in days) of each cycle. A *cycle* is defined as the number of days from the first day of menstral flow in one cycle to the first day of menstral flow in the next cycle.

To determine the days she should abstain from intercourse, a woman should subtract 18 from her shortest cycle; this is the first day she should abstain from intercourse in an upcoming cycle. Then she should subtract

Key Terms

withdrawal (coitus interruptus)
A contraceptive practice in which the erect penis is removed from the vagina before ejaculation.

periodic abstinence
Birth control methods that rely on a couple's avoidance of intercourse during the ovulatory phase of a woman's menstrual cycle; also called *fertility awareness* or *natural family planning.*

calendar method
A form of periodic abstinence in which the variable lengths of a woman's menstrual cycle are used to calculate her fertile period.

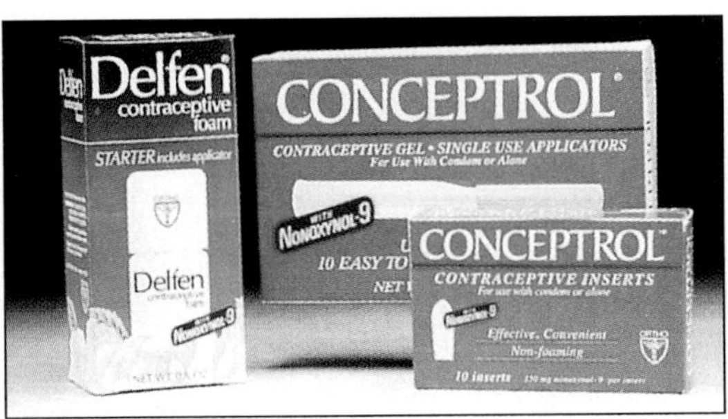

Vaginal spermicide.

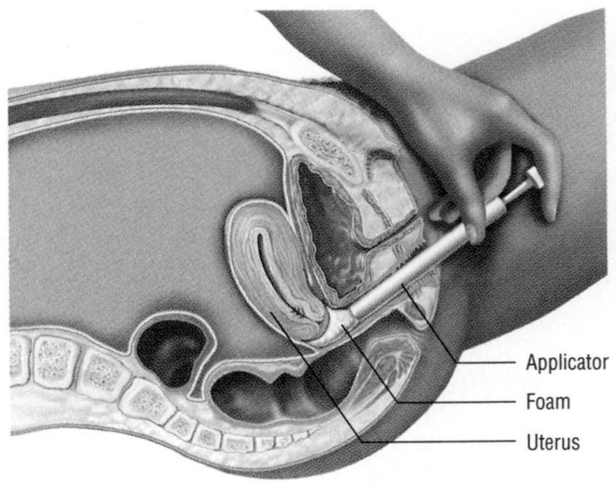

Figure 14-2 Spermicidal foams, gels, and suppositories are placed deep into the vagina in the region of the cervix no longer than 30 minutes before intercourse.

11 from her longest cycle; this is the last day she must abstain from intercourse in an upcoming cycle.

The *basal body temperature method* requires a woman (for about 3 or 4 successive months) to take her body temperature every morning before she rises from bed. A finely calibrated thermometer, available in many drugstores, is used for this purpose.[3] The theory behind this method is that a distinct correlation exists between body temperature and the process of ovulation. Just before ovulation, the body temperature supposedly dips and then rises about 0.5° to 1.0° F for the rest of the cycle. The woman is instructed to refrain from intercourse during the interval when the temperature change takes place.

Drawbacks of this procedure include the need for consistent, accurate readings and the realization that all women's bodies are different. Some women may not fit the temperature pattern projection because of biochemical differences in their bodies. Also, body temperatures can fluctuate because of a wide variety of illnesses and physical stressors.

The *Billings cervical mucus method* is another periodic abstinence technique. Generally used with other periodic abstinence techniques, this method requires a woman to evaluate the daily mucous discharge from her cervix. Users of this method become familiar with the changes in both appearance (from clear to cloudy) and consistency (from watery to thick) of their cervical mucus throughout their cycles. Women are taught that the unsafe days are when the mucus becomes clear and is the consistency of raw egg whites. Such a technique of ovulation determination must be learned from a physician or family planning professional.

The *symptothermal method* of periodic abstinence combines the use of the BBT method and the cervical mucus method. Couples using the symptothermal method are already using a calendar to chart the woman's body changes. Thus some family planning professionals consider the symptothermal method a combination of all of the periodic abstinence approaches.

Vaginal Spermicides

Although they are not recommended as the primary form of fertility control, spermicidal agents are often recommended to be used with other forms of birth control. Alone, **spermicides** offer a reasonable amount of contraceptive protection for the woman who is sexually active on an *infrequent* basis. Spermicides containing nonoxynol-9 do not provide reliable protection against STDs and HIV infection.

Modern spermicides are safe, reasonably effective, reversible forms of contraception that can be obtained without a physician's prescription; they can be purchased in most drugstores and in many supermarkets. Like condoms, spermicides are relatively inexpensive. When used together, spermicides and condoms provide a high degree of contraceptive protection and disease prevention.

Spermicides, which are available in foam, cream, gel, suppository, or film form, are made of water-soluble bases with a spermicidal chemical incorporated in the base. The base material is designed to liquefy at body temperature and distribute the spermicidal component in an even layer over the tissues of the upper vagina (Figure 14-2). The Star Box describes a unique film spermicide.

Spermicides are not specific to sperm cells; they also attack other cells and thus may provide the woman with some additional protection against many STDs and **pelvic inflammatory disease (PID).** However, when used alone, spermicides do not provide sufficient protection against most pathogens, including the virus that causes AIDS.

Condoms

Colored or natural, smooth or textured, straight or shaped, plain or reservoir-tipped, dry or lubricated—the condom is approaching an art form. This is perhaps an exaggeration. Still, the familiar **condom** remains a safe, effective, reversible contraceptive device. All condoms manufactured in the United States must be approved by the FDA.

Vaginal Contraceptive Film

A unique spermicide delivery system developed in England is vaginal contraceptive film (VCF). Vaginal contraceptive film is a sheet containing nonoxynol-9 that is inserted over the cervical opening. Shortly after insertion of the VCF, it dissolves into a gel-like material that clings to the cervical opening. The VCF can be inserted up to an hour before intercourse. Over the course of several hours, the material will be washed from the vagina in the normal vaginal secretions.

This spermicide is a nonprescription form of contraception that is as effective as other spermicidal foams and gels. A box of 12 sheets costs about $12. Like other spermicidal agents, VCF may help in minimizing the risk of some STDs and PID, but when used alone, does not provide reliable protection against all pathogens, including HIV.

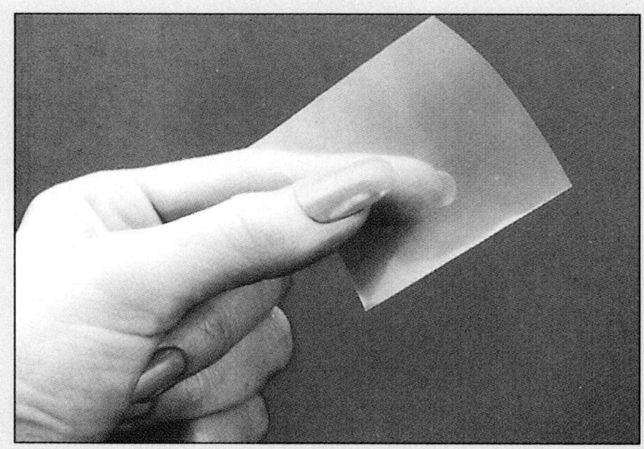

Vaginal contraceptive film.

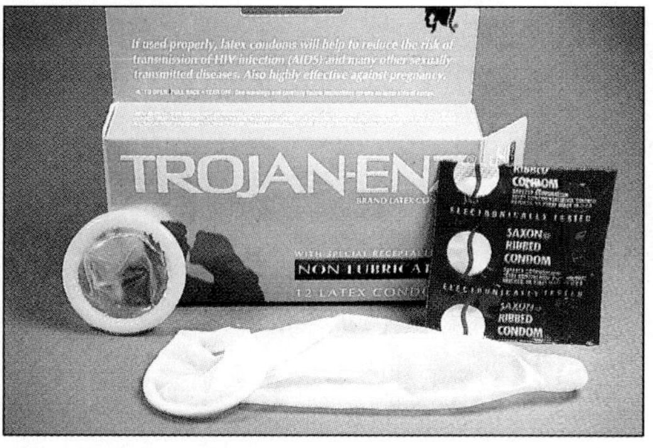

Condoms.

For couples who are highly motivated in their desire to prevent a pregnancy, the effectiveness of a condom can approach that of an oral contraceptive—especially if condom use is combined with a spermicide. (Many lubricated condoms now also contain a spermicide.) For couples who are less motivated or who use condoms on an irregular basis, the condom can be considerably less effective. This readily available and inexpensive method of contraception requires responsible use if it is to achieve a high level of effectiveness (see the Changing for the Better box on p. 354).

The condom offers a measure of protection against STDs. For both the man and the woman, chlamydial infections, gonorrhea, HIV infection, and other STDs are less likely to be acquired when the condom is used. When combined with a spermicide containing nonoxynol-9, condoms may become even more effective against the spread of STDs. Although advertisements suggest that condoms provide protection against the transmission of genital herpes, users of condoms must remember that this protection is limited to the penis and vagina—not to the surrounding genital region, where significant numbers of lesions are found. Like other barrier methods of contraception, the condom is a reasonable choice for couples who are motivated in their desire to prevent a pregnancy and who are willing to assume the level of responsibility required.

The FDA has approved both male and female types of polyurethane condoms. At the time of this writing, at least three brands of polyurethane male condoms and one female condom (Reality) are available as one-time-use condoms. These condoms are good alternatives for people who have an allergic sensitivity to latex. Also, they are thinner and stronger than latex condoms and can be used with oil-based lubricants. Currently, these condoms are believed to provide protection against STDs that is comparable to that of latex condoms.

Key Terms

spermicides
Chemicals capable of killing sperm.

pelvic inflammatory disease (PID)
A generalized infection of the pelvic cavity that results from the spread of an infection through a woman's reproductive structures.

condom
A latex shield designed to cover the erect penis and retain semen on ejaculation; "rubber."

Changing *for the Better*

Maximizing the Effectiveness of Condoms

Putting on a condom seems so easy. Is there anything else I need to know about condom use?

These simple directions for using condoms correctly, in combination with your motivation and commitment to regular use, should provide you with reasonable protection:

- Keep a supply of condoms at hand. Condoms should be stored in a cool, dry place so that they are readily available at the time of intercourse. Condoms that are stored in wallets or automobile glove compartments may not be in satisfactory condition when they are used. Temperature extremes are to be avoided. Check the condom package for the expiration date.
- Do not test a condom by inflating or stretching it. Handle it gently and keep it away from sharp fingernails.
- For maximum effectiveness, put the condom on before genital contact. Either the man or the woman can put the condom in place. Early application is particularly important in the prevention of STDs. Early application also lessens the possibility of the release of preejaculate fluid into the vagina.
- Unroll the condom on the erect penis. For those using a condom without a reservoir tip, a ½-inch space should be left to catch the ejaculate. To leave this space, pinch the tip of the condom as you roll it on the erect penis. Do not leave any air in the tip of the condom (Figure 14-3).
- Lubricate the condom if this has not already been done by the manufacturer. When doing this, be certain to use a water-soluble lubricant and not a petroleum-based product such as petroleum jelly. Petroleum can deteriorate the latex material. Other oil-based lubricants, such as mineral oil, baby oil, vegetable oil, shortening, and certain hand lotions, can quickly damage a condom. Use water-based lubricants only!
- After ejaculation, be certain that the condom does not become dislodged from the penis. Hold the rim of the condom firmly against the base of the penis during withdrawal. Do not allow the penis to become flaccid (soft) while still in the vagina.
- Inspect the condom for tears before throwing it away. If the condom is damaged in some way, immediately insert a spermicidal agent into the vagina.

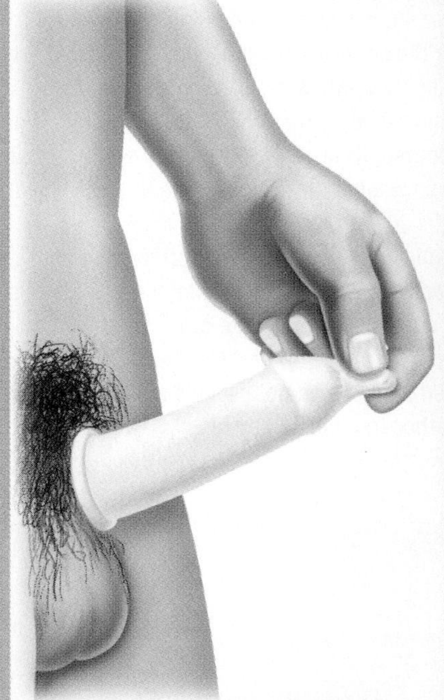

Figure 14-3 Pinch the end of the condom to leave ½ inch of space at the tip.

The Reality female condom is a soft, loose-fitting polyurethane sheath containing two polyurethane rings (see photo). Reality is inserted like a diaphragm to line the inner walls of the vagina. The larger ring remains outside the vagina, and the external portion of the condom provides some protection to the labia and the base of the penis. Reality is coated on the inside with a silicone-based lubricant. Additional lubricant is provided for the outside of the sheath. This lubricant does not contain a spermicide. Female and male condoms should not be used together since they might adhere to each other and cause slippage or displacement.[2] The contraceptive effectiveness of the female condom is not as high as that of the male

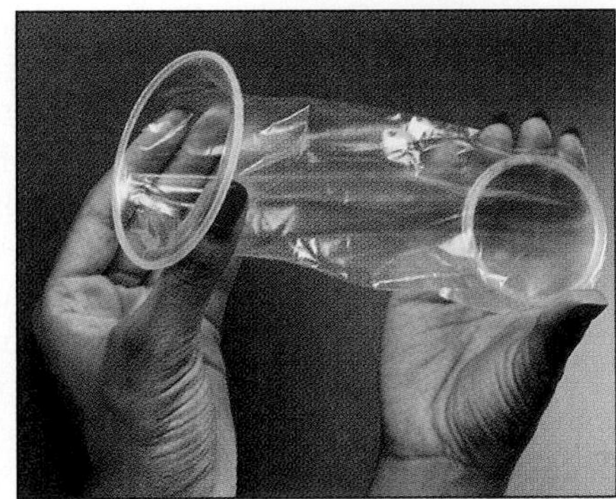

Female condom.

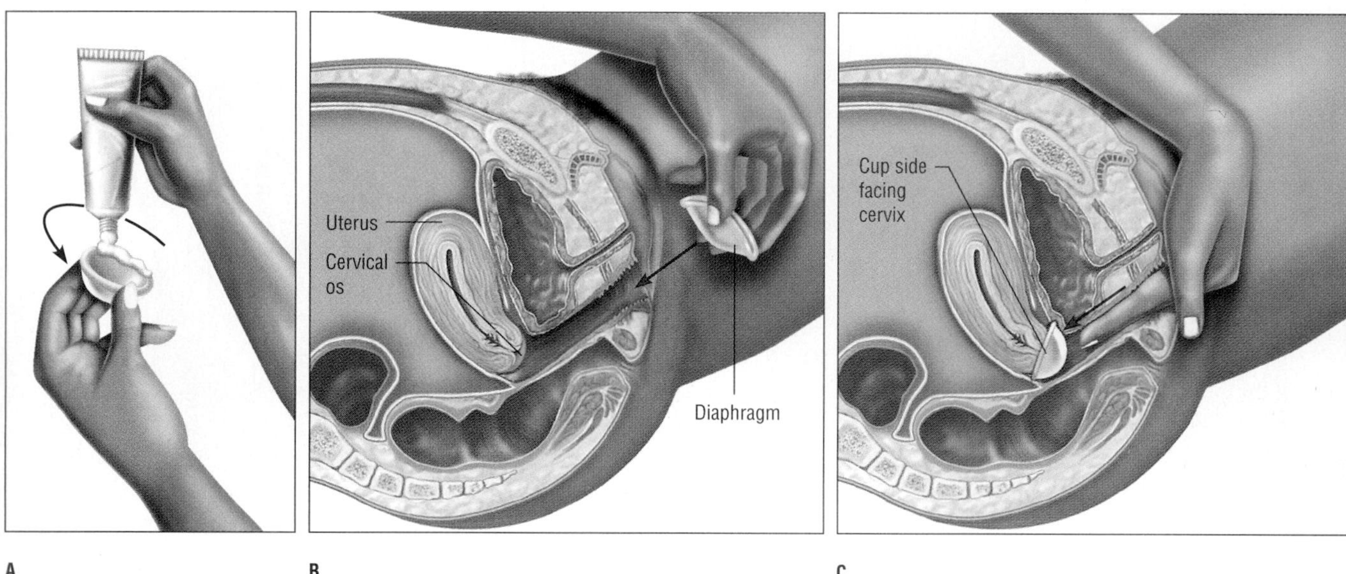

Figure 14-4 **A**, Spermicidal cream or jelly is placed into the diaphragm. **B**, The diaphragm is folded lengthwise and inserted into the vagina. **C**, The diaphragm is then placed against the cervix so that the cup portion with the spermicide is facing the cervix. The outline of the cervix should be felt through the central part of the diaphragm.

condom. However, as people become more familiar with using the female condom, its effectiveness may increase.

Diaphragm

The **diaphragm** is a soft rubber cup with a springlike metal rim that, when properly fitted and correctly inserted by the user, rests in the top of the vagina. In its proper position the diaphragm covers the cervical opening (Figure 14-4). During intercourse the diaphragm stays in place quite well and cannot usually be felt by either the man or the woman.

The diaphragm is always used with a spermicidal cream or jelly. The diaphragm should be covered with an adequate amount of spermicide inside the cup and around the rim. When used properly with a spermicide, the diaphragm is a relatively effective contraceptive, and when combined with the man's use of a condom, its effectiveness is even greater.

Diaphragms must always be fitted and prescribed by a physician. The cost of obtaining a diaphragm and keeping a supply of spermicide may be higher than that of other methods. Also, a high level of motivation to follow the instructions *exactly* is important.

Diaphragms and other vaginal barrier methods, such as the cervical cap, do not provide reliable protection against STDs and HIV infection. If you are concerned about possible infection, either avoid sexual activity or use a latex condom and spermicide in combination.

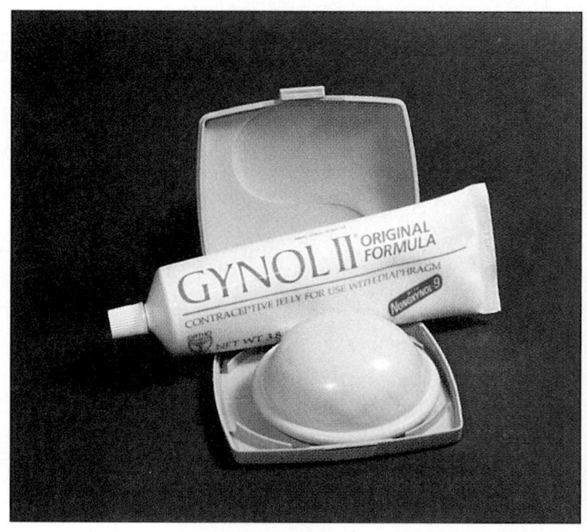

Diaphragm and contraceptive jelly.

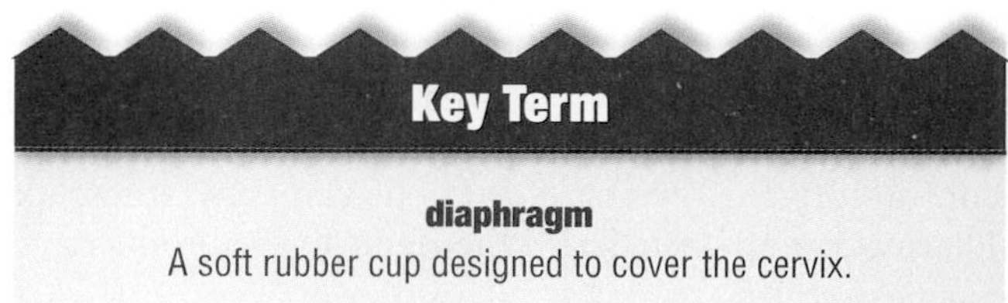

Key Term

diaphragm
A soft rubber cup designed to cover the cervix.

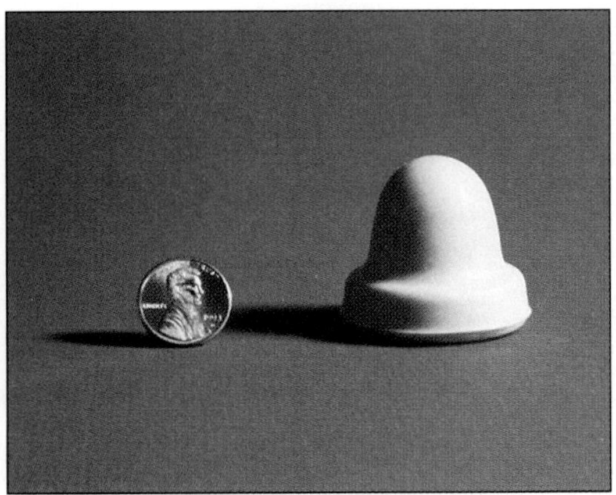

Cervical cap.

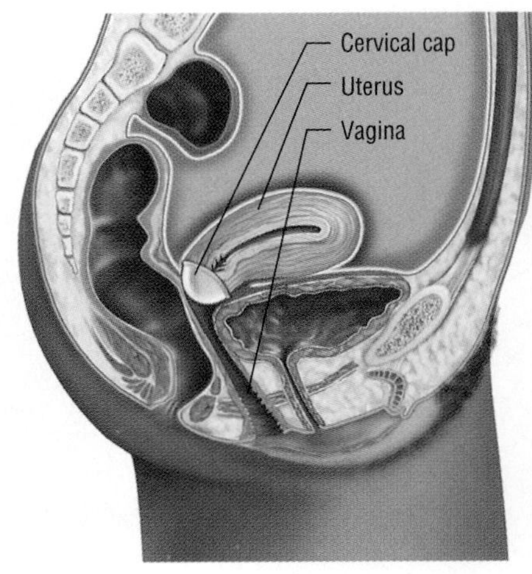

Figure 14-5 After the spermicidal cream or jelly is placed in the cervical cap, the cap is inserted into the vagina and placed against the cervix.

Cervical Cap

The **cervical cap** is a small, thimble-shaped device that fits over the entire cervix. Resembling a small diaphragm, the cervical cap is placed deeper than the diaphragm. The cap is held in place by suction rather than by pushing against anatomical structures (Figure 14-5). As with the diaphragm, a spermicide is used with the cervical cap. Thus it requires many of the same skills for insertion and care as does the diaphragm. The use effectiveness of the cervical cap appears to be approximately equal to that of the diaphragm. As with the diaphragm, the effectiveness of the cervical cap is much higher in women who have never had children. Cervical caps are distributed in the United States through physician prescription.

Contraceptive Sponge

The sponge is a small, pillow-shaped polyurethane device containing nonoxynol-9 spermicide. The sponge is dampened with tap water and inserted deep in the vagina to cover the cervical opening. This device provides contraceptive protection for up to 24 hours, regardless of the number of times intercourse occurs. After intercourse, the device must be left in place for at least 6 hours. Once removed, the sponge must be discarded. The sponge must not be left in place for longer than 24 to 30 hours because of the risk of toxic shock syndrome.[2] Used alone, the sponge does not provide reliable protection against STDs and HIV infection. In women who have not given birth to children, the contraceptive effectiveness of the sponge is similar to that of the diaphragm.

Prior to its removal from the market in 1995, when the manufacturer refused to upgrade its physical plant to meet new government safety regulations, the Today Sponge was the most popular female over-the-counter contraceptive. However, a different company, Allendale Pharmaceuticals, purchased the rights to the product and plans to have the Today Sponge back on the market after FDA approval. For the latest information on this product, see the Allendale website at **www.todaysponge.com.**

Intrauterine Device

The **intrauterine device (IUD)** is a method of birth control that functions in various ways to reduce the likelihood of conception and implantation of fertilized ovum in the uterus. IUDs, especially the ones that contain hormones, thicken cervical mucus and thus, make it difficult for sperm to reach an ovum. Additionally, IUDs seem to alter the uterine lining and make it very difficult for a fertilized ovum to implant itself successfully.

Two types of IUDs are available in the United States: progestin-containing (Progestasert and Mirena) and copper-containing (ParaGard). Progestasert is effective for one year, Mirena for up to five years, and the ParaGard IUD is effective for up to ten years. Only a skilled physician can prescribe and insert an IUD. As with many other forms of contraception, IUDs do not offer protection against STDs or HIV infection.

As Table 14-1 indicates, IUDs are very effective birth control devices, surpassed in effectiveness only by abstinence, sterilization, and oral (or implanted, or injected) contraceptives. Some women using IUDs experience increased menstrual bleeding and cramping. Two uncommon but potentially serious side effects of IUD use are uterine perforation (in which the IUD imbeds itself into the uterine wall) and PID (which is a life-threatening infection of the abdominal cavity). The choice of over 100 million women worldwide, IUDs are used by fewer than 1% of women at risk of pregnancy in the United States.[2]

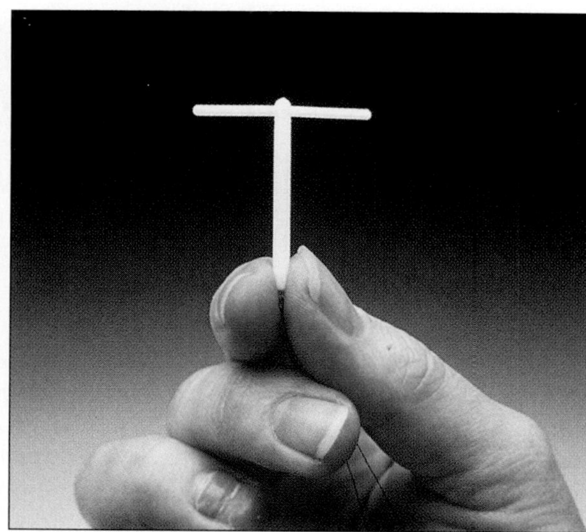

Progestasert IUD.

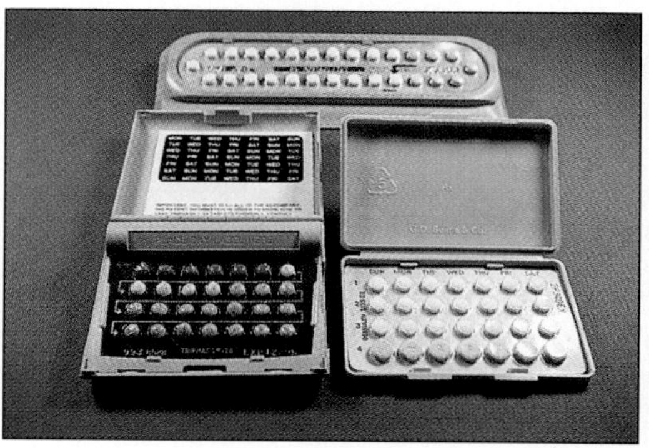

Oral contraceptives.

A woman deciding whether to use an IUD must discuss any concerns openly with her physician. The IUD can be a very acceptable form of contraception, especially for women who are in their middle to late reproductive years, unable to take birth control pills, in a stable monogamous relationship, and not at risk for STDs.

Oral Contraceptives

Introduced in 1960, the **oral contraceptive pill** provides one of the highest effectiveness rates of any single reversible contraceptive method used today. "The pill" is the method of choice for 16 million users in the United States.[2]

Use of the pill requires a physical examination by a physician and a prescription. Since oral contraceptives are available in a wide range of formulas, follow-up examinations are important to ensure that a woman is receiving an effective dosage with as few side effects as possible. Determining the right prescription for a particular woman may require a few consultations.

All oral contraceptives contain synthetic (laboratory-made) hormones. The *combined pill* uses both synthetic estrogen and synthetic progesterone in each of twenty-one pills. In 1984, *triphasic pills* were introduced in the United States. In these pills the level of synthetic progesterone varies every 7 days during the cycle.[2] Estrogen levels remain constant during the cycle. As with many forms of contraception, it must be emphatically stated that *oral contraceptives do not provide protection from the transmission of STDs or HIV infection.* Furthermore, the use of antibiotics lowers the pill's contraceptive effectiveness.

Oral contraceptives function in several ways. The estrogen in the pill tends to reduce ova development and ovulation. The progesterone in the pill helps reduce ovulation (by lowering the release of luteinizing hormone). The progesterone in the pill also causes the uterine wall to develop inadequately and helps thicken cervical mucus, thus making it difficult for sperm to enter the uterus.

The physical changes produced by the oral contraceptive provide some beneficial side effects in women. Since the synthetic hormones are taken for 21 days and then are followed by **placebo pills** or no pills for 7 days, the menstrual cycle becomes regulated. Even women who have irregular cycles immediately become "regular." Since the uterine lining is not developed to the extent seen in a nonuser, the uterus is not forced to contract with the same amount of vigor. Thus menstrual cramping is reduced, and the resultant menstrual flow is diminished. Research indicates that oral contraceptive use may provide protection against anemia, PID, noncancerous breast tumors, recurrent ovarian cysts, ectopic pregnancy, endometrial cancer, and ovarian cancer.[2]

Key Terms

cervical cap
A small, thimble-shaped device designed to fit over the cervix.

intrauterine device (IUD)
A small, plastic, medicated or unmedicated device that prevents continued pregnancy when inserted in the uterus.

oral contraceptive pill
A pill taken orally, composed of synthetic female hormones that prevent ovulation or implantation; "the pill."

placebo pills
Pills that contain no active ingredients.

The negative side effects of the oral contraceptive pill can be divided into two general categories: (1) unpleasant and (2) potentially dangerous. The unpleasant side effects generally subside within 2 or 3 months for most women. A number of women report some or many of the following symptoms:

- Tenderness in breast tissue
- Nausea
- Mild headaches
- Slight, irregular spotting
- Weight gain
- Fluctuations in sex drive
- Mild depression
- More frequent vaginal infections

TALKING POINTS • You've tried two different types of oral contraceptives and had unpleasant side effects with both. Your doctor says you should consider another birth control method, but you disagree. How could you talk to him about this in a matter-of-fact way?

The potentially dangerous side effects of the oral contraceptive pill are most often seen in the cardiovascular system. Blood clotting, strokes, hypertension, and heart attack all seem to be associated with the estrogen component of the combined pill. When compared with the risk to nonusers, the risk of dying from cardiovascular complications is only slightly increased among healthy young oral contraceptive users.

Additionally, the present consensus is that oral contraceptive users place themselves at slightly increased risk of developing breast cancer and cervical cancer.[2] However, it must be emphasized that this risk is quite small. Most health professionals agree that the risks related to pregnancy and childbirth are much greater than those associated with oral contraceptive use. Certainly, a woman who is contemplating the use of the pill must discuss all of the risks and benefits with her physician.

There are some **contraindications** for the use of oral contraceptives. If you have a history of blood clotting, migraine headaches, liver disease, a heart condition, high blood pressure, obesity, diabetes, epilepsy, or anemia, or if you have not established regular menstrual cycles, the pill probably should not be your contraceptive choice. A thorough health history is important before a woman starts to take the pill.

Two additional contraindications are receiving considerable attention by the medical community. Cigarette smoking and advancing age are highly associated with an increased risk of potentially serious side effects. Increasing numbers of physicians are not prescribing oral contraceptives for their patients who smoke. The risk of cardiovascular-related deaths is enhanced in women over age 35. The risk is even higher in female smokers over age 35.

For the vast majority of women, however, the pill, when properly prescribed, is safe and effective. Careful scrutiny of a woman's health history and careful follow-up examinations when a problem is suspected are essential elements that can provide a margin of safety. The ease of administration, the relatively low cost, and the effectiveness of the pill make it a sound choice for many women.

Minipills

Some women prefer not to use the combined oral contraceptive pill. To avoid some of the potentially serious side effects of the combined pill, some physicians are prescribing **minipills.** These oral contraceptives contain no estrogen—only low-dose progesterone. The minipill seems to work by making an unsuitable environment for the transportation and implantation of the fertilized ovum. The effectiveness of the minipill is slightly lower than that of the combined pill. *Breakthrough bleeding* and **ectopic pregnancy** are more common in minipill users than in combined-pill users.

Emergency contraception

Emergency contraception is designed to prevent pregnancy after unprotected vaginal intercourse. This method is also called post-coital or "morning after" contraception. Emergency contraception is available in two forms: emergency hormonal contraception and the insertion of an IUD. Both forms of contraception can be prescribed (or carried out) only by a physician.

Emergency hormonal contraception involves the use of two doses of certain oral contraceptives.[4] The most commonly used oral contraceptives are the combined pills (Preven), which contain both synthetic estrogen and progesterone. The first dose of pills is taken within 72 hours of unprotected intercourse. A second dose is taken 12 hours later. If progesterone-only pills (Plan B) are used for emergency contraception, the first dose must be taken within 48 to 72 hours after unprotected intercourse.

The insertion of an IUD is a less commonly used, but highly effective, form of emergency contraception. To function as a contraceptive, however, the IUD must be inserted within 5 days after unprotected intercourse.

Injectable Contraceptives

In 1992 the FDA approved a form of synthetic progesterone called *Depo-Provera.* This injectable contraceptive provides an extremely high degree of effectiveness for a 3-month period. In October 2000, the FDA also approved Lunelle, a once-a-month injection of estrogen and progestin.[5] Both Depo-Provera and Lunelle have success rates higher than 99%.

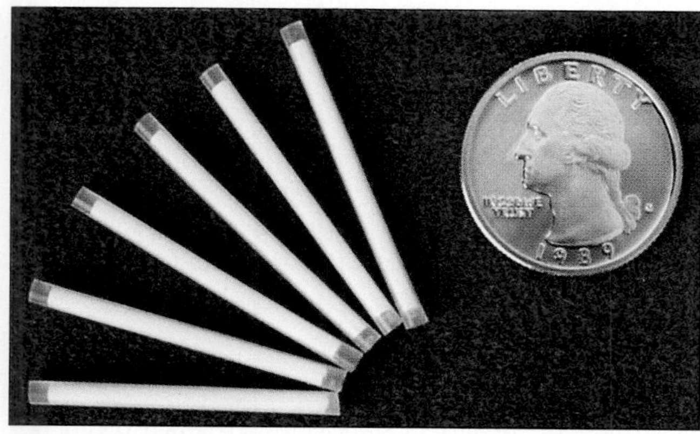

The Norplant subdermal implant.

Weight gain is the major complaint of Lunelle users.[5] New users of Depo-Provera report occasional breakthrough bleeding in the early months of use as the most common unpleasant side effect. After this point, the most commonly reported side effect is amenorrhea (the absence of periods). Many women consider amenorrhea to be a desirable effect of Depo-Provera use. Unlike users of oral contraceptives and subdermal implants, who return to fertility a few months after stopping their use, women who stop using Depo-Provera may experience infertility for a period of up to 1 year.[2]

Subdermal Implants

In late 1990, subdermal implants (Norplant) were approved for use in the United States. This form of contraception involves the use of six silicone rods filled with synthetic progesterone. Using a local anesthetic, the physician implants these rods just beneath the skin of the woman's upper or lower arm. The rods release low levels of the hormone for 5 years. An extremely effective contraceptive, subdermal implants appear to produce minimal side effects. Irregular patterns of menstrual bleeding are the most common side effect. Sometimes the implanted rods are difficult to remove. Norplant implants cost approximately $600 for a 5-year supply.

Sterilization

All of the contraceptive mechanisms or methods already discussed have one quality in common: they are reversible. Although microsurgical techniques are providing medical breakthroughs, **sterilization** should generally be considered an irreversible procedure.[3] When you decide to use sterilization, you are giving up control of your own fertility because you will no longer be able to produce offspring. For this reason, couples considering sterilization procedures usually must undergo extensive discussions with a physician or family planning counselor to identify their true feelings about this finality. People must be aware of the possible changes in self-concept they might have after sterilization. If you are a man who equates fertility with masculinity, you may have trouble accepting your new status as a sterile man. If you are a woman who equates motherhood with femininity, you might have adjustment problems after sterilization.

The male sterilization procedure is called a *vasectomy.* Accomplished with a local anesthetic in a physician's office, this 20- to 30-minute procedure consists of the surgical removal of a section of each vas deferens. After a small incision is made through the scrotum, the vas deferens is located and a small section is removed. The remaining ends are either tied or *cauterized* (Figure 14-6, *A*).

Immediately after a vasectomy, sperm may still be present in the vas deferens. A backup contraceptive is recommended until a physician microscopically examines a semen specimen. This examination usually occurs about 6 weeks after the surgery. After a vasectomy, men can still produce male sex hormones, get erections, have orgasms, and ejaculate. (Recall that sperm account for only a small portion of the semen.) Some men even report increased interest in sexual activity, since their chances of impregnating a woman are virtually nonexistent.

What happens to the process of spermatogenesis within each testicle? Sperm cells are still being produced, but they are destroyed by specialized white blood cells called *phagocytic leukocytes.*

The most common method of female sterilization is *tubal ligation.* During this procedure, the fallopian tubes are cut and the ends are tied back. Some physicians cauterize the tube ends to ensure complete sealing (Figure 14-6, *B*). The fallopian tubes are usually reached through the abdominal wall. In a *minilaparotomy,* a small incision is made through the abdominal wall just below the navel. The resultant scar is quite small and is the basis for the term *band-aid surgery.*

Key Terms

contraindications
Factors that make the use of a drug inappropriate or dangerous for a particular person.

minipills
Low-dose progesterone oral contraceptives.

ectopic pregnancy
A pregnancy in which the fertilized ovum implants at a site other than the uterus, typically in the fallopian tubes.

sterilization
Generally permanent birth control techniques that surgically disrupt the normal passage of ova or sperm.

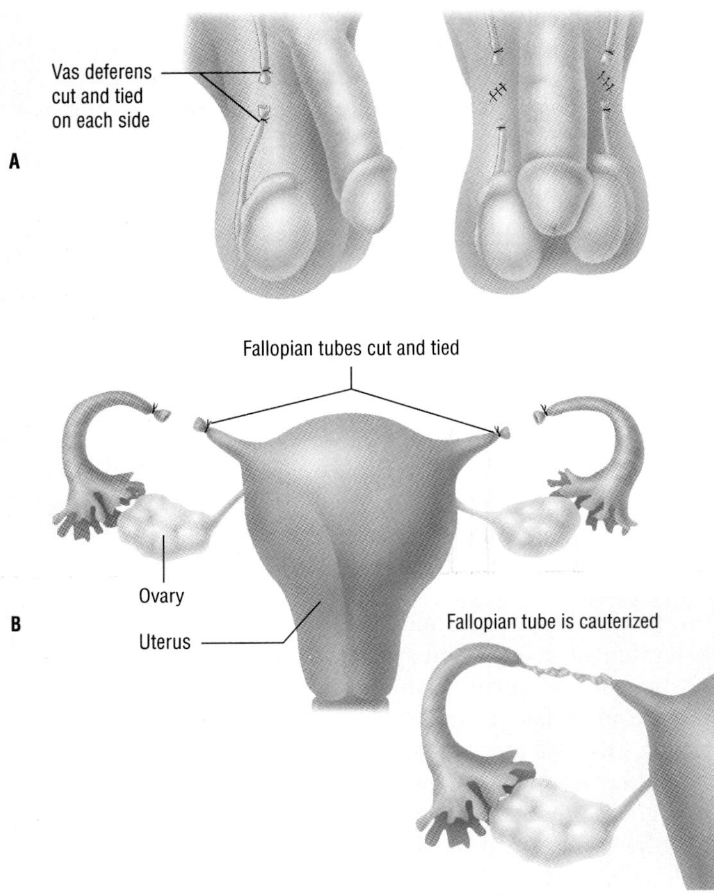

Figure 14-6 The most frequently used forms of male and female sterilization. **A,** Vasectomy. **B,** Tubal ligation.

Female sterilization requires about 20 to 30 minutes, with the patient under local or general anesthesia. The use of a *laparoscope* has made female sterilization much simpler than in the past. The laparoscope is a small tube equipped with mirrors and lights. Inserted through a single incision, the laparoscope locates the fallopian tubes before they are cut, tied, or cauterized. When a laparoscope is used through an abdominal incision, the procedure is called a *laparoscopy.*

Women who are sterilized still produce female hormones, ovulate, and menstruate. However, the ovum cannot move down the fallopian tube. Within a day of its release, the ovum will start to disintegrate and be absorbed by the body. Freed of the possibility of becoming pregnant, many sterilized women report an increase in sex drive and activity.

Two other procedures produce sterilization in women. *Ovariectomy* (the surgical removal of the ovaries) and *hysterectomy* (the surgical removal of the uterus) accomplish sterilization. However, these procedures are used to remove diseased (cancerous, cystic, or hemorrhaging) organs and are not considered primary sterilization techniques.

TALKING POINTS • You and your husband have children, and you'd like to stop taking the pill for health reasons. Your husband says you're pressuring him to have a vasectomy. How can you keep the dialogue going in a cooperative way?

Abortion

Regardless of the circumstances under which pregnancy occurs, women may now choose to terminate their pregnancies. No longer must women who do not want to be pregnant seek potentially dangerous, illegal abortions. On the basis of current technology and legality, women need never experience childbirth. The decision is theirs to make.

Abortion should never be considered a first-line, preferred form of fertility control. Rather, abortion is a final, last-chance undertaking. It should be used only when responsible control of one's fertility could not be achieved. The decision to abort a fetus is a highly controversial, personal one—one that needs serious consideration by each woman.

On the basis of the landmark 1973 U.S. Supreme Court case *Roe v. Wade,* the United States joined many of the world's most populated countries in legalizing abortions within the following guidelines:

1. For the first 3 months of pregnancy (first trimester), the decision to abort lies with the woman and her doctor.
2. For the next 3 months of pregnancy (second trimester), state law may regulate the abortion procedure in ways that are reasonably related to maternal health.
3. For the last weeks of pregnancy (third trimester), when the fetus is judged capable of surviving if born, any state may regulate or even prohibit abortion except where abortion is necessary to preserve the life or health of the mother. If a pregnancy is terminated during the third trimester, a viable fetus would be considered a live birth and would not be allowed to die.

Each year, approximately 1.4 million women in the United States make the decision to terminate a pregnancy.[6] Thousands of additional women probably consider abortion but elect to continue their pregnancies.

Clearly, abortion is a political issue. It will be interesting to see how future abortion-related decisions will unfold. Special interest groups on both sides of the issue, the Supreme Court, state legislatures, federal agencies (such as the FDA and the Department of Health and Human

Services), the Congress, and the president all have a say in the abortion debate in this country. Regardless of the eventual outcomes of this debate, here are the present abortion procedures available in the United States.

TALKING POINTS • **You're unexpectedly pregnant, but abortion doesn't seem like a good choice for you. Your boyfriend, your family, and your friends all have strong but conflicting opinions about the situation. How can you show that you value their advice but still make it clear that the final decision needs to be yours alone?**

First-trimester abortion procedures

Menstrual extraction. Also referred to as *menstrual regulation, menstrual induction,* and *preemptive abortion,* menstrual extraction is a process carried out between the fourth and sixth week after the last menstrual period (or in the days immediately after the first missed menstrual period). This procedure is generally performed in a physician's office with a local anesthetic or *paracervical anesthetic* used. A small plastic *cannula* is inserted through the undilated cervical canal into the cavity of the uterus. Once the cannula is in position, a small amount of suction is applied by a hand-held syringe. By rotating and moving the cannula across the uterine wall, the physician can withdraw the endometrial tissue.

Vacuum aspiration. Induced abortions undertaken during the sixth through ninth weeks of pregnancy are generally done through *vacuum aspiration* of the uterine contents. Vacuum aspiration is the most commonly performed abortion procedure. This procedure is similar in nature to menstrual extraction. Unlike menstrual extraction, however, vacuum aspiration may require **dilation** of the cervical canal and the use of a local anesthetic. In this more advanced stage of pregnancy, a larger cannula must be inserted into the uterine cavity. This process can be accomplished by using metal dilators of increasingly larger sizes to open the canal. After aspiration by an electric vacuum pump, the uterine wall may also be scraped to confirm complete removal of the uterine contents.

Dilation and curettage (D & C). When a pregnancy is to be terminated during the ninth through fourteenth weeks, vacuum aspiration gives way to a somewhat similar procedure labeled **dilation and curettage,** or more familiarly, **D & C.** D & C usually requires a general anesthetic, not a local anesthetic.

Like vacuum aspiration, the D & C involves the gradual enlargement of the cervical canal through the insertion of increasingly larger metal dilators. When the cervix has been dilated to a size sufficient to allow for the passage of a *curette,* the removal of the endometrial tissue can begin. The curette is a metal instrument resembling a spoon, with a cup-shaped cutting surface on its end. As the curette is drawn across the uterine wall, the soft endometrial tissue and fetal parts are scraped from the wall of the uterus. (The D & C is also used in the medical management of certain health conditions of the uterine wall, such as irregular bleeding or the buildup of endometrial tissue.)

As in the case of menstrual extraction, both vacuum aspiration and D & C are very safe procedures for the woman. The need to dilate the cervix more fully in a D & C increases the risk of cervical trauma and the possibility of perforation, but these risks are reported to be low. Bleeding, cramping, spotting, and infections present minimal controllable risks when procedures are done by experienced clinicians under clinical conditions.

Medical abortion. Mifepristone and methotrexate are drugs that a woman can use under medical supervision to induce a medical abortion during the first trimester. Formerly known as RU-486, mifepristone blocks the action of progesterone and causes the uterine lining and any fertilized egg to shed.[2] Under FDA guidelines, women must use mifepristone within 49 days of their last menstrual period. Women take three pills at the first doctor visit and then return 48 hours later to take a second drug, misoprostol, which causes menstruation to occur, usually within about 5 hours. A third visit to a physician is necessary to ensure that the woman is recovering well from the medical abortion. Blood tests or an ultrasound exam will verify that the abortion was successful.

Methotrexate is a drug used since the 1950s for cancer treatment. However, physicians sometimes use this drug in an off-label manner to induce a first term abortion.[2] Typically, a woman receives an injection of methotrexate and, during a second office visit 3 to 7 days later, receives prostoglandin. The fetal contents are expelled, usually within a day, but some methotrexate abortions take up a week to occur. A follow-up office visit is necessary. Medical abortions cost about the same as a first-term surgical abortion ($250–$300).

Key Terms

abortion
Induced premature termination of a pregnancy.

dilation
Gradual expansion of an opening or passageway, such as the cervix.

dilation and curettage (D & C)
A surgical procedure in which the cervical canal is dilated to allow the uterine wall to be scraped.

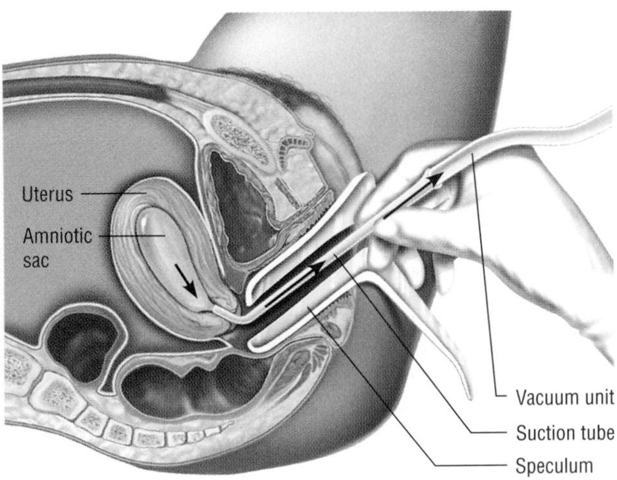

Figure 14-7 During dilation and evacuation, the cervix is dilated and the contents of the uterus are aspirated (removed by suction). This procedure is used to perform abortions up to 16 weeks' gestation.

Second-trimester abortion procedures

When a woman's pregnancy continues beyond the fourteenth week of gestation, termination becomes a more difficult matter. The procedures at this stage are more complicated and take longer to complete. Complications are also more common.

Dilation and evacuation. Vacuum aspiration and D & C can be combined in a procedure called *dilation and evacuation (D & E)* during the earliest weeks of the second trimester (Figure 14-7). The use of D & E increases the likelihood of trauma and postprocedural complications, since larger instruments and greater dilation are required. After about 16 weeks, more intensive procedures will be required to terminate the late second-trimester pregnancy.

Hypertonic saline procedure. From the sixteenth week of gestation to the end of the second trimester, intrauterine injection of a strong salt solution into the amniotic sac is the procedure most frequently used. The administration of intrauterine **hypertonic saline solution** requires a skilled operator so that the needle used to introduce the salt solution enters the amniotic sac. Once the needle is in place, some amniotic fluid is withdrawn, allowing the saline solution to be injected.

Some physicians support the saline procedure by dilating the cervix with *laminaria* or another dilatory product and administering the hormone oxytocin to stimulate uterine contractions. The onset of uterine contractions will expel the dehydrated uterine contents within 24 to 36 hours.

Prostaglandin procedure. The use of prostaglandin is the third type of abortion procedure used during the second trimester. Prostaglandins are hormonelike chemicals that have a variety of useful effects on human tissue. Produced naturally within the body, these substances influence the contractions of smooth muscle. Since the uterine wall is composed entirely of smooth muscle, it is particularly sensitive to the presence of prostaglandins. When prostaglandin is administered in sufficient quantity (through either a uterine intramuscular injection or a vaginal suppository), uterine contractions become strong enough to expel the fetal contents.

Third-trimester abortion procedures

If termination of a pregnancy is required in the latter weeks of the gestational period, a surgical procedure in which the fetus is removed *(hysterotomy)* or a procedure in which the entire uterus is removed *(hysterectomy)* can be undertaken. These procedures are more complicated and involve longer hospitalization, major abdominal surgery, and an extended period of recovery.

In the late 1990s, the U.S. House of Representatives and the U.S. Senate voted to ban a rarely used third-trimester abortion procedure referred to as dilation and extraction. Lawmakers felt that this procedure, also called *partial-birth abortion,* was too gruesome to be permitted. President Clinton vetoed this ban, and because the Senate failed to override his veto, the ban on partial-birth abortion did not become law.

In June 2000, the U.S. Supreme Court invalidated a Nebraska state law that prohibited partial-birth abortions. See Figure 14-8 for a closer look at abortion laws.

Post-Abortion Syndrome

Some women who have an abortion may be faced with the consequence of psychological difficulties in the years that follow the abortion. The term **post-abortion syndrome** refers to "the suggested long-term negative psychological effects of abortion."[7] It is possible that these difficulties may arise soon after the abortion or may not surface until years later. The signs and symptoms of post-abortion syndrome are not unlike those of the more well-known post-traumatic stress disorder. (However, it should be noted that the American Psychiatric Association and other organizations do not recognize post-abortion syndrome as an identifiable illness.)

Women having post-abortion syndrome may experience some or all of the following effects: difficulties with personal relationships, substance abuse problems, nightmares, sexual difficulties, communication problems, damage to self-esteem, and, possibly, suicide.[7] These symptoms may range from mild to severe and may be lengthy in duration.

Do You Know the Abortion Laws in Your State?

State	Requires parents' notification or consent if woman is under 18	Requires counseling or waiting period before abortion	Restricts late-term abortions if no threat to woman's life or health
Alabama	✘		✘
Alaska		✘	
Arizona			✘
Arkansas	✘	✘	✘
California		✘	✘
Colorado			
Connecticut		✘	✘
Delaware	✘		✘
Florida			✘
Georgia	✘		✘
Hawaii			
Idaho	✘	✘	✘
Illinois			✘
Indiana	✘	✘	✘
Iowa	✘		✘
Kansas	✘	✘	✘
Kentucky	✘	✘	✘
Louisiana	✘	✘	✘
Maine		✘	✘
Maryland	✘		✘
Massachusetts	✘		✘
Michigan	✘	✘	✘
Minnesota	✘	✘	✘
Mississippi	✘	✘	
Missouri	✘		✘
Montana			✘
Nebraska	✘	✘	✘
Nevada		✘	✘
New Hampshire			
New Jersey			
New Mexico			
New York			✘
North Carolina	✘		✘
North Dakota	✘	✘	✘
Ohio	✘	✘	✘
Oklahoma	✘		✘
Oregon			
Pennsylvania	✘	✘	✘
Rhode Island	✘	✘	✘
South Carolina	✘	✘	✘
South Dakota	✘	✘	✘
Tennessee	✘		✘
Texas	✘		✘
Utah	✘	✘	✘
Vermont			
Virginia	✘	✘	✘
Washington			✘
West Virginia	✘		
Wisconsin	✘	✘	✘
Wyoming	✘		✘

Figure 14-8 A state-by-state look at abortion laws. Do you know if abortion laws are changing in your state?

Fortunately, there are abortion follow-up services that can be helpful to women who believe they are suffering from the consequences of abortion. Individual and group counseling, as well as post-abortion support groups, can help women cope with difficult, complicated feelings. Look for these services through your medical care provider, or check your local phone book for helpful resources.

PREGNANCY

Pregnancy is a condition that requires a series of complex yet coordinated changes to occur in the female body. This discussion follows pregnancy from its beginning, at fertilization, to its conclusion, with labor and childbirth.

Physiological Obstacles and Aids to Fertilization

Many sexually active young people believe that they will become pregnant (or impregnate someone) only when they want to, despite their haphazard contraceptive practices. Because of this mistaken belief, many young people are not sold on the use of contraceptives. It is important for young adults to remember that from a species survival standpoint, our bodies were designed to promote pregnancy. It is estimated that about 85% of sexually active women of childbearing age will become pregnant within 1 year if they do not use some form of contraception.[2]

With regard to pregnancy, each act of intercourse can be considered a game of physiological odds. There

Key Terms

hypertonic saline solution
A salt solution with a concentration higher than that found in human fluids.

post-abortion syndrome
The long-term negative psychological effects of abortion.

are obstacles that may reduce a couple's chance of pregnancy, including the following:

Obstacles to fertilization

1. *The acidic level of the vagina is destructive to sperm.* The low pH of the vagina will kill sperm that fail to enter the uterus quickly.
2. *The cervical mucus is thick during most of the menstrual cycle.* Sperm movement into the uterus is more difficult, except during the few days surrounding ovulation.
3. *The sperm must locate the cervical opening.* The cervical opening is small compared with the rest of the surface area where sperm are deposited.
4. *Half of the sperm travel through the wrong fallopian tube.* Most commonly, only one ovum is released at ovulation. The two ovaries generally "take turns" each month. The sperm have no way of "knowing" which tube they should enter. Thus it is probable that half will travel through the wrong tube.
5. *The distance sperm must travel is relatively long compared with the tiny size of the sperm cells.* Microscopic sperm must travel about 7 or 8 inches once they are inside the female.
6. *The sperm's travel is relatively "upstream."* The anatomical positioning of the female reproductive structures necessitates an "uphill" movement by the sperm.
7. *The contoured folds of the tubal walls trap many sperm.* These folds make it difficult for sperm to locate the egg. Many sperm are trapped in this maze.

There are also a variety of aids that tend to help sperm and egg cells join. Some of these are listed below.

Aids to fertilization

1. *An astounding number of sperm are deposited during ejaculation.* Each ejaculation contains about a teaspoon of semen.[8] Within this quantity are between 200 and 500 million sperm cells. Even with large numbers of sperm killed in the vagina, millions are able to move to the deeper structures.
2. *Sperm are deposited near the cervical opening.* Penetration into the vagina by the penis allows for the sperm to be placed near the cervical opening.
3. *The male accessory glands help make the semen nonacidic.* The seminal vesicles, prostate gland, and Cowper's glands secrete fluids that provide an alkaline environment for the sperm. This environment helps sperm be better protected in the vagina until they can move into the deeper, more alkaline uterus and fallopian tubes.
4. *Uterine contractions aid sperm movement.* The rhythmic muscular contractions of the uterus tend to cause the sperm to move in the direction of the fallopian tubes.

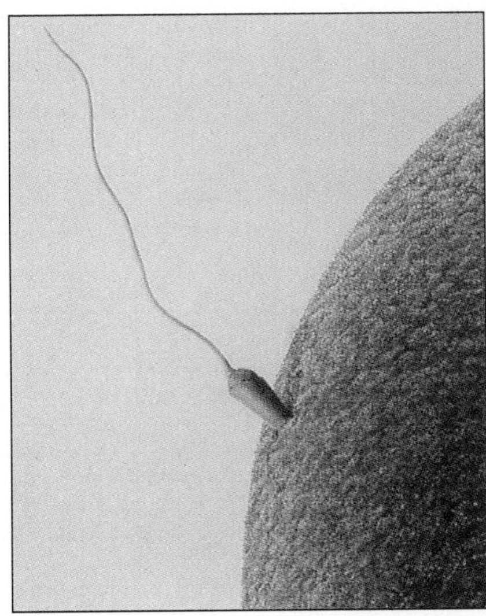

The surface of an ovum is penetrated by sperm at fertilization.

5. *Sperm cells move rather quickly.* Despite their tiny size, sperm cells can move relatively quickly—just about 1 inch per hour. Powered by sugar solutions from the male accessory glands and the whiplike movements of their tails, sperm can reach the distant third of the fallopian tubes in less than 8 hours as they swim in the direction of the descending ovum.
6. *Once inside the fallopian tubes, sperm can live for days.* Some sperm may be viable for up to a week after reaching the comfortable, nonacidic environment of the fallopian tubes. Most sperm, however, will survive an average of 48 to 72 hours. Thus they can "wait in the wings" for the moment an ovum is released from the ovary (Figure 14-9).
7. *The cervical mucus is thin and watery at the time of ovulation.* This mucus allows for better passage of sperm through the cervical opening when the ovum is most capable of being fertilized.

Learning from Our Diversity (p. 366) discusses the particular issues related to pregnancy and parenting after age 40.

Signs of Pregnancy

Aside from pregnancy tests done in a professional laboratory, a woman can sometimes recognize early signs and symptoms. The signs of pregnancy have been divided into three categories:

Presumptive signs of pregnancy

Missed period after unprotected intercourse the previous month

Nausea on awakening (morning sickness)

Increase in size and tenderness of breasts

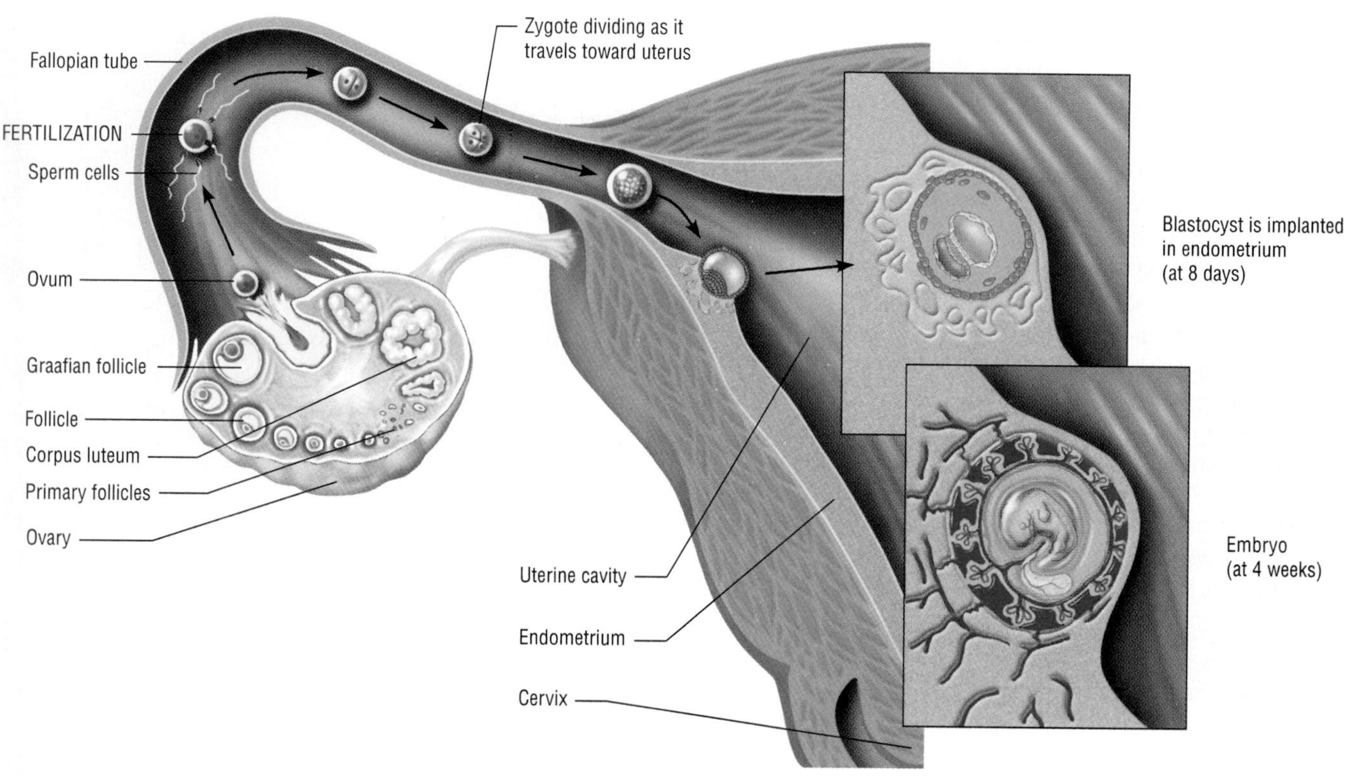

Figure 14-9 After its release from the follicle, the ovum begins its week-long journey down the fallopian tube. Fertilization generally occurs in the outermost third of the tube. Now fertilized, the ovum progresses toward the uterus, where it embeds itself in the endometrium. A pregnancy is established.

Darkening of the areolar tissue surrounding the nipples

Probable signs of pregnancy

Increase in the frequency of urination (the growing uterus presses against the bladder)

Increase in the size of the abdomen

Cervix becomes softer by the sixth week (detected by a pelvic examination by clinician)

Positive pregnancy test

Positive signs of pregnancy

Determination of a fetal heartbeat

Feeling of the fetus moving (quickening)

Observation of fetus by ultrasound or optical viewers

Agents That Can Damage a Fetus

A large number of agents that come into contact with a pregnant woman can affect fetal development. Many of these (rubella and herpes viruses, tobacco smoke, alcohol, and virtually all other drugs) are discussed in other chapters of this text. The best advice for a pregnant woman is to maintain close contact with her obstetrician during pregnancy and to consider carefully the ingestion of any OTC drug (including aspirin, caffeine, and antacids) that could harm the fetus.

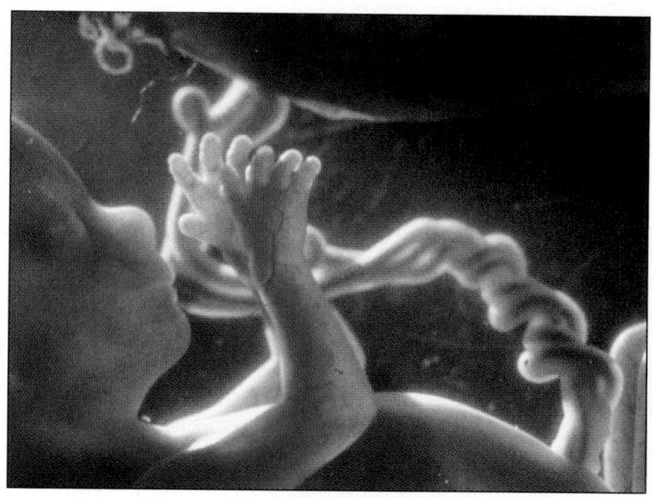

The fetus at 16 weeks' gestation within the amniotic sac.

It is also important for all women to avoid exposure to radiation during the pregnancy. Such exposure, most commonly through excessive X rays or radiation fallout

Learning from Our Diversity

Pregnancy and Parenting after Forty

Women who become pregnant in their forties are not a new phenomenon. Many young people and baby boomers today were delivered by mothers who were 40 or more years old. What *is* new is women becoming pregnant for the first time at an age when many women begin menopause.

The reasons are several. Some couples may have tried to conceive for years and only succeeded when in their forties. Other women and couples delayed pregnancy in order to build their careers, travel, or become more financially secure. In addition, fertility technology, such as in vitro fertilization, microsurgery, and donor eggs or sperm have finally given many couples the baby they long wanted.

The trend of later childbearing began in the late 1970s, when better-educated baby-boom women began entering the work force. For women 40 to 44, the rate of first babies increased from 0.3 to 1.4 per 1,000, still a small percentage but a significant jump.[9]

The common belief that men can father babies well into middle age is supported not only by anecdotal evidence (such as Tony Randall, Larry King, and Anthony Quinn), but also recent research that shows that sperm function in older men does not differ significantly from that of younger men.[10]

Women traditionally were discouraged from becoming pregnant for the first time in their forties because of the health risks to the mother and the risk of birth defects for the baby. It is true that women 40 and older suffer more complications during childbirth, and the risk of having a baby with Down syndrome or another genetic abnormality increases as a mother ages.[9]

The chances of having a cesarean delivery are about 40 percent higher than a younger woman's.[11] The number of women with gestational diabetes and high blood pressure also was higher. Many had more difficulty with labor and delivered babies that were underweight or premature. In addition, the risk of fetal death is higher in women over 35 years old.[12]

Women who want to have a baby should use this information to prevent the problems, however, rather than let it discourage them from having a baby at all, researchers say.

Women who want to start families in their forties should consider the following points:

- Infertility can become a problem with age, but fertility drugs such as Clomid or treatments such as in vitro fertilization can help.
- The rate of miscarriage is higher among older women, so immediate prenatal care is vital.
- Early genetic testing can ease the fears about birth defects. Tests can reveal the presence of Down syndrome, Tay-Sachs disease, cystic fibrosis, and sickle-cell anemia.
- Cesarean sections are more common in older mothers.

On the plus side, another study recently reported that women who are able to give birth after age 40 (not including those who become pregnant through the use of fertility treatments) may be "slow to age" and live longer.[9] This can be good news to older moms who wonder whether they will have the energy to chase a toddler.

from nuclear testing, can irreversibly damage fetal genetic structures.

CHILDBIRTH: THE LABOR OF DELIVERY

Childbirth, or *parturition,* is one of the true peak life experiences for both men and women. Most of the time, childbirth is a wonderfully exciting venture into the unknown. For the parents, this intriguing experience can provide a stage for personal growth, maturity, and insight into a dynamic, complex world.

During the last few weeks of the third **trimester,** most fetuses will move deeper into the pelvic cavity in a process called *lightening.* During this movement, the fetus's body will rotate and the head will begin to engage more deeply into the mother's pelvic girdle. Many women will report that the baby has "dropped."

Another indication that parturition may be relatively near is the increased reporting of *Braxton Hicks contractions.* These uterine contractions, which are of mild intensity and often occur at irregular intervals, may be felt throughout a pregnancy. During the last few weeks of pregnancy *(gestation),* these mild contractions can occur more frequently and may cause a woman to feel as if she is going into labor **(false labor).**

Labor begins when uterine contractions become more intense and occur at regular intervals. The birth of a child can be divided into three stages: (1) *effacement* and dilation of the cervix, (2) delivery of the fetus, and (3) delivery of the placenta (Figure 14-10). For a woman having her

Key Terms

trimester
A 3-month period; human pregnancies encompass three trimesters.

false labor
Conditions that resemble the start of true labor; may include irregular uterine contractions, pressure, and discomfort in the lower abdomen.

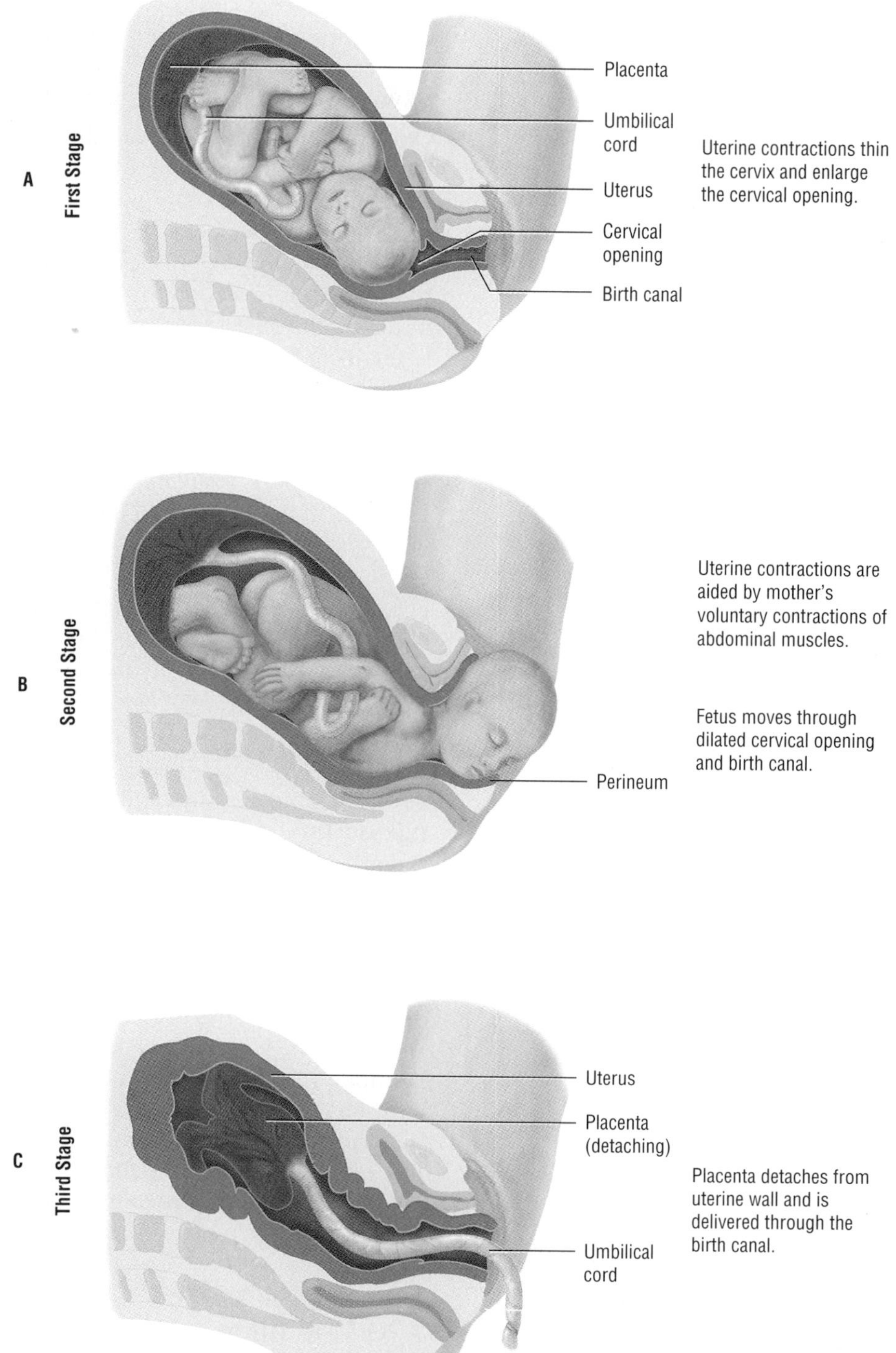
A
First Stage
Placenta
Umbilical cord
Uterus
Cervical opening
Birth canal
Uterine contractions thin the cervix and enlarge the cervical opening.
B
Second Stage
Uterine contractions are aided by mother's voluntary contractions of abdominal muscles.
Fetus moves through dilated cervical opening and birth canal.
Perineum
C
Third Stage
Uterus
Placenta (detaching)
Umbilical cord
Placenta detaches from uterine wall and is delivered through the birth canal.

Figure 14-10 Labor, or childbirth, is a three-stage process. During effacement and dilation, the first stage (**A**), the cervical canal is gradually opened by contractions of the uterine wall. The second stage (**B**), delivery of the fetus, encompasses the actual delivery of the fetus from the uterus and through the birth canal. The delivery of the placenta, the third stage (**C**), empties the uterus, thus completing the process of childbirth.

first child, the birth process lasts an average of 12 to 16 hours. The average length of labor for subsequent births is much shorter—from 4 to 10 hours on the average. Labor is very unpredictable: labors that last between 1 and 24 hours occur daily at most hospitals.

Stage One: Effacement and Dilation of the Cervix

In the first stage of labor the uterine contractions attempt to thin (efface) the normally thick cervical walls and to enlarge (dilate) the cervical opening.[8] These contractions are directed by the release of prostaglandins and the hormone oxytocin into the circulating bloodstream.

The first stage of labor is often the longest. The cervical opening must thin and dilate to a diameter of 10 cm before the first stage of labor is considered complete. Often this stage begins with the dislodging of the cervical mucous plug. The subsequent *bloody show* (mucous plug and a small amount of blood) at the vaginal opening may indicate that effacement and dilation have begun. Another indication of labor's onset may be the bursting or tearing of the fetal amniotic sac. "Breaking the bag of waters" refers to this phenomenon, which happens in various measures in expectant women.

The pain of the uterine contractions becomes more intense as the woman moves through this first stage of labor. As the cervical opening effaces and dilates from 0 to 3 cm, many women report feeling happy, exhilarated, and confident. In the early phase of the first stage of labor, the contractions are relatively short (lasting from 15 to 60 seconds) and the intervals between contractions range from 20 minutes to 5 minutes as labor progresses. However, these rest intervals will become shorter and the contractions more forceful when the woman's uterus contracts to dilate 4 to 7 cm.

In this second phase of the first stage of labor, the contractions usually last about 1 minute each and the rest intervals drop from about 5 minutes to 1 minute over a period of 5 to 9 hours.

The third phase of the first stage of labor is called *transition.* During transition, the uterus contracts to dilate the cervical opening to the full 10 cm required for safe passage of the fetus out of the uterus and into the birth canal (vagina). This period of labor is often the most painful part of the entire birth process. Fortunately, it is also the shortest phase of most labors. Lasting between 15 and 30 minutes, transition contractions often last 60 to 90 seconds each. The rest intervals between contractions are short and vary from 30 to 60 seconds.

An examination of the cervix by a nurse or physician will reveal whether full dilation of 10 cm has occurred. Until the full 10 cm dilation, women are cautioned not to "push" the fetus during the contractions. Special breathing and concentration techniques help many women cope with the first stage of labor.

Stage Two: Delivery of the Fetus

Once the mother's cervix is fully dilated, she enters the second stage of labor, the delivery of the fetus through the birth canal. Now the mother is encouraged to help push the fetus out (with her abdominal muscles) during each contraction. In this second stage the uterine contractions are less forceful than during the transition phase of the first stage and may last 60 seconds each, with a 1- to 3-minute rest interval.

This second stage may last up to 2 hours in first births. For subsequent births, this stage will usually be much shorter. When the baby's head is first seen at the vaginal opening, *crowning* is said to have taken place. Generally the back of the baby's head appears first. (Infants whose feet or buttocks are presented first are said to be delivered in a *breech position.*) Once the head is delivered, the baby's body rotates upward to let the shoulders come through. The rest of the body follows quite quickly. The second stage of labor ends when the fetus is fully expelled from the birth canal.

Stage Three: Delivery of the Placenta

Usually within 30 minutes after the fetus is delivered, the uterus will again initiate a series of contractions to expel the placenta (or *afterbirth*). The placenta is examined by the attending physician to ensure that it was completely expelled. Torn remnants of the placenta could lead to dangerous *hemorrhaging* by the mother. Often the physician will perform a manual examination of the uterus after the placenta has been delivered.

Once the placenta has been delivered, the uterus will continue with mild contractions to help control bleeding and start the gradual reduction of the uterus to its normal, nonpregnant size. This final aspect of the birth process is called **postpartum.** External abdominal massage of the lower abdomen seems to help the uterus contract, as does an infant's nursing at the mother's breast.

Cesarean Deliveries

A **cesarean delivery** (cesarean birth, C-section) is a procedure in which the fetus is surgically removed from the mother's uterus through the abdominal wall. This type of delivery, which is completed in up to an hour, can be performed with the mother having a regional or a general anesthetic. A cesarean delivery is necessary when either the health of the baby or the mother is at risk.

Although a cesarean delivery is considered major surgery, most mothers cope well with the delivery and postsurgical and postpartum discomfort. The hospital stay is usually a few days longer than for a vaginal delivery.

INFERTILITY

Most traditional-age college students are interested in preventing pregnancy. However, increasing numbers of other people are trying to do just the opposite: they are trying to become pregnant. It is estimated that about one in six couples has a problem with *infertility.* These couples wish to become pregnant but are unable to do so.

Why do couples experience infertility? The reasons are about evenly balanced between men and women. About 10% of infertility has no detectable cause. The most common male complication is insufficient sperm production and delivery. A number of approaches can be used to increase sperm counts. Among the simple approaches are the application of periodic cold packs on the scrotum and the replacement of tight underwear with boxer shorts. When a structural problem reduces sperm production, surgery can be helpful. Opinion is divided about whether increased frequency of intercourse improves fertility. Most experts (fertility endocrinologists) suggest that couples have intercourse at least a couple of times in the week preceding ovulation.

Men can also collect (through masturbation) and save samples of their sperm to use in a procedure called *artificial insemination by partner.* Near the time of ovulation, the collected samples of sperm are then deposited near the woman's cervical opening. In the related procedure called *artificial insemination by donor,* the sperm of a donor are used. Donor semen is screened for the presence of pathogens, including the AIDS virus.

Causes of infertility in women center mostly on obstructions in the reproductive tract and the inability to ovulate. The obstructions sometimes result from tissue damage (scarring) caused by infections. Chlamydial and gonorrheal infections often produce fertility problems. In certain women the use of IUDs has produced infections and PID; both of these increase the chances of infertility. Other possible causes of structural abnormalities include scar tissue from previous surgery, fibroid tumors, polyps, and endometriosis. A variety of microsurgical techniques may correct some of these complications.

One of the most recent innovative procedures involves the use of **transcervical balloon tuboplasty.** In this procedure, a series of balloon-tipped catheters are inserted through the uterus into the blocked fallopian tubes. Once inflated, these balloon catheters help open the scarred passageways.

When a woman has ovulation difficulties, pinpointing the specific cause can be very difficult. Increasing age produces hormone fluctuations associated with lack of ovulation. Being significantly overweight or underweight also has a serious effect on fertility. However, in women of normal weight who are not approaching menopause, it appears that ovulation difficulties are caused by lack of synchronization between the hormones governing the menstrual cycle. Fertility drugs can help alter the menstrual cycle to produce ovulation. Clomiphene citrate (Clomid), in oral pill form, and injections of a mixture of LH and FSH taken from the urine of menopausal women (Pergonal) are the most common fertility drugs available. Both are capable of producing multiple ova at ovulation.

For couples who are unable to conceive after drug therapy, surgery, and artificial insemination, the use of *in vitro fertilization and embryo transfer (IVF-ET)* is another option. This method is sometimes referred to as the "test tube" procedure. Costing up to $10,000 per attempt, IVF-ET consists of surgically retrieving fertilizable ova from the woman and combining them in a glass dish with sperm. After several days, the fertilized ova are transferred into the uterus.

A newer test tube procedure is called *gamete intrafallopian transfer (GIFT).* Similar to IVF-ET, this procedure involves depositing a mixture of retrieved eggs and sperm directly into the fallopian tubes.

Fertilized ova (zygotes) can also be transferred from a laboratory dish into the fallopian tubes in a procedure called *zygote intrafallopian transfer (ZIFT).* One advantage of this procedure is that the clinicians are certain that ova have been fertilized before the transfer to the fallopian tubes.

Surrogate parenting is another option that has been explored in the last decade, although the legal and ethical issues surrounding this method of conception have not been fully resolved. Surrogate parenting exists in a number of forms. Typically, an infertile couple will make a contract with a woman (the surrogate parent), who will then be artificially inseminated with semen from the expectant father. In some instances the surrogate will receive an embryo from the donor parents. In some cases, women have served as surrogates for their close relatives. The surrogate

Key Terms

postpartum
The period after the birth of a baby, during which the uterus returns to its prepregnancy size.

cesarean delivery
Surgical removal of a fetus through the abdominal wall.

transcervical balloon tuboplasty
The use of inflatable balloon catheters to open blocked fallopian tubes; a procedure used for some women with fertility problems.

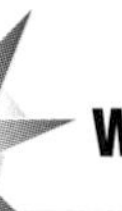

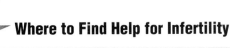

Where to Find Help for Infertility

These agencies can provide you with information about infertility and give referrals to specialists in your area:

American Society for Reproductive Medicine
1209 Montgomery Highway
Birmingham, AL 35216-2809
(205) 978-5000
www.asrm.com

Planned Parenthood Federation of America
810 Seventh Avenue
New York, NY 10019
(800) 829-7732
www.plannedparenthood.org

RESOLVE
1310 Broadway
Somerville, MA 02144
(617) 623-0744
www.resolve.org

These agencies can provide help to prospective adoptive parents:

The National Adoption Center
1500 Walnut Street
Suite 701
Philadelphia, PA 19102
(215) 735-9988
www.adopt.org

The National Council for Adoption
1930 17th Street, N.W.
Washington, DC 20009
(202) 328-8072
www.ncfa-usa.org

Children's Hope International
9229 Lackland
St. Louis, MO 63114
(314) 890-0086
www.childrenshopeint.org

Adoptive Families of America, Inc.
2309 Como Ave.
St. Paul, MN 55108
(800) 372-3300
Publishes OURS Magazine (Organization for United Response)
www.adoptivefam.org

will carry the fetus to term and return the newborn to the parents. Because of the concerns about true "ownership" of the baby, surrogate parenting may not be a particularly viable or legal option for many couples.

The process of coping with infertility problems can be an emotionally stressful experience for a couple. Hours of waiting in physicians' offices, having numerous examinations, scheduling intercourse, producing sperm samples, and undergoing surgical or drug treatments place multiple burdens on a couple. Knowing that other couples are able to conceive so effortlessly adds to the mental strain. Fortunately, support groups exist to assist couples with infertility problems. Some of these groups are listed in the Star Box above.

What can you do to reduce the chances of developing infertility problems? Certainly avoiding infections of the reproductive organs is one crucial factor. Barrier methods of contraception (condoms, diaphragm) with a spermicide reportedly cut the risk of developing infertility in half. The use of an IUD should be carefully considered, and the risk from multiple partners should encourage responsible sexual activity. Men and women should be aware of the dangers from working around hazardous chemicals or consuming psychoactive drugs. Maintaining overall good health and having regular medical (and, for women, gynecological) checkups are also good ideas. Finally, since infertility is linked with advancing age, couples may not want to indefinitely delay having children.

SUMMARY

- *Birth control* refers to all of the procedures that can prevent the birth of a child.
- *Contraception* refers to any procedure that prevents fertilization.
- Each birth control method has both a theoretical-effectiveness rate and a use-effectiveness rate. For some contraceptive approaches, these rates are similar (such as hormonal methods), and for others the rates are very different (such as condoms, diaphragms, and periodic abstinence).
- Many factors should be considered when deciding which contraceptive is best for you.

- Sterilization (vasectomy and tubal ligation) is generally considered an irreversible procedure.
- Currently, abortion remains a woman's choice under the guidelines of the 1973 *Roe v. Wade* decision and various state restrictions.
- Abortion procedures vary according to the stage of the pregnancy.
- There are numerous obstacles and aids to fertilization that influence the likelihood of pregnancy.
- Childbirth takes place in three distinct stages: effacement and dilation of the cervix, delivery of the fetus, and delivery of the placenta.
- Infertility is an important concern for some couples. Various technologies are improving infertile couples' chances of having children.

REVIEW QUESTIONS

1. Explain the difference between the terms *birth control* and *contraception.* Give examples of each.
2. Explain the difference between theoretical and use-effectiveness rates. Which one is always higher? Why is it important to know the difference between these two rates?
3. Identify some of the factors that should be given careful consideration when selecting a contraceptive method. Explain each factor.
4. For each of the methods of birth control, explain how it works and its advantages and disadvantages.
5. How do minipills differ from the combined oral contraceptive? What is a morning-after pill? How do subdermal implants (Norplant) differ from Depo-Provera and Lunelle?
6. Identify and describe the different abortion procedures that are used during each trimester of pregnancy. When is the safest time for an abortion?
7. What are some obstacles and aids to fertilization presented in this chapter? Can you think of others?
8. Identify and describe the events that occur during each of the three stages of childbirth. Approximately how long is each stage?
9. What can be done to reduce chances of infertility? Explain IVF-ET, GIFT, and ZIFT procedures.

THINK ABOUT THIS . . .

- What factors would be most important to you in selecting an appropriate contraceptive method?
- How well do you think college students understand that oral contraceptives do not protect against STDs or HIV infection?
- Under what circumstances, if any, do you believe abortion is acceptable? Unacceptable?
- Will you or your partner someday undergo sterilization? If so, which of you will have the surgery?
- Can you identify locations at or near your college where professional family-planning services are available?
- What effects do you think starting parenthood at a later age has on the parent and on the child?
- How do you feel about a couple's choice not to have children?
- If a woman should not smoke, drink, or use other drugs during pregnancy, should these limitations also be placed on the father? Why or why not?
- To what extent should fathers participate in the birth experience?
- Do you plan to become a parent? If so, when?

REFERENCES

1. Crooks R, Baur K: *Our sexuality,* ed 7, 1998, Brooks/Cole Publishing.
2. Hatcher RA et al: *Contraceptive technology,* ed 17, rev, 1998, Ardent Media, Inc.
3. Allgeier ER, Allgeier AR: *Sexual interactions,* ed 5, 2000, Houghton Mifflin.
4. Planned Parenthood Federation of America: PPFA website, **www. plannedparenthood.org.** Accessed September 21, 2001.
5. Monthly injection provides new contraceptive choice, *FDA Consumer,* 35(1):5, 2001.
6. U.S. Bureau of the Census: *Statistical abstract of the United States: 2000,* ed 120, 2000, U.S. Government Printing Office.
7. Blonna R, Levitan J: *Healthy sexuality,* 2000, Morton Publishing Co.
8. Hyde JS, Delamater JD: *Understanding human sexuality,* ed 6, 1997, McGraw-Hill.
9. Blackburn B: Moms starting families in 40s test odds, *USA Today,* September 24, 1977, 14A.
10. Haidl G, Jung A, Schill WB: Aging and sperm function, *Hum Reprod* 1996:11(3):558–560.
11. Later age pregnancy: Preparing for the happy, healthy event after 40, *Health Oasis,* Mayo Clinic, 1998, **www.mayohealth.org/mayo/9708/htm/aged_p.htm**
12. Fretts RC et al: Increased maternal age and risk of fetal death, *N Engl J Med* 1995:333(15):953–957.

SUGGESTED READINGS

Bullough VL, Bullough B: *Contraception: a guide to birth control methods,* ed 2, 1997, Prometheus Books.
Written for the general reader interested in knowing about a wide range of contraceptive options, this book contains information about the history of contraception and probable future developments in the field.

Peoples D, Ferguson HR: *What to expect when you're experiencing infertility: how to cope with the emotional crisis and survive,* 2000, W.W. Norton & Co.
This book helps couples cope with one of the most difficult emotional, medical, and financial crises—infertility. Written in a question-and-answer format, the book offers practical advice about the uncertainties of infertility. It can help couples communicate more clearly and face the disappointments of miscarriages and failed treatments.

Runkle A: *In good conscience: a practical, emotional, and spiritual guide to deciding whether to have an abortion,* 1998, Jossey-Bass Publishers.
Cutting through the religious and political rhetoric surrounding abortion, this book presents solid information on the subject. Written in a compassionate tone, it is directed toward women who want to make this decision themselves.

Stern DN: *The birth of a mother: how the motherhood experience changes you forever,* 1998, Basic Books.
Written by a well-known psychiatrist, this book describes the tremendous transformation that takes place in many women when they become mothers. It focuses on the positive, powerful psychological growth experienced by these women.

Stewart J: *1001 African names: first and last names from the African continent,* 1996, Citadel Press.
Julia Stewart identifies names for African Americans who want to give their children African names or who want to change their own Western names. This book describes the origins of African naming practices and explains the meanings behind the names.

As we go to Press...

In November 2001, the Food and Drug Administration (FDA) approved the manufacturing and marketing of the nation's first contraceptive patch. This device, called EVRA and manufactured by Ortho-McNeil Pharmaceutical, contains both synthetic estrogen and progesterone, and is delivered in week-long dosages by a patch just under three inches square—somewhat similar to patches already approved for nicotine and nitroglycerin delivery.

EVRA is thought to be especially effective for women who have difficulty remembering to take oral contraceptive pills consistently on a daily basis. Patch users apply a fresh contraceptive patch each week for three weeks and then have a patch-free week (during which menstruation will occur). The contraceptive patch can be applied to a woman's buttocks, upper arm, lower abdomen, and upper chest (but not on her breast).

Name ______________________ **Date** __________ **Section** __________

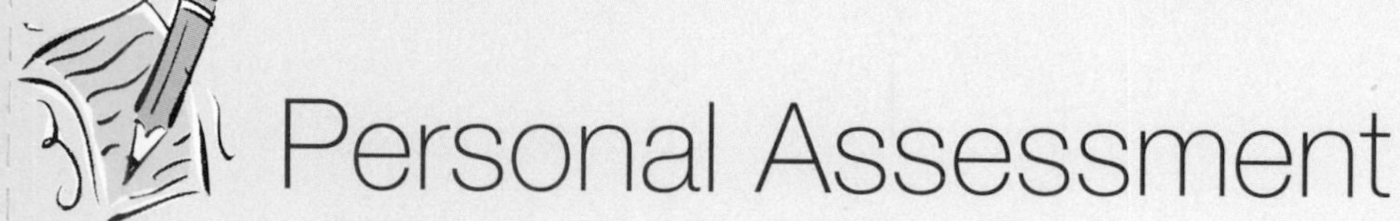

Personal Assessment

Which Birth Control Method Is Best for You?

To assess which birth control method would be best for you, answer the following questions, and check the interpretation below.

Do I:	*Yes*	*No*
1. Need a contraceptive right away?		
2. Want a contraceptive that can be used completely independent of sexual relations?		
3. Need a contraceptive only once in a great while?		
4. Want something with no harmful side effects?		
5. Want to avoid going to the doctor?		
6. Want something that will help protect against sexually transmitted diseases?		
7. Have to be concerned about affordability?		
8. Need to be virtually certain that pregnancy will not result?		
9. Want to avoid pregnancy now but want to have a child sometime in the future?		
10. Have any medical condition or lifestyle that may rule out some form of contraception?		

Interpretation

If you have checked *Yes* to number:

1. Condoms and spermicides may be easily purchased without prescription in any pharmacy.
2. Sterilization, oral contraceptives, hormone implants or injections, cervical caps, and periodic abstinence techniques do not require that anything be done just before sexual relations.
3. Diaphragms, condoms, or spermicides can be used by people who have coitus only once in a while. Periodic abstinence techniques may also be appropriate but require a high degree of skill and motivation.
4. IUDs should be carefully discussed with your physician. Sometimes the use of oral contraceptives or hormone products results in some minor discomfort and may have harmful side effects.
5. Condoms and spermicides do not require a prescription from a physician.
6. Condoms and, to a lesser extent, spermicides and the other barrier methods may help protect against some sexually transmitted diseases. No method (except abstinence) can guarantee complete protection.
7. Be a wise consumer: check prices, ask pharmacists and physicians. The cost of sterilization is high, but there is no additional expense for a lifetime.
8. Sterilization provides near certainty. Oral contraceptives, hormone implants or injections, or a diaphragm-condom-spermicide combination also give a high measure of reliable protection. Periodic abstinence, withdrawal, and douche methods should be avoided. Outercourse may be a good alternative.
9. Although it is sometimes possible to reverse sterilization, it requires surgery and is more complex than simply stopping use of any of the other methods.
10. Smokers and people with a history of blood clots should probably not use oral contraceptives or other hormone approaches. Some people have an allergic reaction to a specific spermicide and should experiment with another brand. Some women cannot be fitted with a diaphragm or cervical cap because of the position of the uterus. The woman and her health care provider will then need to select another suitable means of contraception.

To Carry This Further . . .

There may be more than one method of birth control suitable for you. Always consider how a method you select can also help you avoid an STD. Study the methods suggested above, and consult Table 14-1 to determine what techniques may be most appropriate.

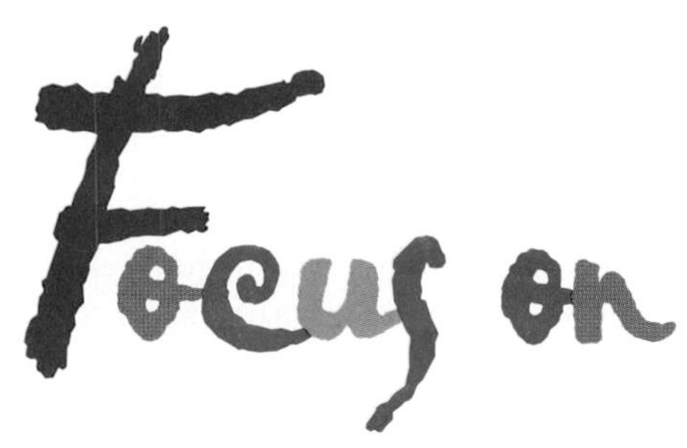

SUPERTWINS: THE BOOM IN MULTIPLE BIRTHS

During World War II their parents gave them patriotic names, such as Franklin, Delano, and Roosevelt, or Franklin D. (for Roosevelt) and Winnie C. (a girl named for Winston Churchill).[1] You may know them as Rachel, Richard, Rebecca, and Ryan or Courtney, Britanny, and Tiffany. They're supertwins—multiple-birth siblings such as triplets, quadruplets, quintuplets, and even sextuplets and more. From 1989 to 1993, an average of 1,057 sets of triplets, 241 sets of quads, and 32 sets of quints were born each year in the United States.[1] More recently, the McCaugheys of Iowa gave birth to septuplets on November 19, 1997. All of their septuplets are home and doing well. Nkem Chukwu and her husband Lyke Louis Udobi of Texas were not as lucky with their octuplets. One of the eight died shortly after delivery in 1998.

Such multiple births are controversial for several reasons, including the increased risk they bring to the mother and the fetuses.

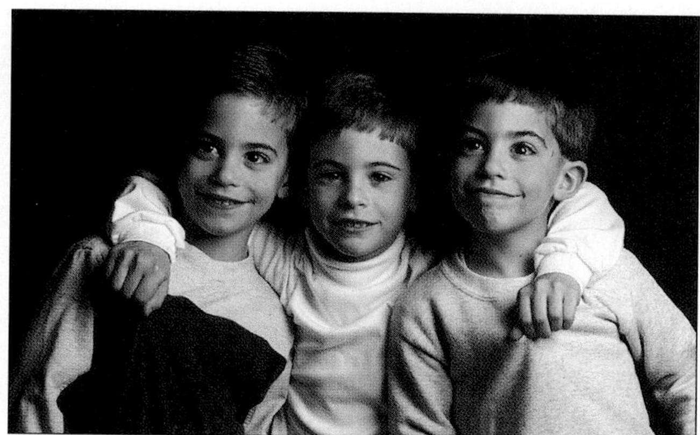

The increased use of fertility drugs and techniques has caused a boom in multiple births. More than 1,000 sets of triplets are born each year in the United States.

The Good, the Bad, and the Unusual

A special type of bonding occurs among multiple-birth siblings that ranges from reading one another's moods to saving another's life, as in the case of twin girls Brielle and Kyrie.[1,2] Kyrie, at 2 pounds 3 ounces, was doing well, but Brielle, the smaller twin, at 2 pounds, had had trouble breathing, an irregular heart rate, and a low blood oxygen level since birth. Then Brielle's condition suddenly became critical. The hospital staff tried every medical procedure they thought might help, to no avail. As a last resort, they put the girls in the same incubator, as some European hospitals do. Amazingly, Brielle's condition immediately improved and within minutes her blood oxygen level was the best it had been since birth. Studies have confirmed that double bedding of multiple-birth babies reduces the length of their hospital stay.[2]

On the darker side, sometimes multiple births, or the prospect of them, are exploited by parents. The Dionne quintuplets, now 60 years old, were the middle 5 of 13 children. When their father sold the rights to exhibit his daughters, the Ontario government made them wards of the state. But the government ended up exploiting them in a bizarre glass playground Quintland-type display, which attracted 10,000 visitors a month. When they were returned to their parents, they were made to feel guilty for their unusual birth and the ensuing familial discord.[3] The surviving quints have written a book about their experiences and have helped teach the world that multiples are not something to be exploited.

Recently, in England, a woman abused fertility drugs by taking them even though she was already fertile and ignoring her physician's instructions while on the drugs. She became pregnant with eight fetuses. She refused to undergo multifetal pregnancy reduction, which would have given the remaining fetuses a better chance of survival, because she had sold her story to a tabloid and would get more money for each baby born. All eight fetuses died at 19 weeks' gestation.[4]

Fertility Drugs and Techniques

Since the birth of the first "test tube baby" (conceived by in vitro fertilization) in 1978, the number of assisted pregnancies and multiple births has escalated. The use of fertility drugs and techniques that stimulate ovulation sometimes causes the release of multiple eggs per cycle.[1,5]

The infertility rate among married couples is 8.5 percent. While this rate has remained relatively constant in recent years, the number of couples seeking help for infertility has tripled.[6] Less than half of the couples who receive fertility treatment ever give birth, but one-fourth of those who *do* achieve a pregnancy give birth to more than one child.[1,6] This happens for a number of reasons. First, some fertility drugs are so strong that they cause multiple eggs to be released during one cycle. Second, some treatments are developed too quickly and are administered under too little supervision.[7] And third, fertility services are so competitive and lucrative ($67,000 to $114,000 per delivery[3]) that many clinics go to great lengths to increase the likelihood of pregnancy, such as implanting up to eight embryos in a woman's uterus. In the United Kingdom, a doctor can lose his or her license for implanting more than three embryos, but no such laws have been passed in the United States.[8] Usually, few or no embryos develop; if too many develop, however, multifetal pregnancy reduction is often suggested.[7] This abortion procedure is usually performed by injecting potassium chloride into the most accessible embryos to increase the odds of survival for the others.[9]

The whole process of fertility treatment has been described as an emotional roller coaster.[1] The parents often want children desperately but can't conceive naturally. The drugs and hormones women are given to promote pregnancy can cause great emotional distress. If a couple does achieve a pregnancy, exhilaration can turn to fear when they find out how many embryos are developing. Will they be able to care for that many children? What if some or all of the babies are sick, or die? Should some be aborted to give the others a better chance? Many fertility clinics do an unsatisfactory job of counseling couples about the likelihood of success and the risks associated with the procedures, so couples often must answer these tough questions without all the information they need.[7]

Medical Complications

After conception, the fertility specialist's job is finished. Everything that goes on during the course of pregnancy and delivery is in the hands of another physician, usually an obstetrician with a specialty in high-risk pregnancy. These physicians must discuss with the parents any risks and concerns that were not addressed earlier.[7]

Each additional fetus shaves roughly 3.5 weeks off the normal 40-week gestation period.[9] Prematurity brings with it a host of problems. The babies are about a third of the weight or less of single babies and much more likely to be ill. The death rate before or soon after birth is 19 times higher for triplets than single babies.[1] From birth to 28 days, the death rate for multiples is still 7 times higher than for singles.[7] Surviving babies suffer higher rates of cerebral palsy and other neurological problems.[10]

Of course, multiple babies have longer hospital stays and are more likely to require intensive care during their stay than single babies. Although the issue of "drive-through" deliveries, in which mother and baby are released within 24 hours, has become a controversial topic lately, the average stay for a single baby is 4.6 days, compared with 8.2 days for twins and 34 days for triplets.[1,6] During their stays, 15 percent of single infants need intensive care, while 50 percent of twins and 75 percent of triplets, quads, and quints require this level of care.[6] Research has shown that most of the heavy use of medical resources in multiple births is due to lower gestational age and lower birth weight.[11]

Multiple births also increase the mother's need for care. The risks of cesarean delivery, anemia, hypertension, postpartum hemorrhage, and kidney failure are all greater in mothers of supertwins.[1,6] And this specialized care is extremely expensive: The estimated cost of a single birth is $9,850, compared with $37,950 for twins and $109,764 for triplets.[6] Hospital costs for quints can easily exceed half a million dollars.[1] If an insurance company covers this cost, we all pay in the form of increased premiums and deductibles. If they do not pay, it can spell financial ruin for the family. And these medical and financial complications all occur even before the newborns come home.

Public and Private Life

Parents of supertwins say the stress kicks in after about six months. Until then, they're busy just trying to meet their constant needs, which during the first three months involves feeding each of three to six babies seven to eight times per day.[1] Because of the stress of the babies' medical problems, financial strain, and pure exhaustion, child abuse is 2.5 to 9 times more likely in families with twins, compared with singles, and parents of supertwins are more likely to divorce.[1,7]

However, some people take it all in stride. One father of quintuplets regards the parenting of his five 3½ and one 7-month-old babies as character building. He's manufactured his own stairstep stroller, and he and his wife handle the 20 minutes of buckling, toy stowing, negotiating with the kids, and answering the questions of strangers whenever they go somewhere, with smiles of their faces.[1]

Some strangers beam at the sight of this unusual family, while others grimace and turn away. When people lightly tell their mother, "I'm glad it's you and not me," she answers in all seriousness, "Me too." The father sums up their situation this way: "Sure, it's a lifestyle change, but you take one day at a time, people help, and things work out."[1]

Family, friends, strangers, and even local and national companies do help out. Discounts on diapers and baby food, two years' worth of free formula, a night's stay at a local motel, discounts on vans, and money to start college funds are examples of public generosity to the families of quads and quints. But along with public generosity comes public nosiness. One family answered a knock on the door from a senior citizens' tour bus group that wanted the parents to wake up the kids for a picture. More commonly, strangers think they can touch the children or ask personal questions of the parents, such as "Are they natural?" and "So, have you had your tubes tied?" and so on.[1]

Two nonprofit support groups help families cope with the unique stressors that multiple-birth families face. The

Triplet Connection, based in California, and Mothers of Supertwins (MOST), based in New York, were both founded in the 1980s by triplet moms to provide reliable, accessible information to the families of supertwins.[1] With the sincere help of most people and organizations like these, parents can increase the odds that the more will truly be the merrier.

For Discussion . . .

Do you know any sets of twins or supertwins? How are their lives and those of their parents different from other families? What would you do if you or your partner were pregnant with supertwins? Do you think society has an obligation to help support supertwin families?

References

1. Jackson DD. People say, you poor thing and I'm thinking I have four healthy kids. *Smithsonian* 27(6):30–39, 1996.
2. Sheehan N. A sister's helping hand. *Reader's Digest* 148(889):155–156, 1996.
3. Came B. A family tragedy. *Maclean's* 107:40–43, 1994.
4. Luscombe B. Eight at once is too many. *Time* 148(18):103, 1996.
5. Anonymous. Where are they now? *Time* 148(7):18, 1996.
6. Anonymous. The high cost of having some babies gets higher by the numbers. *Science News* 146(6):95, 1994.
7. Anonymous. And baby makes three or more: the ethics of fertility treatment are mainly a private matter. *The Economist* 340(7979):16, 1996.
8. Seligmann J. Fewer bundles of pain. Fertility doctors introduce reforms to reduce premature and multiple births. *Newsweek* 127(10):63, 1996.
9. Cowley G, Springen K. More is not merrier: when fertility drugs work too well. *Newsweek* 128(9):49, 1996.
10. Doyle P. The outcome of multiple pregnancy. *Hum Reprod* (11 Suppl) 4:110–117, 1996.
11. Ettner SL, Christiansen CL, Callahan TL, Hall JE. How low birth weight and gestational age contribute to increased inpatient costs for multiple births. *Inquiry* 34(4):325–339, 1997–1998.

part 6

Consumer and Safety Issues

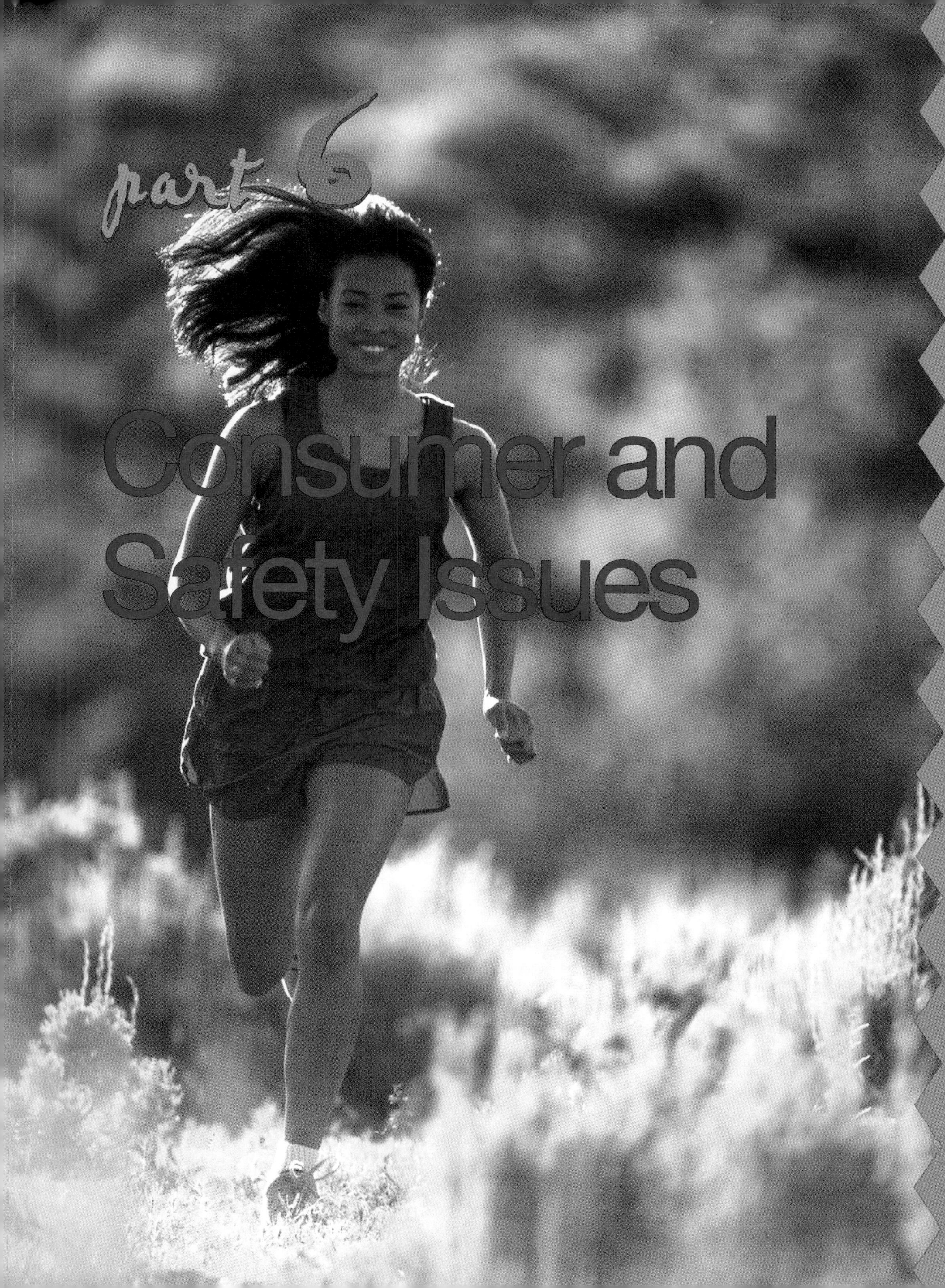

chapter **15**

Becoming an Informed Health-Care Consumer

Online Learning Center Resources

www.mhhe.com/hahn6e

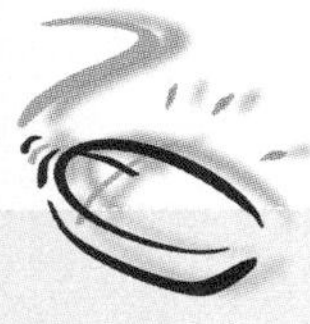

Log on to our Online Learning Center (OLC) for access to these additional resources:

- Chapter key terms and definitions
- Learning objectives
- Additional behavior change objectives
- Student interactive question-and-answer sites
- Self-scoring chapter quiz

The OLC also offers web links for study and exploration of health topics. Here are some examples of what you'll find:

- **www.reutershealth.com** Check the validity of studies, research, treatment, and medicines, and look for valuable women's health information.
- **www.pitt.edu/~cbw/altm.html** Use this jumpsite for links to the latest information on complementary and alternative medicine.
- **www.quackwatch.com** Beware of quacks: this is the premiere site for evaluating health information.

Taking Charge of Your Health

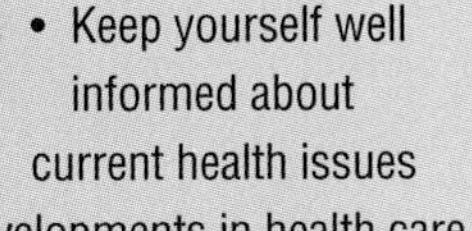

- Keep yourself well informed about current health issues and new developments in health care.
- Analyze the credibility of the health information you receive before putting it into practice.
- Select your health-care providers by using a balanced set of criteria (see p. 386).
- Explore alternative forms of health care, and consider using them as a complement to traditional health care.
- In selecting a health-care plan, compare various plans on the basis of several key factors, not simply cost (see p. 393).
- Assemble a complete personal/family health history as soon as possible. Be sure to include information from older family members.
- Comply with all directions regarding the appropriate use of prescription and OTC medications.

Eye on the Media

The Internet—Your New Health Superstore

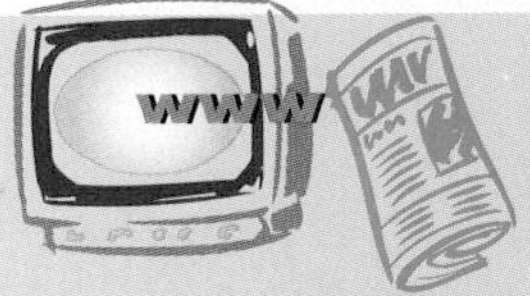

In 2001, an estimated 60 million Americans explored the Internet in search of information, products, and services related to their health (Figure 15-1). A majority will search for information about specific conditions, such as cancer or hypertension. Smaller but still impressive percentages of people will look for information about dieting and nutrition, fitness, women's health, and pharmaceuticals.

The biggest challenge for you as a health consumer is determining the credibility of the information you find on the Internet. How can you know that this information (and accompanying products or services) is trustworthy, motivated by concern for your health and well-being rather than just by profit? A recent study found that the majority of health-related sites were, in fact, accurate but incomplete in the information provided.[1] Recognized authorities offer these guidelines to help you:

- Who does the website belong to? Is it sponsored by an institution of higher education, a professional society, a

Eye on the Media *continued*

government or not-for-profit agency, or a recognized pharmaceutical company? If not, who is responsible for the information? Remember, virtually anyone can develop a web page and begin disseminating information.

- Is the information carefully referenced, showing sources such as government reports, professional journal articles, or respected reference publications? Are the references clearly documented and current? Is the web page updated regularly? Does the information appear to agree with the titles of its own references?
- Does the content of the information seem to have a critical or negative bias toward a particular profession, institution, or treatment method? Is the information more discrediting of others than supportive of itself?
- Are "significant breakthroughs" promised in a way that suggests that only this source has the "ultimate answer" to certain problems? Does this answer involve throwing out your prescriptions, going against your physician's orders, or considering suicide as a way of escaping the pain and difficulties associated with your illness?

If you are skeptical about the credibility of any health-care information you find online, submit the information to a respected health-care professional or organization for assessment. If you and your physician find suspicious information or fraudulent health claims, report this to the Federal Trade Commission. Today, most health-care practitioners feel comfortable with well-informed patients. Many will welcome the chance to learn about your sources of information and share with you any concerns they might have about them.

Once you feel secure about distinguishing reliable and valid information from questionable or fraudulent information, you will be able to make better judgments and choices. Together, you and your health-care provider can use that information in the management of your health care and in planning your approach to a healthier lifestyle.

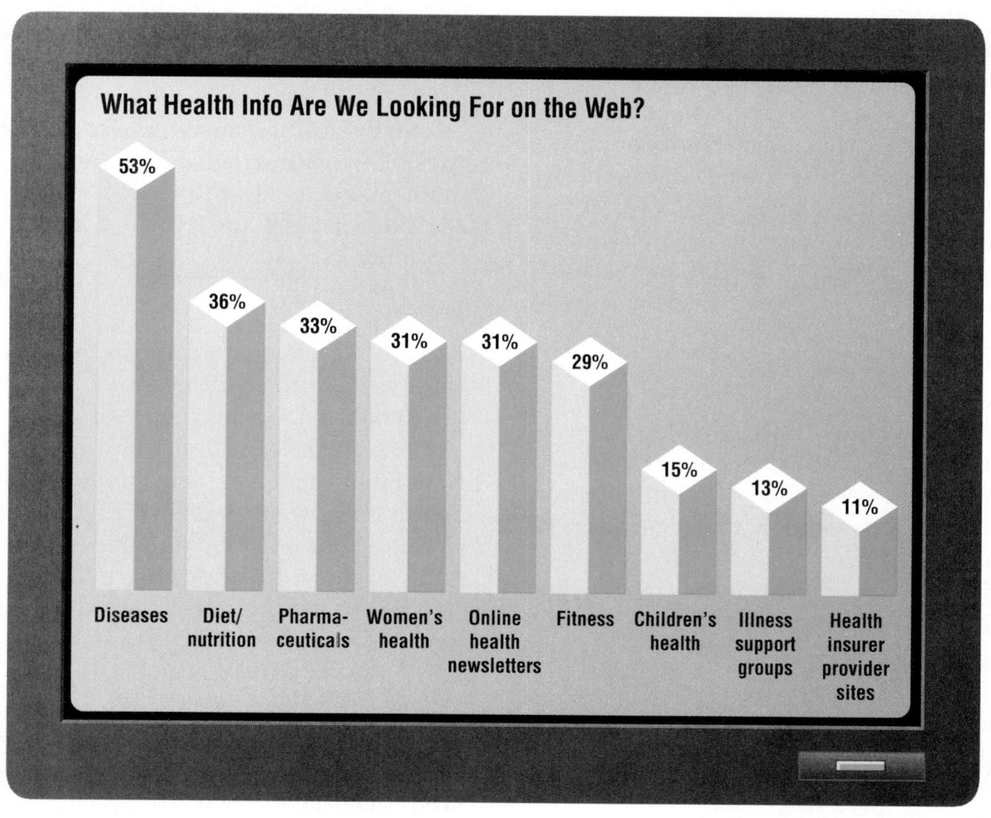

Figure 15-1 Have you used the web lately to find health information?

Health-care providers often evaluate you by criteria pertaining to their area of expertise. The nutritionist knows you by the food you eat. The physical fitness professional knows you by your body type and activity level. In the eyes of the expert in health-care consumerism, you are the product of the health information you believe, the health-influencing services you use, and the products you consume. When your decisions about health information, services, and products are made after careful study and consideration, your health will probably be improved. However, when your decisions lack insight, your health, as well as your pocketbook, may suffer.

HEALTH INFORMATION

The Informed Consumer

To be an informed consumer, you need to learn about services and products that can influence your health. Practitioners, manufacturers, advertisers, and sales personnel use a variety of approaches to try to convince you to buy their products or use their services. Because your health is potentially at stake when you buy into these messages, being an informed consumer is important. Complete the Personal Assessment on p. 399 to rate your own skills as a health-care consumer.

Sources of Information

The sources of health information available to you are as diverse as the people you know, the publications you read, and the experts you see or hear. At present, no single agency or profession regulates the quantity or quality of the health information you receive. The section that follows takes a look at many different sources of information. You will quickly recognize that all are familiar and that some provide more accurate and honest information than others.

Family and friends

From a health-care consumerism point of view, the accuracy of information provided by a friend or family member may be questionable. Too often the information provided by family and friends is based on common knowledge that is wrong. In addition, family members or friends may provide information they believe is in your best interest rather than giving factual information that may have a more negative effect on you.

TALKING POINTS • A family member considers herself good at diagnosing health problems. Since she hasn't been wrong in years, she no longer relies on physicians. What questions could you ask her to point out the dangers associated with her approach?

Today more than ever, family and friends may provide health information as a part of their involvement in the pyramid sales of health products. Strong encouragement toward the use of a particular line of food supplements or vitamins could lead to a forceful sales pitch or even the offer of an opportunity to be a part of their sales team.

Advertisements and commercials

Many people spend a good portion of every day watching television, listening to the radio, and reading newspapers or magazines. Since many advertisements are health oriented, you shouldn't be surprised to learn that these are significant sources of information. Remember that the primary purpose of advertising is to sell products or services. Consider the currently popular "infomercials" in which a compensated studio audience watches a skillfully produced program designed to inform them about the benefits of a particular product or service.

Labels and directions

Federal law requires that many consumer product labels, including many kinds of food (see Chapter 5) and all medications, contain specific information. For example, when a prescription medication is dispensed by a pharmacist, a detailed information sheet describing the drug should be given along with the medication. This insert contains information about the medication's appropriate use, side effects, precautions and contraindications, and interactions with any other medications being used. In addition, it provides instruction for appropriate storage of the medications, as well as directions regarding missed doses.

Many health-care providers and agencies provide consumers with detailed directions about their health problem. Generally, information from these sources is accurate, current, and provided with the health of the consumer in mind.

Folklore

Because it is often passed down from generation to generation, folklore about health is the primary source of health information for some people.

The truthfulness of health information obtained from family members, neighbors, and coworkers is difficult to evaluate. As a general rule, however, use caution concerning its scientific soundness. A blanket criticism is not warranted, however, since folk wisdom is on occasion supported by scientific evidence. Also, the emotional support provided by the suppliers of this information could be the best medicine for some people.

Testimonials

People feel strongly about sharing information that has been beneficial to them. The recommendations made by other people concerning a particular practitioner or health-care product may at first appear to be nothing more than testimonials. Since they are frequently the basis for decision making by others, we assign a small

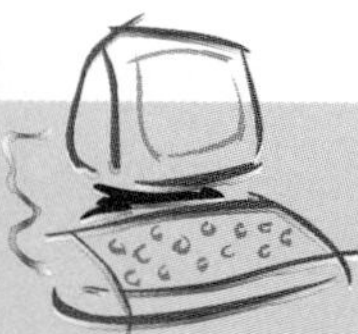

OnSITE/InSIGHT

Learning to Go: Health

Are you a smart health-care consumer? Click on the Motivator icon to see what these lessons have to say about consumer education:

Lesson 45: Become an informed health-care consumer.
Lesson 47: Consider trying alternative medicine.
Lesson 49: Shop for affordable health insurance.

STUDENT POLL

Interested in exploring different health-care options? Go to the Online Learning Center at **www.mhhe.com/hahn6e**. Then go to Student Resources, where you'll find the Student Poll. Answer the following questions and then see what other students said.

1. Do you try to keep up to date with health information?
2. Do you use the Internet to find health information?
3. Do you currently have a physician or health-care provider?
4. Are you covered by health insurance?
5. Have you ever been a victim of health-care quackery?
6. Do you take vitamins or minerals on a regular basis?
7. Have you ever had chiropractic treatment?
8. Have you ever had acupuncture?
9. Do you believe in herbalism as a form of healing?
10. Are you currently taking any prescription medication?
11. Do you prefer to take prescription drugs (vs. over-the-counter) for your illnesses?
12. Do you read medication labels carefully, noting possible side effects?
13. Have you ever purchased drugs over the Internet with approval from your health-care provider?
14. Do you ask for generic prescription brands to save on expenses?
15. Do you think commercials advertising new drugs are effective marketing tools?

measure of importance to them as sources of health information. However, the exaggerated testimonials that accompany the sales pitches of the medical quack or the "satisfied" customers appearing in advertisements and on commercials and infomercials should never be interpreted as valid endorsements.

Mass media

Health programming on cable television stations, lifestyle sections in newspapers, health-care correspondents appearing on TV news shows, and a growing number of health/fitness magazines are examples of health information in the mass media.

Although health information is generally presented well, it is sometimes so brief or superficial that it is of limited use. However, the consumer who wants more complete coverage of a health topic can obtain it by combining sources. The mass media topics most frequently sought out by today's consumers include dietary supplements, nutrition, alternative health maintenance approaches (such as exercise), and cancer. At the same time, however, this information is often viewed as confusing.[2]

Practitioners

The health-care consumer also receives much information from individual health practitioners and their professional associations. In fact, patient education is so clearly provided by today's health-care practitioner that finding one who does not exchange some information with a patient would be unusual. Education enhances patient **compliance** with health-care directives, which is important to the practitioner and the consumer.

An important development in the area of practitioner-provided information and patient education is the evolution of the hospital as an educational institution. Wellness centers, chemical dependence programs, sports medicine centers, and community-based outreach centers have become more common.

On-line computer services

The development of computer technology has created new sources of health information. Today, an estimated 68.5 million Americans subscribe to on-line services and 40% of this group access the Web for health information. Information delivered by experts from major medical centers and local hospitals is perceived by web users as more accurate, timely, and objective than similar information provided by pharmaceutical companies or disease-oriented national agencies.[3] Careful assessment of

Key Term

compliance
Willingness to follow the directions provided by another person, such as a physician.

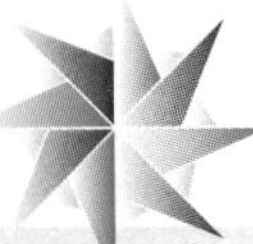

Consumer Protection Agencies and Organizations

Federal Agencies

Office of Consumer Affairs, Food and Drug Administration
U.S. Department of Health and Human Services
5600 Fishers Lane
Rockville, MD 20857
(301) 827-5006
www.fda.gov/oca/aboutoca.htm

Federal Trade Commission
Consumer Inquiries
Public Reference Branch
6th Street and Pennsylvania Avenue
Washington, DC 20580
(202) 326-2222
www.ftc.gov

Fraud Division
Chief Postal Inspector
U.S. Postal Inspection Service
475 L'Enfant Plaza
Washington, DC 20260-2166
(202) 268-4299
www.usps.gov

Consumer Information Center
Pueblo, CO 81009
(719) 948-3334
www.pueblo.gsa.gov

U.S. Consumer Product Safety Commission Hotline
(800) 638-CPSC

Consumer Organizations

Consumers Union of the U.S., Inc.
101 Truman Avenue
Yonkers, NY 10703
(914) 378-2000
www.consumerreports.org

Professional Organizations

American Medical Association
515 N. State St.
Chicago, IL 60610
(312) 464-5000
www.ama-assn.org

American Hospital Association
1 N. Franklin St.
Chicago, IL 60606
(312) 422-3000
www.aha.org

American Pharmaceutical Association
2215 Constitution Avenue, NW
Washington, DC 20037
(202) 628-4410
www.aphanet.org

the health information about a particular form of cancer which was provided on-line has raised questions about the validity of some information offered via the Internet.[4]

Health reference publications

It is now believed that a substantial portion of households own or subscribe to a health reference publication, such as the *The Johns Hopkins Medical Handbook* or the *Physicians' Desk Reference (PDR)*, or a newsletter such as *The Mayo Clinic Health Letter*.

Personal computer programs and videocassettes featuring health information are important sources of information for some consumers.

Reference libraries

Even though a large percentage of households possess health reference material and health-care professionals are dispensing more and more information to the consumer, public and university libraries continue to be much-used sources of health information. Reference librarians can be consulted, and audiovisual and printed materials can be checked out. More and more of these holdings are becoming available through home computer–based on-line services.

Consumer advocacy groups

A variety of nonprofit consumer advocacy groups patrol the health-care marketplace, particularly in relation to services and products (see the Star Box above). These groups produce and send out information designed to aid the consumer in recognizing questionable services and products. Large well-organized groups, such as The National Consumers' League and Consumers' Union, and smaller groups at the state and local levels champion the right of the consumer to receive valid and reliable information about health-care products and services.

Voluntary health agencies

Volunteerism and the traditional approach to health-care and health promotion are virtually inseparable. Few countries besides the United States boast so many national voluntary organizations, with state and local affiliates, dedi-

Learning from Our Diversity

Americans with Disabilities Act—New Places to Go

Although federal laws designed to end discrimination on the basis of gender and race were enacted in the United States decades ago, a law designed to address discrimination on the basis of physical and mental disabilities was not enacted until 1990. This law, the *Americans with Disabilities Act (1990),* has done a great deal to level the playing field for the disabled, both on college campus and in the larger community. On campuses today, it's common to see students whose obvious disabilities would have prevented them from attending college before this law was enacted. Students with cerebral palsy, spina bifida, spinal cord injuries, sensory impairments, and orthopedic disabilities share living quarters, lecture hall seats, and recreational facilities with their nondisabled classmates.

Equally important are those students whose disabilities are largely unobservable. Students with learning disabilities, mental disabilities, and subtle but disabling chronic health conditions such as Crohn's disease, lupus, and fibromyalgia may pass unnoticed. Yet their lives are equally challenged.

The Americans with Disabilities Act does not suggest that preferential treatment be given to students with disabilities, nor does it allow students to be unaccountable for their behavior. Instead, it seeks to create an environment—on the college campus and beyond—where people, regardless of disability, can learn new things, form meaningful relationships, and develop independence.

This law has the power to remove the physical and emotional barriers that can hinder a person with a disability from succeeding. For the first time, it allows students with disabilities to go where everyone else can—and beyond.

cated to the enhancement of health through research, service, and public education. The American Cancer Society, the American Red Cross, and the American Heart Association are all voluntary (not-for-profit) health agencies. Consumers can, in fact, expect to find a voluntary health agency for virtually every health problem.

Government agencies

Government agencies are effective providers of information to the public. Through meetings and the release of information to the media, agencies such as the Food and Drug Administration, Federal Trade Commission, United States Postal Service, and Environmental Protection Agency contribute to public awareness of health issues. Particularly through labeling, advertising, and the distribution of information through the mail, government agencies also control the quality of information sent out to the buying public. The various divisions of the National Institutes of Health regularly release research findings and recommendations about clinical practices, which in turn reach the consumer through clinical practitioners.

Despite their best intentions, federal health agencies are often less effective than what the public deserves. A variety of factors, including inadequate staff, poor administration, and lobbying by special interest groups, prevent these federal agencies from enforcing the consumer protection legislation that exists. As a result, the public is left with a sense of false confidence regarding the consumer protection provided by the federal government.

State government also provides the public with health information. State agencies are primary sources of information, particularly in the areas of public health and environmental protection.

One striking example of how health-care activism has achieved significant and lasting results is the Americans with Disabilities Act (see Learning from Our Diversity above).

Qualified health educators

Health educators work in a variety of settings and provide their services to diverse groups of individuals. Community health educators work with virtually all of the agencies mentioned above; patient educators function in primary care settings; and school health educators are found at all educational levels. Increasingly, health educators are being employed in a wide range of wellness-based programs in community, hospital, corporate, and school settings.

HEALTH-CARE PROVIDERS

The types and sources of health information just discussed can contribute greatly to the decisions you make as an informed consumer. The choices you make about physicians, health services, and medical payment plans will reflect your commitment to remain healthy and your trust in specific people who are trained in keeping you healthy. Refer to the Changing for the Better box on p. 386 for tips on choosing a physician.

Physicians and Their Training

In every city and many smaller communities, the local telephone directory shows the many types of physicians engaged in the practice of medicine. These health-care providers hold the academic degree of Doctor of Medicine (MD) or Doctor of Osteopathy (DO).

Changing *for the Better*

Choosing a Physician

I need to find a doctor for myself. What specific things should I be looking for, and what questions should I ask?

When choosing a physician, plan to obtain answers to the following questions during your initial visit:

- Obtain a description of the physician's medical background, such as education, residencies, and specialty areas.
- What are the normal office hours? What should be done if help is needed outside of normal office hours?
- What is included in a comprehensive physical examination?
- How does the physician feel about second and third opinions?
- Which hospitals is the physician affiliated with in your area?
- Is the physician comfortable referring patients to specialists when the complexity of a condition warrants their expertise?
- With which specialists is the physician associated?
- What is the physician's fee schedule?

Ask yourself the following questions after your visit:

- Was I comfortable with the physician's age, gender, race, and national origin?
- Was I comfortable with the physician's demeanor? Did I find communication with the physician to be understandable and reassuring? Were all my questions answered?
- Did the physician seem interested in having me as a patient?
- Are the physician's training and practice speciality in an area most closely associated with my present needs and concerns?
- Does the physician have staff privileges at a hospital of my preference?
- Does the physician's fee-for-service policy in any way exclude or limit my ability to receive necessary services?
- Did the physician take a complete medical history as a part of my initial visit? Was prevention, health promotion, or wellness addressed by the physician at any point during my visit?
- Did I at any point during my visit sense that the physician was unusually reluctant or anxious to try new medical procedures or medications?
- When the physician is unavailable, are any colleagues on call for 24 hours? Did I feel that telephone calls from me would be welcomed and responded to in a reasonable period?

If you have answered yes to most of these questions, you have found a physician with whom you should feel comfortable. If you have been using the services of a particular physician but are becoming dissatisfied, how could you resolve this dissatisfaction?

At one time, **allopathy** and **osteopathy** were clearly different health-care professions regarding their healing philosophies and modes of practice. Today, however, MDs and DOs receive similar educations and engage in very similar forms of practice. Both can function as **primary care physicians** or as board-certified specialists. One difference is that that osteopathic physicians are more likely to use techniques of manipulation in treating health problems. Additionally, DOs perceive themselves as being more holistically oriented than MDs.

The training of medical and osteopathic physicians is a long process. Usually, 4 years of initial undergraduate preparation is required. There is strong emphasis on the sciences—biology, chemistry, mathematics, anatomy, and physiology. Most undergraduate schools have preprofessional courses of study for students interested in medical or osteopathic schools.

Once accepted into professional schools, students generally spend 4 years or more in intensive training, which includes advanced study in the preclinical medical sciences and clinical practice. When this phase of training is completed, the students are awarded the MD or DO degree. Next, they take the state medical license examination. Most newly licensed physicians complete a residency at a hospital. During this period, physicians gain experience in various clinical areas and begin specialized programs. Residency programs vary in length from 3 to 4 years. At the conclusion of residency programs, board-eligible or board-certified status is granted. Interestingly, since the late 1990s, applications for medical schools have been in a state of decline.[5] This previously unseen trend suggests several factors at play, including attractive options in the job market and changes in admission practices.

Complementary (Alternative) Practitioners

Several forms of health care offer complementary or alternative approaches within the large health-care market. Examples include chiropractic, acupuncture, reflexology, homeopathy, naturopathy, herbalism, and ayurveda. Although the traditional medical community has long scoffed at these alternatives as ineffective and unscientific, many people use these forms of health care and believe strongly that they are as effective as (or more effective than) allopathic and osteopathic medicine.

Chiropractic

This system is based on manual manipulation of the spine to correct misalignments. Recent studies have

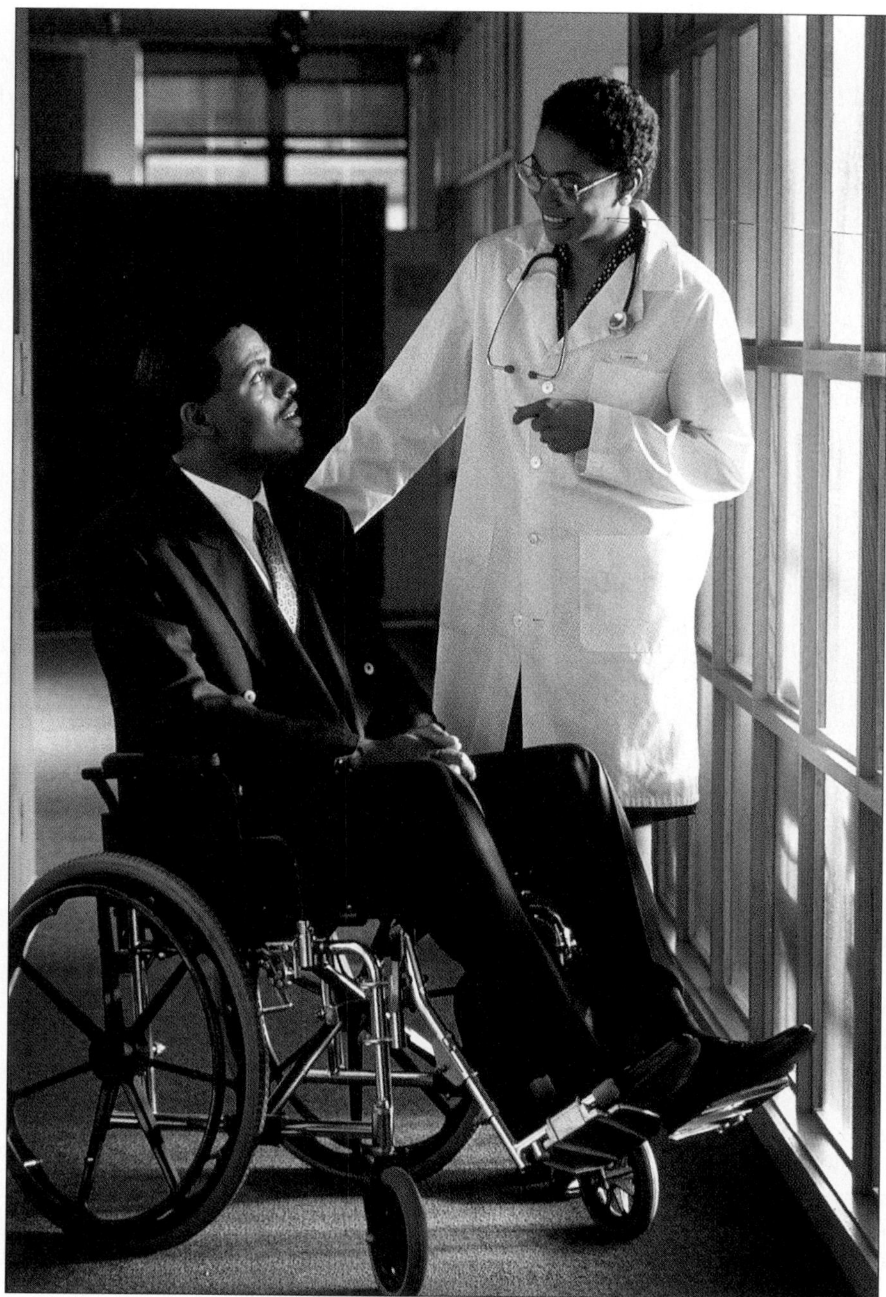

It's important to have a good relationship with the people who help keep us healthy.

Key Terms

allopathy (ah LOP ah thee)
System of medical practice in which specific remedies (often pharmaceutical agents) are used to produce effects different from those produced by a disease or injury.

osteopathy (os tee OP ah thee)
System of medical practice that combines allopathic principles with specific attention to postural mechanics of the body.

Key Terms

primary care physician
The physician who sees a patient on a regular basis, rather than a specialist who sees the patient only for a specific condition or procedure.

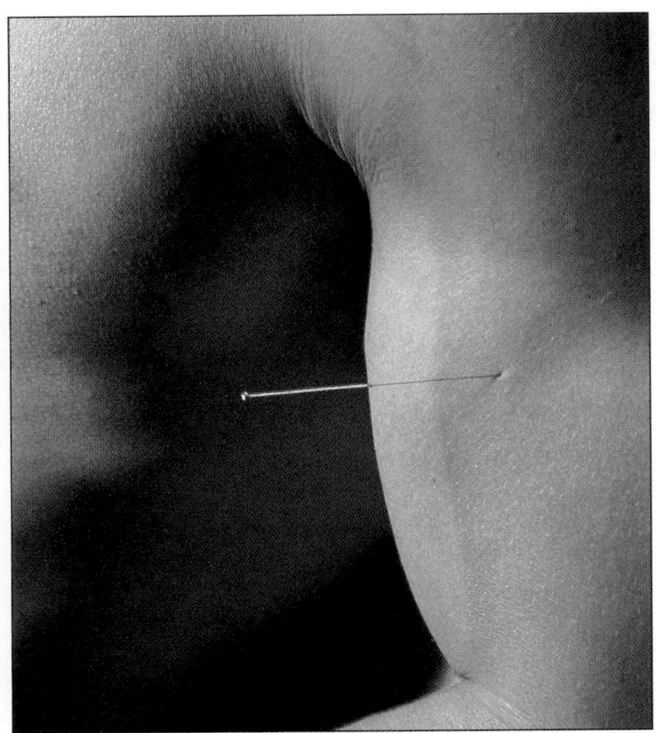

Acupuncture has received increasing acceptance within the Western medical community.

shown that **chiropractic** treatment of some types of low-back pain can be more effective than conventional care. With about 50,000 practitioners in the United States, chiropractic is the third-largest health profession, used by 15 to 20 million people.

Acupuncture

Acupuncture is, for Americans, the most familiar component of the 3000-year-old Chinese medical system. This system is based on balancing the active and passive forces with the patient's body to strengthen the chi ("chee"), or life force. Acupuncturists place hair-thin needles at certain points in the body to stimulate the patient's chi.

Of all the Chinese therapies, acupuncture is the most widely accepted in the West. Researchers have produced persuasive evidence of acupuncture's effectiveness as an anesthetic and as an antidote to chronic pain, migraines, dysmenorrhea, and osteoarthritis.[6] In addition, some studies have found that acupuncture can help patients overcome addictions to alcohol, drugs, and tobacco. Conversely, research funded by the federal government shows that acupuncture is far more than a placebo but is not superior to standard pain management care.[7]

Reflexology

Reflexology uses principles similar to those of acupuncture but focuses on treating certain disorders through massage of the soles of the feet.

Homeopathy

Homeopathy uses infinitesimal doses of herbs, minerals, or even poisons to stimulate the body's curative powers. The theory on which homeopathy is based, called the *Law of Similars,* is that if large doses of a substance can cause a problem, tiny doses can trigger healing of that same problem. In three carefully controlled studies involving inner ear dysfunction, general pain management, and the treatment of common warts, homeopathic medications were found to be no more effective than placeboes.[8] In the inner ear study, the homeopathic preparation was, however, as effective as one histamine-based medication.

Naturopathy

Proponents of **naturopathy** believe that when the mind and the body are in balance and receiving proper care, with a healthy diet, adequate rest, and minimal stress, the body's own vital forces are sufficient to fight off disease. Getting rid of an ailment is only the first step toward correcting the underlying imbalance that allowed the ailment to take hold, naturists believe. Correcting the imbalance might be as simple as rectifying a shortage of a particular nutrient or as complex as reducing overlong work hours, strengthening a weakened immune system, and identifying an inability to digest certain foods.

Herbalism

Herbalism may be the world's oldest and most widely used healing form. Herbalists make herbal brews for treating a variety of ills, such as depression, anxiety, and hypertension. In some cases, scientific research supports the herbalists' beliefs. For example, several studies have found St. John's wort to be more effective than a placebo in alleviating mild depression.[9]

Ayurveda

Even older than Chinese medicine, India's **ayurveda** takes a preventive approach and focuses on the whole person. This system employs diet, tailored to the patient's constitutional type, or "dosha"; herbs; yoga and breathing exercises; meditation; massages; and purges, enemas, and aromatherapy. Research has shown ayurveda to be effective in treating rheumatoid arthritis, headaches, and chronic sinusitis.

If you'd like to consult a practitioner in one of the alternative disciplines but don't know where to start, see the Changing for the Better box on p. 389 for some tips on choosing a provider in alternative medicine.

At the urging of many people in both the medical and alternative health-care fields, the National Institutes of Health agreed to establish an Office of Complementary and Alternative Medicine to serve as a funding agency for carefully controlled research into a wide array

Changing *for the Better*

Choosing the Best Complementary Medical Practitioner for You

I'm interested in exploring complementary approaches to medicine, but I feel uncertain about how to proceed. What steps should I take?

Perhaps you are one of the millions of people who feel that their doctors don't encourage them to ask questions, don't seek their opinion about their medical condition, or don't take a thorough medical history. Perhaps you want advice on improving your health rather than just a quick diagnosis and prescription.

For whatever reasons, millions of Americans are turning to complementary medical practitioners, such as doctors of naturopathy, Chinese medicine, or ayurveda. Unfortunately, the patient looking for these alternatives faces other problems: practitioners' training may be weak, they might not be licensed or covered by insurance, they are hard to find, and they usually are not permitted to prescribe drugs unless they also happen to be medical doctors. This means that you must do some legwork to find a good provider who can meet your needs.

Consider the following tips for finding the practitioner who is right for you.

- *Don't forget the family doctor.* Family-practice medicine is enjoying a surge in the United States and many of these doctors tend to think holistically.
- *Find a doctor who believes in complementary therapies.* Your doctor's attitude toward the treatment can be just as important as your own.
- *Give the treatment time.* Complementary therapies encourage the body to do its own healing. This often takes time. Seek a doctor who is confident in your self-healing ability, so you won't become discouraged if it takes some time.
- *Request natural healing.* Natural healing tends to change the internal conditions so that pathogens are less likely to gain a foothold; conventional medicine seeks to destroy the pathogen. Natural healing searches for the causes of symptoms, while conventional medicine treats symptoms.
- *Know your disease.* Find books that describe your conditions and offer complementary as well as conventional treatments. This way you can discuss your treatment with your doctor and can create an effective treatment plan.
- *Treat yourself.* Don't overuse your health-care provider, whether conventional or complementary. For many conditions, you can be your own best doctor; of course, persistent or severe symptoms should send you to the doctor.
- *Learn whether the treatment is covered by insurance.* Coverage of complementary treatment differs sharply by state. Some insurance groups are beginning to pay for more complementary medicine, and HMOs are hiring some complementary specialists.
- *Talk to professional associations.* Most of the more established complementary fields have associations that can give you a list of providers. Use it as a start.
- *Get a brochure.* The doctor's literature can tell you a lot about his or her outlook and experience.
- *Interview the doctor.* Before making an appointment, talk with the doctor over the telephone. Then, in the doctor's office, take notes, even use a tape recorder, to make certain you understand. Watch for a doctor who is a good listener, a good communicator, and open-minded.

Key Terms

chiropractic
Manipulation of the vertebral column to relieve pressure and cure illness.

acupuncture
Insertion of fine needles into the body to alter electroenergy fields and cure disease.

reflexology
Massage applied to specific areas of the feet to treat illness and disease in other areas of the body.

Key Terms

homeopathy (ho mee OP ah thee)
The use of minute doses of herbs or minerals to stimulate healing.

naturopathy (nay chur OP ah thee)
A system of treatment that avoids drugs and surgery and emphasizes the use of natural agents to correct underlying imbalances.

herbalism
An ancient form of healing in which herbal preparations are used to treat illness and disease.

ayurveda (ai yur VEY da)
Traditional Indian medicine based on herbal remedies.

of alternative healing arts and to act as a clearinghouse for information on these forms of health care. An initial publication in 1994, *Alternative Medicine: Expanding Medical Horizons*,[10] established a benchmark for the work of the organization. Today, more than $100 million of funded research is ongoing, and gradually credible evidence is being collected and disseminated. A quarterly newsletter and a variety of on-line reports and news releases are accessible on the Internet.

TALKING POINTS • A friend tells you she is planning to try a "high colonic" procedure offered at a local spa. How would you explain that there are risks associated with this practice?

Restricted-Practice Health-Care Providers

Much of your health care is provided by medical physicians. However, you probably also use the services of various health-care specialists who have advanced graduate level training. Among these professionals are dentists, psychologists, podiatrists, and optometrists.

Dentists (Doctor of Dental Surgery, DDS) are trained to deal with a wide range of diseases and impairments of the teeth and oral cavity. Dentists undergo undergraduate predental programs that emphasize the sciences, followed by 4 additional years of graduate study in dental school and, with increasing frequency, an internship program. State licensure examinations are required. Like medical physicians, dentists can also specialize by completing a postdoctoral master's degree in fields such as oral surgery, **orthodontics,** and **prosthodontics.** Dentists are also permitted to prescribe therapy programs (such as appliances for the treatment of temporomandibular joint dysfunction) and drugs that pertain to their practices (primarily analgesics and antibiotics).

Psychologists provide services related to an understanding of behavior patterns or perceptions. Over forty states have certification or licensing laws that prohibit unqualified people from using the term *psychologist.* The consumer should examine the credentials of a psychologist. Legitimate psychologists have received advanced graduate training (often leading to a PhD or EdD degree) in clinical, counseling, industrial, or educational psychology. Furthermore, these practitioners will have passed state certification examinations and, in many states, will have met further requirements that allow them to offer health services to the public. Psychologists may have special interests and credentials from professional societies in individual, group, family, or marriage counseling. Some are certified as sex therapists.

Unlike *psychiatrists,* who are medical physicians, psychologists cannot prescribe or dispense drugs. They may refer to or consult with medical physicians about clients who might benefit from drug therapy.

Podiatrists are highly trained clinicians who practice podiatric medicine, or care of the feet (and ankles). Although not MDs or DOs, doctors of podiatric medicine (DPM) treat a wide variety of conditions related to the feet, including corns, bunions, warts, bone spurs, hammertoes, fractures, diabetes-related conditions, athletic injuries, and structural abnormalities. Podiatrists perform surgery, prescribe medications, and apply orthotics (supports or braces), splints, and corrective shoes for structural abnormalities of the feet.

Doctors of podiatric medicine follow an educational path similar to that taken by MDs and DOs, consisting of a 4-year undergraduate preprofessional curriculum, 4 additional years of study in a podiatric medical school, and an optional residency of 1 or 2 years. Board-certified areas of specialization include surgery, orthopedics, and podiatric sports medicine. Hospital affiliation generally requires board certification in a specialized area.

Optometrists are eye specialists who deal primarily with vision problems associated with **refractory errors.** They examine the eyes and prescribe glasses or contact lenses to correct visual disorders. Most recently, optometrists have been permitted to prescribe medications appropriate to the scope of their professional practice. They also are attempting to correct certain ocular muscle imbalances with specific exercise regimens. Optometrists must complete undergraduate training and additional years of coursework at one of sixteen accredited colleges of optometry in the United States, one of two in Canada, or one in Puerto Rico before taking a state licensing examination.

Opticians are technicians who manufacture and fit eyeglasses or contact lenses. Although they are rarely licensed by a state agency, they perform the important function of grinding lenses to the precise prescription designated by an optometrist or *ophthalmologist* (physicians who have specialized in vision care). To save money and time, many consumers take an optometrist's or ophthalmologist's prescription for glasses or contact lenses to optician-staffed retail stores that deal exclusively with eyewear products.

Nurse Professionals

Nurses constitute a large group of health professionals who practice in a variety of settings. Frequently, the responsibilities of nurses vary according to their academic preparation. Registered nurses (RNs) are academically prepared at two levels: (1) the technical nurse, and (2) the professional nurse. The technical nurse is educated in a 2-year associate degree program. The professional nurse receives 4 years of education and earns a bachelor's degree. Both technical and professional nurses must successfully complete state licensing examinations before they can practice as RNs.

Many professional nurses continue their education and earn master's and doctoral degrees in nursing or other health fields. Some professional nurses specialize in a clinical area (such as pediatrics, gerontology, public health, or school health) and become certified as *nurse practitioners.* Working under the supervision of physicians, nurse practitioners perform many of the diagnostic and treatment procedures performed by physicians. The ability of these highly trained nurses to function at this level provides communities with additional primary care providers, as well as freeing physicians to deal with more complex cases. Many college health centers employ nurse practitioners because of their ability to deliver high-quality care at a low cost to the institution.

Licensed practical nurses (LPNs) are trained in hospital-based programs ranging from 12 to 18 months. Because of their brief training, LPNs' scope of practice is limited. Most LPN training programs are gradually being phased out.

Allied Health-Care Professionals

Our primary health-care providers are supported by a large group of allied health-care professionals, who often take the responsibility for highly technical services and procedures. Such professionals include respiratory and inhalation therapists, radiological technologists, nuclear medicine technologists, pathology technicians, general medical technologists, operating room technicians, emergency medical technicians, registered nurse midwives, physical therapists, occupational therapists, clinical social workers, family therapists, cardiac rehabilitation therapists, dental technicians, physician assistants, and dental hygienists. Depending on the particular field, the training for these specialty support areas can take from 1 to 5 years of post–high school study. Programs include hospital-based training leading to a diploma through associate, bachelor's, and master's degrees. Most allied health-care professionals must also pass state or national licensing examinations.

SELF-CARE

The emergence of the **self-care movement** suggests that many people are becoming more responsible for the maintenance of their health. They are developing the expertise to prevent or manage numerous types of illness, injuries, and conditions. They are learning to assess their health status and treat, monitor, and rehabilitate themselves in a way that was once thought possible only with the direct help of a physician or other health-care specialist.

The benefits of this movement are that self-care can (1) lower health-care costs, (2) be effective for particular conditions, (3) free physicians and other health-care specialists to spend time with other patients, and (4) enhance interest in health activities.

Self-care is an appropriate alternative to professional care in three areas. First, self-care may be appropriate for certain acute conditions that have familiar symptoms and are of limited duration and seriousness. Common colds and flu, many home injuries, sore throats, and nonallergic insect bites are often easily managed with self-care.

A second area in which self-care might be appropriate is therapy. For example, many people are now administering injections for allergies and migraine headaches and continuing physical therapy programs in their homes. Asthma, diabetes, and hypertension are also conditions that can be managed or monitored with self-care.

A third area in which self-care has appropriate application is health promotion. Weight-loss programs, physical conditioning activities, and stress-reduction programs are particularly well suited to self-care.

Although self-care is sometimes appropriate, visiting a physician to obtain a diagnosis is often a wise choice. Additionally, some self-care skills should (or must) be first practiced under the supervision of a health-care professional before being implemented at home. In fact, some conditions that can be managed on a daily basis, such as diabetes, require regular assessment by a physician to ensure that management criteria are being met on a consistent basis.

People interested in practicing more self-care must be skilled consumers. The self-care marketplace is growing very rapidly and is expected to be a multibillion-dollar industry by the end of the decade. Equipment such as blood pressure–measuring instruments, stethoscopes, and screening kits for cholesterol, HIV, and pregnancy, as well as OTC drugs, can represent significant investments. Clearly, your money, time, and willingness to develop expertise are important factors in this growing area of health-care consumerism. See Exploring Your Spirituality on p. 392 for a discussion of how taking charge of your own health can be an empowering experience.

Key Terms

orthodontics
Dental specialty that focuses on the proper alignment of the teeth.

prosthodontics
Dental specialty that focuses on the construction and fitting of artificial appliances to replace missing teeth.

refractory errors
Incorrect patterns of light wave transmissions through the structures of the eye.

self-care movement
Trend toward individuals taking increased responsibility for prevention or management of certain health conditions.

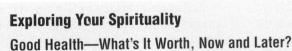

Exploring Your Spirituality

Good Health—What's It Worth, Now and Later?

The average life expectancy for women in the United States today is 80 years. For men, it's 76 years. That's a dramatic change from just a few generations ago. Thanks to tremendous advances in medical science and technology, many people are enjoying healthy, happy, and spiritually fulfilling lives well into their final years.

But this longevity comes with a price tag. It means that making healthful choices every day—including a balanced diet, exercise, adequate rest, and opportunities for emotional and spiritual expression—takes on new importance. If you're going to live 10 "extra" years, what do you want to do with that time? Probably many of the things you're doing now, plus some different ones. Are you going to be able to meet the challenge—healthwise?

Taking charge of your health right now, when you're young and healthy, can be one of the most empowering things you do. By consciously choosing a healthy lifestyle—limiting your intake of alcohol, avoiding drugs and cigarette smoking, and limiting your sexual partners—you are building the foundation for good health in your later years.

If you should ever have a serious health problem, you'll be better equipped to handle it if you're used to taking care of yourself. You'll feel comfortable being involved in your treatment decisions and doing whatever you can to control the quality of your life. You'll see your health crisis as a challenge you need to deal with, instead of viewing yourself as a helpless victim.

Taking charge of your own health—by being an informed health-care consumer, by choosing a healthy lifestyle, and by fostering a positive attitude—brings a sense of peace. It's knowing that you're doing everything you can to take care of yourself. It's enhancing the quality of your life today and preparing for an active and rewarding tomorrow.

HEALTH INSURANCE

A wide array of professionals is required to deliver highly sophisticated health care, and the demand for such care is growing because of our large aging population. Therefore the cost of health care, which now exceeds $1 trillion per year, is higher in the United States than anywhere else in the world. For the majority of Americans, who have not reached the age of retirement, such care is affordable only through participation in group or individual health-care insurance plans.

Health insurance is a financial agreement between an insurance company and an individual or group for the payment of health costs. After paying a premium to an insurance company, the policyholder is covered for specific benefits. Each policy is different in terms of coverage for illnesses and injuries. Merely having an insurance policy does not mean that all health-care expenses will be covered. Most health insurance policies require various forms of payments on the part of the policyholder, which include provisions for deductible amounts, fixed indemnity benefits, coinsurance, and exclusions.

A *deductible* amount is an established amount that the insuree must pay before the insurer reimburses for services. For example, many policies require that a family pays the first $200 or $400 of expense for that year before it begins to reimburse its percentage (coinsurance) of subsequent expenses. Usually, the lower the deductible amount is, the higher the premium will be.

A policy with *fixed indemnity* benefits will pay only a specified amount for a particular procedure or service. If the policy pays only $1000 for an appendectomy and the actual cost of the appendectomy was $1500, then the policy owner will owe the health-care provider $500. A policy with *full-service* benefits, which pays the entire cost of a particular procedure or service, may be worth the extra cost.

Policies that have *coinsurance* features require that the policy owner and the insurance company share the costs of certain covered services, usually on a percentage basis. One standard coinsurance plan requires that the policyholder pay 20% of the costs above a deductible amount, and the company pays the remaining 80%.

An *exclusion* refers to a service or expense that is not covered by the policy. Elective or cosmetic surgery procedures, unusual treatment protocols, prescription drugs, and certain kinds of consultations are common exclusions in many policies. Illness and injuries that already exist at the time of purchase (preexisting conditions) are often excluded. Also, injuries incurred during high-risk activities (ice hockey, hang gliding, mountain climbing, intramural sports) might not be covered by a policy.

Health insurance can be obtained through individual policies or group plans. Group health insurance plans usually offer the widest range of coverage at the least expensive price and are often purchased cooperatively by companies and their employees. In 1998, the average employer's portion of an employee's health insurance plan was $4,208.[11] Fortunately, no employee is refused entry into a group insurance program. A federal law allows health insurance to be transferred when a person changes employment, without losing coverage because of a preexisting condition. Today, as many large American companies downsize, tens of thousands of employees can lose, their affordable group health insurance, virtually without warning.

Changing *for the Better*

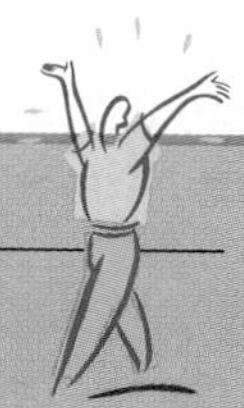

Selecting a Health Insurance Policy

I'm looking into getting health insurance for myself. Right now, I feel overwhelmed by all the information I've gathered. How can I make an intelligent choice?

Before you purchase a health insurance policy, ask yourself the following questions. The more questions you can answer with a "yes," the better you should feel that the policy you select is right for you.

General Questions

- Do I really need an individual insurance policy?
- Am I already covered by a group insurance policy?
- Is the insurance company I'm considering rated favorably by *Best's Insurance Reports* or my state insurance department?
- Have I compared health insurance policies from at least two other companies?
- Does this company have a "return rate" of 50% or more?
- Can I afford this insurance policy?
- Do I understand the factors that might raise the cost of this policy?

Specific Questions

- Do I clearly understand which health conditions are covered and which are not?
- Do I clearly understand whether I have fixed indemnity benefits or full-service benefits?
- Do I clearly understand the deductible amounts of this policy?
- Do I clearly understand when the major medical portion of this policy starts?
- Do I clearly understand all information in this policy that refers to exclusions and preexisting conditions?
- Do I clearly understand any disability provisions of this policy?
- Do I clearly understand all information concerning both cancellation and renewal of this policy?

Individual policies can be purchased by one person (or a family) from an insurance company. These policies are often much more expensive than group plans and may provide much less coverage. People who do not have access to a group plan should still attempt to secure individual policies, since the financial burdens resulting from a severe accident or illness that is not covered by some form of health insurance can be devastating. Many colleges and universities offer annually renewable health insurance policies that students can purchase. The Changing for the Better box above gives the consumer some questions to consider before purchasing a health insurance policy.

TALKING POINTS • **In a conversation with your parents, you learn that their health insurance plan will not provide coverage for you after you turn 23, even though you'll still be a full-time student. How could you suggest an arrangement that would benefit both parties?**

HEALTH-RELATED PRODUCTS

Prescription and OTC drugs constitute an important part of any discussion of health-care products.

Prescription Drugs

Caution: Federal law prohibits dispensing without prescription.

This FDA warning appears on the labels of approximately three-fourths of all medications. Prescription drugs must be ordered for patients by a licensed practitioner. Because these compounds are legally controlled and may require special skills for their administration, access to these drugs is limited.

Although the *Physicians' Desk Reference* lists more than 2500 compounds that can be prescribed, only 200 drugs make up most of the 2.84 billion prescriptions (new and refills) dispensed by 31,000 pharmacies in 2000. Total retail prescription sales of $131.8 billion for 2000 represent an 9% increase over the previous year's sales. It is projected that by the year 2005 approximately 4 billion prescriptions will be filled annually.[12] The rapid expansion of on-line pharmacies noted in 1999 is unlikely to influence the number of prescriptions filled. Instead, their presence is more likely to affect the sales of "brick and mortar" drugstore chains.

Research and development of new drugs

As consumers of prescription drugs, you may be curious about how drugs gain FDA approval for marketing. The rigor of this process may be why fewer than 100 new drugs are added to the list of approved drugs each year.

On a continuous basis, the nation's pharmaceutical companies are exploring the molecular structure of various chemical compounds in an attempt to discover important new compounds with desired types and levels of biological activity. Once these new compounds are identified, extensive in-house research with computer simulations and animal testing is required to determine whether clinical trials involving humans are warranted. Of the 125,000 or more compounds under study each year, only a few thousand receive such extensive preclinical evaluation. Even fewer of these are then passed on to the FDA to undergo the evaluation process necessary to gain approval for further research with humans. Once a drug is approved for clinical trials, the pharmaceutical companies can secure a patent, which prevents the drug from being manufactured by other companies for the next 17 years.

The $500 million price tag for bringing a new drug into the marketplace reflects this slow, careful process. If this 7-year period of development goes well, a pharmaceutical company will benefit from 10 years of legally protected retail sales before generic versions of the drug can be offered by other companies.

Generic versus brand-name drugs

When a new drug comes into the marketplace, it carries with it three names: its **chemical name,** its **generic name,** and its **brand name.** While the 17-year patent is in effect, no other drug with the same formulation can be sold. When the patent expires, other companies can manufacture a drug of chemical and therapeutic equivalence and market it under the brand-name drug's original generic name. Because extensive research and development are not necessary at this point, the production of generic drugs is far less costly than the initial development of the brand-name drug. Nearly all states allow pharmacists to substitute generic drugs for brand-name drugs, as long as the prescribing physician approves.

At the time of this writing, the pharmaceutical industry is actively attempting to extend the patent protection on several of the most profitable drugs on the market because their period of protected sales is expiring. In some cases the manufacturers have appealed directly to Congress for waivers to the current patent law, contending that they need additional time to recoup research and development costs. Other manufacturers have quietly "layered" additional patents onto their products to prevent manufacturers of generic versions from using the same shape or color used in brand-name versions, even though the chemical formulations are no longer protected. In another approach, manufacturers of highly profitable brand-name drugs have offered to pay manufacturers of generic drugs to not make generic versions of their products once the patent protection has expired.

TALKING POINTS • On a visit to your campus health center, you get a prescription with "Do Not Substitute" indicated. You happen to know that a generic form is available and that generics often cost 40% to 70% less than brand-name drugs. How could you ask the physician why he or she specified that you should buy the name brand?

Over-the-Counter Drugs

When people are asked when they last took some form of medication, many say that they took aspirin, a cold pill, or a laxative that very morning. In making this decision, these individuals made a self-diagnosis, determined a course of self-treatment, self-administered that treatment, and freed a physician to serve people whose illnesses are more serious than theirs. None of this would have been possible without readily available, inexpensive, and effective OTC drugs.

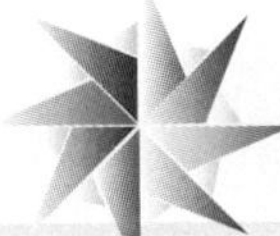

Categories of Over-the-Counter (OTC) Products

- Antacids
- Antimicrobials
- Sedatives and sleep aids
- Analgesics
- Cold remedies and antitussives
- Antihistamines and allergy products
- Mouthwashes
- Topical analgesics
- Antirheumatics
- Hematinics
- Vitamins and minerals
- Antiperspirants
- Laxatives
- Dentrifices and dental products
- Sunburn treatments and preventives
- Contraceptive and vaginal products
- Stimulants
- Hemorrhoidals
- Antidiarrheals
- Dandruff and athlete's foot preparations

In comparison with the 2500 prescription drugs available, there are as many as 300,000 different OTC products, routinely classified into twenty-six different families (see the Star Box above). Like prescription drugs, nonprescription drugs are regulated by the FDA. However, for OTC drugs, the marketplace is a more powerful determinant of success.

The regulation of OTC drugs is based on a provision in a 1972 amendment to the 1938 Food, Drug, and Cosmetic Act. As a result of that action, OTC drugs were placed in three categories (I, II, and III) on the basis of the safety and effectiveness of their active ingredient(s). Today, only category I OTC drugs that are safe, effective, and truthfully labeled can be sold. The FDA's drug classification process also allows (1) some OTC drugs to be made stronger and (2) some prescription drugs to become nonprescription drugs if their strength is reduced through reformulation. Today, more than 650 products (containing over fifty-six active ingredients) that were once available only by prescription have FDA approval for OTC sale. As many as twenty-five additional such products reach the market each year.

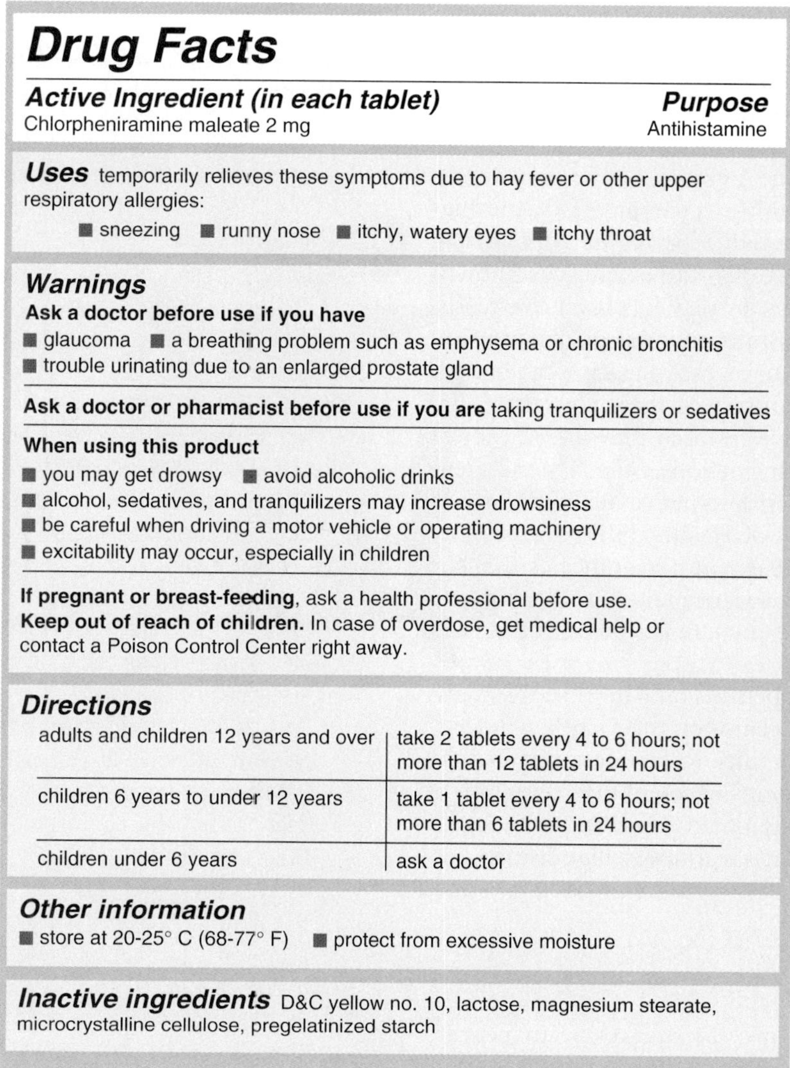

Drug Facts

Active Ingredient (in each tablet) — **Purpose**
Chlorpheniramine maleate 2 mg — Antihistamine

Uses temporarily relieves these symptoms due to hay fever or other upper respiratory allergies:
■ sneezing ■ runny nose ■ itchy, watery eyes ■ itchy throat

Warnings
Ask a doctor before use if you have
■ glaucoma ■ a breathing problem such as emphysema or chronic bronchitis
■ trouble urinating due to an enlarged prostate gland

Ask a doctor or pharmacist before use if you are taking tranquilizers or sedatives

When using this product
■ you may get drowsy ■ avoid alcoholic drinks
■ alcohol, sedatives, and tranquilizers may increase drowsiness
■ be careful when driving a motor vehicle or operating machinery
■ excitability may occur, especially in children

If pregnant or breast-feeding, ask a health professional before use.
Keep out of reach of children. In case of overdose, get medical help or contact a Poison Control Center right away.

Directions

adults and children 12 years and over	take 2 tablets every 4 to 6 hours; not more than 12 tablets in 24 hours
children 6 years to under 12 years	take 1 tablet every 4 to 6 hours; not more than 6 tablets in 24 hours
children under 6 years	ask a doctor

Other information
■ store at 20-25° C (68-77° F) ■ protect from excessive moisture

Inactive ingredients D&C yellow no. 10, lactose, magnesium stearate, microcrystalline cellulose, pregelatinized starch

Figure 15-2 The FDA will soon require over-the-counter drugs to carry standardized labels, such as the one above. A version of the label for OTC drugs shown above should begin appearing by 2004.

Like the proposed label shown above (Figure 15-2), current labels reflect FDA requirements. The labels must clearly state the type and quantity of active ingredients, alcohol content, side effects, instructions for appropriate use, warnings against inappropriate use, and risks of using the product with other drugs (polydrug use). Unsubstantiated claims must be carefully avoided in advertisements for these products.

Dietary Supplements

Currently, more than 60 million Americans are using a vast array of vitamins, minerals, herbal products, hormones, and amino acids in their quest for improved health. Possible reasons for this trend include the following: Baby Boomers are now in middle age and have increasing concerns about illness and premature death; Americans increasingly view traditional Western medicine as impersonal; some people are seeking an alternative to prescription medications; and many people want a greater sense of control over their bodies and health. As a result, we are now spending more than $12 billion on *dietary supplements.* These products are not subject to

Key Terms

chemical name
Name used to describe the molecular structure of a drug.

generic name
Common or nonproprietary name of a drug.

brand name
Specific patented name assigned to a drug by its manufacturer.

the demanding clinical studies required for prescription medications or even the "safe and effective" standards that OTC products must meet.

However, the traditional medical community is showing increasing interest in the potential health benefits of dietary supplements. A growing number of teaching hospitals are establishing departments of complementary medicine, and medical students are learning about the documented role (to the extent it is known) that dietary supplements can play in preventive medicine. Additionally, major international pharmaceutical companies are beginning to market dietary supplements. The reputations and resources of these companies are likely to generate extensive research into the efficacy of these products. Also, the formation of the National Center for Complementary and Alternative Medicine (as part of the National Institutes of Health [NIH]), with more than $100 million in research funds, indicates that the contribution that dietary supplementation can make to high-level health will be the subject of carefully controlled studies.

At this time the FDA permits only three supplements to include specific health claims on their labels. These include folic acid and its ability to facilitate neural tube closure, calcium and its contribution to the prevention of osteoporosis, and a highly qualified claim for omega-3 fatty acids in the reduction of cardiovascular disease.

Changing *for the Better*

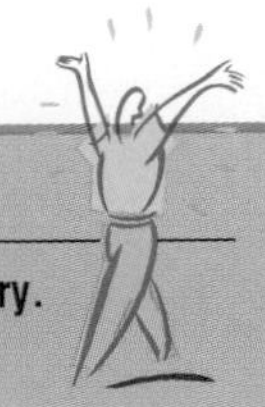

Recognizing Quackery

I don't want to get taken in by health-care quackery. What should I be on the lookout for?

"Duck" when you encounter these!

- Makes promises of quick, dramatic, simple, painless, or drugless treatment or cures
- Uses anecdotes, case histories, or testimonials to support claims
- Displays credentials or uses titles that might be confused with those of the scientific or medical community, such as Stan Smith, Ph.D. (in result)
- Claims a product or service provides treatment or cure for multiple or all illnesses and conditions
- States that this treatment or cure is either secret or not yet available in the United States
- States that medical doctors should not be trusted because they do more harm than good with their approaches to diagnosis and treatment
- Reports that most disease is due to a faulty diet and can be treated with nutritional supplements
- Promotes the use of hair analysis to diagnose illnesses or deficiencies
- Claims that "natural" products are superior to those sold in drugstores or dispensed by physicians
- Supports the "freedom of choice" concept that should allow you to try something even though it has not been proved safe and effective

HEALTH-CARE QUACKERY AND CONSUMER FRAUD

A person who earns money by marketing inaccurate health information, unreliable health care, or ineffective health products is called a fraud, quack, or charlatan. **Consumer fraud** flourished with the old-fashioned medicine shows of the late 1880s. Unfortunately, consumer fraud still flourishes (see the Focus on article on p. 403). Look no further than large city newspapers to see questionable advertisements for disease cures and weight-loss products. In health and illness, quacks have found the perfect avenues to realize maximum gain with minimum effort.

When people are in poor health, they may be afraid of dying. So powerful is their desire to live and be relieved of their suffering that they may be especially vulnerable to promises of improved health and longer life. Even though many people have great faith in their physicians, they also would like to have access to experimental treatments or products touted as being superior to currently available therapies. When tempted with the promise of real help, people are sometimes willing to set aside traditional medical care. Of course, quacks recognize this vulnerability and present a variety of "reasons" to take their advice (see the Changing for the Better box above).[13] Gullibility, blind faith, impatience, superstition, ignorance, or hostility toward professional expertise eventually carry the day. In spite of the best efforts of agencies at all levels, no branch of government can protect consumers from their own errors of judgment that so easily play into the hands of quacks and charlatans.

Regardless of the specific motivation that leads people into consumer fraud, the outcome is frequently the same. First, the consumer suffers financial loss. The services or products provided are grossly overpriced, and the consumers have little recourse to help them recover their money. Second, the consumers often feel disappointed, guilty, and angered by their own carelessness as consumers. Far too frequently, consumer fraud may lead to unnecessary suffering.

Key Term

consumer fraud
Marketing of unreliable and ineffective services, products, or information under the guise of curing disease or improving health; quackery.

SUMMARY

- Sources of health information include family, friends, commercials, labels, and information supplied by health professionals.
- Physicians can be either Doctors of Medicine (MDs) or Doctors of Osteopathy (DOs). They receive similar training and engage in similar forms of practice.
- Although alternative health-care providers, including chiropractors, naturopaths, and acupuncturists, meet the health-care needs of many people, systematic study of these forms of health care is only now under way.
- Restricted-practice health-care providers play important roles in meeting the health and wellness needs of the public.
- Nursing at all levels is a critical health-care profession.
- Self-care is often a viable approach to preventing illness and reducing the use of health-care providers.
- Health insurance is critical in our ability to afford modern health-care services.
- The development of prescription medication is a long and expensive process for pharmaceutical manufacturers.
- More than 60 million Americans use some type of dietary supplement. Federally sponsored research is under way to determine the efficacy of supplements in the treatment and prevention of illness.
- Critical health consumerism, including the avoidance of health quackery, requires careful use of health-related information, products, and services.

REVIEW QUESTIONS

1. Determine how you would test the accuracy of the health-related information you have received in your lifetime.
2. Identify and describe some sources of health-related information presented in this chapter. What factors should you consider when using these sources?
3. Point out the similarities between allopathic and osteopathic physicians. What is an alternative health-care practitioner? Give examples of each type of alternative practitioner.
4. Describe the services that are provided by the following restricted-practice health-care providers: dentists, psychologists, podiatrists, optometrists, and opticians. Identify several allied health-care professionals.
5. In what ways is the trend toward self-care evident? What are some reasons for the popularity of this movement?
6. What is health insurance? Explain the following terms relating to health insurance: deductible amount, fixed indemnity benefits, full-service benefits, coinsurance, exclusion, and preexisting illness.
7. What do the chemical name, brand name, and generic name of a prescription drug represent? OTC drugs are categorized according to what two factors?
8. In comparison with prescription medications and OTC products, what regulatory control does the FDA exercise over dietary supplements?
9. What is health-care quackery? What responsibilities have been given to the FDA? What can a consumer do to avoid consumer fraud?

THINK ABOUT THIS . . .

- How do you rate yourself as an informed consumer of health information, services, and products?
- Are there any types of providers mentioned in this chapter whom you would not choose to consult? Explain your answer.
- To what extent and in what ways have you engaged in self-care?
- Many insurance companies exclude certain kinds of illness (such as AIDS) from coverage and will not pay for the needed drugs. Who then should cover the cost? Under what circumstances do you think that expensive medications should be prescribed for terminally ill patients?
- Is life insurance more important than health insurance for young adults? Explain your answer.
- Why do you think it is difficult to get people to seek help for preventive care even though it is usually less expensive than treatment services?
- When you read a newspaper or magazine, do some health-rated advertisements seem questionable to you?

REFERENCES

1. Information on the Internet found to be usually accurate but also incomplete, *Qual Lett Healthc Lead* 13(7):11–12, 2001.
2. *Confusing health news,* Princeton Research Associates, 1999, Rodale Press.
3. *Trusted for on-line health,* MSB Associates, cyberdialogue/findsvp, February, 1999.

4. Hoffman-Toetz L, Clarke JN: Quality of breast cancer sites on the World Wide Web, *Can J Public Health* 91(4):281–284, 2000.
5. Tieman J: Med school downer. Applications decline for third year in a row, experts cite anti-affirmative action initiatives, *Mod Health* 30(38):18–19, 2000.
6. National Institutes of Health: Consensus Conference. Acupuncture, *JAMA* 280(17):1518–1524, 1998.
7. Acupuncture effective for certain medical conditions, panel says, *CAM Newsletter,* January 1998. **nccam.nih.gov/nccam/cam/jan/1.htm**
8. Studies evaluated homeopathy. *Complementary and Alternative Medicine at the NIH,* 5(3), 1998.
9. Verbach EU et al: Efficacy and tolerability of St. John's wort extract LI 160 versus imipramine in patients with severe depression episodes according to ICD-20, *Pharmacopsychiatry* 30 (suppl 2):81–85, 1997.
10. *Alternative medicine: expanding medical horizons—a report to the National Institutes of Health on alternative medical systems in the United States.* NIH Pub. No. 94-066, 1994.
11. Kaiser Family Foundation (KFF) state health facts online: 50 state comparison: average annual total employment-based premiums, 1998.
12. Industry facts-at-a-glance. National Association of Chain Drug Stores (NACDS), 2001.
13. Cornacchia HJ, Barrett S: *Consumer health: a guide to intelligent decisions,* ed 6, 1997, Mosby.

SUGGESTED READINGS

Brill D: *Cliffs Notes understanding health insurance,* 1999, IDG Books Worldwide.

There are *Cliffsnotes* for every other topic imaginable, so why not for health insurance? Regardless of whether you're taking an insurance class for college credit or you're a recent graduate looking for group or individual health insurance, this handy little book with the familiar yellow and black cover provides the basics. Money saved by having access to this book before purchasing health insurance might represent your first "great investment."

Edmunds M, Coye MJ (eds): *America's children: health insurance and access to care,* 1998, National Academy Press.

Over 40 million Americans, including children, have no health insurance. For them, the reality of illness and injury presents challenges in securing care, something that people who are insured take for granted. Reliance on Medicaid, the overuse of emergency rooms, and the absence of care altogether follows the children of the uninsured into the classroom and onto the playground. Students majoring in social work and early childhood education will find this book helpful in increasing their understanding of the stressors faced by many of their youngest clients and students.

Molony D: *The American Association of Oriental Medicine's complete guide to Chinese herbal medicine: how to treat illness and maintain wellness with Chinese herbal medicine,* 1998, Berkeley Publishing.

This book reviews the 4000-year-old history of Chinese medicine and explains the underlying principles of using herbs to promote inner balance. The author also details the efficacy and methods of use of 170 herbs, alone and in combination. The book includes a list of conditions that can be safely and effectively treated with herbs, a helpful glossary of terms, and the location of reputable suppliers of medicinal herbs.

Rappaport K (ed): *Directory of schools for alternative and complementary health care,* 1998, Orxy Press.

For people who are interested in entering the field of complementary health care, this book offers help in finding acceptable programs in the United States and Canada. It presents a wide array of information, including names, locations, telephone and fax numbers, courses of study, admission requirements, costs, and accessibility to people with disabilities. Although the programs are not ranked, background information is provided for accreditation, certification of graduates, and professional associations. A glossary of alternative medical terms appears at the end of the book.

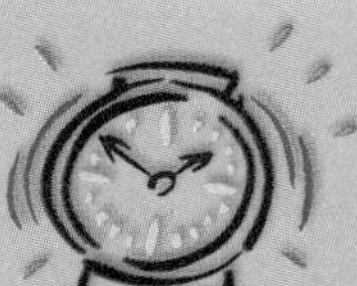

As we go to Press...

The practice of medicine is both an art and a science, and each is at times imperfect in its expression. This underlies the estimated 100,000 premature deaths that occur annually in America's hospitals, nursing homes, and physicians' offices. Clearly, prescription errors, nosocomial infections, inaccurately written orders, and surgical mistakes each hold the potential to cause deaths among hospital patients. But are there truly 100,000 such deaths each year?

In an article appearing in *Journal of the American Medical Association,* it was found that 100,000 deaths per year due to medical error is greatly inflated. Rather, an estimate of 10,000 and 15,000 has been suggested as more realistic. This considerably smaller number suggests that earlier figures were inflated due to the failure of earlier researchers to take into consideration those patients who would have died regardless of treatment and/or the absence of a common definition for what constitutes a medical error.

Name ______________________ **Date** __________ **Section** __________

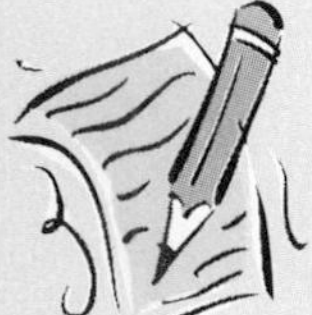

Personal Assessment

Are You a Skilled Health Consumer?

Circle the selection that best describes your practice. Then total your points for an interpretation of your health consumer skills.

1 Never
2 Occasionally
3 Most of the time
4 All of the time

1. I read all warranties and then file them for safekeeping.
   1 2 3 4
2. I read labels for information pertaining to the nutritional quality of food.
   1 2 3 4
3. I practice comparative shopping and use unit pricing, when available.
   1 2 3 4
4. I read health-related advertisements in a critical and careful manner.
   1 2 3 4
5. I challenge all claims pertaining to secret cures or revolutionary new health devices.
   1 2 3 4
6. I engage in appropriate medical self-care screening procedures.
   1 2 3 4
7. I maintain a patient-provider relationship with a variety of health-care providers.
   1 2 3 4
8. I inquire about the fees charged before using a health-care provider's services.
   1 2 3 4
9. I maintain adequate health insurance coverage.
   1 2 3 4
10. I consult reputable medical self-care books before seeing a physician.
    1 2 3 4
11. I ask pertinent questions of health-care providers when I am uncertain about the information I have received.
    1 2 3 4
12. I seek second opinions when the diagnosis of a condition or the recommended treatment seems questionable.
    1 2 3 4
13. I follow directions pertaining to the use of prescription drugs, including continuing their use for the entire period prescribed.
    1 2 3 4
14. I buy generic drugs when they are available.
    1 2 3 4
15. I follow directions pertaining to the use of OTC drugs.
    1 2 3 4
16. I maintain a well-supplied medicine cabinet.
    1 2 3 4

YOUR TOTAL POINTS __________

Interpretation

16–24 points	A very poorly skilled health consumer
25–40 points	An inadequately skilled health consumer
41–56 points	An adequately skilled health consumer
57–64 points	A highly skilled health consumer

To Carry This Further. . .

Could you ever have been the victim of consumer fraud? What will you need to do to be a skilled consumer?

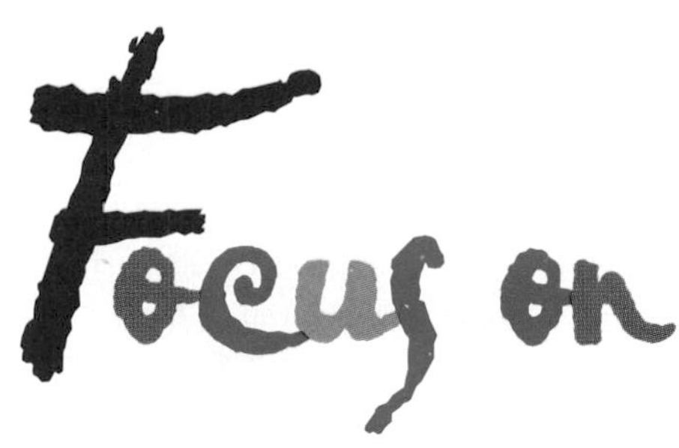

FACT OR FICTION? USING HEALTH INFORMATION ON THE INTERNET

So you want to find some information on health. Maybe you have a paper due in this class. Maybe you need more information on a condition that you or a loved one has. Or maybe you simply want to take advantage of the latest information on fitness and nutrition to make healthful decisions. No matter what information you're looking for, you can probably find it on the Internet. But be wary as you search—a great deal of misinformation is also available, and it may be hard for you to separate health fact from health fiction.

You can be relatively certain that government sites and links contain reliable information. In fact, the U.S. Department of Health and Human Services has established a site to provide consumer information. It can be accessed under Health/General Health or directly at **www.healthfinder.gov.** This site was launched in April 1997 to improve consumer access to federal health information online. As Healthfinder points out in its introductory paragraph, information alone can't take the place of health care you may need. But it can make you an informed partner in your own health care. This site leads you to selected on-line publications, databases, websites, support and self-help groups, government agencies, not-for-profit organizations, and universities that provide reliable health information to the public.[1]

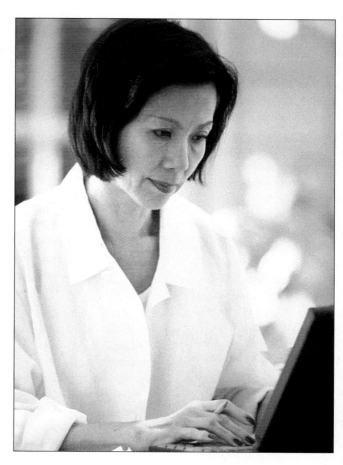

Using health information from reliable websites can help you become an active participant in your own health care.

Unfortunately, the government does not have the resources to filter out all false and misleading health-care information that appears on the Internet. Many people mistakenly believe that advertising claims must be true or advertisers would not be allowed to continue making them. Not enough time, money, and regulators are available to assess the validity of each and every health claim. However, health-care professionals and consumer advocates can give us the tools we need to determine the reliability of health information for ourselves.

What Is Quackery and How Can You Spot It?

One prominent consumer advocate is Stephen Barrett, a retired physician and nationally renowned author (with forty-five books to his credit).[2] In 1969 he founded the Lehigh Valley Committee against Health Fraud, which recently changed its name to Quackwatch. Investigation of questionable claims, answering of inquiries, distribution of reliable publications, reporting of illegal marketing, and improvement of the overall quality of health information on the Internet are all tasks that this group takes on.

Quackery is more difficult to spot than most people think.[3] Fraud is deliberate deception and is more easily recognized and corrected. Quackery involves the use of methods that are not scientifically valid,[4] therefore, information purveyed by quacks cannot be scientifically confirmed or denied. This is where the problem arises. There is no way to separate the good from the bad or the harmful from the benign or helpful.

Anecdotes and Testimonials

Some alternative health-care methods have been accepted by the scientific community, having met reliable criteria for safety and effectiveness; other methods are in the experimental stages. These methods are unproven but are based on plausible, rational principles and are undergoing responsible testing. But many other alternative health remedies are groundless and completely lack scientific rationale. Instead of scientific tests, people who promote these methods rely on anecdotes and testimonials to "prove" the effectiveness of their products. Much of the "success" of these products is due to the placebo effect; no cause-and-effect relationship has been established between use of the product and abatement of symptoms. People who use the remedies either get better coincidentally or think that their condition has improved simply because they're taking something for it.

Intelligent Consumer Behavior

Americans waste $50 million to $150 million per year on bogus mail-order health remedies.[5] Many of these products are now available on the Internet. You can avoid wasting your money in this way by not buying any of these products without medical advice from your physician or other health-care professional. And don't be fooled by money-back guarantees; they're usually as phoney as the products that they back.

Be wary of characteristic quackery ploys. Purveyors of quackery may say that they care about you, but their care, even if it were sincere, can't make useless medicine work. These products are commonly touted as having no side effects. If this is true, then the product is too weak to have any effect at all. Quacks will encourage you to jump on the bandwagon of their time-tested remedy, as if popularity and market longevity are surrogates for effectiveness. When they do claim that their products are backed by scientific studies, these studies turn out to be untraceable, misinterpreted, irrelevant, nonexistent, or based on poorly designed research.

The costs of buying into health-care quackery are more than financial. The psychological effects of disillusionment and the physical harm caused by the method itself or by abandoning more effective care are much worse.

HONcode Principles

Any reputable health information site on the Internet subscribes to the HONcode Principles. These principles are put forth and monitored by the Geneva-based Health On the Net Foundation and have arisen from input from webmasters and medical professionals in several countries.[6] According to these principles, any medical advice appearing at a site must meet the following requirements:

- It must be given by medically trained and qualified professionals unless a clear statement is made that the information comes from a nonmedically qualified individual or organization.
- The information must be intended to support, not replace, the physician-patient relationship.
- Data relating to individual patients and visitors to a medical website are confidential.
- Site information must have clear references to source data, and, where possible, specific links to that data.
- Claims related to the benefit or performance of a treatment, product, or service must be supported by appropriate, balanced evidence.
- The webmaster's e-mail address should be clearly displayed throughout the website.
- Commercial and noncommercial support and funding for the site should be clearly revealed.
- There must be a clear differentiation between advertising at the site and the original material created by the institution operating the site.

Be skeptical about any health information you find on the Internet that does not meet these criteria. Ask your physician whether the information is accurate, or move on to a more reliable site.

Assessing Health-Care Information

The Internet is a valuable health-care tool. Reliable information is supplied by government health agencies, research universities, hospitals, disease foundations, and other experts. However, not all health sites are reputable. As the saying goes, you can't believe everything you read, even if it's on the Internet. Anyone can create an on-line resource that looks professional. Ordinary people who believe they've been helped by a product, companies trying to sell products and services, and even cheats and quacks are all out there spouting their information. To protect yourself, you must be an informed consumer of information. To evaluate the credibility of an on-line source, ask yourself the following questions:[7]

1. Who is sponsoring the site?
2. Who manages this site?
3. What are the credentials of the sponsor and manager?
4. Who is the site's content intended for?
5. Does there appear to be any vested interests involving the site's sponsorship and management and the content of the site? (For example, is this a pharmaceutical manufacturer's site with content related to studies supported by the manufacturer?)
6. Is the information provided current and is the last updating posted on the site?
7. If opinionated statements are made, are they identified as such?

Although the Internet cannot and should not replace visits with a physician, reliable information obtained on the Net can make us more active partners in our own health-care. It can give us information we can use to stay healthy and prevent disease. It can help us to ask our doctors the right questions and educate us so that we're not afraid to ask them. It can connect us to people who are experiencing the same things as we are. It can help us learn about our health, receive support from others, and make sound health-care decisions based on fact—not fiction.

For Discussion . . .

Which health sites have you visited on the Internet? Did you find them informative? reliable? fun? What could be done to improve the status of health information on the Internet?

References

1. U.S. Department of Health and Human Services, 1999, **www.healthfinder.gov**
2. Rosen M: *Biography magazine interview of Dr. Stephen Barrett, M.D.*, November 17, 1998. **www.quackwatch.com/10Bio/biography.html**
3. Barrett S: *Common misconceptions*, 1997. **www.quackwatch.com/01QuackeryRelatedTopics/miscon.html**
4. Barrett S: *Quackery: how should it be defined*, 1997. **www.quackwatch.com/quackdof.html**
5. Barrett S: *Mail-order quackery*, 1996. **www.com/01QuackeryRelatedTopics/mailquack.html**
6. *Health On the Net Foundation. HONcode principles.* 1997 **www.quackwatch.com/00AboutQuackwatch/honcode.html**
7. Miller L: How to diagnose good sites, *USA Today*, July 14, 1999, p 5D.

chapter **16**

Protecting Your Safety

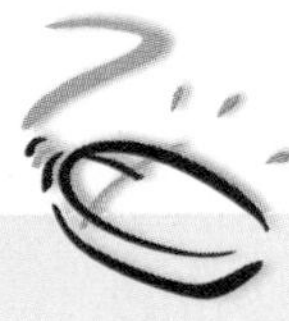

Online Learning Center Resources

www.mhhe.com/hahn6e

Log on to our Online Learning Center (OLC) for access to these additional resources:

- Chapter key terms and definitions
- Learning objectives
- Additional behavior change objectives
- Student interactive question-and-answer sites
- Self-scoring chapter quiz

The OLC also offers web links for study and exploration of health topics. Here are some examples of what you'll find:

- **www.drivers.com** Read up on traffic safety issues, get tips for new drivers, and learn how to deal with road rage.
- **www.jointogether.org** Get the facts about substance abuse and gun violence from people who are working to solve these problems in their own communities.
- **www.cybergrrl.com/planet/dv** Learn about domestic violence and how this problem affects children, the elderly, teenagers, and pregnant women.

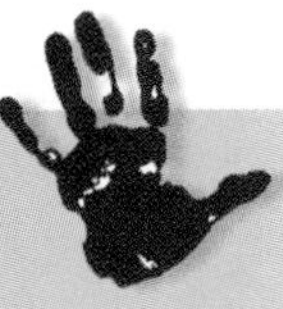

Taking Charge of Your Health

- Use the Personal Assessment on p. 423 to determine how well you manage your own safety.
- Assess your behaviors and those of your dating partners for signs of potential date rape by reviewing the "Avoiding Date Rape" box on p. 415
- Check you residence for the safety strategies listed on p. 416. Make the necessary changes to correct any deficiencies.
- Review the motor vehicle safety tips on p. 417. If you need to make changes to your car or your driving, begin working on them at once.
- Check the recommendations for recreational safety on p. 416, and put them into practice. Be assertive about using these measures when you are participating in activities with others.
- Find out about the security services available on your campus, and take advantage of them. Post the 24-hour-help phone number in your room and carry it with you.

Eye on the Media

Images of Terrorism: The World Trade Center Disaster

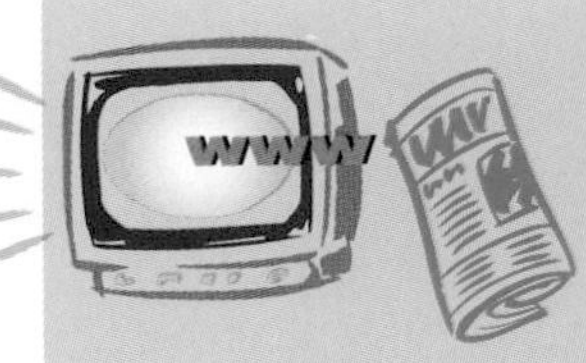

When terrorists attacked the world Trade Center in New York City on Tuesday, September 11, 2001, Americans—and the rest of the world—watched in horror as a plane struck one of the twin towers. Within minutes another plane crashed into the second tower. Two hours later, both towers had fallen. TV viewers saw Manhattan office workers running for their lives. They watched a person falling to his death. They saw firemen and other rescue workers going back into buildings that were clearly unsound to look for people who might still be alive.

For three full days the major TV networks suspended their regular programming to cover the disaster in depth. No commercials, no sitcoms, no soap operas, and no David Letterman or Jay Leno for days. When Letterman returned to the air, it wasn't to tell jokes but to have Dan Rather talk about the tragic events, and viewers saw the normally staunch newsman's eyes fill with tears. When *Saturday Night Live* featured New York Major Rudolph Giuliani, it was as a respected guest, not as a target for a spoof. By Saturday morning the cartoons were back—for the children.

Eye on the Media *continued*

Many people who were on their way to work or at home in their apartments in lower Manhattan on September 11, saw the events unfold before their eyes. For most Americans, who watched the real-life drama on TV, the effect was powerful. It was almost impossible not to watch what was happening. Some people who hadn't yet heard the news thought they were seeing a disaster movie.

In the days, weeks, and months that followed, the horrific nature of the terrorist attack began to take its toll. For the people who lost relatives or friends, uncertainty and disbelief were followed be denial and grief. But for the majority of Americans, who didn't know anyone personally who died in the World Trade Center disaster, there was still an enormous sadness and a general sense of unease.

People lost sleep and felt depressed. Some worried about having to get on an airplane again. Young children had an especially difficult time—wondering why this happened and whether *they* would be victims of a terrorist attack. Some children touched buildings to make sure they were "safe" before going inside.

Many worried about the future—about further attacks, about biological terrorism, and about this event as the beginning of a long, unconventional war against an elusive enemy. Most disturbing was the feeling that the United States would never be the same again, that Americans could never feel safe again. It wasn't the first time that Americans had seen themselves portrayed as a hated enemy. But the TV images of people in Afghanistan and Pakistan celebrating at our tragic misfortune took on new meaning and power. Why do these people hate us so much?—we wondered.

Where were you on the morning of September 11, 2001, when disaster struck? How did you hear the news—on TV, on the radio, or from a friend? Do you view your personal safety in a different way today?

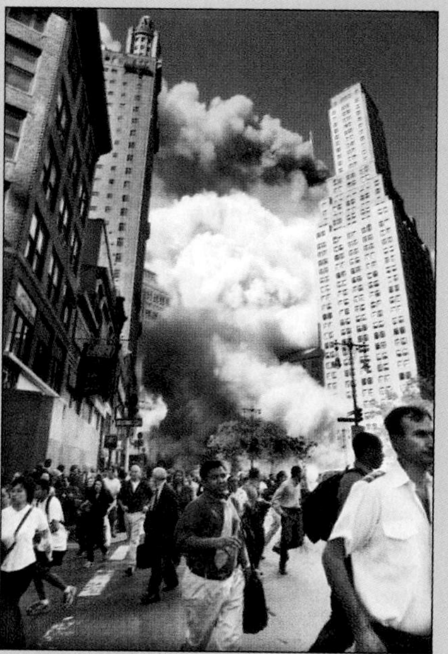

These people fleeing from the World Trade Center on the morning of September 11, 2001, were eye witnesses to the destruction of the landmark's south tower following a terrorist attack that resulted in the loss of thousands of lives.

As recently as 20 years ago, the suspicious disappearance of a school-aged child or the death of a bystander during a drive-by shooting was virtually unheard of. However, violent crimes are committed so frequently in the United States that it is difficult to watch a television news report or read a newspaper without seeing headlines announcing some heinous murder or other senseless act of violence, including terrorist acts.

Although the overall crime rate has dropped in the last decade, domestic violence continues to be directed at women and children, and many people fear being a random victim of a homicide, robbery, or carjacking. Law enforcement officials contend that gang activities and hard-core drug involvement are significant factors related to continued violent behavior in our society.

Although violence may seem to be focused in urban areas, no community is completely safe. Even people who live in small towns and rural areas now must lock their doors and remain vigilant about protecting their safety. Crime on college campuses remains a threat for all students. Complete the Personal Assessment on p. 423 to see whether you are adequately protecting your own safety.

INTENTIONAL INJURIES

Intentional injuries are injuries that are committed on purpose. Except for suicide (which is self-directed), intentional injuries reflect violence committed by one person acting against another person. Examples include homicide, robbery, rape, suicide, assault, child abuse, spouse abuse, and elder abuse. Each year in the United States, intentional injuries cause about 50,000 deaths and another 2 million nonfatal injuries.[1]

In 1999, nearly 29 million crimes were committed against U.S. residents age 12 and older, according to data collected by the National Crime Victimization Survey. More recently, the U.S. Bureau of Justice Statistics reported that the violent crime rate in the United States dropped 15% between 1999 and 2000.[2] This drop continued a downward trend in the violent crime rate since 1994.

Homicide

Homicide, or murder, is the intentional killing of one person by another. The United States leads the industrialized world in homicide rates. The 1999 murder rate was 5.7 per 100,000 inhabitants. Fortunately, this rate reflected an annual decline since 1991. In fact, this rate was the lowest since the late 1960s.[2]

Criminal justice experts are trying to pinpoint why U.S. homicide rates are dropping. No one answer has emerged, but speculation centers on better community policing efforts; the 1994 passage of the broad Federal Crime Bill; recent legislation, such as the Brady Law; and a variety of tough state laws, such as the "three strikes and you're out" provisions, that mandate life sentences without parole for repeat violent offenders. If recent incarceration rates do not change, an estimated 1 in 20 people (5.1%) will serve time in a state or federal prison. The chances of going to prison are higher for men (9%) than for women (1.1%).[3]

One continuing phenomenon is the extent to which illegal drug activity is related to homicide. A variety of research studies from large cities indicate that 25% to 50% of all homicides are drug related.[4] Most of these murders are associated with drug trafficking, including disputed drug transactions. Additionally, high percentages of both homicide assailants and victims have drugs in their systems at the time of the homicide.[4]

Handguns continue to be the weapon of choice for homicides. It was the proliferation of handguns and their use in violent crimes that led to the passage of the so-called Brady Law.

Domestic Violence

Domestic violence refers to criminal acts of violence committed within a home or homelike setting by people that have some type of relationship with the victim. This text will discuss three forms of domestic abuse: intimate abuse, child abuse, and elder abuse.

Intimate abuse

Intimate abuse refers to violence committed by a current or former spouse or boyfriend or girlfriend.[5] (This is the term currently used by the U.S. Department of Justice and is similar to *partner abuse.*) Intimate violence can include murder, rape, sexual assault, robbery, aggravated assault, and simple assault. Violent acts that constitute abuse range from a slap on the face to murder.

A 1998 report released by the Bureau of Justice Statistics revealed some slightly encouraging findings.[5] The report indicated that intimate nonlethal violence had declined somewhat since 1993. For example, in 1996, there were 840,000 female survivors of nonlethal violent crime, compared with 1.1 million female survivors in 1993. Nonlethal intimate violence against males remained steady between 1993 and 1996, at about 150,000 male survivors annually.

Cell Phone Safety While Driving

Cell phones that fit easily into a pocket or purse are being used in every place imaginable, including restaurants, theaters, subways, parks, golf courses, and, of course, in cars. And it's in cars that the use of cellular phones is most controversial. A variety of studies and reports indicate a four- to nine-fold increase in the potential for car crashes associated with the driver's use of a cell phone. In July 2001, the state of New York passed the country's first *statewide ban* on the use of hand-held cellular phones while driving. Violators of this ban are subject to a $100 fine for the first offense.

Research suggests the use of a cell phone decreases driver concentration and delays driver reaction time. The use of mounted, hands-free phones may improve safety, although the safety benefit has been controversial. Experts in traffic safety are careful to point out that there are too many other factors associated with driving to make it fair to blame behind-the-wheel phone use for all or most accidents. These complicating factors include adverse weather conditions, the structural integrity of the cars, the age and health of the drivers, radio, CD, or cigarette use, and interactions between drivers and passengers. The influence of other drivers on the road must also be considered.

If you must use your cell phone in a car, consider these commonsense rules: Get off the main road to a safe parking area to make your call, especially if the call is an important one or one that might upset you. If you must talk while driving, opt for a hands-free phone. Dial when your car is stopped. Keep calls very brief. Don't try to dial or talk in heavy traffic. Keep your eyes on the road. (Or, let a passenger make the call!)

Murders by intimates in 1996 reached the lowest levels since 1976. Intimate murders in 1996 were approximately 1800, whereas nearly 3000 such murders took place in 1976. As has been the case for many years, three of every four survivors of intimate murder in 1996 were female.[5]

One serious issue related to domestic violence is the vast underreporting of this crime to law enforcement authorities. The U.S. Department of Justice estimates that about half of the survivors of domestic violence do not report the crime to police. Too many survivors view these violent situations as private or personal matters and not actual crimes. Despite painful injuries, many survivors view the offenses against them as minor.

It's easy to criticize the survivors of domestic violence for not reporting the crimes committed against them, but this may be unfair. Why do women stay in abusive relationships? Many women who are injured may fear being killed if they report the crime. They may also fear for the safety of their children. Women who receive economic support from an abuser may worry about being left with no financial resources.

However, help is available for victims of intimate abuse. Most communities have family support or domestic violence hot lines that abused people can call for help. Many have shelters where abused women and their children can seek safety while their cases are being handled by the police or court officials. If you are being abused or know of someone who is being injured by domestic violence, don't hesitate to use the services of these local hot lines or shelters. Also, check the resources listed in the Health Reference Guide at the back of this text.

TALKING POINTS • A close friend confides that her boyfriend sometimes "gets rough" with her. She's afraid to talk to him about it because she thinks that will make things worse. What immediate steps would you tell her to take?

Child abuse

Like intimate abuse, **child abuse** tends to be a silent crime. It is estimated that about 1 million children are survivors of child abuse and neglect each year. Some children are survivors of repeated crimes, and since many survivors do not report these crimes, the actual incidence of child abuse is difficult to determine.

Children are abused in various ways.[6] Physical abuse reflects physical injury, such as bruises, burns, abrasions, cuts, and fractures of the bones and skull. Sexual abuse includes acts that lead to sexual gratification of the abuser. Examples include fondling, touching, and various acts involved in rape, sodomy, and incest. Child neglect is also a form of child abuse and includes an extreme failure to provide children with adequate clothing, food, shelter, and medical attention. A strong case can also be made for psychological abuse as a form of child abuse. Certainly, children are scarred by family members and others who routinely damage their psychological development. However, this form of abuse is especially difficult to identify and measure.

The most common form of child abuse is neglect.[6] The incidence of child neglect is approximately three times that of physical abuse and about seven times the incidence of child sexual abuse. Each form of abuse can have devastating consequences for the child—both short term and long term.

Research studies in child abuse reveal some noteworthy trends. Abused children are much more likely than nonabused children to grow up to be child abusers themselves. Abused children are also more likely to suffer from poor educational performance, increased health problems, and low levels of overall achievement. Recent research points out that abused children are significantly more likely than nonabused children to become involved in adult crime and violent criminal behavior.[6]

It is beyond the scope of this book to discuss the complex problem of reducing child abuse. However, the violence directed against children can likely be lessened through a combination of early identification measures and violence prevention programs. Teachers, friends, relatives, social workers, counselors, psychologists, police, and the court system must not hesitate to intervene as soon as child abuse is suspected. The later the intervention, the more likely that the abuse will have worsened. Once abuse has occurred, it is likely to happen again.

Violence prevention programs can help parents and caregivers learn how to resolve conflicts, improve communication, cope with anger, improve parenting skills, and challenge the view of violence presented in movies and television. Such programs may help stop violence before it begins to damage the lives of young children. Figure 16-1 provides simple alternatives parents can choose to avoid hitting a child.[7]

Elder abuse

Among the nation's 31 million elderly people, 1.5 million are survivors of neglect and abuse. Particularly vulnerable are women over the age of 75 years. Often, the abusers are the adult children of the victims.

Many elderly people are hit, kicked, attacked with knives, denied food and medical care, and have their Social Security checks and automobiles stolen. This problem reflects a combination of factors, particularly the stress of caring for failing older people by middle-aged children who are also faced with the demands of dependent children and careers. In many cases, the middle-aged children were themselves abused, or there may be a chemical dependence problem. The alternative, institutionalization, is so expensive that it is often not an option for either the abused or the abusers.

Key Terms

intentional injuries
Injuries that are purposely committed by a person.

homicide
The intentional killing of one person by another person.

intimate abuse
Violence committed against a person by her or his current or former spouse, boyfriend, or girlfriend.

child abuse
Harm that is committed against a child; usually referring to physical abuse, sexual abuse, or child neglect.

12 alternatives to lashing out at your child.

The next time everyday pressures build up to the point where you feel like lashing out—STOP! And try any of these simple alternatives.

You'll feel better . . . and so will your child.

1. Take a deep breath. And another. Then remember you are the adult . . .
2. Close your eyes and imagine you're hearing what your child is about to hear.
3. Press your lips together and count to 10. Or better yet, to 20.
4. Put your child in a time-out chair. (Remember the rule: one time-out minute for each year of age.)
5. Put yourself in a time-out chair. Think about why you are angry: is it your child, or is your child simply a convenient target for your anger?
6. Phone a friend.
7. If someone can watch the children, go outside and take a walk.
8. Take a hot bath or splash cold water on your face.
9. Hug a pillow.
10. Turn on some music. Maybe even sing along.
11. Pick up a pencil and write down as many helpful words as you can think of. Save the list.
12. Write for parenting information: Parenting, Box 2866, Chicago, IL 60690.

Take Time Out. Don't Take It Out On Your Child.

® National Committee for Prevention of Child Abuse

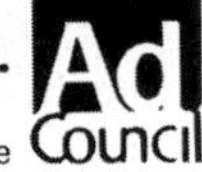

CHILD ABUSE PREVENTION CAMPAIGN
MAGAZINE AD NO. CA-2835-90—7" x 10"
Volunteer Agency: Lintas: Cambell-Ewald, Campaign Director: Beth M. Pritchard, S.C. Johnson & Son, Inc.

Figure 16-1 Alternatives to abusing your child.

Although protective services are available in most communities through welfare departments, elder abuse is frequently unseen and unreported. In many cases, the elderly people themselves are afraid to report their children's behavior because of the fear of embarrassment that they were not good parents to their children. Regardless of the cause, however, elder abuse must be reported to the appropriate protective service so that intervention can occur.

Gangs and Youth Violence

In the last 30 years, gangs and gang activities have been increasingly responsible for escalating violence and criminal activity. Before that time, gangs used fists, tire irons, and, occasionally, cheap handguns ("Saturday night specials"). Now, gang members don't hesitate to use AK-47s (semiautomatic military assault weapons) that have the potential to kill large groups of people in a few seconds.

Most, but not all, gangs arise from big city environments, where many socially alienated, economically disadvantaged young people live. Convinced that society has no significant role for them, gang members can receive support from an association of peers that has well-defined lines of authority. Rituals and membership initiation rites are important in gang socialization. Gangs often control particular territories within a city. Frequently, gangs are involved in criminal activities, commonly illicit drug trafficking and robberies.

Youth violence is also spreading from the inner cities to the suburbs. Public health officials and law enforcement personnel claim that youth violence is growing in epidemic proportions.

Attempting to control gang and youth violence is expensive for communities. For every gang-related homicide, there are about 100 nonfatal gang-related intentional injuries, so gang violence becomes an expensive health-care proposition. Furthermore, gang and youth violence takes an enormous financial and human toll on law enforcement, judicial, and corrections departments. Reducing gang and youth violence is a daunting task for the nation.

Gun Violence

The tragic effect of gun violence has already been touched on throughout this chapter. Guns are being used more than ever in our society and in other parts of the world. Gun violence is a leading killer of teenagers and young men, especially African American men, and the use of semiautomatic assault weapons by individuals and gang members continues. Accidental deaths of toddlers and young children from loaded handguns is another dimension of the violence attributable to guns in our society. In addition, guns are often used in **carjackings** (see the Changing for the Better box on p. 410).

The growing use of firearms has prompted serious discussions about enactment of gun control laws. For years, gun control activists have been in opposition with the National Rifle Association (NRA) and its congressional supporters. Gun control activists want fewer guns manufactured and greater controls over the sale and possession of handguns. Gun supporters believe that such controls are not necessary and that people (criminals) are responsible for gun deaths, not simply the guns. This debate will certainly continue.

TALKING POINTS • At a campus talk on carjacking, one college student announced that he planned to carry a registered gun to protect himself. How would you respond to his position?

Learning from Our Diversity

Violence against the Disabled

No one is totally free from the risk of senseless violence—children, adults, or college students. No single group, however, is a more tragic target of violence than the disabled. Despite the protective efforts of laws such as the Fair Housing Amendments Act, the Americans with Disabilities Act, and the Rehabilitation Act, the disabled remain an easily victimized segment of the population.

Because of the high level of vulnerability that disabled persons face, national advocacy groups, such as All Walks Of Life, are working to assist the disabled, their caregivers, and the general population in reducing the risk of violence to this group. However, much can also be accomplished on an individual basis. If you are an able-bodied college student, you can probably implement the following suggestions on your campus:

- Encourage your disabled peers to remain vigilant by staying tuned in to their environment. Remind them that simply because they appear disabled does not guarantee that they will be protected from harm.
- Support your disabled friends in the challenges imposed by their limitations, particularly when they are in unfamiliar environments or experiencing unusual situations.
- Suggest that your peers with disabilities carry, or wear a personal alarm device. Such devices, also frequently carried by able-bodied students, can be purchased in bookstores or sporting goods stores.
- Remind your disabled friends to inform others about their schedule plans, for example, when they will be away from school and when they are likely to return.
- Encourage people with disabilities to seek the assistance of an escort (security personnel) when leaving a campus building or a shopping mall to enter a large parking area.
- Be an advocate for your disabled friends. For example, if residence hall room doors do not have peepholes at wheelchair height, find out if the doors can be modified.

One additional approach remains controversial. That is the teaching of self-defense techniques to people with disabilities. Groups that advocate instruction to the disabled in the martial arts, such as judo, remind us that "doing nothing will produce nothing." Others contend that a limited ability to use a martial art leads to a false sense of confidence that encourages a disregard for other forms of protection. They further argue that if disabled persons try to counter aggression with ineffectively delivered martial arts techniques, they may anger their attacker and actually increase the aggression against themselves.

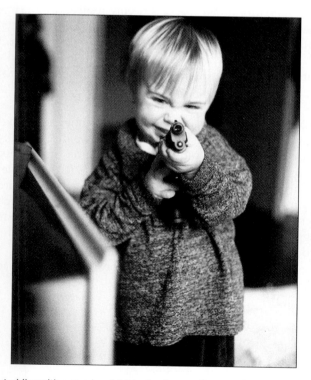

A toddler with a gun is a frightening image. Guns and ammunition should be stored separately in locked containers, and children should be taught that guns are not toys.

Bias and Hate Crimes

One sad aspect of any society is how some segments of the majority treat certain people in the minority. Nowhere is this more obvious than in **bias and hate crimes.** These crimes are directed at individuals or groups of people solely because of a racial, ethnic, religious, or other difference attributed to these minorities. The targeted individuals are often verbally and physically attacked, their houses are spray painted with various slurs, and many are forced to move from one neighborhood or community to another.

Key Terms

carjacking
A crime that involves a thief's attempt to steal a car while the owner is behind the wheel; carjackings are usually random, unpredictable, and frequently involve handguns.

bias and hate crimes
Criminal acts directed at a person or group solely because of a specific characteristic, such as race, religion, ethnic background, or political belief.

Changing *for the Better*

Preventing Carjacking

There have been several carjacking incidents in my area recently. What can I do to avoid this problem without carrying a gun?

In the last 10 years a new form of violence has reached the streets of America. This crime is commonly called *carjacking.* Unlike auto theft, in which a car thief attempts to steal an unattended parked car, carjacking involves a thief's attempt to steal a car with a driver still behind the wheel.

Most carjacking attempts begin when a car is stopped at an intersection, usually at a traffic light. A carjacker will approach the driver and force him or her to give up the car. Resisting an armed carjacker can be extremely dangerous. Law enforcement officials offer the following tips to prevent carjacking:

- Drive only on well-lit and well-traveled streets, if possible.
- Always keep your doors locked when driving your car.
- Observe traffic that may be following you. If you think that something suspicious is happening, try to locate a police officer or a busy, populated area to seek help.
- If someone approaches your car and you cannot safely drive away, roll the window down only slightly and leave the car running and in gear. If the situation turns bad, use your wits and quickly flee the scene, either in the car or on foot. Remember: your life is worth more than your car.
- If another car taps the rear bumper of your car (a common carjacking maneuver to get you to exit your car) and you feel uncomfortable about getting out of your car, tell the other driver that you are driving to the police station to complete the accident report.

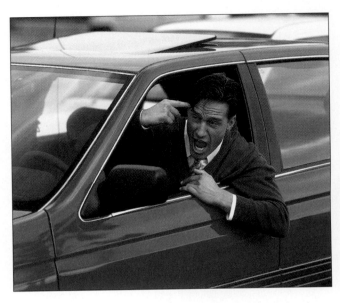

The stresses of home, work, and commuting, the anonymity of driving, and other factors can add up to road rage.

According to Federal Bureau of Investigation (FBI) statistics, there are about 8000 hate crime incidents in the United States each year.

Typically, the offenders in bias or hate crimes are fringe elements of the larger society who believe that the mere presence of someone with a racial, ethnic, or religious difference is inherently bad for the community, state, or country. Examples in the United States include skinheads, the Ku Klux Klan, and other white supremacist groups. (The case of Matthew Shepard [see the Star Box on p. 411] drew worldwide attention to hate crimes.) Increasingly, state and federal laws have been enacted to make bias and hate crimes serious offenses.

Road Rage

Within the last 10 years, a phenomenon called "road rage" has been on the rise on the streets and highways of the United States. This violence occurs when a driver becomes enraged at the driving behavior of others—cutting off someone, driving too slowly, going through yellow lights and red lights, playing loud music, passing a long line of cars on the shoulder, playing "chicken" as two lanes merge into one. Toss in horn-honking, four-letter words, and hand gestures, and you have all the elements of the daily commute.

Sometimes road rage has deadly results. It's not unusual for road ragers to force other cars into accidents. Since some drivers carry guns, they may injure or kill other drivers. These tragedies usually are not premeditated. They often happen when a driver loses control under the pressure of a triggering incident.

There is no typical profile of a person who expresses road rage. Although road ragers are frequently young-adult, aggressive males, road rage can be displayed by anyone who drives and is stressed by time constraints, family problems, or job difficulties. One quick way to determine if you are prone to road rage is to tape record your voice while you're driving. If you hear yourself screaming and complaining, you could be considered an aggressive driver. You will need to find ways to calm yourself during your commute.

To avoid becoming a perpetrator or a victim of road rage, follow these recommendations:

- Avoid making hand gestures
- Use your horn sparingly
- Allow plenty of time to reach your destination
- Imagine yourself being videotaped while driving
- Avoid blocking the passing lane
- Avoid switching lanes without signaling
- Use only one parking place
- Avoid parking in a space for disabled people, unless you are disabled

Violence Based on Sexual Orientation

Recent news reports indicate that violence based on sexual orientation continues to occur in the United States. Nowhere is this more clear than in the case of Matthew Shepard, an openly gay University of Wyoming freshman who was murdered in October 1998. Shepard was lured from a Laramie, Wyoming, bar by two young adult men posing as homosexuals. These men beat Shepard severely, stole $20 from him, and tied him to a fence post, where he was left to die. The men were later convicted of kidnapping and murder.

In July 1999, Barry Winchell, an Army private at Fort Campbell, Kentucky, was bludgeoned to death with a bat wielded by fellow private Calvin Glover. Glover, who said he was intoxicated when he committed the crime, was later convicted of premeditated murder in a military court and sentenced to life in prison, with the possibility of parole. Another soldier, charged as an accessory to the crime, apparently had spread rumors among members of the Army unit that Winchell was gay.[9] This accomplice also tried to clean up the scene of the crime. He was sentenced to 12 years in prison.

The murder of Private Winchell prompted calls for a reevaluation of the military's 1993 "don't ask, don't tell" policy concerning homosexuals.[10] Under this policy, gays can serve in the military as long as they do not disclose their sexual orientation. Superiors in the military cannot investigate or expel personnel who keep their sexual orientation to themselves. Some believe this "don't ask, don't tell" policy prevents military authorities from investigating complaints of harassment based on sexual orientation. This policy came up in the year 2000 presidential campaign and could be revised in the future.

Both of these deaths served as a reminder that the federal government has not yet passed the Hate Crimes Prevention Act. Supported by President Clinton, but not passed by Congress at the time of this writing, this proposed legislation would add acts of hatred motivated by sexual orientation, gender, and disability to the list of hate crimes already covered by federal law. Among these crimes already covered are ones motivated by prejudice based on race, religion, color, or national origin.

It will be interesting to see whether this proposed federal legislation will be enacted soon. The public outcry following the deaths of Matthew Shepard and Barry Winchell indicates that much support exists for some version of a Hate Crimes Prevention Act.

- Refrain from tailgating
- Do not allow your door to hit the parked car next to you
- If you drive slowly, pull over and let others pass
- Avoid the unnecessary use of high-beam headlights
- Do not talk on a car phone while driving
- Avoid making eye contact with aggressive drivers
- Keep your music volume under control

Always drive defensively. Assume that a difficult situation may get out of hand, so conduct yourself in a calm, courteous manner. It's better to swallow your pride and preserve your health than to risk unnecessary danger to yourself or other people on the road.

TALKING POINTS • You're in a car with a friend when another driver starts tailgating you very closely. Your friend (the driver) slows down to annoy the tailgater. How would you convince your friend that his action is dangerous?

Stalking

In recent years the crime of stalking has received considerable attention. **Stalking** refers to an assailant's planned efforts to pursue an intended victim. Most stalkers are male. Many stalkers are excessively possessive or jealous and pursue people with whom they formerly had a relationship. Other stalkers pursue people with whom they have had only an imaginary relationship.

Stalkers often go to great lengths to locate their intended victims and frequently know their daily whereabouts. Although not all stalkers plan to batter or kill the person they are pursuing, their presence and potential for violence can create an extremely frightening environment for the intended victim and family. Some stalkers serve time in prison for their offense, waiting years to "get back at" their victims.

Virtually all states have enacted or tightened their laws related to stalking and have created stiff penalties for offenders. In many areas the criminal justice system is proactive in letting possible victims of stalking know, for example, when a particular prison inmate is going to be released. In other areas, citizens are banding together to provide support and protection for people who may be victims of stalkers.

Key Term

stalking
A crime involving an assailant's planned efforts to pursue an intended victim.

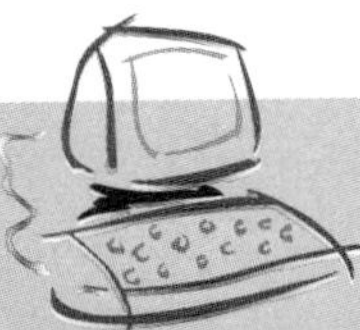

OnSITE/InSIGHT

Learning to Go: Health

Are you proactive about your personal safety? Click on the Motivator icon to check out the following lessons:

Lesson 46: Protect yourself from rape and sexual assault.
Lesson 48: Avoid becoming a victim of crime.
Lesson 50: Keep yourself safe at home.
Lesson 51: Play it safe when you're having fun.
Lesson 52: Drive safely and defensively.
Lesson 53: Shield yourself from road rage.

STUDENT POLL

Is personal safety an ongoing concern of yours? Go to the Online Learning Center at **www.mhhe.com/hahn6e**. Access student Resources to find the Student Poll. Answer these questions and then check out how other students responded.

1. Do you feel safe in your home?
2. Do you feel safe in your work or school environment?
3. Are you trained in first aid or CPR?
4. Do you often experience road rage?
5. Have you ever physically taken your anger out on someone?
6. Do you practice techniques to help control your emotions (time-out, walks, etc.)?
7. Have you ever witnessed abuse, or known about it, and not reported it?
8. Have you ever suffered from domestic violence?

If you think you are or someone you know is being stalked, contact the police (or a local crisis intervention hot line number) to report your case and follow their guidance. Be on the alert if someone from a past relationship suddenly reappears in your life or if someone seems to be irrationally jealous of you or overly obsessed with you. Report anyone who continues to pester or intimidate you with phone calls, notes or letters, e-mails, or unwanted gifts. Report people who persist in efforts to be with you after you have told them you don't want to see them. Until the situation is resolved, be alert for potentially threatening situations and keep in close touch with friends. Exploring Your Spirituality (p. 413) features the question of dealing with fear in our lives.

TALKING POINTS • You suspect that someone is stalking you, but your friends think you're being dramatic. How would you get objective advice on what to do?

SEXUAL VICTIMIZATION

Ideally, sexual intimacy is a mutual, enjoyable form of communication between two people. Far too often, however, relationships are approached in an aggressive, hostile manner. These sexual aggressors always have a victim—someone who is physically or psychologically traumatized. *Sexual victimization* occurs in many forms and in a variety of settings. This section takes a brief look at sexual victimization as it occurs in rape and sexual assault, sexual abuse of children, sexual harassment, and the commercialization of sex.

Rape and Sexual Assault

As violence in our society increases, the incidence of rape and sexual assault correspondingly rises. The victims of these crimes fall into no single category. Victims of *rape* and *sexual assault* include young and old, male and female. They can be the mentally retarded, prisoners, hospital patients, and college students. We all are potential victims, and self-protection is critical. Read the Star Box on p. 414 concerning myths about rape.

Sometimes a personal assault begins as a physical assault that turns into a rape situation. Rape is generally considered a crime of sexual aggression in which the victim is forced to have sexual intercourse. Current thought about rape characterizes this behavior as a violent act that happens to be carried out through sexual contact. (See the Changing for the Better boxes on p. 413 and 414 on rape awareness guidelines and help for the rape survivor.)

Acquaintance and date rape

In recent years, closer attention has been paid to the sexual victimization that occurs during relationships. *Acquaintance rape* refers to forced sexual intercourse between individuals who know each other. *Date rape* is a form of acquaintance rape that involves forced sexual intercourse by a dating partner. Studies on a number of campuses suggest that about 20% of college women reported having experienced date rape. An even higher percentage of women report being kissed and touched against their will. Alcohol is frequently a significant contributing factor in these rape situations. (See Chapter 8 concerning alcohol's role in campus crime.) Some men have reported being psychologically coerced into intercourse by their female dating partners. In many cases the aggressive partner will display

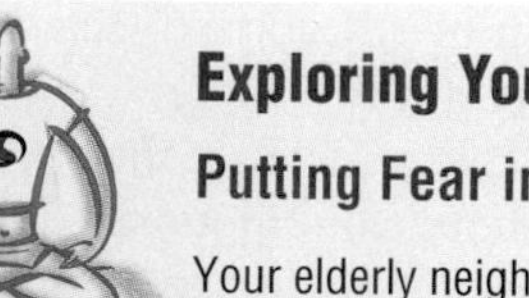

Exploring Your Spirituality

Putting Fear in Perspective

Your elderly neighbor stays locked in her house all day, afraid to open the door to anyone. Too many hours of watching local TV news, you think. But it's not just older people who are living in fear. Parents, women, gays, and minorities are all looking over their shoulders.

Some parents who walked to school when they were children wouldn't think of letting their kids do that. What about child molesters and kidnappers? A young woman at a party guards her drink all night—afraid that someone might put a drug in it. She's afraid of being raped. The gay person who goes to his old neighborhood to visit his grandmother feels uneasy. Is it his imagination, or are people looking at him in a threatening way? An African American man walking down the street hears a racial slur. Should he ignore it, or stop and say something?

All of these situations call for caution. If you're a parent, you need to be careful about your child's safety. But your child can walk to school—accompanied by you, another parent, or an older child. If you're a woman, you can keep an eye on your drink at a party without making that the focus of your attention. If you're a gay man who feels uncomfortable in an unfamiliar part of town, stay focused on where you're going. Walk quickly and confidently, without being intimidated. If you're a minority who's being taunted, keep your dignity and remain calm.

Putting fear in perspective takes practice. First, stay reasonable. Recognize that acts of violence represent the extreme elements of society. There's a good reason you probably haven't met many (or any) murderers, robbers, or rapists. They make up a small segment of society. The people you usually encounter, who are basically good, represent the large majority. Second, be aware. Pay attention to what's going on around you. See things in a neutral way. If you do, you'll realize when an argument is about to turn into a fistfight or worse. Third, use common sense. Don't put yourself at risk, but don't stop living. You can't build your life around avoiding a potential act of violence. Fourth, trust your senses. If someone is walking too close to you and you feel uncomfortable, cross the street and go into a store. Last, practice what-if situations. For example, what would you do if you were in your car at a stoplight and someone held a gun up to your window? Considering your possible actions ahead of time, without dwelling on them, is one way of preparing yourself for real-life threats.

Living in fear is something that happens gradually—as fear takes control of a person's life. But that doesn't need to happen to you. You can take control of fear in a healthy, positive way—to build a life of rich experiences balanced by caution and good sense.

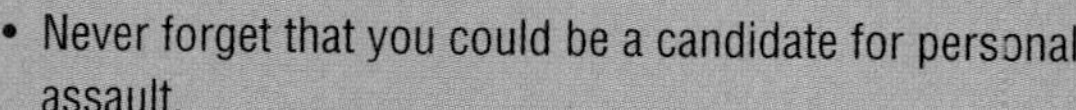

Changing *for the Better*

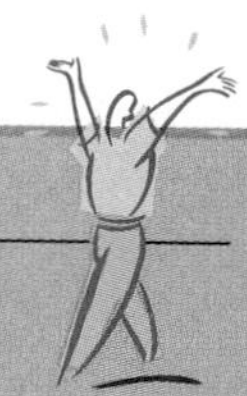

Rape Awareness Guidelines

I don't want to live in fear, but I have a special concern about the potential for rape. What common sense things should I be doing to avoid this possibility?

- Never forget that you could be a candidate for personal assault.
- Use approved campus security or escort services, especially at night.
- Think carefully about your patterns of movement to and from class or work. Alter your routes frequently.
- Walk briskly with a sense of purpose. Try not to walk alone at night.
- Dress so that the clothes you wear do not unnecessarily restrict your movement or make you more vulnerable.
- Always be aware of your surroundings. Look over your shoulder occasionally. Know where you are so that you won't get lost.
- Avoid getting into a car if you do not know the driver well.
- If you think you are being followed, look for a safe retreat. This might be a store, a fire or police station, or a group of people.
- Be especially cautious of first dates, blind dates, or people you meet at a party or bar who push to be alone with you.
- Let trusted friends know where you are and when you plan to return.
- Keep your car in good working order. Think beforehand how you would handle the situation should your car break down.
- Limit, and even avoid, alcohol to minimize the risk of rape.
- Trust your best instincts if you are assaulted. Each situation is different. Do what you can to protect your life.

Myths about Rape

Despite the fact that we are all potential victims, many of us do not fully understand how vulnerable we are. Rape, in particular, has associated with it a number of myths (false assumptions), including the following:

- Women are raped by strangers. In approximately half of all reported rapes, the victim has some prior acquaintance with the rapist. Increasingly, women are being raped by husbands, dating partners, and relatives.
- Rapes almost always occur in dark alleys or deserted places. The opposite is true. Most rapes occur in or very near the victim's residence.
- Rapists are easily identified by their demeanor or psychological profile. Most experts indicate that rapists do not differ significantly from nonrapists.
- The incidence of rape is overreported. Estimates are that only one in five rapes is reported.
- Rape happens only to people in low socioeconomic classes. Rape occurs in all socioeconomic classes. Each person, male or female, young or old, is a potential victim.
- There is a standard way to escape from a potential rape situation. Each rape situation is different. No one method to avoid rape can work in every potential rape situation. Because of this, we encourage personal health classes to invite speakers from a local rape prevention services bureau to discuss approaches to rape prevention.

certain behaviors that can be categorized (see the Changing for the Better box on p. 415).

Psychologists believe that aside from the physical harm of date rape, a greater amount of emotional damage may occur. Such damage stems from the concept of broken trust. Date rape victims feel particularly violated because the perpetrator was not a stranger: it was someone they initially trusted, at least to some degree. Once that trust is broken, developing new relationships with other people becomes much more difficult for the date rape victim.

Nearly all victims of date rape seem to suffer from *post-traumatic stress syndrome.* They may have anxiety, sleeplessness, eating disorders, and nightmares. Guilt concerning their own behavior, loss of self-esteem, and judgment of other people can be overwhelming, and the individual may require professional counseling. Because of the seriousness of these consequences, all students should be aware of the existence of date rape.

Date rape drugs

As you may recall from Chapter 7, Rohypnol, GHB (liquid ecstasy, G), and ketamine (K, Special K, and Cat) have joined alcohol as forms of date rape intoxicants. For their own safety, students must be vigilant about being duped into consuming substances that increase the likelihood of sexual assault and violence.

Sexual Abuse of Children

One of the most tragic forms of sexual victimization is the sexual abuse of children. Children are especially vulnerable to sexual abuse because of their dependent relationships with parents, relatives, and caregivers (such as babysitters, teachers, and neighbors). Often, children are unable to readily understand the difference between appropriate and inappropriate physical contact. Abuse may range from blatant physical manipulation, including fondling, to oral sex, sodomy, and intercourse.

Changing *for the Better*

Help for the Rape Survivor

If I should be in a position to help someone who has been raped, what information do we both need to know?

- *Call the police immediately to report the assault.* Police can take you to the hospital and start gathering information that may help them apprehend the rapist. Fortunately, many police departments now use specially trained officers (many of whom are female) to work closely with rape victims during all stages of the investigation.
- If you do not want to contact the police immediately, *call a local rape crisis center.* Operated generally on a 24-hour hot line basis, these centers have trained counselors to help the survivor evaluate her options, contact the police, escort her to the hospital, and provide aftercare counseling.
- *Do not alter any potential evidence related to the rape.* Do not change your clothes, douche, take a bath, or rearrange the scene of the crime. Wait until all the evidence has been gathered.
- *Report all bruises, cuts, and scratches, even if they seem insignificant.* Report any information about the attack as completely and accurately as possible.
- *You will probably be given a thorough pelvic examination.* You may have to ask for STD tests and pregnancy tests.
- Although it is unusual for a rape victim's name to appear in the media, you might *request that the police withhold your name* as long as is legally possible.

Changing *for the Better*

Avoiding Date Rape

I've heard that there are warning signs for date rape. What signs should I be alert for?

First, consider your partner's behaviors. Many, but not all, date rapists show one or more of the following behaviors: a disrespectful attitude toward you and others, lack of concern for your feelings, violence and hostility, obsessive jealousy, extreme competitiveness, a desire to dominate, and unnecessary physical roughness. Consider these behaviors as warning signs for possible problems in the future. Reevaluate your participation in the relationship.

Below are some specific ways both men and women can avoid a date rape situation:

Men

- *Know your sexual desires and limits.* Communicate them clearly. Be aware of social pressures. It's OK not to score.
- *Being turned down when you ask for sex is not a rejection of you personally.* Women who say no to sex are not rejecting the person; they are expressing their desire not to participate in a single act. Your desires may be beyond control, but your actions are within your control.
- *Accept the woman's decision.* "No" means "No." Don't read other meanings into the answer. Don't continue after you are told "No!"
- *Don't assume that just because a woman dresses in a sexy manner and flirts that she wants to have sexual intercourse.*
- *Don't assume that previous permission for sexual contact applies to the current situation.*
- *Avoid excessive use of alcohol and drugs.* Alcohol and other drugs interfere with clear thinking and effective communication.

Women

- *Know your sexual desires and limits.* Believe in your right to set those limits. If you are not sure, STOP and talk about it.
- *Communicate your limits clearly.* If someone starts to offend you, tell him so firmly and immediately. Polite approaches may be misunderstood or ignored. Say "No" when you mean "No."
- *Be assertive.* Often men interpret passivity as permission. Be direct and firm with someone who is sexually pressuring you.
- *Be aware that your nonverbal actions send a message.* If you dress in a sexy manner and flirt, some men may assume you want to have sex. This does not make your dress or behavior wrong, but it is important to be aware of a possible misunderstanding.
- *Pay attention to what is happening around you.* Watch the nonverbal clues. Do not put yourself into vulnerable situations.
- *Trust your intuitions.* If you feel you are being pressured into unwanted sex, you probably are.
- *Avoid excessive use of alcohol and drugs.* Alcohol and other drugs interfere with clear thinking and effective communication.

Because of the subordinate role of children in relationships involving adults, sexually abusive practices often go unreported. Sexual abuse can leave emotional scars that make it difficult to establish meaningful relationships later in life. For this reason, it is especially important for people to pay close attention to any information shared by children that could indicate a potentially abusive situation. Most states require that information concerning child abuse be reported to law enforcement officials.

Sexual Harassment

Sexual harassment consists of unwanted attention of a sexual nature that creates embarrassment or stress. Examples of sexual harassment include unwanted physical contact, excessive pressure for dates, sexually explicit humor, sexual innuendos or remarks, offers of job advancement based on sexual favors, and overt sexual assault. Unlike more overt forms of sexual victimization, sexual harassment may be applied in a subtle manner and can, in some cases, go unnoticed by coworkers and fellow students. Still, sexual harassment produces stress that cannot be resolved until the harasser is identified and forced to stop. Both men and women can be victims of sexual harassment.

Sexual harassment can occur in many settings, including employment and academic settings. On the college campus, harassment may be primarily in terms of the offer of sex for grades. If this occurs to you, think carefully about the situation and document the specific times, events, and places where the harassment took place. Consult your college's policy concerning harassment. Next, you could report these events to the appropriate administrative officer (perhaps the affirmative action officer, dean of academic affairs, or dean of students). You may also want to discuss the situation with a staff member of the university counseling center.

If harassment occurs in the work environment, the victim should document the occurrences and report them to the appropriate management or personnel official. Reporting procedures will vary from setting to setting. Sexual harassment is a form of illegal sex discrimination and violates Title VII of the Civil Rights Act of 1964.

In 1986 the U.S. Supreme Court ruled that the creation of a "hostile environment" in a work setting was sufficient evidence to support the claim of sexual harassment. This action served as an impetus for thousands of women to step forward with sexual harassment allegations. Additionally, some men are also filing sexual harassment lawsuits against female supervisors.

Not surprisingly, this rising number of complaints has served as a wake-up call for employers. From university settings to factory production lines to corporate board rooms, employers are scrambling to make certain that employees are fully aware of actions that could lead to a sexual harassment lawsuit. Sexual harassment workshops and educational seminars on harassment are now common and serve to educate both men and women about this complex problem.

Violence and the Commercialization of Sex

It is beyond the scope of this book to explore whether sexual violence can be related to society's exploitation or commercialization of sex. However, sexually related products and messages are intentionally placed before the public to try to sway consumer decisions. Do you believe that there could be a connection between commercial products, such as violent pornography in films and magazines, and violence against women? Does prostitution lead directly to violence? Do sexually explicit "900" phone numbers or Internet pornography cause an increase in violent acts? Can the sexual messages in beer commercials lead to acquaintance rape? What do you think?

UNINTENTIONAL INJURIES

Unintentional injuries are injuries that have occurred without anyone intending that any harm be done. Common examples include injuries resulting from car crashes, falls, fires, drownings, firearm accidents, recreational accidents, and residential accidents. Each year, unintentional injuries account for over 150,000 deaths and millions of nonfatal injuries.

Unintentional injuries are very expensive for our society, both from a financial standpoint and from a personal and family standpoint. Fortunately, to a large extent it is possible to avoid becoming a victim of an unintentional injury. By carefully considering the tips presented in the safety categories that follow, you will be protecting yourself from many preventable injuries.

Since this section of the chapter focuses on a selected number of safety categories, we encourage readers to consider some additional, related activities. For further information in the area of safety, consult a safety textbook (one of which is listed in the references for this chapter).[8] Finally, we encourage you to take a first aid course from the American Red Cross. American Red Cross first aid courses incorporate a significant amount of safety prevention information along with the teaching of specific first aid skills.

Residential Safety

Many serious accidents and personal assaults occur in dorm rooms, apartments, and houses. As a responsible adult, you should make every reasonable effort to prevent these tragedies from happening. One good idea is to discuss some of the following points with your family or roommates and implement needed changes:

- Fireproof your residence. Are all electrical appliances and heating and cooling systems in safe working order? Are flammable materials safely stored?
- Prepare a fire escape plan. Install smoke or heat detectors.
- Do not give personal information over the phone.
- Use initials for first names on mailboxes and in phone books.
- Install a peephole and deadbolt locks on outside doors.
- If possible, avoid living in first floor apartments. Change locks when moving to a new apartment or home.
- Put locks on all windows.
- Require repair people or delivery people to show valid identification.
- Do not use an elevator if it is occupied by someone who makes you feel uneasy.
- Be cautious around garages, laundry rooms, and driveways (especially at night). Use lighting for prevention of assault.

Recreational Safety

The thrills we get from risk-taking are an essential part of our recreational endeavors. Sometimes we can get into serious accidents because we fail to consider important recreational safety information. Do some of the following recommendations apply to you?

- Seek appropriate instruction for your intended activity. Few skill activities are as easy as they look.
- Always wear your automobile seat belt.
- Make certain that your equipment is in excellent working order. Use specific safety gear designed for cycling, in-line skating, and scooter use.
- Involve yourself gradually in an activity before attempting more complicated, dangerous skills.
- Enroll in an American Red Cross first aid course to enable you to cope with unexpected injuries.
- Remember that alcohol use greatly increases the likelihood that people will get hurt.
- Protect your eyes from serious injury.
- Learn to swim. Drowning occurs most frequently to people who never intended to be in the water.

- Obey the laws related to your recreational pursuits. Many laws are directly related to the safety of the participants.
- Be aware of weather conditions. Many outdoor activities turn to tragedy with sudden shifts in the weather. Always prepare yourself for the worst possible weather.

Firearm Safety

Each year about 13,000 Americans are murdered with guns and another 2000 die in gun-related accidents. Most murders are committed with handguns. (Shotguns and rifles tend to be more cumbersome than handguns and thus are not as frequently used in murders, accidents, or suicides.) Over half of all murders result from quarrels and arguments between acquaintances or relatives. With many homeowners arming themselves with handguns for protection against intruders, it is not surprising that over half of all gun accidents occur in the home. Children are frequently involved in gun accidents, often after they discover a gun they think is unloaded. Handgun owners are reminded to adhere to the following safety reminders:

- Make certain that you follow the gun possession laws in your state. Special permits may be required to carry a handgun.
- Make certain that your gun is in good mechanical order.
- If you are a novice, enroll in a gun safety course.
- Consider every gun to be a loaded gun, even if someone tells you it is unloaded.
- Never point a gun at an unintended target.
- Keep your finger off the trigger until you are ready to shoot.
- When moving with a handgun, keep the barrel pointed down.
- Load and unload your gun carefully.
- Store your gun and ammunition safely in a locked container. Use a trigger lock on your gun when not in use.
- Take target practice only at approved ranges.
- Never play with guns at parties. Never handle a gun when intoxicated.
- Educate children about gun safety and the potential dangers of gun use. Children must never believe that a gun is a toy.

Motor Vehicle Safety

The greatest number of accidental deaths in the United States take place on highways and streets. Young people are most likely to die from a motor vehicle accident (Figure 16-2). According to Bever,[8] the following is a description of a prime candidate for such a death:

> a male, 15 to 24 years of age, driving on a two-lane, rural road between the hours of 10 PM and 2 AM on a Saturday night. If he has been drinking and is driving a subcompact car or motorcycle, the likelihood that he and his passengers will have a fatal accident is even more pronounced.

Motor vehicle accidents also cause disabling injuries. With nearly 2 million such injuries each year, concern for the prevention of motor vehicle accidents should be important for all college students, regardless of age. With this thought in mind, we offer some important safety tips for motor vehicle operators:

- Make certain that you are familiar with the traffic laws in your state.
- Do not operate an automobile or motorcycle unless it is in good mechanical order. Regularly inspect your brakes, lights, and exhaust system.
- Do not exceed the speed limit. Observe all traffic signs.
- Always wear safety belts, even on short trips. Require your passengers to buckle up. Always keep small children in child restraints.
- Never drink and drive. Avoid horseplay inside a car.
- Be certain that you can hear the traffic outside your car. Keep the car's radio/music system at a reasonable decibel level.
- Give pedestrians the right-of-way.
- Drive defensively at all times. Do not challenge other drivers. Refrain from drag racing.
- Look carefully before changing lanes.
- Be especially careful at intersections and railroad crossings.
- Carry a well-maintained first aid kit that includes flares or other signal devices.
- Alter your driving behavior during bad weather.
- Do not drive when you have not had enough sleep (see the Focus on box, p. 425).

Home Accident Prevention for Children and the Elderly

Approximately 1 person in 10 is injured each year in a home accident. Children and the elderly spend significantly more hours each day in a home setting than do young adults and midlife people. It is especially important that accident prevention be given primary consideration for these groups (see the Changing for the Better box on p. 419). Here are some important tips to remember. Can you think of others?

Key Term

unintentional injuries
Injuries that have occurred without anyone's intending that harm be done.

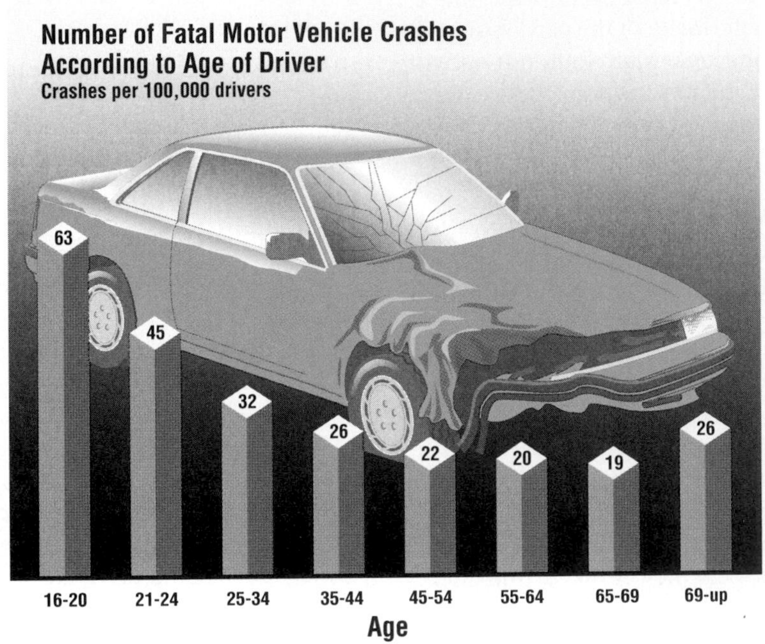

Figure 16-2 Driving is a dangerous activity for those under age 25. What could be done to reduce the number of driving fatalities among this age group?

For everyone

- Be certain that you have adequate insurance protection.
- Install smoke detectors appropriately.
- Keep stairways clear of toys and debris. Install railings.
- Maintain electrical and heating equipment.
- Make certain that inhabitants know how to get emergency help.

For children

- Know all the ways to prevent accidental poisoning.
- Use toys that are appropriate for the age of the child.
- Never leave young children unattended, especially infants.
- Keep any hazardous items (guns, poisons, etc.) locked up.
- Keep small children away from kitchen stoves.

For the elderly

- Protect from falls.
- Be certain that elderly people have a good understanding of the medications they may be taking. Know the side effects.
- Encourage elderly people to seek assistance when it comes to home repairs.
- Make certain that all door locks, lights, and safety equipment are in good working order.

Refer to pp. 407–408 for additional information related to the protection of older adults.

CAMPUS SAFETY AND VIOLENCE PREVENTION

Although many of the topics in this chapter are unsettling, students and faculty must continue to lead normal lives in the campus environment despite potential threats to our health. The first step in being able to function adequately is knowing about these potential threats. You have read about these threats in this chapter; now you must think about how this information applies to your campus situation.

The campus environment is no longer immune to many of the social ills that plague our society. At one time the university campus was thought to be a safe haven from the real world. Now there is plenty of evidence to indicate that significant intentional and unintentional injuries can happen to anyone at any time on the college campus.

For this reason, you must make it a habit to think constructively about protecting your safety. In addition to the personal safety tips presented earlier in this chapter, remember to use the safety assistance resources available on your campus. One of these might be your use of university-approved escort services, especially in the evenings as you move from one campus location to another. Another resource is the campus security department (campus police). Typically, campus police have a

Changing *for the Better*

Making Your Home Safe, Comfortable, and Secure

I take a common sense approach to safety, but I worry sometimes that I haven't thought about something important. What's the basic checklist for different areas?

Entry

- Install a deadbolt lock on the front door and locks or bars on the windows.
- Add a peephole or small window in the front door.
- Trim bushes so burglars have no place to hide.
- Add lighting to the walkway and next to the front door.
- Get a large dog.

Bedroom and Nursery

- Install a smoke alarm and a carbon monoxide detector.
- Remove high threshold at doorway to avoid tripping.
- Humidifiers can be breeding grounds for bacteria; use them sparingly and follow the manufacturer's cleaning instructions.
- In the nursery, install pull-down shades or curtains instead of blinds with strings that could strangle a child.

Living Room

- Secure loose throw rugs or use ones with nonskid backing.
- Remove trailing wires where people walk.
- Cover unused electrical outlets if there are small children in the home.
- Provide additional lighting for reading, and install adjustable blinds to regulate glare.

Kitchen

- To avoid burns, move objects stored above the stove to another location.
- Install ceiling lighting and additional task lighting where food is prepared.
- Keep heavy objects on bottom shelves or countertops; store lightweight or seldom-used objects on top shelves.
- Promptly clean and store knives.
- Keep hot liquids such as coffee out of children's reach, and provide close supervision when the stove or other appliances are in use.
- To avoid food-borne illness, thoroughly clean surfaces that have come into contact with raw meat.

Bathroom

- A child can drown in standing water; keep the toilet lid down and the tub empty.
- Clean the shower, tub, sink, and toilet regularly to remove mold, mildew, and bacteria that can contribute to illness.
- Store medications in their original containers in a cool, dry place out of the reach of children.
- Add a bath mat or nonskid strips to the bottom of the tub.
- Add grab bars near the tub or shower and toilet, especially if there are elderly adults in the home.
- Keep a first-aid kit stocked with bandages, first-aid ointment, gauze, pain relievers, syrup of Ipecac, and isotonic eyewash; include your physician's and a nearby emergency center's phone numbers.

Stairway

- Add a handrail for support.
- Remove all obstacles or stored items from stairs and landing.
- Repair or replace flooring material that is in poor condition.
- Add a light switch at the top of the stairs.
- If there is an elderly person in the home, add a contrasting color strip to the first and last steps to identify the change of level.

Fire Prevention Tips

- Install smoke detectors on every level of your home.
- Keep fire extinguishers handy in the kitchen, basement, and bedrooms.
- Have the chimney and fireplace cleaned by a professional when there is more than ¼ inch of soot accumulation.
- Place space heaters at least 3 feet from beds, curtains, and other flammable objects.
- Don't overload electrical outlets, and position drapes so that they don't touch cords or outlets.
- Recycle or toss combustibles, such as newspapers, rags, old furniture, and chemicals.
- If you smoke, use caution with cigarettes and matches; never light up in bed.
- Plan escape routes and practice using them with your family.

24-hour emergency phone number. If you think you need help, don't hesitate to call this number. Campus security departments frequently offer short seminars on safety topics to student organizations or residence hall groups. Your counseling center on campus might also offer programs on rape prevention and personal protection.

If you are motivated to make your campus environment safer, you might wish to contact an organization that focuses on campus crime. Safe Campuses Now is a nonprofit student group that tracks legislation, provides educational seminars, and monitors community incidents involving students. For information about Safe Campuses Now, including how to start a chapter on your campus, call (706) 354-1115, or see their web page at **www.uga.edu\~safe-campus.** We encourage you to become active in making your campus a safer place to live.

SUMMARY

- Everyone is a potential victim of violent crime.
- Each year in the United States, intentional injuries cause about 50,000 deaths and another 2 million nonfatal injuries.
- Handguns are the weapon of choice for homicides.
- Domestic violence includes intimate abuse, child abuse, and elder abuse.
- Forms of child abuse include physical abuse, sexual abuse, and child neglect. Child neglect is the most common form.
- Youth violence is a serious social problem, and much of the violence is related to gang activities.
- Bias and hate crimes, crimes based on sexual orientation, and stalking are increasingly recognized as serious violent acts.
- Rape and sexual assault, acquaintance rape, date rape, and sexual harassment are forms of sexual victimization in which victims often are both physically and psychologically traumatized.
- Unintentional injuries are injuries that occur accidentally. The numbers of fatal and nonfatal unintentional injuries are exceedingly high.

REVIEW QUESTIONS

1. Identify some of the categories of intentional injuries. How many people are affected each year by intentional injuries?
2. What are some of the most important facts concerning homicide in the United States? How are most homicides committed?
3. Identify the three types of domestic violence discussed in the chapter.
4. What reasons might explain why so many people do not report domestic violence?
5. Aside from the immediate consequences of child abuse, what additional problems do many abused children face in the future?
6. Explain why gangs and gang activities have increased tremendously over the last 30 years. What effect do gangs have on a community?
7. List some examples of groups that are known to have committed bias or hate crimes.
8. Identify some general characteristics of a typical stalker.
9. Explain some of the myths associated with rape. How can date rape be prevented?
10. Identify some examples of behaviors that could be considered sexual harassment. Why are employers especially concerned about educating their employees about sexual harassment?
11. Identify some common examples of unintentional injuries. Point out three safety tips from each of the safety areas listed at the end of this chapter.

THINK ABOUT THIS . . .

- To what extent are you concerned about your personal safety? Are you comfortable with your level of concern? Or do you think you should be more or less concerned?
- Has there been any gun violence at your college? Are you aware of any students carrying guns or other concealed weapons on your campus?
- Do you know of educational programs on your campus that have dealt with rape prevention or sexual harassment? Where can you go on your campus to seek help for crises related to these issues?
- Is there a particular place on your campus where you believe that your personal safety is threatened? If so, how do you cope with this threat?

REFERENCES

1. McKenzie JF, Pinger RR, Kotecki JE: *An introduction to community health,* ed 3, 1999, Jones & Bartlett.
2. Bureau of Justice Statistics: *National Crime Victimization Survey,* U.S. Department of Justice, January 2001, **www.ojp.usdoj.gov.**
3. Bureau of Justice Statistics: *Criminal offenders statistics: lifetime likelihood of going to state or federal prison,* U.S. Department of Justice, December 11, 1999, **www.ojp.usdoj.gov.**
4. Bureau of Justice Statistics: *Drugs, crime and the justice system: a national report,* U.S. Department of Justice, December 1992, U.S. Government Printing Office.
5. U.S. Department of Justice: *Murder by intimates declined 36 percent since 1976,* press release, March 16, 1998, p. 1.
6. Widom CS: The cycle of violence, *Research in Brief,* National Institute of Justice, U.S. Department of Justice, U.S. Government Printing Office, 1992.

7. National Committee for Prevention of Child Abuse: *12 alternatives for whacking your kid,* undated pamphlet.
8. Bever, DL: *Safety: a personal focus,* ed 4, 1996, Mosby.
9. Soldier gets life with parole; apologizes to slaying victim's parents, December 9, 1999, **www.cnn.com.**
10. President seeks better implementation of "don't ask, don't tell," December 11, 1999, **www.cnn.com.**

SUGGESTED READINGS

Brandenburg, JB: *Confronting sexual harassment: what schools and colleges can do,* 1997, Teachers College Press.
This book explains the origins and scope of the problem of sexual harassment on campus. The author discusses ways to develop policies and grievance procedures, examines legal issues, and suggests useful education programs and strategies.

Giggans PO, Levy B: *50 ways to a safer world: everyday actions you can take to prevent violence in neighborhoods, schools, and communities,* 1997, Seal Press Feminist Publications.
This handbook offers practical advice in an easy-to-read format. It suggests simple, logical ways to prevent violence in the home, on the streets, and in schools. Each of the 50 actions is clearly explained in this 144-page publication.

Goold GB: *First aid in the workplace: what to do in the first five minutes,* ed 2, 1998, Prentice-Hall.
This book covers all essential elements required by OSHA's current guidelines. It's designed for a 6- to 8-hour first aid course for people with little or no first aid training. Presenting information clearly and concisely, it details basic first aid procedures for a number of injuries that can occur in the workplace. Photographs are used to illustrate specific skills.

Marques L, Carter L, Nelson M: *Child safety made easy,* 1998, Screamin' Mimi Publications.
Illustrated with cartoon characters, this humorous book presents hundreds of important safety tips for various people who care for small children. The writing style is straightforward, and explanations are concise. This book would be especially useful for first-time parents.

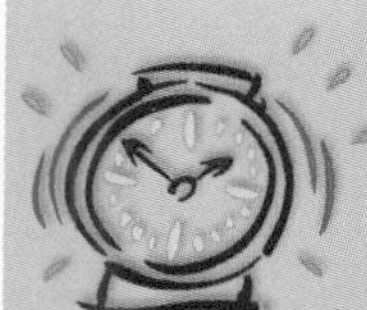

As we go to Press...

The tragic terrorist events that happened in New York City, Washington D.C., and rural Pennsylvania on September 11, 2001 immediately changed the way government regulators and airline companies focused their safety efforts. Airline customers are now being told to arrive at the ticket counter two hours prior to their domestic flights and three hours prior to international flights. Paper tickets are now required by some airlines instead of electronic tickets. Some airports do not permit curbside check-in of luggage. Generally, passengers must check baggage at the ticket counter. All airports are tightening the security and video surveillance operations in the terminals and in the parking lots. Multiple forms of personal identification are required before being allowed to embark on a plane.

Common items that many people routinely carry are no longer permitted through the passenger security stations. Aerosol containers (e.g., hair spray, shaving cream), pen knives, corkscrews, scissors, disposable razors, syringes, tweezers and any other items deemed capable of becoming a weapon are not permitted in carry-on bags or purses. These items must now be stored in checked baggage. On board eating utensils, especially steak knives, are being replaced by safer, plastic items.

As we go to press, the best advice is for travelers to check with their airlines well in advance of their travel dates. Airline websites provide clear instructions for passengers.

Additionally, the Federal Aviation Administration and various federal law enforcement officials are considering placing armed U.S. marshals aboard domestic flights. Also being considered is the use of an impenetrable door to the cockpit area, so terrorists could not have access to the pilot compartment. These, and other possible changes, will significantly alter the way Americans travel.

Name ______________________ **Date** ____________ **Section** ____________

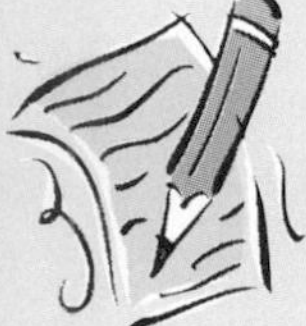

Personal Assessment

How Well Do You Protect Your Safety?

This quiz will help you measure how well you manage your personal safety. For each item below, circle the number that reflects the frequency with which you do the safety activity. Then, add up your individual scores and check the interpretation at the end.

3 I regularly do this

2 I sometimes do this

1 I rarely do this

1. I am aware of my surroundings and do not get lost.
   3 2 1
2. I avoid locations in which my personal safety could be compromised.
   3 2 1
3. I intentionally vary my daily routine (such as walking patterns to and from class, parking places, and jogging or biking routes) so that my whereabouts are not always predictable.
   3 2 1
4. I walk across campus at night with other people.
   3 2 1
5. I am careful about disclosing personal information (address, phone number, social security number, my daily schedule, etc.) to people I do not know.
   3 2 1
6. I carefully monitor my alcohol intake at parties.
   3 2 1
7. I watch carefully for dangerous weather conditions and know how to respond if necessary.
   3 2 1
8. I do not keep a loaded gun in my home.
   3 2 1
9. I know how I would handle myself if I were to be assaulted.
   3 2 1
10. I maintain adequate insurance for my health and my property.
    3 2 1
11. I keep emergency information numbers near my phone.
    3 2 1
12. I keep my first aid skills up-to-date.
    3 2 1
13. I use deadbolt locks on the doors of my home.
    3 2 1
14. I use the safety locks on the windows at home.
    3 2 1
15. I check the batteries used in my home smoke detector.
    3 2 1
16. I have installed a carbon monoxide detector in my home.
    3 2 1
17. I use adequate lighting in areas around my home and garage.
    3 2 1
18. I have the electrical, heating, and cooling equipment in my home inspected regularly for safety and efficiency.
    3 2 1
19. I use my car seat belt.
    3 2 1
20. I drive my car safely and defensively.
    3 2 1
21. I keep my car in good mechanical order.
    3 2 1
22. I keep my car doors locked.
    3 2 1
23. I have a plan of action if my car should break down while I am driving it.
    3 2 1
24. I use appropriate safety equipment, such as flotation devices, helmets, and elbow pads, in my recreational activities.
    3 2 1
25. I can swim well enough to save myself in most situations.
    3 2 1
26. I use suggestions for personal safety each day.
    3 2 1

TOTAL POINTS ________

Interpretation

Your total may mean that:

72–78 points	You appear to carefully protect your personal safety.
65–71 points	You adequately protect many aspects of your personal safety.
58–64 points	You should consider improving some of your safety-related behaviors.
Below 58 points	You must consider improving some of your safety-related behaviors.

To Carry This Further . . .

Although no one can be completely safe from personal injury or possible random violence, there are ways to minimize the risks to your safety. Scoring high on this assessment will not guarantee your safety, but your likelihood for injury should remain relatively low. Scoring low on this assessment should encourage you to consider ways to make your life more safe. Refer to the text and this assessment to provide you with useful suggestions to enhance your personal safety. Which safety tips will you use today?

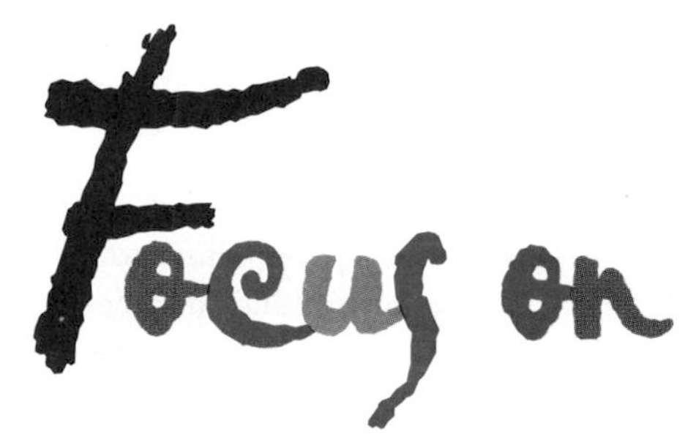

DROWSY DRIVING

Dean was driving home from college late on a moonlit Friday night. His on-campus job kept him working until 9 PM after a day of classes. He had stopped to shoot pool with some friends after work and started his hour-long trek home at about 11:30. Just after midnight, Dean turned onto a 15-mile stretch of perfectly straight highway that cut through pastures and fields. The summer night was crystal clear. The radio was playing loudly, there were few oncoming cars, and visibility was good.

"I felt fine," Dean recalled later. "I was a little run down, but I wasn't sleepy at all. I was cruising along listening to tunes, and the next thing I knew I was surrounded by corn. The sound of the stalks hitting the car must have woken me up. It scared the hell out of me. I guess I fell asleep for a few seconds, but I don't know how it could have happened."

The Danger of Driving While Sleepy

Dean experienced a phenomenon that is too often ignored. Falling asleep at the wheel is something that no one thinks will happen to them, yet drowsy driving is estimated to cause up to 200,000 accidents per year on American roads.[1,2] Dean was lucky. His car veered right where a dirt tractor path connected with the road, and he missed a deep ditch by only a few feet. He avoided power poles, trees, and oncoming traffic as well. "Since then, I've put off several late-night trips when I thought I might be too tired. I even took a nap once on an overnight drive when I felt myself drifting," Dean said. "If I hadn't fallen asleep at the wheel before, I probably would have kept driving."

Sleepiness is a significant cause of traffic fatalities. Up to 3% of all yearly vehicular deaths in the United States can be attributed to driving while drowsy, yet Americans remain woefully uneducated to this problem.[1]

Sleepiness undermines a person's ability to make sound decisions and reduces attention span considerably.[2] Any condition that impairs the judgment of drivers should be taken seriously. It has been estimated that 100 million Americans fail to get enough sleep and that up to 50% of all accident-related fatalities (not just driving fatalities) can be attributed to sleep deprivation.[3]

Early Warning Signs

Drivers are often not aware that they are in need of sleep until after they get behind the wheel, or they ignore the signs of sleep deprivation and drive anyway. When drowsiness sets in, drivers are often caught by surprise, and they can fall asleep without realizing it. Being able to recognize the signs of sleep deprivation before we fall victim to it is therefore important. Some of the symptoms of sleep deprivation you should watch out for are:[1,2]

- Struggling against fatigue throughout the day
- Needing caffeine to stay alert, especially on a daily basis
- Falling asleep quickly (within 5 minutes) after stopping to rest
- Having an irritable or argumentative attitude without knowing why
- Needing an alarm clock to wake up in the morning (well-rested people wake up on time naturally)

Tips to Avoid Drowsy Driving

Because of the stealthy manner in which sleep can overtake you, it is important to evaluate your condition before getting behind the wheel and also while you are on the road. It is also important to prevent regular sleep deprivation. We must reduce the risk of falling asleep while driving by using common sense. The following suggestions should help reduce your chances of driving while drowsy:[1]

- Get plenty of sleep. About 8 hours of sleep per night is desirable. If this is not practical, try to catch up on sleep when possible (take naps, sleep more on weekends, etc.).
- Take breaks while driving. Stop at least every 2 hours on long trips. If possible, avoid driving alone so the driving duties can be split. Don't eat heavy meals, and avoid too much caffeine.
- Stay alert. Talk, listen to the radio, sing, or do whatever you can to keep from drifting off. Don't let all of the passengers in the car sleep; having someone to converse with can help keep the driver alert.
- Don't get too comfortable. Getting too relaxed can promote dozing off. Avoid using cruise control. Reduce use of the heater, and keep the windows open when possible.
- Don't drink and drive. This is true anytime, but even a small amount of alcohol in the system can intensify the effects of fatigue on the body.
- If you feel yourself drifting off or you think you may be in danger of falling asleep, stop driving. Dozing off for a few seconds (a phenomenon known as microsleep) is a significant warning sign of fatigue. Don't try to fight through fatigue while driving. Pull off the road at a safe place and take a nap if you need to.

Take time to heed the warning signs of fatigue. Remember that dozing off at the wheel creates a potentially dangerous situation for both yourself and others on or near the road. Being able to recognize when you are at risk of falling asleep and taking steps to avoid driving while drowsy are more than just common sense; they're a necessity for your own and others' personal safety. Getting a few extra winks of sleep and taking the time to ensure you are alert before you get into the driver's seat could save lives.

The National Heart, Lung, and Blood Institute (NHLBI), one of the National Institutes of Health, oversees the National Center on Sleep Disorders Research. This center is an excellent resource for current information, research results, and reports concerning drowsy driving. You can look for links to drowsy driving at the website **www.nhlbi.nih.gov.**

For Discussion . . .

How much sleep do you get each night on average? Do you regularly experience any of the signs of fatigue mentioned in this article? Do you experience fatigue more often during certain times of the day or week? If so, can you think of ways to increase the amount of sleep you get? What would you have to give up to accomplish this goal?

References

1. Matson M: Forgotten menace on our highways, *Reader's Digest,* 144(86), June 1994.
2. Toufexis A: Drowsy America, *Time,* 136(26), Dec 17, 1990.
3. Bennett G: Why you must get more sleep, *McCall's,* 122(3), Dec 1994.

part 7

The Life Cycle

chapter **17**

Accepting Dying and Death

Online Learning Center Resources

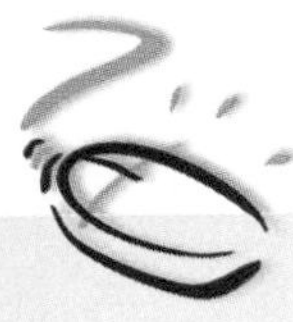

www.mhhe.com/hahn6e

Log on to our Online Learning Center (OLC) for access to these additional resources:

- Chapter key terms and definitions
- Learning objectives
- Additional behavior change objectives
- Student interactive question-and-answer sites
- Self-scoring chapter quiz

The OLC also offers web links for study and exploration of health topics. Here are some examples of what you'll find:

- **www.livingbank.org** Go to this site to find out what's involved in giving "the gift of life." Check out the organ donation facts.
- **www.choices.org** Learn how to foster communication about end-of-life decisions, and access educational information and advice about legal issues.
- **www.medbroadcast.com** Explore the Death and Dying section here to learn about the grieving process and why some elderly adults choose suicide.

Taking Charge of Your Health

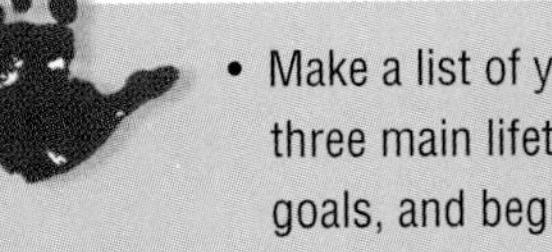

- Make a list of your three main lifetime goals, and begin taking steps toward reaching them.
- Talk to family members and friends about their thoughts on death to broaden your views on this subject.
- Review the steps in planning for organ donation, and make this commitment.
- Set up a realistic timetable for planning death-related issues, such as having a will drawn up and arranging for an advance medical directive.
- Begin a weekly journal for recording your thoughts on living and dying. Review your entries periodically to see how your opinions may change over time.
- Explore your current feelings about living and dying by answering the three important questions on p. 440.

Eye on the Media

Finding Grief Support Online

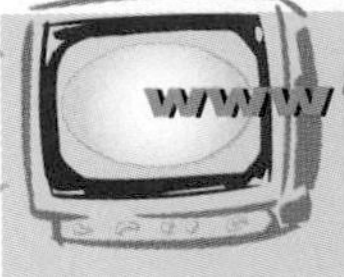

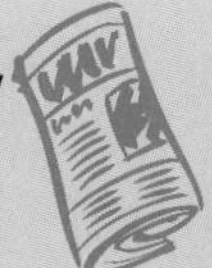

If you were grieving over the death of a loved one, getting out of bed in the morning might take all the physical and mental energy you could muster. Going across campus to talk to a counselor might be just too hard. The problem is you could go for weeks or months without talking about your feelings.

With access to the web, there's an alternative—on-line grief support groups. This approach offers some real advantages. First of all, it's easy. You don't need to leave your room, where you feel safe and comfortable. It's also anonymous. You don't have to give your real name, and you can reveal as much or as little as you want. You can move through the grief process at your own pace, too. Most important, it's a way of connecting with people who are going through some of the same feelings you are. You'll feel less alone and isolated. You can open up completely and begin the healing process by making your feelings concrete.

The disadvantages? Going on-line for support could be a way of avoiding the people you care about most (who also care about you). There's no

Eye on the Media *continued*

substitute for human contact at a time of loss. Yes, you need space and time alone. But you may also need to cry with someone near you and have that person hold you. Depending on the type of on-line group you try, you may not find what you're looking for. Some sites are built around testimonials to loved ones who have died. Others are just a place to talk. Pouring out your heart will help—and is actually necessary—but you also need guidance and direction. So look for a support group sponsored by a qualified person, such as a psychologist trained in grief support. Many support groups feature a religious slant, which may or may not match your beliefs. Others want you to donate to their organization.

GriefNet (**www.griefnet.org**) is based on the philosophy that healing is a natural process. With more than thirty-five e-mail support groups and two websites, GriefNet is a nonprofit corporation that operates under the name Rivendell Resources. It is supervised by Cendra Lynn, PhD, a clinical grief psychologist, death educator, and traumatologist who has worked in the field of grief/dying for more than thirty years. Each of the support groups is monitored, and some problems are forwarded to Dr. Lynn for feedback. This site offers a newsletter; a library link for articles on death and dying; a listing of books, videotapes, and audiocassettes for purchase; resource listings for organizations and people in your community who offer aid, such as hospice programs, support groups, and counselors; and memorials. Its companion linked site is called KIDSAID, which is aimed at kids (and their parents) who are going through grief.

Healing Hearts (**www.healinghearts.net**) is centered on retreats as a way of working through the grieving process. It also offers on-line answers to commonly asked questions about death and dying. The cofounders, Linda Hardy and Fran Kirkham, have both worked with Children to Children, a program for grieving children, as well as with adult groups.

Professional Counseling Services (**www.hoyweb.com**) is a Christian-oriented site that features a wide variety of support groups. It offers a free initial counseling consultation with Lynette J. Hoy, NCC, LCPC. In the area of grief and loss, this site lists Compassionate Friends, the Grief Recovery Institute, and GriefShare (**info@griefshare.org**).

Such on-line support groups are suggested as a possible resource during times of grief. They are not meant to replace the support of your family and friends. As with all on-line connections, caution and common sense should be used.

The primary goal of this chapter is to help people realize that the reality of death can serve as a focal point for a more enjoyable, productive, and contributive life. Each day in our lives becomes especially meaningful only after we have fully accepted the reality that someday we are going to die. We can then live each day to its fullest, as if it were our last day.

Our mortality provides us with a framework from which to appreciate and conduct our lives. It should help us prioritize our activities so that we can accomplish our goals (in our academic work, our relationships with others, and our recreation) before we die. Quite simply, death gives us our only absolute reason for living.

DYING IN TODAY'S SOCIETY

Since shortly after the turn of the 20th century, the manner in which people experience death in this society has changed significantly. Formerly, most people died in their own homes, surrounded by family and friends. Young children frequently lived in the same home with their aging grandparents and saw them grow older and eventually die. Death was seen as a natural extension of life. Children grew up with a keen sense of what death meant, both to the dying person and to the grieving survivors.

Times have indeed changed. Today approximately 70% of people die in hospitals, nursing homes, and extended care facilities, not in their own homes. The extended family is seldom at the bedside of the dying person.[1] Frequently, frantic efforts are made to keep a dying person from death. Although medical technology has improved our lives, some people believe that it has reduced our ability to die with dignity. Many are convinced that our way of dying has become more artificial and less civilized than it used to be. The trend toward hospice care may be a positive response to this high-tech manner of dying (see p. 434).

DEFINITIONS OF DEATH

Before many of the scientific advancements of the past 30 years, death was relatively easy to define. People were considered dead when a heartbeat could no longer be detected and when breathing ceased. Now, with the technological advancements made in medicine, especially emergency medicine, some patients who give every indication of being dead can be resuscitated. Critically ill people, even those in comas, can now be kept alive for years with many of their bodily functions maintained by medical devices, including feeding tubes and respirators.

Thus death can be a very difficult concept to define.[2] Numerous professional associations and ad hoc interdisciplinary committees have struggled with this problem and have developed criteria by which to establish death. Some of these criteria have been adopted by state legislatures, although there is certainly no consensus definition of death that all states embrace.

Clinical determinants of death refer to measures of bodily functions. Often judged by a physician, who can then sign a legal document called a *medical death certificate,* these clinical criteria include the following:

1. Lack of heartbeat and breathing.
2. Lack of central nervous system function, including all reflex activity and environmental responsiveness. Often this can be confirmed by an **electroencephalograph** reading. If there is no brain wave activity after an initial measurement and a second measurement after 24 hours, the person is said to have undergone *brain death.*
3. The presence of **rigor mortis,** indicating that body tissues and organs are no longer functioning at the cellular level. This is sometimes referred to as *cellular death.*

The *legal determinants* used by government officials are established by state law and often adhere closely to the clinical determinants already listed. A person is not legally dead until a death certificate has been signed by a physician, **coroner,** or health department officer.

EUTHANASIA

There are two types of euthanasia for desperately ill people: they are either intentionally put to death (**direct [active] euthanasia**) or allowed to die without being subjected to heroic lifesaving efforts (**indirect [passive] euthanasia**). Direct euthanasia usually involves the administration of large amounts of depressant drugs, which eventually causes all central nervous system functions to stop. Although direct euthanasia is commonly practiced on housepets and laboratory animals, it is illegal for humans in the United States, Canada, and other developed countries. However, in 1992, the Netherlands became the first developed country to enact legislation that permits euthanasia under strict guidelines.

Indirect euthanasia is increasingly occurring in a number of hospitals, nursing homes, and medical centers. Physicians who withhold heroic lifesaving techniques or drug therapy treatments or who disconnect life support systems from terminally ill patients are practicing indirect euthanasia. Although some people still consider this form of euthanasia a type of murder, indirect euthanasia seems to be gaining legal and public acceptance for people with certain terminal illnesses—near-death cancer patients, brain-dead accident victims, and hopelessly ill newborn babies. Physicians' orders of *do not resuscitate (DNR)* and *comfort measures only (CMO)* are examples of passive euthanasia that are familiar to hospital personnel.

TALKING POINTS • You're having a class discussion on euthanasia. How would you argue different viewpoints—including euthanasia as murder and euthansia as an act of mercy?

PHYSICIAN-ASSISTED SUICIDE

In recent years, physician-assisted suicide has been the focus of three important news stories. In July 1997, the U.S. Supreme Court unanimously ruled that dying people have no fundamental constitutional right to physician-assisted suicide. In effect, this ruling left the decision to individual states to permit or prohibit physician-assisted suicide.

By April 1999, more than thirty states had enacted laws prohibiting assisted suicide, and many other states had essentially prohibited it through common law.[3] Only the state of Oregon had passed a law that legalized assisted suicide, including specific guidelines and limiting its use to people with less than 6 months to live.

The third major news story concerned the April 1999 Michigan conviction of Dr. Jack Kevorkian, a retired pathologist who had aided in the suicides of over 100 people. Kevorkian was convicted of second-degree murder and delivery of a controlled substance in the assisted suicide of Thomas Youk, a 52-year-old patient with

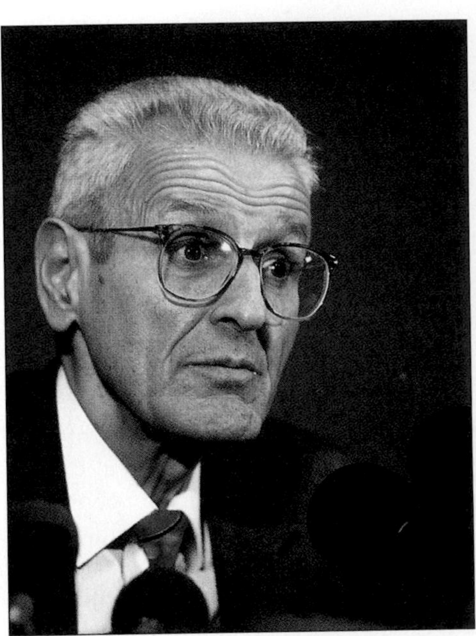

Dr. Jack Kevorkian was convicted of murder in 1999. How do you stand on the issue of physician-assisted suicide?

Lou Gehrig's disease. This suicide had been televised on the CBS show "60 Minutes." Kevorkian is serving a 10- to 25-year sentence at a prison in Jackson, Michigan.

ADVANCE MEDICAL DIRECTIVES

Because some physicians and families find it difficult to support indirect euthanasia, many people are starting to use legal documents called *advance medical directives.*[4] One of these medical directives is the living will (see the Star Box on p. 432). This is a document that confirms a dying person's desire to be allowed to die peacefully and with a measure of dignity if a time should arise when there is little hope for recovery from a terminal illness or severe injury. Living will statutes exist in all fifty states and the District of Columbia. The living will requires that physicians or family members carry out a person's wishes to die naturally, without receiving life-sustaining treatments. An estimated 25% of U.S. adults have signed living wills.[5]

A second important document that can assist terminally ill or incapacitated patients is the **medical power of attorney for health care** document. This legal document authorizes another person to make specific health-care decisions about treatment and care under specified circumstances, most commonly when patients are in long-term vegetative states and cannot communicate their medical wishes. This document helps inform hospitals and physicians which person will help make the critical medical decisions. Usually this person is a loving relative. It is recommended that people complete both a living will and a medical power of attorney for health-care document.

EMOTIONAL STAGES OF DYING

A process of self-adjustment has been observed in people who have a terminal illness. The stages in this process have helped form the basis for the modern movement of death education. An awareness of these stages may help you understand how people adjust to other important losses in their lives.

Perhaps the most widely recognized name in the area of death education is Dr. Elisabeth Kübler-Ross. As a psychiatrist working closely with terminally ill patients at the University of Chicago's Billings Hospital, Kübler-Ross was able to observe the emotional reactions of dying people. In her classic book *On Death and Dying,* Kübler-Ross summarized the psychological stages that dying people often experience.[6]

- *Denial.* This is the stage of disbelief. Patients refuse to believe that they actually will die. Denial can serve as a temporary defense mechanism and can allow patients the time to accept their prognosis on their own terms.
- *Anger.* A common emotional reaction after denial is anger. Patients can feel as if they have been cheated. By expressing anger, patients are able to vent some of their fears, jealousies, anxieties, and frustrations. Patients often direct their anger at relatives, physicians and nurses, religious symbols, and normally healthy people.
- *Bargaining.* Terminally ill people follow the anger stage with a stage characterized by bargaining. Patients who desperately want to avoid their inevitable deaths attempt to strike bargains—often with God or a church leader. Some people undergo religious conversions. The goal is to buy time by promising to repent for past sins, to restructure and rededicate their lives, or to make a large financial contribution to a religious cause.
- *Depression.* When patients realize that, at best, bargaining can only postpone their fate, they may begin an unpredictable period of depression. In a sense, terminally ill people are grieving for their own anticipated death. They may become quite withdrawn and refuse to visit with close relatives and friends. Prolonged periods of silence or crying are normal components of this stage and should not be discouraged.
- *Acceptance.* During the acceptance stage, patients fully realize that they are going to die. Acceptance ensures a relative sense of peace for most dying people. Anger, resentment, and depression are usually gone. Kübler-Ross describes this stage as one without much feeling. Patients feel neither happy nor sad. Many are calm and introspective and prefer to be left either alone or with a few close relatives or friends.

Key Terms

electroencephalograph
An instrument that measures the electrical activity of the brain.

rigor mortis
Rigidity of the body that occurs after death.

coroner
An elected legal official empowered to pronounce death and to determine the official cause of a suspicious or violent death.

direct (active) euthanasia
The process of inducing death, often through the injection of lethal drugs.

indirect (passive) euthanasia
The process of allowing a person to die by disconnecting life support systems or withholding lifesaving techniques.

medical power of attorney for health care
A legal document that designates who will make health-care decisions for people unable to do so for themselves.

The Living Will

The living will is a legally binding document in all fifty states and the District of Columbia. This document allows individuals to express their wishes concerning dying with dignity. When such a document has been drawn, families and physicians are better able to deal with the wishes of people who are near death from conditions from which there is no reasonable expectation of recovery. Figure 17-1 is a sample living will for the state of Florida. However, people should use a living will that is specific for the state in which they live. For additional information and materials, contact the Partnership for Caring organization by using the toll-free number 1-800-989-9455 or by visiting Partnership for Caring website (**www.partnershipforcaring.org**). At this site, you can download state-specific packages for free.

Instructions	**Florida Living Will**
Print the date	Declaration made this ______ day of ____________, ______ . (day) (month) (year)
Print your name	I, ______________________________, willfully and voluntarily make known my desire that my dying not be artificially prolonged under the circumstances set forth below, and I do hereby declare that:
Please initial each that applies	If at any time I am incapacitated and _____ I have a terminal condition, or _____ I have an end-stage condition, or _____ I am in a persistent vegetative state
	and if my attending or treating physician and another consulting physician have determined that there is no reasonable medical probability of my recovery from such condition, I direct that life prolonging procedures be withheld or withdrawn when the application of such procedures would serve only to prolong artificially the process of dying, and that I be permitted to die naturally with only the administration or the performance of any medical procedure deemed necessary to provide me with comfort care or to alleviate pain. It is my intention that this declaration be honored by my family and physician as the final expression of my legal right to refuse medical or surgical treatment and to accept the consequences for such refusal. In the event that I have been determined to be unable to provide express and informed consent regarding the withholding, withdrawal, or continuation of life-prolonging procedures, I wish to designate, as my surrogate to carry out the provisions of the declarations:
Print the name, home address and telephone number of your surrogate	Name: ______________ Address: ______________ ______________ Zip Code: ______ Phone: ______________
© 2000 Partnership for Caring, Inc.	

	Florida Living Will—Page 2 of 2
	I wish to designate the following person as my alternate surrogate to carry out the provisions of this declaration should my surrogate be unwilling or unable to act on my behalf:
Print name, home address and telephone number of your alternate surrogate	Name: ______________ Address: ______________ ______________ Zip Code: ______ Phone: ______________
Add personal instructions (if any)	Additional instructions (optional):
	I understand the full import of this declaration, and I am emotionally and mentally competent to make this declaration.
Sign the document	Signed: ______________
Witnessing Procedure	Witness 1: Signed: ______________ Address: ______________
Two witnesses must sign and print their addresses	Witness 2: Signed: ______________ Address: ______________
© 2000 Partnership for Caring, Inc.	*Courtesy of* **Partnership for Caring, Inc.** 1035 30th Street, NW Washington, DC 20007 800-989-9455 6/00

Figure 17-1 A sample living will.

One or two additional points should be made about the psychological stages of dying. Just as each person's life is totally unique, so is each person's death. Unfolding deaths vary as much as do unfolding lives. Some people move through Kübler-Ross's stages of dying very predictably, but others do not. It is not uncommon for some dying people to avoid one or more of these stages entirely.

The second important point to be made about Kübler-Ross's stages of dying is that the family members or friends of dying people often pass through similar stages as they observe their loved ones dying. When informed that a close friend or relative is dying, many people will also experience varying degrees of denial, anger, bargaining, depression, and acceptance. Because of this, as caring people we need to recognize that the emotional needs of the living must be fulfilled in ways that do not differ appreciably from those of the dying.

TALKING POINTS • You and your brother are grieving over the recent death of your father in an auto crash. You're getting back to normal gradually, but he is in serious depression—having trouble functioning at work and at home. How would you recommend professional counseling to your brother without making him feel worse?

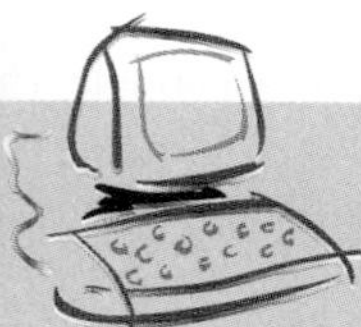

OnSITE/InSIGHT

Learning to Go: Health

Do you think it's too soon to think about death and dying? Click on the Motivator icon to explore this topic in the following lessons:

Lesson 54: Come to terms with death and dying.
Lesson 55: Express your wants in a living will.
Lesson 56: Cope with grief when you lose a loved one.

STUDENT POLL

What are your thoughts on dying and death? Go to the Online Learning Center at **www.mhhe.com/hahn6e**. Click on Student Resources, where you'll find the Student Poll. Answer these questions and then see how other students responded.

1. Do you avoid talking or thinking about death?
2. Are you afraid of dying?
3. Have you had to deal with the death of a loved one?
4. Have you ever lost a loved one who is younger than you?
5. Did you ever have to deal with the death of a loved one when you were a teenager or younger?
6. Do you support euthanasia?
7. Do you support physician-assisted suicide?
8. Do you know someone who is in hospice care?
9. Would you agree to being placed in a nursing home facility in your late adulthood?
10. Have you thought about your own funeral service?
11. Do you have a will?
12. Would you consider being an organ donor?
13. Have you ever sought therapy after the death of a loved one?
14. Do you have difficulty developing close relationships with others for fear of losing them some day?

NEAR-DEATH EXPERIENCES

As Bob lay on the gymnasium floor in apparent cardiac arrest, he watched from above as the team trainer and coaches performed CPR. After observing his own attempted resuscitation, he began walking in the direction of his uncle's voice. The last time he had heard his uncle's voice was a few days before his death 4 years earlier. Suddenly, his uncle instructed Bob to stop and turn back because Bob was not yet ready to join him. Over 24 hours later, Bob regained consciousness in the cardiac intensive care unit of The Ohio State University Hospital.

Death brings an end to our physical existence. Perhaps this is the ultimate connection between death and our physical dimension of health. Many people believe that, in a positive sense, death brings with it a sense of relief and comfort—two qualities that may be most needed when one is dying. The classic work of Raymond Moody,[7] who examined reports of people who had near-death experiences, suggests that we may have less to fear about dying than we have generally thought.

In a comprehensive study of more than 100 people who had near-death experiences, Kenneth Ring[8] reported that these people shared a core experience. This experience was composed of some or all of the following stages:

1. A sense of well-being and peace
2. An out-of-body experience in which the dying person floats above his or her body and is able to witness the activities that are occurring
3. A movement into extreme blackness or darkness
4. A shaft of intense light that generally leads upward or lies in the distance
5. A decision to enter into the light

Central to this experience is the need to make a decision to move toward death or to return to the body that has been temporarily vacated.

Experts are not in agreement as to whether near-death experiences are truly associated with death or more closely associated with the depersonalization that is experienced by some people during particularly frightening situations. In a scientific sense, near-death experiences are impossible to prove. Science can neither verify nor deny the existence of out-of-body experiences.[1]

Regardless, for those who have had near-death experiences, simply knowing that death might not be such an unpleasant experience appears to be comforting. Most seem to have formed a new orientation toward living.

INTERACTING WITH DYING PEOPLE

Facing the impending death of a friend, relative, or loved one is a difficult experience. If you have yet to go through this situation, be assured that, as you grow older, your opportunities will increase. This is part of the reality of living.

Most counselors, physicians, nurses, and ministers who spend time with terminally ill people suggest that you display one quality when interacting with dying people: honesty. Just the thought of talking with a dying person may make you feel uncomfortable. (Most of us have had no training in this sort of thing.) Sometimes, to make ourselves feel less anxious or depressed, we may tend to deny that the person we are with is dying. Our words and nonverbal behavior indicate that we prefer not to face the truth. Our words become stilted as we gloss over the facts and merely attempt to cheer up both our dying friend and ourselves. This behavior is rarely beneficial or supportive—for either party.

As much as possible, we should attempt to be genuine and honest. We should not try to avoid crying if we feel the need to cry. At the same time, we can provide emotional support for dying people by allowing them to express their feelings openly. We should resist the temptation of trying to pull someone out of the denial, anger, or depression. We should not feel obliged to talk constantly and to fill long pauses with idle talk. Sometimes nonverbal communication, including touching, may be much more appreciated than mere talk. Since our interactions with dying people help fulfill our needs, we too should express our emotions and concerns as openly as possible.

TALKING WITH CHILDREN ABOUT DEATH

Because most children are curious about everything, it is not surprising that they are also fascinated about death. From very young ages, children are exposed to death through mass media (cartoons, pictures in newspapers and magazines, and news reports), adult conversations ("Aunt Emily died today," "Uncle George is terminally ill"), and their discoveries (a dead bird, a crushed bug, a dead flower). The manner in which children learn about death will have an important effect on their ability to recognize and accept their own mortality and to cope with the deaths of others.

Psychologists encourage parents and older friends to avoid shielding children from or misleading children about the reality of death. Young children need to realize that death is not temporary and it is not like sleeping. Parents should make certain they understand children's questions about death before they give an answer. Most children want simple, direct answers to their questions, not long, detailed dissertations, which often confuse the issues. For example, when a 4-year-old asks her father, "Why is Tommy's dog dead?" an appropriate answer might be, "Because he got very, very sick and his heart stopped beating." Getting involved in a lengthy discussion about "doggy heaven" or the causes of specific canine diseases may not be necessary or appropriate.

Parents should answer questions when they arise and always respond with openness and honesty. In this way, young children can learn that death is a real part of life and that sad feelings are a normal part of accepting the death of a loved one.

TALKING POINTS • Your 6-year-old child's favorite teacher has died of cancer, and she is having trouble accepting that her teacher is gone forever. How would you explain the reality of the situation in a positive way?

DEATH OF A CHILD

Adults face not only the death of their parents and friends but perhaps also the death of a child. Whether because of sudden infant death syndrome (SIDS), chronic illness, accident, or suicide, children die and adults are forced to grieve the loss of someone who was "too young to die" (see "Focus on" Death of an Infant or Unborn Child" at the end of this chapter).

Coping with the death of a child presents adults with a difficult period of adjustment, particularly when the death was unexpected. Experts agree that grieving adults, particularly the parents, should express their grief fully and proceed cautiously on their return to normal routines. Many pitfalls can be avoided. Adults who are grieving for dead children should do the following:

- *Avoid trying to cope by using alcohol or drugs.*
- *Make no important life changes.* Moving to a different home, relocating, or changing jobs usually doesn't help parents deal any better with the grief they are experiencing.
- *Share their feelings with others.* Grieving adults should share their feelings particularly with other adults who have experienced a similar loss. Group support is available in many communities.
- *Avoid trying to erase the death.* Giving away clothing and possessions that belonged to the child cannot erase the memories the adult has of the child.
- *Give themselves the time and space to grieve.* On the anniversary of the child's death or on the child's birthday, grievers should give themselves special time just for grieving.
- *Don't attempt to replace the child.* Do not quickly have another child or use the deceased child's name for another child.

For most adults, grief over the death of a child will require an extended period. Eventually, however, life can return to normal.

HOSPICE CARE FOR THE TERMINALLY ILL

The thought of dying in a hospital ward, with spotless floors, pay television, and strict visiting hours, leaves many people with a cold feeling. Perhaps this thought alone has helped encourage the concept of **hospice care.** Hospice care provides an alternative approach to dying

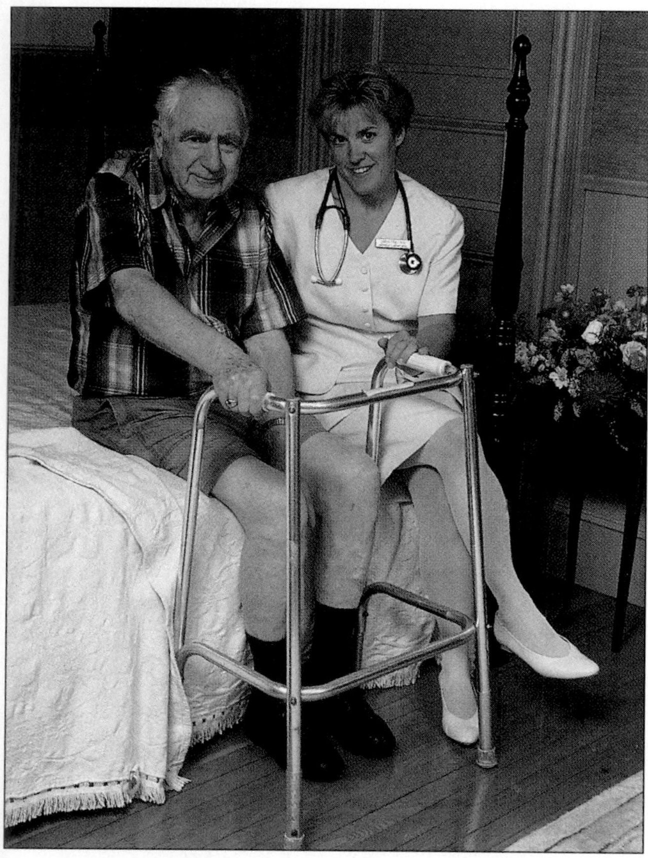

Hospice care allows terminally ill patients to spend their last days in a warm, homelike setting.

for terminally ill patients and their families. The goal of hospice care is to maximize the quality of life for dying people and their family members. Popularized in England during the 1960s, yet derived from a concept developed during the Middle Ages (where *hospitable lodges* took care of weary travelers), the hospice helps people die comfortably and with dignity by using one or more of the following strategies:

- *Pain control.* Dying people are not usually treated for their terminal disease; they are provided with appropriate drugs to keep them free from pain, alert, and in control of their faculties. Drug dependence is of little concern, and patients can receive pain medication when they feel they need it.
- *Family involvement.* Family members and friends are trained and encouraged to interact with the dying person and with each other. Family members often care for the dying person at home. If the hospice arrangement includes a hospice ward in a hospital or a separate building (also called a hospice), the family members have no restrictions on visitation.
- *Multidisciplinary approach.* The hospice concept promotes a team approach.[9] Specially trained physicians, nurses, social workers, counselors, and volunteers work with the patient and family to fulfill important needs. The needs of the family receive nearly the same priority as those of the patient.
- *Patient decisions.* Contrary to most hospital approaches, hospice programs encourage patients to make their own decisions. The patient decides when to eat, sleep, go for a walk, and just be alone. By maintaining a personal schedule, the patient is more apt to feel in control of his or her life, even as that life is slipping away.

Another way in which the hospice differs from the hospital approach concerns the care given to the survivors. Even after the death of the patient, the family receives a significant amount of follow-up counseling. Helping families with their grief is an important role for the hospice team.

The number of hospices in the United States has climbed quickly to well over 3300.[10] People seem to be convinced that the hospice system does work effectively. Part of this approval may be the cost factor. The cost of caring for a dying person in a hospice is usually less than the cost of full (inpatient) services provided by a hospital. Although insurance companies are delighted to see the lower cost for hospice care, many are still uncertain as to how to define hospice care. Thus not all insurance companies are fully reimbursing patients for their hospice care. Before discussing the possibility of hospice care for members of your family, you should consider the extent of hospice coverage in your health insurance policy.

GRIEF AND THE RESOLUTION OF GRIEF

The emotional feelings that people experience after the death of a friend or relative are collectively called *grief. Mourning* is the process of experiencing these emotional feelings in a culturally defined manner. See the Star Box on p. 436 for more information about the grieving process. The expression of grief is seen as a valuable process that gradually permits people to detach themselves from the deceased. Expressing grief, then, is a sign of good health.

Although people experience grief in remarkably different ways, most people have some of the following sensations and emotions:

Key Term

hospice care (HOS pis)
An approach to caring for terminally ill patients that maximizes the quality of life and allows death with dignity.

The Grieving Process

The grieving process consists of four phases, each of which is variable in length and unique in form to the individual. These phases are composed of the following:

1. *Internalization of the deceased person's image.* By forming an idealized mental picture of the dead person, the grieving person is freed from dealing too quickly with the reality of the death.
2. *Intellectualization of the death.* Mental processing of the death and the events leading up to its occurrence move the grieving person to a clear understanding that death has occurred.
3. *Emotional reconciliation.* During this third and often delayed phase, the grieving person allows conflicting feelings and thoughts to be expressed and eventually reconciled with the reality of the death.
4. *Behavioral reconciliation.* Finally, the grieving person is able to comfortably return to a life in which the death has been fully reconciled. Old routines are reestablished and new patterns of living are adopted where necessary. The grieving person has largely recovered.

A mistake that might be made by the friends of a grieving person is encouraging a return to normal behavior too quickly. When friends urge the grieving person to return to work right away, make new friends, or become involved in time-consuming projects, they may be preventing necessary grieving from occurring. It is not easy or desirable to forget about the fact that a spouse, friend, or child has recently died.

- *Physical discomfort.* Shortly after the death of a loved one, grieving people display a rather similar pattern of physical discomfort. This discomfort is characterized by "sensations of somatic distress occurring in waves lasting from 20 minutes to an hour at a time, a feeling of tightness in the throat, choking with shortness of breath, need for sighing, and an empty feeling in the abdomen, lack of muscular power, and an intense subjective distress described as a tension or mental pain. The patient soon learns that these waves of discomfort can be precipitated by visits, by mentioning the deceased, and by receiving sympathy."[11]
- *Sense of numbness.* Grieving people may feel as if they are numb or in a state of shock. They may deny the death of their loved one.
- *Feelings of detachment from others.* Grieving people see other people as being distant from them, perhaps because the others cannot feel the loss. A person in grief can feel very lonely. This is a common response.
- *Preoccupation with the image of the deceased.* The grieving person may not be able to complete daily tasks without constantly thinking about the deceased.
- *Guilt.* The survivor may be overwhelmed with guilt. Thoughts may center on how the deceased was neglected or ignored. Sensitive survivors feel guilt merely because they are still alive. Indeed, guilt is a common emotion.
- *Hostility.* Survivors may express feelings of loss and remorse through hostility, which they direct at other family members, physicians, lawyers, and others.
- *Disruption in daily schedule.* Grieving people often find it difficult to complete daily routines. They can suffer from an anxious type of depression. Seemingly easy tasks take a great deal of effort. Initiation of new activities and relationships can be difficult. Social interaction skills can be lost.
- *Delayed grief.* In some people, the typical pattern of grief can be delayed for weeks, months, and even years.

The grief process will continue until the bereaved person can establish new relationships, feel comfortable with others, and look back on the life of the deceased person with positive feelings (see the Changing for the Better box on p. 437). Although the duration of the grief resolution process will vary with the emotional attachments one has to a deceased person, grief usually lasts from a few months to a year. Professional help should be sought when grieving is characterized by unresolved guilt, extreme hostility, physical illness, significant depression, and a lack of other meaningful relationships. Trained counselors, physicians, and hospice workers can all play significant roles in helping people through grief. Exploring Your Spirituality (p. 438) shows how handling grief can vary greatly from one individual to another.

TALKING POINTS • The boyfriend of one of your best friends recently drowned. Your friend has withdrawn from her family and friends in her grief. How could you help her get professional counseling without making her family feel that you are interfering?

RITUALS OF DEATH

Our society has established a number of rituals associated with death that help the survivors accept the reality of death, ease the pain associated with the grief process, and provide a safe disposal of the body (see the Learning from Our Diversity box on p. 439). Our rituals give us the chance to formalize our goodbyes to a person and to receive emotional support and strength from family members and friends. In recent years, more of our rituals seem to be celebrating the life of the deceased. In doing this, our rituals also reaffirm the value of our own lives.

Changing *for the Better*

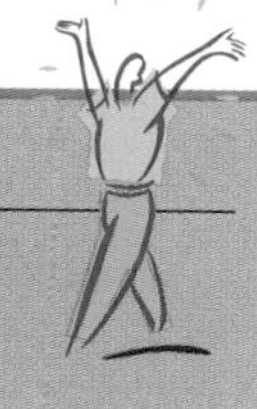

Helping the Bereaved

I know someone whose brother just died. I want to help without getting in the way at this difficult time. What's the best approach?

Leming and Dickinson[1] point out that the peak time of grief begins in the week after a loved one's funeral. Realizing that there is no one guaranteed formula for helping the bereaved, you can help by performing some or all of the following:

- Make few demands on the bereaved; allow him or her to grieve.
- Help with the household tasks.
- Recognize that the bereaved person may vent anguish and anger and that some of it may be directed at you.
- Recognize that the bereaved person has painful and difficult tasks to complete; mourning cannot be rushed or avoided.
- Do not be afraid to talk about the deceased person; this lets the bereaved know that you care for the deceased.
- Express your own genuine feelings of sadness, but avoid pity. Speak from the heart.
- Reassure bereaved people that the intensity of their emotions is very natural.
- Advise the bereaved to get additional help if you suspect continuing severe emotional or physical distress.
- Keep in regular contact with the bereaved; let him or her know you continue to care about them.

Most of our funeral rituals take place in funeral homes, churches, and cemeteries. *Funeral homes* (or *mortuaries*) are business establishments that provide a variety of services to the families of dead people. The services are carried out by funeral directors, who are licensed by the state in which they operate. Most funeral directors are responsible for preparing the bodies for viewing, filing death certificates, preparing obituary notices, establishing calling hours, assisting in the preparation and details of the funeral, casket selection, transportation to and from the cemetery, and family counseling. Although licensing procedures vary from state to state, most new funeral directors must complete 1 year of college, 1 year of mortuary school, and 1 year of internship with a funeral home before taking a state licensing examination.

TALKING POINTS • **How would you approach your parents to learn about their wishes concerning their own deaths, a subject they have never brought up?**

Full Funeral Services

An ethical funeral director will attempt to follow the wishes of the deceased's family and provide only the services requested by the family. Most families want traditional **full funeral services.** Three significant components of the full funeral services are as follows.

Embalming

Embalming is the process of using formaldehyde-based fluids to replace the blood components. Embalming helps preserve the body and return it to a natural look. Embalming permits friends and family members to view the body without being subjected to the odors associated with tissue decomposition. Embalming is often an optional procedure, except when death results from specific communicable diseases or when body *disposition* (disposal) is delayed.

Calling hours

Sometimes called a *wake,* this is an established time when friends and family members can gather in a room to share their emotions and common experiences about the dead person. Generally in the same room, the body will be in a casket, with the lid open or closed. Open caskets assist some people to confirm that death truly did occur. Some families prefer not to have any calling hours, sometimes called *visiting hours.*

Funeral service

Funeral services vary according to religious preference and the emotional needs of the survivors. Although some services are held in a church, most funeral services today take place in a funeral home, where a special room might serve as a chapel. Some services are held at the graveside. Families may also choose to have a simple *memorial service* within a few days after the funeral. Completing the Personal Assessment on p. 445 will help you think about what kind of funeral arrangements you would prefer for yourself. As the Star Box illustrates on page 440, some people choose some highly unusual ways to honor the memory of their loved ones.

Disposition of the Body

Bodies are disposed of in one of four ways. *Ground burial* is the most common method. About 75% of all bodies are placed in ground burial. The casket is almost always

Key Term

full funeral services
All of the professional services provided by funeral directors.

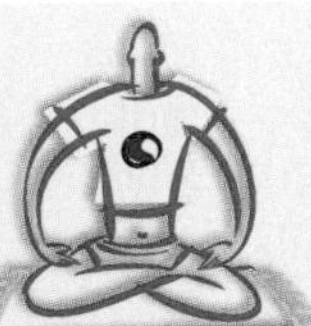

Exploring Your Spirituality

Will I Ever Get Over Losing My Friend?

The news that one of your close friends committed suicide came as a shock. Jack was a social guy who was liked by everyone. His girlfriend recently broke up with him, but he seemed to be taking it all right. He talked to you about the situation—seemed disappointed but not despairing. He mentioned that he was still in touch with his former girlfriend and seemed glad about that.

That's why his suicide is so hard to comprehend. Were there warning signs you missed? If you had done more to support him during the breakup, would he still be here? Did you talk to him enough? Did you really listen to him? How could you be a good friend and not know that he was despondent? You feel guilty every time you think of Jack.

It's hard to come to terms with any death—even one that's expected, such as when the person is sick or old. But Jack was healthy and young, just about your age. That makes it harder to accept his death. Still, you need to come to terms with it—let yourself feel sad about it, reflect on your friendship with him, and, ultimately, get on with your own life. What can you do to cope?

- *Don't blame yourself.* If Jack was sending out signals for help, you were not alone in missing them. His whole network of family and friends did, too. Whatever your friend's mental state was at the time of his death, it was his decision to take his own life.
- *Talk about the problem.* You and your friends are all feeling sad and guilty, missing Jack, and confused about his death. So try to support one another. Take the time to listen to them and share your own feelings. Recognize that it's going to take time to deal with this death. Not facing it now will only delay the grieving process.
- *Take solace in your religious or spiritual beliefs.* Talk to your clergyman, if you have one, about what you're going through. An objective listener can help you put your thoughts and feelings in perspective. Ask your congregation's prayer group to add your friend's name (and his family's) to their remembrance list.
- *Do something positive.* Consider doing volunteer work for a suicide hotline in your community. You can't bring Jack back, but you may be able to help keep someone else from making the fatal choice he did.

Your friend's death could be a turning point for you. Examine your own life—how you're living now and what you hope to accomplish in the future. Start taking action on your lifetime goals. Show your love for others. Make a difference on campus and in your community. Make the world a better place for yourself and for others.

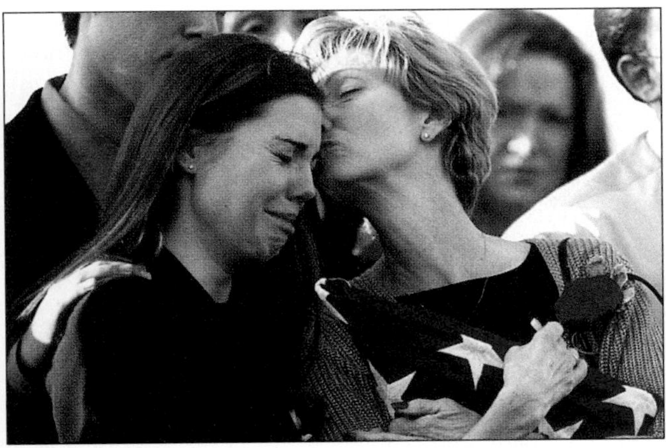

Grief is even harder to bear when loss happens suddenly, such as when a person commits suicide or dies in an accident. Marilyn Thompson, wife of Alaska Airlines Captain Ted M. Thompson, comforts her daughter, Beth, after a memorial service for the crew of Alaska Airlines Flight 261, which crashed off the coast of California on February 5, 2000, killing all 88 people aboard.

placed in a metal or concrete vault before being buried. The vault serves to further protect the body (a need only of the survivors) and to prevent collapse of ground because of the decaying of caskets. Use of a vault is required by most cemeteries.

A second type of disposition is *entombment.* Entombment refers to nonground burial, most often in structures called **mausoleums.** A mausoleum has a series of shelves where caskets can be sealed in vaultlike areas called *niches.* Entombment can also occur in the basements of buildings, especially in old, large churches. The bodies of famous church leaders are sometimes entombed in vaultlike spaces called **crypts.**

Cremation is a third type of body disposition. In the United States, 25% of all bodies are cremated.[12] This practice is increasing. Generally both the body and casket (or cardboard cremation box) are incinerated so that only the bone ash from the body remains. The body of an average adult produces about 5 to 7 pounds of bone ash. These ashes can then be placed in containers called urns, and then buried, entombed, or scattered, if permitted by state law. The cost of cremation (from $200 to $500) is much less than ground burial. Some families choose to cremate after having full funeral services.[13]

Learning from Our Diversity

Hospice: Spiritual Healing for the Dying

Once considered a radical approach to caring for people with terminal illness, the hospice movement has been experiencing increasing popularity in the United States over the past two decades. Founded in England by Dr. Cicely Saunders, the modern hospice movement seeks to provide comfort and relief of physical pain to the dying without seeking a cure or using heroic measures to sustain life. Whereas some patients choose to live in a hospice facility, the majority remain in their homes, where care is provided by family and friends under the guidance of hospice health-care professionals. Whether in a facility or at home, hospice patients have chosen to accept the reality of their terminal illness and to forgo medical care that is aimed at prolonging life or achieving a cure.[14]

In addition to physical pain relief, a less well known but equally important goal of hospice care is to alleviate "spiritual pain," which Cicely Saunders identifies as part of the "total pain" of dying. This is the pain of the whole person and is the overlapping of the physical, psychological, social, and spiritual. One physician experienced in hospice care identified these elements of spiritual pain: "the experiences of disconnection, disharmony, non-alignment, and disintegration."

Dr. Saunders recognized in the dying the presence of spiritual pain, and she directed the resources of hospice professionals to alleviate this special kind of distress. This pain is a combined fear of dying, guilt and regret about one's life, and sadness about the imminent separation from spouse, children, or friends. Such distress comes from the awareness that life is almost over and death is near. Although medical skills can help patients live longer and more comfortably with physical pain, spiritual pain can be more intense and last longer.

The "why" questions—such as "Why me?" and "Why now?" are indicators of spiritual pain. The feelings expressed are despair, fear, guilt, failure, and hopelessness. Sometimes, according to one expert, listening is enough to bring about some spiritual peace and quiet, which he describes as "experiences such as connection, alignment, harmony, and meaningfulness."

Sometimes, he says, healing and spiritual peace and quiet just happen on their own. To realize that spiritual healing sometimes "just happens" is important because, even though those who care for the dying can help in healing, it is the dying who heal themselves. One caution he gives is that "our own personal answers" about life and our own religious beliefs should not be given in an effort to heal someone. Caregivers should always offer words of encouragement, he says; these words, along with the loving way that medical and nursing care is given, can, as Cicely Saunders says, reach the most hidden places in the person's spirit.

Have you known a dying person who chose to spend his or her last days in hospice care instead of a hospital? What is your impression of that person's experience with hospice? Which choice do you think you would make for yourself: hospice care or hospital?

A fourth method of body disposition is *anatomical donation.* Separate organs (such as corneal tissue, kidneys, or the heart) can be donated to a medical school, research facility, or organ donor network. Certain states permit people to indicate on their driver's licenses that they wish to donate their organs. However, family consent (by next of kin) is also required at the time of death for organ or tissue donation to occur. Recently, hospitals have been required by federal law to inform the family of a deceased person about organ donation at the time of his or her death. The need for donor organs is far greater than the current supply. For some, the decision to donate body tissue and organs is rewarding and comforting. Organ donors understand that their small sacrifice can help give life or improve the quality of life for another person. In this sense, their death can mean life for others. To become an organ donor, you must fill out a uniform organ donor card like the one in Figure 17-2 on page 441.

Some people choose to donate their entire body to medical science. Often this is done through prior arrangements with medical schools. Bodies still require embalming. After they are studied, the remains are often cremated and returned to the family, if requested.

Costs

The full funeral services offered by a funeral home average from $2000 to $3000, and other expenses must be added to this price. Casket prices vary significantly, with the average cost between $1500 and $2500. If the family chooses an especially fancy casket, then the costs could spiral up to $10,000 or more. Costs that extend beyond these expenses include (should one choose them) those shown in the Star Box on page 440. When all of the expenses associated with a typical funeral are added up, the average cost is between $5500 and $7000.

Key Terms

mausoleum (moz oh LEE um)
An above-ground structure, which frequently resembles a small stone house, into which caskets can be placed for disposition.

crypts
Burial locations generally underneath churches.

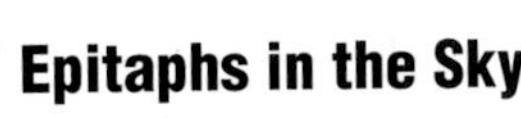

Epitaphs in the Sky

Two interesting (and to some people, amusing) postmortem options have become available to those who want to connect with the cosmos. The first is the naming of distant celestial stars for people who have died. For a designated fee, ranging from about $100 to $500, a person, or his or her loved ones, can purchase the rights to name a star. The extent to which this naming is a legally binding arrangement between the payee and the "owner" of the star is subject to debate. However, this process seems to give some measure of comfort to the living.

The second new adventure in postmortem arrangements is the rocketing of ashes into outer space. For a fee approaching $5000, Celestis, Inc., of Houston, Texas, will launch a cremated person's remains into orbit. However, only a small portion of the person's ashes—enough to fill a lipstick-size vial—will make the voyage. The ashes will be sent with about 100 other vials in a single launch. The Celestis company (**www.celestis.com or 1-800-ORBIT-11**) believes that these ash vials will orbit the Earth for 18 months to 10 years, when they will vaporize on reentry into the atmosphere.

Would you consider one of these two unusual options for yourself or a family member?

Regardless of the rituals you select for the handling of your body (or the body of someone in your care), most educators are encouraging people to prearrange their plans. Before you die, you can save your survivors a lot of misery by putting your wishes in writing. *Funeral prearrangements* relieve the survivors of many of the details that must be handled at the time of your death. You can gather much of the information for your obituary notice and your wishes for the disposition of your body. Prearrangements can be made with a funeral director, family member, or attorney. Many individuals also prepay the costs of their funeral. By making arrangements in advance of need, you can enhance your own peace of mind. Currently about 30% to 40% of funerals are preplanned or prepaid or both. Interestingly, in the 1960s, nearly all funerals were planned by relatives at the time of a person's death.

PERSONAL PREPARATION FOR DEATH

This chapter is designed to help you discover some new perspectives about death and develop your own personal death awareness. Remember that the ultimate goal of death education is a positive one—to help you best use and enjoy your life. Becoming aware of the reality of your own mortality is a step in the right direction. Reading about the process of dying, grief resolution, and the rituals surrounding death can also help you imagine that someday you too will die.

There are some additional ways in which you can prepare for the reality of your own death. Preparing a will, purchasing a life insurance policy, making funeral prearrangements, preparing a living will, and considering an anatomical or organ donation are measures that help you prepare for your own death (see the Changing for the Better box on p. 441). At the appropriate time, you might also wish to talk with family and friends about your own death. You may discover that an upbeat, positive discussion about death can help relieve some of your apprehensions and those of others around you.

Another suggestion to help you emotionally prepare for your own death is to prepare an *obituary notice* or **eulogy** for yourself. Include all the things you would like to have said about you and your life. Now compare your obituary notice and eulogy with the current direction your life seems to be taking. Are you doing the kinds of activities for which you want to be known? If so, great! If not, perhaps you will want to consider why your current direction does not reflect how you would like to be remembered. Should you make some changes to restructure your life's agenda in a more personally meaningful fashion?

Another suggestion to help make you aware of your own eventual death is to write your own **epitaph.** Before doing this, you might want to visit a cemetery. (Unfortunately, most of us visit cemeteries only when we are forced to.) Reading the epitaphs of others may help you develop your own epitaph.

Further awareness of your own death might come from attempting to answer these questions in writing (since this pushes you beyond mere thinking): (1) If I

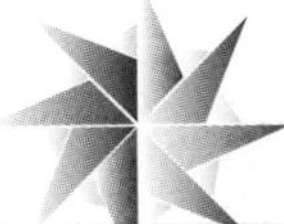

Estimated Funeral Costs

Cemetery lot	$400–$1200
Opening and closing of grave	$300–$800
Vault	$350–$1000
Mausoleum space	$1500–$5000
Honorarium for minister	$75–$100
Organist and vocalists	$50–$75 each
Flowers over casket	$100+
Grave marker	$500–$1500+
Beautician services	$75+

Changing *for the Better*

Planning an Organ Donation

I've thought about organ donation for a long time, and now I'm ready. What steps do I need to take to do this?

This is one of the most compassionate, responsible acts a person can do. Here are the simple steps that are involved:

1. You must complete a uniform donor card (Figure 17–2 see below). Obtain a card from a physician, a local hospital, or the nearest regional transplant or organ bank.
2. Print or type your name on the card.
3. Indicate which organs you wish to donate. You may also indicate your desire to donate all organs and tissues.
4. Sign your name in the presence of two witnesses, preferably your next of kin.
5. Fill in any additional information (for example, date of birth, city and state in which the card is completed, and date the card is signed).
6. Tell others about your decision to donate. Some donor cards have detachable portions to give to your family.
7. Always carry your card with you.
8. If you have any questions, you can call the United Network for Organ Sharing (UNOS) at 1-888-TXINFO1, or visit this organization's website at **www.unos.org.**

Uniform Donor Card

Of ____________________

(print or type name of donor)

In the hope that I may help others, I hereby make this anatomical gift, if medically acceptable, to take effect upon my death. The words and marks below indicate my wishes.

I give: ☐ any needed organs or parts

☐ only the following organs or parts

____

specify the organ(s), tissue(s), or part(s)

for the purposes of transplantation, therapy, medical research or education:

☐ my body for anatomical study if needed.

Limitations or special wishes, if any: ____________________

National Kidney Foundation

Please detach and give this portion of the card to your family.

This is to inform you that, should the occasion ever arise, I would like to be an organ and tissue donor. Please see that my wishes are carried out by informing the attending medical personnel that I have indicated my wishes to become a donor. Thank you.

____

Signature *Date*

For further information write or call:

National Kidney Foundation

30 East 33rd Street, New York, NY 10016

(800)-622-9010

Figure 17-2 Signing a uniform organ donor card allows you to donate your organs to a research facility, medical school, or organ donor network.

had only one day to live, how would I spend it? (2) What one accomplishment would I like to make before I die? (3) Once I am dead, what two or three things will people miss most about me? By answering these questions and accomplishing a few of the tasks suggested in this section, you will have a good start on accepting your own death and understanding the value of life itself.

Key Terms

eulogy
A composition or speech that praises someone; often delivered at a funeral or memorial service.

epitaph
An inscription on a grave marker or monument.

SUMMARY

- Personal death awareness encourages you to live a meaningful life.
- Death is determined primarily by clinical and legal factors.
- Euthanasia can be undertaken with either direct or indirect measures.
- The most current advance medical directives are the living will and the medical power of attorney for health care.

Both documents permit critically ill people (especially those who cannot communicate) to die with dignity.
- Denial, anger, bargaining, depression, and acceptance are the five classic psychological stages that dying people commonly experience, according to Kübler-Ross.
- Hospice care provides an alternative approach to dying for terminally ill people and their families.
- The expression of grief is a common experience that can be expected when a friend or relative dies. The grief process can vary in intensity and duration.
- Death in our society is associated with a number of rituals to help survivors cope with the loss of a loved one and to ensure proper disposal of the body.

REVIEW QUESTIONS

1. How does the experience of dying today differ from that in the early 1900s?
2. Identify and explain the clinical and legal determinants of death and indicate who establishes each of them.
3. Explain the difference between direct and indirect euthanasia.
4. How does a living will differ from a medical power of attorney for health-care document? Why are these advance medical directives becoming increasingly popular?
5. Identify the five psychological stages that dying people tend to experience. Explain each stage.
6. Identify and explain the four strategies that form the basis of hospice care. What are the advantages of hospice care for the patient and the family?
7. Explain what is meant by the term grief. Identify and explain the sensations and emotions most people have when they experience grief. When does the grieving process end? How can adults cope with the death of a child? How can we assist grieving people?
8. What purposes do the rituals of death serve? What are the significant components of the full funeral service? What are the four ways in which bodies are disposed?
9. What activities can we undertake to become better aware of our own mortality?

THINK ABOUT THIS . . .

- How were issues related to death handled in your family when you were growing up?
- Will hospice care be an option you might choose someday?
- Have you or any of your relatives prepared a living will or a medical power of attorney for health-care document?
- At your death, would you want your organs or body tissue donated to help another person? Are there any organs you would prefer not to donate?
- If you found out you were going to die tomorrow, what would you do today?
- If it were determined that you were in a persistent vegetative state, would you want your life support to be disconnected?

REFERENCES

1. Leming MR, Dickinson GE: *Understanding dying, death, and bereavement,* ed 5, 2001, Harcourt.
2. Kastenbaum RJ: *Death, society, and human experience,* ed 6, 1998, Allyn and Bacon.
3. **www.pbs.org/wgbh/pages/frontline/kevorkian/law,** The law on assisted suicide, December 16, 1999.
4. Partnership for Caring: *Advance directives,* www.partnershipforcaring.org, accessed Sept 24, 2001.
5. Partnership for Caring: Personal correspondence, Sept 20, 2001.
6. Kübler-Ross E: *On death and dying,* reprint ed, 1997, Collier Books.
7. Moody RA: *The last laugh: a new philosophy of near-death experiences, apparitions, and the paranormal,* 1999, Hampton Roads Publishing Co.
8. Ring K: *Life at death: a scientific investigation of the near-death experience,* 1980, Coward, McCann & Geoghegan.
9. DeSpelder LA, Strickland AL: *The last dance: encountering death and dying,* ed 5, 1999, Mayfield.
10. National Hospice and Palliative Care Organization: *NHPCO facts and figures,* www.mhpco.org, accessed Sept 26, 2001.
11. Lindemann E: Symptomology and management of acute grief. In Fulton et al, editors: *Death and dying: challenge and change,* 1978, Addison-Wesley.
12. Cremation Association of North America (CANA): *2000 data and projections to the year 2025,* Aug 29, 2001, pp. 1–4.
13. Bowman J (Licensed Funeral Director): Personal correspondence, Sept 25, 2001.
14. Carr W: Spiritual pain and healing in the hospice, *America,* 173(4):26, 1995.

SUGGESTED READINGS

Berman PL: *The journey home: what near-death experiences and mysticism teach us about the gift of life,* 1998, Pocket Books.

Respected Harvard theologian Philip Berman analyzes his experiences, his beliefs, and the views of others to conclude that near-death experiences are relevant to people's lives. Berman expands beyond near-death experiences to examine other mystical experiences and their effect on the lives of the living.

Green R: *The Nicholas effect: a boy's gift to the world,* 1999, O'Reilly and Associates.

This is the true story of the death of Nicholas Green, a 7-year-old American tourist in Italy who was killed in a botched robbery. It tells how his courageous parents coped with this tragedy by opening their hearts to others. Nicholas's parents decided to donate his organs to seven Italian citizens. Their act inspired a worldwide increase in organ donations.

James JW, Friedman R: *The grief recovery handbook: the action program for moving beyond death, divorce, and other losses,* revised ed, 1998, HarperCollins.

This is a revised edition of a highly successful book that has helped people progress after a serious loss. Readers will come to realize that the passage of time alone rarely heals, but charting a specific course of action can provide a positive recovery. This book can help people rediscover joy in their lives.

Loving C: *My son, my sorrow: a mother's plea to Dr. Kevorkian,* 1998, New Horizon Press.

Carol Living's 27-year-old son begged her to help him die as he developed more and more serious complications from Lou Gehrig's disease. Confronting this dilemma, Loving turned to Dr. Kevorkian for assistance. This book illuminates one side of the debate about physician-assisted suicide.

As we go to Press...

In the weeks and months after the September 11, 2001 terrorist attacks on the World Trade Center and the Pentagon, law enforcement agencies were still trying to determine the total number of bodies expected to be found. As we go to press, the number of expected deaths is thought to be approximately 4,000. This figure includes bodies from the fourth airplane crash site in rural Pennsylvania.

The horrific nature of the terrorist attack has created real difficulties for many American citizens. Certainly, family members and friends of the victims are still grieving, but so are many persons who do not know anyone lost in the attack. People are losing sleep, feeling depressed, and many are worried about flying on an airplane again. Some children are having an especially difficult time, wondering why this happened and whether *they* will also become victims of a terrorist attack.

Psychologists remind us that these feeling are to be expected, given the magnitude of the September 11 tragedy. Twenty-four-hour television radio news coverage of the attack has only added to the anxiety that many people feel, especially as they wonder about the future. Many Americans are worried that this attack is only the beginning of a long, unconventional war against an elusive target. Despite a dramatic outpouring of patriotic feelings, they worry about how many American troops will be killed in the war on terrorism. They already feel sympathy and compassion for the innocent people who will likely die in the crossfire.

Name ______________________ **Date** __________ **Section** __________

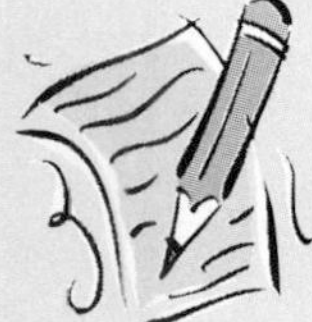

Personal Assessment

Planning Your Funeral

In line with this chapter's positive theme of the value of personal death awareness, here is a funeral service assessment that we frequently give to our health classes. This inventory can help you assess your reactions and thoughts about the funeral arrangements you would prefer for yourself.

After answering each of the following questions, you might wish to discuss your responses with a friend or close relative.

1. Have you ever considered how you would like your body to be handled after your death?
   _____ Yes _____ No
2. Have you already made funeral prearrangements for yourself?
   _____ Yes _____ No
3. Have you considered a specific funeral home or mortuary to handle your arrangements?
   _____ Yes _____ No
4. If you were to die today, which of the following would you prefer?
   _____ Embalming _____ Ground burial
   _____ Cremation _____ Entombment
   _____ Donation to medical science
5. If you prefer to be cremated, what would you want done with your ashes?
   _____ Buried _____ Entombed
   _____ Scattered
   _____ Other; please specify __________
6. If your funeral plans involve a casket, which of the following ones would you prefer?
   _____ Plywood (cloth covered)
   _____ Hardwood (oak, cherry, mahogany, maple, etc.)
   _____ Steel (sealer or nonsealer type)
   _____ Stainless steel
   _____ Copper or bronze
   _____ Other; please specify __________
7. How important would a funeral service be for you?
   _____ Very important
   _____ Somewhat important
   _____ Somewhat unimportant
   _____ Very unimportant
   _____ No opinion
8. What kind of funeral service would you want for yourself?
   _____ No service at all
   _____ Visitation (calling hours) the day before the funeral service; funeral held at church or funeral home
   _____ Graveside service only (no visitation)
   _____ Memorial service (after body disposition)
   _____ Other; please specify __________
9. How many people would you want to attend your funeral service or memorial service?
   _____ I do not want a funeral or memorial service
   _____ 1–10 people
   _____ 11–25 people
   _____ 26–50 people
   _____ Over 51 people
   _____ I do not care how many people attend
10. What format would you prefer at your funeral service or memorial service? Select any of the following that you would like.

	Yes	No
Religious music	_____	_____
Nonreligious music	_____	_____
Clergy present	_____	_____
Flower arrangements	_____	_____
Family member eulogy	_____	_____
Eulogy by friend(s)	_____	_____
Open casket	_____	_____
Religious format	_____	_____

Other; please specify __________

11. Using today's prices, how much would you expect to pay for your total funeral arrangements, including cemetery expenses (if applicable)?
   _____ Less than $4500
   _____ Between $4501 and $6000
   _____ Between $6001 and $7500
   _____ Between $7501 and $9000
   _____ Above $9000

To Carry This Further . . .

Which items had you not thought about before? Were you surprised at the arrangements you selected? Will you share your responses with anyone else? If so, whom?

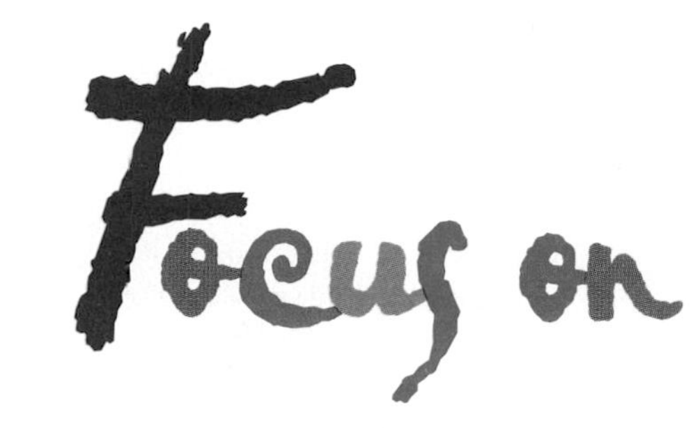

DEATH OF AN INFANT OR UNBORN CHILD

Life is fragile at all stages but especially so during the prenatal and early formative years. Indeed, from conception through development, birth, infancy and childhood, humans require an amazing amount of parental care and nurturing. Few other organisms are so dependent on others for their safety and well-being during the early months of life. Thus parents and children are tied together by a physical and emotional bond like no other. When that bond is severed by the tragic death of a young child, the pain and anguish the parents feel can be too much to bear. Getting through such a traumatic experience can be one of life's toughest challenges.[1]

Most pregnancies progress to full term and result in the birth of a healthy child. However, researchers now believe that about one third of pregnancies end in miscarriage. Since the development of accurate home-pregnancy tests, many women are finding out early in the first trimester that they are pregnant. Thus, rather than mistaking the miscarriage for a late heavy menstrual period, more women are now aware that their pregnancy has ended. Most then go through the grieving process discussed here. In addition, other complications occur in a small number of cases. These problems can sometimes cause termination of the pregnancy (miscarriage or elective abortion), death of the baby during birth, or death during infancy. Though most people know that such things can happen, many feel that such tragedies happen only to others. When faced with the death or potential loss of a child, parents often find their belief system shaken and their faith tested.[2]

The Mourning Process

The process of grieving is different for each family. There are no set rules for getting over the loss of a child. There is no right way to mourn and no time limit for the mourning process. The first days, months, and years may seem meaningless, and parents may find themselves living day to day with no real purpose or focus.[3]

Despite the pain each individual in the family feels, care must be taken to preserve family unity. Each person must realize that other family members may grieve in different ways. Wives and husbands may grieve differently, and this can cause strain in their marriage. If one parent seems quiet or preoccupied, the other should not mistake this behavior for a lack of emotion. Parents should also make sure that they do not ignore the feelings of other children in the family. Sometimes the mourning parents become wrapped up in their own grief and forget that the tragedy affects their other children as well. Siblings should be encouraged to discuss their feelings to help with their own grief and to reaffirm their importance within the family.[3]

The way a baby dies can affect the mourning process. Whether the child is lost before birth (miscarriage, abortion), during birth (stillbirth, trauma), or in infancy (sudden infant death syndrome [SIDS], accident, birth defect) can affect how the parents deal with the loss. It can also have an effect on how family and friends provide support for the parents.

Death of an Unborn Child

Miscarriage can be especially difficult to deal with for the woman involved. The baby has been lost within the mother's womb, and she may blame herself for the loss as a result. She may think that something she did (or did not do) has caused the miscarriage.[2,4] "One night just before I found out I was pregnant, I went out with friends and had a few beers," recalls Gabrielle, who had a miscarriage when she was 26.[5] "I didn't know I was pregnant. I was late with my period but didn't suspect I was pregnant until later. I can't help but wonder if the alcohol caused it (the miscarriage)." Consumption of alcohol or over-the-counter medications before a woman knows she is pregnant is a common cause of guilt after a miscarriage. An exact cause of a miscarriage may never be determined, and the woman needs to be reassured that she did not cause any abnormalities in the fetus.[2]

A miscarriage can be painful, embarrassing, and stressful for the woman. Physical symptoms may not occur when the baby dies but may be delayed for some time. Rosalinda became pregnant in the first month after she stopped taking her birth control pills. About 3 weeks into the pregnancy, "I found myself crying uncontrollably while driving home from work," she recalls. "Although I had no visible signs of miscarriage, I was sure something was wrong." Rosalinda had always been successful in other endeavors, but she started to fear that she would fail in her attempts to bring a baby into the world. "At 11 weeks my fears came true. We were on a much-needed vacation in Las Vegas. Two days of cramping turned into uncontrollable hemorrhaging." She and her husband wound up in the hotel lobby trying to get a cab to the hospital.

"You can imagine my utter embarrassment as I'm holding a towel in front of me to hide the blood as my husband is haggling with the bellman to let us go to the front of the line."[6]

Sometimes parents find out about a potentially fatal or severely debilitating problem with the fetus before the child is born. In these situations the parents are faced with the choice of continuing the pregnancy or terminating it. Hearing such a diagnosis, taking in all available information, and reaching a decision can be a traumatic experience. Parents must weigh many factors when making this decision, including their spiritual beliefs, potential suffering of the baby (if the long-term prognosis is poor), effects on the family of having a child with special needs, and financial considerations. If a decision is made to terminate the pregnancy (or if a continued pregnancy may result in miscarriage or stillbirth), the couple must be prepared for the sadness and trauma of parting with their baby.[4]

Death during the Birthing Process

In some instances, the parents know beforehand that the baby has a poor chance of surviving through birth, so they have a chance to prepare for this occurrence. For others, however, the baby's death is totally unexpected. Parents who thought they would be bringing home a healthy baby end up dealing with the devastation of losing their child. "The worst part was returning home," recalls Marcus, whose wife delivered a stillborn child after complications during birth. "The nursery was all set up . . . that brought back all of the feelings we had initially experienced after the birth."[7]

In the past, babies with lethal birth defects were often quickly taken away from their mothers, but today many parents are being given the option of spending time holding and saying good-bye to their baby, and medical personnel are encouraged to accommodate the parents and support their wishes in this regard.[4]

Losing a Baby after It Is Born

Even after a baby is delivered, there are health risks. After her miscarriage, Gabrielle gave birth to a seemingly healthy daughter, only to lose her 5 months later. "She just stopped breathing," Gabrielle recalls. "We had all been asleep, and when we went in to check on her she wasn't moving or breathing. We tried to wake her . . . she wasn't face down or anything like that. The doctors had no reason for it. They said it was SIDS."

The loss of a second child was devastating for Gabrielle, and it nearly ruined her marriage. "We were both very tense. We thought about trying again, but we felt jinxed. We fought a lot in the weeks after it happened." Gabrielle and her husband received counseling and eventually began to realize that they were not at fault for their tragic losses. They now have a healthy 3-year-old daughter. "We got up the courage to try one more time, thank God," she says.[5]

Dealing with the Loss of a Baby

Support of family and friends is especially important when trying to recover from the death of a child. Friends and coworkers can help by acknowledging the death of the child and offering support.[3] Often people will not mention the baby because they feel that the parents will become upset by bringing up the subject, but not talking about the baby can cause pain for the parents.[3] Showing up in person (as opposed to just calling or sending a card) to offer support can also help.[8]

While the mother is still in the hospital, medical personnel should be made aware of what the mother has been through. Sometimes a mother who has lost her baby will remain in the maternity wing of the hospital. A discreet notice posted on the door of her room will alert personnel that the room's occupant has lost her child, thus preventing any unfortunate assumptions.[2]

Tactful language can also help prevent unpleasant feelings for the parents. If an unhealthy fetus were miscarried or had to be aborted, sometimes people would try to rationalize the loss for the parents by saying it was "nature's way" of preventing the birth of an imperfect child.[8] Such comments are not only insensitive, but they imply that the parents should be grateful that they lost the baby. Even seemingly innocent comments can cause pain in the wrong context. Rosalinda wondered why she had continued to gain weight for 2 months even though the doctor said the baby had probably died only 3 or 4 weeks into her pregnancy. " 'It's probably just pizza,' my husband said. The doctor laughed and agreed." Rosalinda felt that her husband's attempt to lighten the situation was "probably the most insensitive statement I've ever heard him make . . . my opinion of the doctor also dropped dramatically at that point."[6] She later underwent a D & C (dilation and curettage) but was asked to sign a form giving her permission for an abortion even though she had already miscarried. She was "deeply humiliated to have to sign this. Didn't they realize how much I had already been through?"

Often parents will want to hold on to the memory of the child. Such feelings are quite normal and do not mean that the parents are holding on to their grief or are neurotic.[3] Remembering the child can give a sense of meaning to parents' lives. Often parents will do something constructive to help them remember their baby and get over the death. Putting together a scrapbook, donating the baby's clothes and toys to charity, writing memoirs, or setting up a place for remembrance can help the family keep memories of the baby.[3,8,9]

Eventually the grief should lose its intensity. It may flare up again around "anniversaries" (the baby's due date or birthday, the day of the baby's death), but gradually things should become bearable. The family will be forever changed by the experience. The death of a child can cause the value system of the parents to change, and their spiritual beliefs may be shaken as well.[3] But if the parents receive support from medical staff, family, and friends, ultimately the devastation can be overcome. It is hoped that such tragedies, while terribly unfortunate, can make these families stronger and bring them closer together.

For Discussion . . .

What are the differences in dealing with losing a child before, during, or after it is born? If you were faced with the choice of giving birth to a child with severe birth defects or terminating the pregnancy, which would you choose? If you lost a baby, would you try again to have one?

References

1. DeSpelder LA, Strickland AL: *The last dance: encountering death and dying,* ed 5, 1999, Mayfield.
2. Hitchcock Pappas DJ, McCoy MC: Grief counseling. In Kuller JA et al, editors: *Prenatal diagnosis and reproductive genetics,* 1995, Mosby.
3. Cole D: When a child dies, *Parents' Magazine,* p. 3, March 1994.
4. Salmon DK: Coping with miscarriage, *Parents' Magazine,* p. 5, May 1991.
5. Anonymous: Personal communication, April 1996.
6. Anonymous: Personal communication, March 1996.
7. Anonymous: Personal communication, Dec 1995.
8. Allison C: For Felicity, *Reader's Digest,* p. 199, Jan 1993.
9. Robb DB: Moving on, *Reader's Digest,* p. 223, Jan 1995.

appendix

Mental Disorders

CATEGORIES OF MENTAL DISORDERS

Anxiety Disorders

Anxiety disorders are characterized by a fear that leads to overarousal of heartbeat, muscle tension, and shakiness.

- *Phobic disorder.* Excessive irrational fears. Examples are agoraphobia (fear of open places), claustrophobia (fear of enclosed places), and acrophobia (fear of heights).
- *Panic disorder.* Overwhelming fear of losing control or going crazy. Panic attacks can last from a minute to an hour or more. No clear reason exists as to why panic attacks occur.
- *Generalized anxiety disorder.* Continued, free-floating anxiety that lasts for at least 1 month.
- *Obsessive-compulsive disorder.* Obsessive behavior is characterized by recurring irrational thoughts that remain out of control. Compulsive behavior reflects an irresistible urge to act repeatedly.

Dissociative Disorders

Dissociative disorders are those in which there is a sudden, temporary change in consciousness or self-identity.

- *Psychogenic amnesia.* Inability to recall a stressful event.
- *Psychogenic fugue.* Disorder in which a person loses memory of his or her past, moves to another locale, and takes on a new identity.
- *Multiple personality.* Disorder characterized by several distinct personalities occupying the same person.

Somatoform Disorders

People with somatoform disorders complain of a physical ailment, yet no physical abnormality can be found.

- *Conversion disorder.* Severe, unexplained loss of some physical ability (such as eyesight or use of the legs).
- *Hypochondriasis.* The belief that one is sick, although no medical evidence can be found.

Affective Disorders

In affective disorders a disturbance exists in a person's ability to express emotions.

- *Dysthymic disorder.* Persistent feelings (lasting for at least 2 years) characterized by lack of energy, loss of self-esteem, pessimistic outlook, inability to enjoy other people or pleasurable activities, and thoughts about suicide. The disorder is likely the most common psychological problem in humans.
- *Major depressive disorder.* Depression more severe than dysthymic disorder. Evidenced by poor appetite and significant weight loss, psychomotor symptoms, impaired reality testing, and recurrent thoughts of suicide.
- *Bipolar disorder.* Mood swings from elation to depression (formerly known as manic-depression).

Schizophrenic Disorders

Schizophrenic disorders are largely recognized by a person's verbal behavior. These disorders are characterized by disturbances in thought, perception, and attention. Schizophrenic patients may speak in a meaningless fashion, switch from topic to topic, and convey little important information. They may have delusions of grandeur or persecution, hallucinations, or excited or slowed motor activity. Usually schizophrenic patients do not think that their thoughts and actions are abnormal.

- *Disorganized type.* Characterized by disorganized delusions and frequent hallucinations that may be sexual or religious in nature. Exaggerated social impairment is common.
- *Catatonic type.* Characterized by a marked impairment in motor activity. May hold one body position for hours and not respond to the speech of others.
- *Paranoid type.* Characterized by delusions of persecution, often ones that are complex and systemized. Paranoid schizophrenic patients may experience vivid hallucinations that support their delusions.

THERAPEUTIC APPROACHES TO MENTAL DISORDERS

A variety of approaches can be used to help people who have mental disorders. These approaches involve psychotherapy or the use of biological therapies. A brief outline of the more widely known strategies follows, since a comprehensive presentation on this topic is beyond the scope of this appendix.

Insight-Oriented Therapies

Underlying this category of therapeutic approaches is the belief that the client must gain insight into the experiences that led up to his or her problem or maladaptive behavior. By being able to recognize the underlying motives for one's behavior, a client will be better able to objectively view his or her beliefs, feelings, and thinking patterns. These underlying motives often are beneath the person's level of consciousness. Insight-oriented forms of psychotherapy include cognitive therapy, psychoanalysis, person-centered therapy, transactional analysis, and gestalt therapy.

Behavior Therapy

Discussed briefly in Chapter 6, behavior therapy (also called *behavior modification*) attempts to produce behavior change in a client by using scientifically tested principles of classical and operant conditioning and observational learning. Techniques of behavior therapy include operant conditioning (behavior reinforcement), aversive conditioning, systematic desensitization, assertiveness training, and self-control techniques.

Group Therapy

This form of therapy involves a therapist and several clients who have similar problems. Examples might be group therapy for people with eating disorders, smoking concerns, sexual problems, family problems, or relationship concerns. By meeting together and working to resolve their similar concerns, clients often receive support from other group members. With multiple members, a larger volume of pertinent information exists for clients to share. In a practical sense, group therapy is usually less expensive than individual therapy and the therapist can reach more clients at once.

Biological Therapies

Psychiatrists and other physicians are qualified to approach mental disorders from a medical framework. They are able to use chemotherapy (tranquilizers, antidepressants, lithium), electroconvulsive therapy (ECT or shock therapy), and even psychosurgery (brain surgery). Often these approaches are used with clients who have especially serious psychiatric disorders or who do not respond well to psychotherapy.

Glossary

A

abortion induced premature termination of a pregnancy

absorption passage of nutrients or alcohol through the walls of the stomach or intestinal tract into the bloodstream

abuse any use of a legal or illegal drug that is detrimental to health

acid-base balance acidity-alkalinity of body fluids

acquaintance rape forced sexual intercourse between individuals who know each other

acquired immunity (AI) significant component of the immune system associated with the formation of antibodies and specialized blood cells that are capable of destroying pathogens

ACTH (adrenocorticotropic hormone) hormone produced in the pituitary gland and transmitted to the cortex of the adrenal glands; stimulates production and release of corticoids

activity requirement calories required for daily physical work

acupuncture insertion of fine needles into the body to alter electroenergy fields and cure disease

acute alcohol intoxication potentially fatal elevation of the blood alcohol concentration, often resulting from rapid consumption of large amounts of alcohol

acute rhinitis the common cold; the sudden onset of nasal inflammation

adaptive thermogenesis physiological response of the body to adjust its metabolic rate to the presence or absence of calories

addiction term used interchangeably with physical dependence

adrenal glands paired triangular endocrine glands situated above each kidney; site of epinephrine and corticoid production

adrenaline powerful stress response hormone (*see* epinephrine)

adrenocorticotropic hormone (ACTH) hormone produced in the pituitary gland and transmitted to the cortex of the adrenal glands; stimulates production and release of corticoids

aerobic energy production body's production of energy when the respiratory and circulatory systems are able to process and transport a sufficient amount of oxygen to muscle cells

agent causal pathogen of a particular disease

AIDS acquired immunodeficiency syndrome; viral-based destruction of the immune system, leading to illness and death from opportunistic infections

alcoholism primary chronic disease with genetic, psychosocial, and environmental factors influencing its development and manifestations

allergens environmental substances to which people may be hypersensitive; allergens function as antigens

allopathy system of medical practice in which specific remedies (often pharmaceutical agents) are used to produce effects different from those produced by a disease or injury

alveoli thin, saclike terminal ends of the airways; the sites at which gases are exchanged between the blood and inhaled air

Alzheimer's disease gradual development of memory loss, confusion, and loss of reasoning; will eventually lead to total intellectual incapacitation, brain degeneration, and death

amenorrhea cessation or lack of menstrual periods

amino acids chief components of protein; synthesized by the body or obtained from dietary sources

amotivational syndrome behavioral pattern characterized by widespread apathy toward productive activities

anabolic steroids drugs that function like testosterone to produce increases in weight, strength, endurance, and aggressiveness

anaerobic energy production body's production of energy when needed amounts of oxygen are not readily available

analgesic drugs drugs that reduce the sensation of pain

anaphylactic shock life-threatening congestion of the airways resulting from hypersensitivity to a foreign protein

androgyny the blending of both masculine and feminine characteristics

anemia condition reflecting abnormally low levels of hemoglobin

aneurysm a ballooning or outpouching on a weakened area of an artery

angina pectoris chest pain that results from impaired blood supply to the heart muscle

angioplasty surgical insertion of a balloon-tipped catheter into the coronary artery to open areas of narrowing

anorexia nervosa emotional disorder in which appetite and hunger are suppressed and marked weight loss occurs

anovulatory not ovulating

antagonistic effect effect produced when one drug nullifies (reduces, offsets) the effects of a second drug

anti-angiogenesis drug-based therapy that prevents cancerous tumors from developing an enriching blood supply

antibodies chemical compounds produced by the immune system to destroy antigens and their toxins

arrhythmias irregularities of the heart's normal rhythm or beating pattern

arteriosclerosis calcification of an artery's wall that makes the vessel less elastic, more brittle, and more susceptible to bursting; hardening of the arteries

artificial insemination depositing of sperm in the female reproductive tract in an attempt to impregnate; sperm may be those of the partner or of a donor

artificially acquired immunity (AAI) type of acquired immunity resulting from the body's response to pathogens introduced into the body through immunizations

asbestos fibrous material found in insulation and many other building materials; causes asbestosis

asphyxiation death resulting from lack of oxygen to the brain

atherosclerosis the buildup of plaque on the inner walls of arteries

attention deficit hyperactivity disorder (ADHD) inability to concentrate well on a specified task; often accompanied by above-normal physical movement; also called *hyperactivity*

autoimmune immune response against the cells of a person's own body

axon portion of a neuron that conducts electrical impulses to the dendrites of adjacent neurons; neurons typically have one axon

ayurveda traditional Indian medicine based on herbal remedies

AZT (azidothymidine) the first drug approved for use in the treatment of AIDS; capable of reducing symptoms and possibly extending life of a person with AIDS

B

balanced diet diet featuring food selections from each of the five food groups

ballistic stretching a "bouncing" form of stretching in which a muscle group is lengthened repetitively to produce multiply quick, forceful stretches

basal cells foundation cells that underlie the epithelial cells

basal metabolic rate (BMR) the amount of energy (in calories) your body requires to maintain basic functions

behavior modification behavioral therapy designed to change the learned behavior of an individual

benign noncancerous; tumors that do not spread

beta blockers drugs that prevent overactivity of the heart, which results in angina pectoris

bias and hate crimes criminal acts directed at a person or group solely because of a specific characteristic, such as race, religion, ethnic background, or political beliefs

binge drinking alcohol use characterized by periods of intense alcohol consumption; for example, drinking heavily on the weekend

bioavailability speed and extent to which a drug becomes biologically active within the body; bioavailability for a drug varies among individuals and within a given individual over time

biofeedback self-monitoring of physiological processes as they occur within the body

biological sexuality male and female aspects of sexuality

birth control all of the procedures that can prevent the birth of a child

bisexual choosing members of both genders as one's sexual preference

blackout temporary state of amnesia experienced by a drinker; an inability to remember events that occur during a period of alcohol use

blood alcohol concentration (BAC) percentage of alcohol in a measured quantity of blood

blood analysis chemical analysis of various substances in the blood; helps determine changes and possible disturbances in the body

BOD POD body composition system used to measure body fat through air displacement

bodybuilding sports activity in which the participants train their bodies to reach desired goals of muscular size, symmetry, and proportion

body fat analysis determination of the percentage of body tissue composed of fat

body image subjective perception of how one's body appears

body mass index (BMI) numerical expression of body weight based on height and weight

body wrapping a nonsurgical form or body contouring in which the body is tightly wrapped with damp strips of cloth until dehydration of underlying tissues occurs

bonding important initial sense of recognition established between the newborn and those adults on whom the newborn will depend

brain death the absence of brain wave activity after an initial measurement followed by a second measurement 24 hours later

brand name specific name assigned to a patented drug or product by its manufacturer

Braxton Hicks contractions false labor contractions; mild and of irregular spacing

breakthrough bleeding midcycle uterine bleeding; spotting

breech position birth position in which the baby's feet or buttocks are presented first

brown fat specialized body fat capable of dispersing excess calories as heat

bulimia nervosa binge eating followed by purging the body of the food

C

calcium channel blockers drugs that prevent arterial spasms; used in the longterm management of angina pectoris

calendar method form of periodic abstinence in which the variable lengths of a woman's menstrual cycle are used to calculate her fertile period

calipers device to measure the thickness of a skinfold from which percent body fat can be calculated

caloric balance caloric input equals caloric output; weight remains constant

calories units of heat (energy); specifically, 1 calorie equals the heat required to raise 1 kilogram of water 1° C

cannula hollow metal or plastic tube through which materials can be aspirated

carbohydrates chemical compounds comprised of sugar or saccharide units; the body's primary source of energy

carbon monoxide chemical compound (CO) that can inactivate red blood cells

carcinogenic related to the production of cancerous changes; property of environmental agents, including drugs, that may stimulate the development of cancerous changes within cells

carcinoma in situ cancer at its site of origin

cardiac pertaining to the heart

cardiac muscle specialized smooth muscle tissue that forms the middle (muscular) layer of the heart wall

cardiogram reading of heart and lung function from a cardiograph machine

cardiorespiratory endurance ability of the body to process and transport oxygen required by muscle cells so that these cells can continue to contract

cardiovascular pertaining to the heart (cardio) and blood vessels (vascular)

carjacking a crime that involves a thief's attempt to steal a car while the owner is behind the wheel; carjackings are usually random and unpredictable and often involve handguns

catabolism metabolic process of breaking down tissue for the purpose of converting it to energy

CT scan computerized axial tomography; x-ray procedure designed to visualize structures within the body that would not normally be seen through conventional x-ray procedures

cauterize to apply a small electrical current and permanently close a tube or vessel; to burn

celibacy self-imposed avoidance of sexual intimacy

central nervous system the brain and spinal cord

cereal germ highly nutritious portions of the cereal grain, often removed during milling

cerebral cortex outer covering of the brain; site of intellect, memory, thought processes, and rationalization

cerebral hemorrhage bleeding from the cerebral arteries within the brain

cerebrovascular accident stroke; brain tissue damage resulting from impaired circulation of blood vessels in the brain

cerebrovascular occlusion blockage to arteries supplying blood to the cerebral cortex of the brain; resulting in a stroke

cervical cap small, thimble-shaped contraceptive device designed to fit over the cervix

cesarean delivery surgical removal of a fetus through the abdominal wall

chemical name name used to describe the molecular structure of a drug

chemoprevention the safe and effective use of dietary supplements in the prevention of illness and disease

child abuse harm committed against a child; usually refers to physical abuse, sexual abuse, or child neglect

chiropractic manipulation of the vertebral column to relieve pressure and cure illness

chlamydia the most prevalent sexually transmitted disease; caused by a nongonococcal bacterium

cholesterol a primary form of fat found in the blood; lipid material manufactured within the body, as well as derived through dietary sources

chronic develops slowly and persists for a long period of time

chronic bronchitis persistent inflammation and infection of the smaller airways within the lungs

chronic disorder condition that develops and progresses slowly over an extended period of time

chronic fatigue syndrome (CFS) illness that causes severe exhaustion, fatigue, aches, and depression; mostly affects women in their thirties and forties

cilia small, hairlike structures that extend from cells that line the air passage

cirrhosis condition characterized by pathological changes to the liver resulting from chronic heavy alcohol consumption; a frequent cause of death among heavy alcohol users

clitoris small shaft of erectile tissue located in front of the vaginal opening; the female homolog of the male penis

codependence unhealthy relationship in which one person is addicted to alcohol or another drug and a person close to him or her is "addicted" to the alcoholic or drug user

cohabitation sharing of a residence by two unrelated, unmarried people; living together

coitus penile-vaginal intercourse

coitus interruptus (withdrawal) a contraceptive practice in which the erect penis is removed from the vagina before ejaculation

cold turkey immediate, total discontinuation of use of tobacco or other addictive substances

coliform bacteria intestinal tract bacteria whose presence in a water supply suggests contamination by human or animal waste

collateral circulation ability of nearby blood vessels to enlarge and carry additional blood around a blocked blood vessel

companionate love friendly affection and deep attachment, based on extensive familiarity with another person

compliance willingness to follow the directions provided by another person

condom latex shield designed to cover the erect penis and retain semen on ejaculation

confrontation an approach to convince drug-dependent people to enter treatment

congestive heart failure inability of the heart to pump out all the blood that returns to it; can lead to dangerous fluid accumulation in veins, lungs, and kidneys

consumer fraud marketing of unreliable and ineffective services, products, or information under the guise of curing disease or improving health; quackery

contact inhibition ability of a tissue, on reaching its mature size, to suppress additional growth

contraception any procedure that prevents fertilization

contraindications factors that make the use of a drug inappropriate or dangerous for a particular person

cooldown stretching and walking after exercise

coronary arteries vessels that supply oxygenated blood and nutrients to heart muscle

coronary artery bypass surgery surgical procedure designed to improve blood flow to the heart by providing alternative routes for blood around points of blockage

coroner an elected legal official empowered to pronounce death and to determine the official cause of a suspicious or violent death

corpus luteum cellular remnant of the graafian follicle after the release of an ovum

corticoids hormones generated by the adrenal cortex; corticoids influence the body's control of glucose, protein, and fat metabolism

CPR cardiopulmonary resuscitation; first aid procedure designed to restore breathing and heart function

crack a crystalline form of cocaine that is smoked; has an instantaneous effect and is highly dependence-producing

creativity innovative ability; insightful capacity to solve problems; ability to move beyond analytical or logical approaches to experiences

cross-tolerance transfer of tolerance from one drug to another within the same general category

crosstraining use of more than one aerobic activity to achieve cardiovascular fitness

cruciferous vegetables vegetables that have flowers with four leaves in the pattern of a cross

crypts burial locations generally located beneath churches

CT scan computed tomography scan; an x-ray procedure that is designed to visualize structures within the body that would not normally be seen through conventional x-ray procedures

cunnilingus oral stimulation of the vulva or clitoris

cystitis infection of the urinary bladder

D

date rape a form of acquaintance rape that involves forced sexual intercourse by a dating partner

dehydration abnormal depletion of fluids from the body; severe dehydration can lead to death

delirium tremens (DTs) uncontrollable shaking associated with withdrawal from heavy chronic alcohol use

dendrite portion of a neuron that receives electrical stimuli from adjacent neurons; neurons typically have several such branches or extensions

denial in this case, the failure to acknowledge that alcohol or drug use seriously affects one's life

dependence general term that reflects the need to keep consuming a drug for psychological or physical reasons, or both

depressants the psychoactive drugs that reduce the function of the central nervous system

designated driver a person who abstains from or carefully limits alcohol use to drive others safely

designer drugs drugs that chemically resemble drugs on the FDA Schedule 1

desirable weight weight range deemed appropriate for people of a specific gender, age, and frame size

diaphragm soft rubber vaginal cup designed to cover the cervix

diastolic pressure blood pressure against blood vessel walls when the heart relaxes

dilation gradual expansion of an opening or passageway

dilation and curettage (D & C) surgical procedure in which the cervical canal is dilated to allow the uterine wall to be scraped

dilation and evacuation (D & E) surgical procedure using cervical dilation and vacuum aspiration to remove uterine wall material and fetal parts

direct (active) euthanasia process of inducing death, often through the injection of lethal drugs

distress stress that diminishes the quality of life; commonly associated with disease, illness, and maladaptation

diuresis increased discharge of fluid from the body; frequent urination

diuretic drugs drugs that aid the body in removing excess fluid

drug synergism enhancement of a drug's effect as a result of the presence of additional drugs within the system

duration length of time one needs to exercise at the target heart rate to produce the training effect

dynamic in a state of change; health is dynamic in the sense that it is influenced by factors from both within and outside the individual

dysplastic nevi small moles whose presence may indicate a high likelihood of developing malignant melanoma

E

ECG electrocardiograph; an instrument to measure and record the electrical activity within the heart

echocardiography procedure that uses high-frequency sound waves to visualize the structure and function of the heart

ectopic pregnancy a pregnancy wherein the fertilized ovum implants at a site other than the uterus, typically in the fallopian tube

effacement a thinning and pulling back of the cervical opening to allow movement of the fetus from the uterus

electrical impedance method of testing the percentage of body fat using an electrical current

electroencephalograph instrument that measures the electrical activity of the brain

embolism potentially fatal situation in which a circulating blood clot lodges itself in a smaller vessel

empower the ability to make choices and take responsibility for oneself

enabling in this case, the inadvertent support that some people provide to alcohol or drug abusers

endometrium innermost lining of the uterus, broken down and discharged during menstruation

enriched process of returning to foods some of the nutritional elements (B vitamins and iron) removed during processing

environmental tobacco smoke tobacco smoke that is diluted and stays within a common source of air

enzymes organic substances that control the rate of physiological reactions but are not themselves altered in the process

epinephrine powerful adrenal hormone whose presence in the bloodstream prepares the body for maximal energy production and skeletal muscle response

episodic medicine medical practice centered on the diagnosis and treatment of illness or injury at the time of its occurrence or the appearance of symptoms

epitaph inscription on a grave marker or monument

erection the engorgement of erectile tissue with blood; characteristic of the penis, clitoris, nipple, labia minora, and scrotum

ergogenic aids supplements that are taken to improve athletic performance

erotic dreams dreams whose content elicits a sexual response

Escherichia coli (E. coli) a bacterium found in food or water that indicates contamination by animal or human excrement

essential amino acids nine amino acids that can be obtained only from dietary sources

essential hypertension hypertension (high blood pressure) resulting from chronic widespread constriction of arterioles

estrogen ovarian hormone that initiates the development of the uterine wall

eulogy a composition or speech that praises someone; often delivered at a funeral or memorial service

eustress stress that enhances the quality of life

excitement stage initial arousal stage of the sexual response pattern

exhibitionism exposure of one's genitals for the purpose of shocking other people

F

faith the purposes and meaning that underlie an individual's hopes and dreams

fallopian tubes paired tubes that allow passage of ova from the ovaries to the uterus; the oviducts

false labor conditions that tend to resemble the start of true labor; may include irregular uterine contractions, pressure, and discomfort in the lower abdomen

fast foods convenience foods; foods featured in a variety of restaurants, including hamburgers, pizza, and tacos

fat density percent of the total calories in a food item derived from fat

FDA Schedule 1 list comprising drugs that hold a high potential for abuse but have no medical use

fecundity the ability to produce offspring

fellatio oral stimulation of the penis

femininity behavioral expressions traditionally observed in females

fermentation chemical process whereby plant products are converted into alcohol by the action of yeast on carbohydrates

fertility ability to reproduce

fetal alcohol effects developmental impairment in a child linked to a mother's use of alcohol during pregnancy

fetal alcohol syndrome characteristic birth defects noted in the children of some women who consume alcohol during their pregnancies

fiber plant material that cannot be digested; found in cereal, fruits, and vegetables

fight-or-flight response the reaction to a stressor by confrontation or avoidance (sometimes called the fight, fright, flight, or folly [or 4F] response)

flaccid nonerect; the state of erectile tissue when vasocongestion is not occurring

flashback unpredictable return of a psychedelic trip

flexibility ability of joints to function through an intended range of motion

follicle-stimulating hormone (FSH) gonadotropic hormone required for initial development of ova (in the female) and sperm (in the male)

food additives chemical compounds that are intentionally or unintentionally added to our food supply that change some property of the food such as color or texture

foreplay activities, often involving touching and caressing, that prepare individuals for sexual intercourse

freebase altered form of cocaine that can be smoked

frequency number of times per week one should exercise to achieve a training effect

full funeral services all of the professional services provided by funeral directors

functional foods foods capable of contributing to the improvement/prevention of specific health problems

G

gait pattern of walking

gaseous phase portion of tobacco smoke containing carbon monoxide and many other physiologically active gaseous compounds

gateway drugs easily obtained legal or illegal drugs (alcohol, tobacco, marijuana) whose use may precede the use of less common illegal drugs

gender general term reflecting a biological basis of sexuality; the male gender or the female gender

gender adoption lengthy process of learning the behaviors that are traditional for one's gender

gender identification achievement of a personally satisfying interpretation of one's masculinity or feminity

gender identity recognition of one's gender

gender preference emotional and intellectual acceptance of one's gender

gender schema mental image of the cognitive, affective, and performance characteristics appropriate to a particular gender; a mental picture of being a man or a woman

general adaptation syndrome sequenced physiological response to the presence of a stressor; the alarm, resistance, recovery, and exhaustion stages of the stress response

generativity midlife developmental task; repaying society for its support through contributions associated with parenting, creativity, and occupation

generic name common or nonproprietary name of a drug

genetic counseling medical counseling regarding the transmission and management of inherited conditions

genetic predisposition inherited tendency to develop a disease process if necessary environmental factors exist

glucose blood sugar; the body's primary source of energy

gonads male or female sex glands; testes produce sperm and ovaries produce eggs

H

hallucinogens psychoactive drugs capable of producing hallucinations (distortions of reality)

hashish resins collected from the flowering tops of marijuana plants

health claims statements attesting to a food's contribution to the improvement/prevention of specific health problems

health promotion movement in which knowledge, practices, and values are transmitted to people for their use in lengthening their lives, reducing the incidence of illness, and feeling better

healthy body weight body weight within a weight range appropriate for a person with an acceptable waist-to-hip ratio

heart catheterization procedure wherein a thin catheter is introduced through an arm or leg artery into the coronary circulation to visualize areas of blockage

heart-lung machine device that oxygenates and circulates blood during bypass surgery

hemorrhaging bleeding; often implies profuse bleeding

herbalism an ancient form of healing in which herbal preparations are used to treat illness and disease

heterosexual having a sexual preference for a member of the opposite gender

high-density lipoprotein (HDL) the type of lipoprotein that transports cholesterol from the bloodstream to the liver where it is eventually removed from the body; high levels of HDL are related to a reduction in heart disease

HIV human immunodeficiency virus

holistic health broadest view of the composition of health; views health in terms of its physical, emotional, social, intellectual, spiritual, and occupational makeup

homeopathy the use of minute doses of herbs or minerals to stimulate healing

homicide the intentional killing of one person by another

homosexual choosing a member of one's own gender as one's sexual preference

hormone replacement therapy (HRT) medically administered estrogen and progestin to replace hormones lost at menopause

hospice care approach to caring for terminally ill patients that maximizes the quality of life and allows death with dignity

host an infected person capable of infecting others

host negligence a legal term that reflects the failure of a host to provide reasonable care and safety for people visiting the host's residence or business

hot flashes temporary feelings of warmth experienced by women during and after menopause; caused by blood vessel dilation

Human Genome Project international quest by geneticists to identify the location and composition of every gene within the human cell

human papillomavirus (HPV) sexually transmitted virus capable of causing precancerous changes in the cervix; causative agent for genital warts

hypercellular obesity form of obesity seen in individuals who possess an abnormally large number of fat cells

hyperglycemia elevated blood glucose levels; an important indicator of diabetes mellitus

hyperparathyroidism condition reflecting the overactive production of parathyroid hormone by the parathyroid glands

hypertonic saline solution salt solution with a concentration higher than that found in human fluids

hypertrophic obesity form of obesity in which fat cells are enlarged, but not excessive in number

hypochondriasis neurotic conviction that one is ill or afflicted with a particular disease

hysterectomy surgical removal of the uterus

I

immune system system of biochemical and cellular elements that protect the body from invading pathogens and foreign materials

immunizations laboratory-prepared pathogens that are introduced into the body for the purpose of stimulating the body's immune system

incest marriage or coitus (sexual intercourse) between closely related individuals

incubation stage time required for a pathogen to multiply significantly enough for signs and symptoms to appear

indirect (passive) euthanasia process of allowing a person to die by disconnecting life support systems or withholding lifesaving techniques

infatuation a relatively temporary, intensely romantic attraction to another person

infertility inability of a male to impregnate or of a female to become pregnant

inhalants psychoactive drugs that enter the body through inhalation

inhibitions inner controls that prevent a person's engaging in certain types of behavior

insulin pancreatic hormone required by the body for the effective metabolism of glucose (blood sugar)

insulin-dependent (type 1) diabetes mellitus form of diabetes generally seen for the first time in childhood or adolescence; juvenile onset diabetes

intensity level of effort one puts into an activity

intentional injuries injuries that are purposely inflicted on one person by another person

interstitial cells specialized cells within the testicles that on stimulation by ICSH produce the male sex hormone testosterone

interstitial cell stimulating hormone (ICSH) a gonadotropic hormone of the male required for the production of testosterone

intimacy any close, mutual verbal or nonverbal behavior within a relationship

intimate abuse violence committed against a person by her or his current or former spouse, boyfriend, or girlfriend

intrauterine device (IUD) small plastic medicated or unmedicated device that when inserted in the uterus prevents continued pregnancy

in vitro fertilization and embryo transfer (IVF-ET) laboratory fertilization of an ovum taken from the woman with subsequent return of the developing embryo into the woman's uterus

ionizing radiation form of radiation capable of releasing electrons from atoms

isokinetic exercises muscular strength training exercises that use machines to provide variable resistances throughout the full range of motion

isometric exercises muscular strength training exercises that use a resistance so great that the resistance object cannot be moved

L

labia majora larger, more external skin folds that surround the vaginal opening

labia minora small, liplike folds of skin immediately adjacent to the vaginal opening

lactating breastfeeding; nursing

lactovegetarian diet vegetarian diet that allows for the consumption of milk and dairy products

laminaria plugs made of seaweed that on exposure to moisture expand and dilate the canal into which they have been placed

larynx the anatomical voice box; the structure in which the vocal cords are located

legumes peas and beans; plant sources high in the essential amino acids

lesbianism female homosexuality

lightening movement of fetus deeper into the pelvic cavity before the onset of the birth process

lipoprotein proteinlike structure in the bloodstream to which circulating fatty materials attach; associated with cardiovascular disease

living will document confirming a person's desire to be allowed to die peacefully and with a measure of dignity in case of terminal illness or major injury

low-density lipoprotein (LDL) the type of lipoprotein that transports the largest amount of cholesterol in the bloodstream; high levels of LDL are related to heart disease

luteinizing hormone (LH) female gonadotropic hormone required for fullest development and release of ova; ovulating hormone

Lyme disease systemic bacterial infection transmitted by deer ticks

M

macrobiotic diet vegetarian diet composed almost entirely of brown rice

mainstream smoke the smoke inhaled and then exhaled by a smoker

mammogram x ray examination of the breast

masculinity behavioral expressions traditionally observed in males

masochism sexual excitement while being injured or humiliated

mastectomy removal of breast tissue

masturbation self-stimulation of the genitals

maternal supportive tissues general term referring to the development of the placenta and other tissues specifically associated with pregnancy

mausoleum above-ground structure into which caskets can be placed for disposition and that frequently resembles a small stone house

maximum heart rate maximum number of times the heart can beat per minute

medical power of attorney for health care a legal document that designates who will make health-care decisions for people unable to do so for themselves

menarche time of a female's first menstrual cycle

menopause decline and eventual cessation of hormone production by the reproductive system

menstrual extraction procedure using vacuum aspiration to remove uterine wall material within 2 weeks after a missed menstrual period

menstrual phase phase of the menstrual cycle during which the broken-down lining of the uterus (endometrium) is discharged from the body

menstruation the cyclic buildup and destruction of the uterine wall

metabolic rate rate or intensity at which the body uses energy

metabolite breakdown product of a drug

metastasis spread of cancerous cells from their site of origin to other areas of the body

migraine headaches severe, recurrent headaches, usually affecting one side of the head

minerals chemical elements that serve as structural elements within body tissue or participate in physiological processes

minipills low-dose progesterone oral contraceptives

misuse inappropriate use of legal drugs intended to be medications

monogamous paired relationship with one partner

mononuclear leukocytes large white blood cells that have only one nucleus

mononucleosis ("mono") viral infection characterized by weakness, fatigue, swollen glands, and low-grade fever

monounsaturated fats fats made of compounds in which one hydrogen-bonding position remains to be filled; semisolid at room temperature; derived primarily from peanut and olive oils

morbidity illness or disease

morning-after pill high-dose combination oral contraceptive used to terminate a possible pregnancy

mortality death

MRI scan magnetic resonance imaging; an imaging procedure that uses a giant magnet to generate an image of body tissue

mucus clear, sticky material produced by specialized cells within the mucous membranes of the body; mucus traps much of the suspended particulate matter from tobacco smoke

multiorgasmic capacity potential to have several orgasms within a single period of sexual arousal

murmur an atypical heart sound that suggests a backwashing of blood into a chamber of the heart from which it has just left

muscular endurance ability of a muscle or muscle group to function over time; depends on well-developed respiratory and circulatory systems

muscular strength ability to contract skeletal muscles to engage in work

myelin white, fatty insulating material that surrounds the axons of many nerve cells

myocardial infarction heart attack; the death of heart muscle as a result of a blockage in one of the coronary arteries

myotonia buildup of neuromuscular tonus within a particular tissue

N

narcolepsy sleep-related disorder in which a person has a recurrent, overwhelming, and uncontrollable desire to sleep

narcotics psychoactive drugs derived from the oriental poppy plant; narcotics relieve pain and induce sleep

naturally acquired immunity (NAI) type of acquired immunity resulting from the body's response to naturally occurring pathogens

naturopathy a system of treatment that avoids drugs and surgery and emphasizes the use of natural agents to correct underlying imbalances

nerve blockers drugs that can stop the flow of electrical impulses through the nerves into which they have been injected

neuromuscular tonus level of nervous tension within the muscle

neuron nerve cell; the structural unit of the nervous system

neurophysiological nervous system function; processes through which the body senses and responds to its internal and external environments

neurotransmitters chemical messengers released by neurons that permit electrical impulses to be transferred from one nerve cell to another

neutraceuticals functional foods packaged to resemble medications

nicotine physiologically active, dependence-producing drug found in tobacco

night-eating syndrome a dietary pattern in which excessive eating occurs before bedtime or during the night

nitroglycerin a blood vessel dilator used by some cardiac patients to relieve angina

nocturnal emission ejaculation that occurs during sleep; "wet dream"

nodes in this case, the electrical centers found in cardiac muscle

nomogram graphic means of finding an unknown value

non–insulin-dependent (type 2) diabetes mellitus form of diabetes generally seen for the first time in people 35 years of age and older; adult-onset diabetes

nonoxynol 9 a spermicide commonly used with contraceptive devices

nontraditional-age students administrative term used by colleges and universities for students who, for whatever reason, are pursuing undergraduate work at an age other than that associated with traditional college years (18-24)

norepinephrine adrenaline-like neurotransmitter produced within the nervous system

nurse practitioners registered nurses who have taken specialized training in one or more clinical areas and are able to engage in limited diagnosis and treatment of illnesses

nutrients elements in foods that are required for the growth, repair, and regulation of body processes

O

obesity condition in which overweight is the result of excess body fat

oncogenes genes that are believed to activate the development of cancer

oogenesis production of ova in a biologically mature female

oral contraceptive pill taken orally, composed of synthetic female hormones that prevent ovulation or implantation; "the pill"

orgasmic platform expanded outer third of the vagina that during the plateau phase of the sexual response grips the penis

orgasmic stage third stage of the sexual response pattern; the stage during which neuromuscular tension is released

orthodontics dental specialty that focuses on the proper alignment of the teeth

osteoarthritis arthritis that develops with age; largely caused by weight-bearing and deterioration of joints

osteopathy system of medical practice that combines allopathic principles with specific attention to postural mechanics of the body

osteoporosis the loss of calcium from the bone caused by the inability of the body to use dietary calcium; seen primarily in postmenopausal women

outercourse sexual activity that does not involve intercourse

ovary female reproductive structure that produces ova and the female gonadal sex hormones estrogen and progesterone

overload principle principle whereby a person gradually increases the resistance load that must be moved or lifted

overweight condition in which body weight is above desirable weight

ovolactovegetarian diet diet that excludes the use of all meat but does allow the consumption of eggs and dairy products

ovulation the release of a mature egg from the ovary

oxidation in this case, the process that removes alcohol from the bloodstream

oxygen debt physical state that occurs when the body can no longer process and transport sufficient amounts of oxygen for continued muscle contraction

P

pacemaker sinoatrial or SA node; an area of cells within the heart that controls its electrical activity

Pap test a cancer screening procedure in which cells are removed from the cervix and examined for precancerous changes

paracervical anesthetic anesthetic injected into tissues surrounding the cervical opening

paraphilia a preference for unusual sexual practices

particulate phase portion of tobacco smoke composed of small suspended particles

partner abuse violence committed against a domestic partner

parturition childbirth

passionate love state of extreme absorption in another; tenderness, elation, anxiety, sexual desire, and ecstasy

passive smoking inhalation of air that is heavily contaminated with tobacco smoke

passively acquired immunity (PAI) temporary immunity achieved by providing antibodies to a person exposed to a particular pathogen

pathogen disease-causing agent

peak stage stage of an infectious disease at which symptoms are most fully expressed; acute stage

pedophilia sexual contact with children as a source of sexual excitement

pelvic inflammatory disease (PID) acute or chronic infections of the peritoneum or lining of the abdominopelvic cavity; associated with a variety of symptoms and a potential cause of sterility

periodic abstinence birth control methods that rely on a couple's avoidance of intercourse during the ovulatory phase of a woman's menstrual cycle; also called *fertility awareness* or *natural family planning*

periodontal disease destruction of soft tissue and bone that surround the teeth

peritonitis inflammation of the pertoneum or lining of the abdominopelvic cavity

phen-fen an abbreviation for the names of two drugs (phentermine and fenfluramine) once used to promote weight loss

phenylpropanolamine (PPA) active chemical compound once found in most over-the-counter diet products

physical dependence need to continue using a drug to maintain normal body function and to avoid withdrawal illness; also called *addiction*

pituitary gland "master gland" of the endocrine system; the wide variety of hormones produced by the pituitary are sent to structures throughout the body

placebo medications that contain no active ingredients

placenta structure through which nutrients, metabolic wastes, and drugs (including alcohol) pass from the bloodstream of the mother into the bloodstream of the developing fetus

plateau stage second stage of the sexual response pattern; a leveling off of arousal immediately before orgasm

platelet adhesiveness tendency of platelets to clump together, thus enhancing speed at which the blood clots

platonic close association between two people that does not include a sexual relationship

podiatrists specialists who treat a variety of ailments of the feet

polyunsaturated fats fats composed of compounds in which multiple hydrogen-bonding positions remain open; these fats are liquids at room temperature; derived from a variety of vegetable sources

positive caloric balance caloric intake greater than caloric expenditure

post-abortion syndrome long-term negative psychological effects of abortion

postpartum period of time after the birth of a baby during which the uterus returns to its prepregnancy size

potentiated effect phenomenon whereby the use of one drug intensifies the effect of a second drug

primary care physician the physician who sees a patient on a regular basis, rather than a specialist who sees the patient only for a specific condition or procedure

problem drinking alcohol use pattern in which a drinker's behavior creates personal difficulties or difficulties for other people

procreation reproduction

prodromal stage stage of an infectious disease process in which only general symptoms appear

professional nurses registered nurses who hold a bachelor's degree in nursing from a college or university

progesterone ovarian hormone that continues the development of the uterine wall that was initiated by estrogen

progressive resistance exercises muscular strength training exercises that use traditional barbells and dumbbells with fixed resistances

proof twice the percentage of alcohol by volume in a beverage; 100 proof alcohol is 50% alcohol

prophylactic mastectomy elective (voluntary) removal of the breast or breasts to prevent the development of breast cancer

prostaglandin inhibitors drugs that block the production of prostaglandins, thus eliminating the hormonal stimulation of smooth muscles

prostaglandins chemical substances that stimulate smooth muscle contractions

prosthodontics dental specialty that focuses on the construction and fitting of artificial appliances to replace missing teeth

proteins compounds composed of chains of amino acids; primary components of muscle and connective tissue

protooncogenes normal genes that hold the potential of becoming cancer-causing oncogenes

psychoactive drug any substance capable of altering one's feelings, moods, or perceptions

psychogenic disorders illnesses with observable symptoms that are generated by stress but are not associated with tissue change

psychological dependence need to consume a drug for emotional reasons; also called *habituation*

psychoneuroimmunology a newly emerging field of human biology and clinical medicine that studies the functional interfaces among the mind, nervous system, and immune system

psychosocial sexuality masculine and feminine aspects of sexuality

psychosomatic disorders physical illnesses of the body generated by the effects of stress

puberty achievement of reproductive ability

pulmonary emphysema irreversible disease process of the lungs in which the alveoli are destroyed

pulmonary hypertension a serious form of high blood pressure that affects lung vessels

purging use of vomiting or laxatives to remove undigested food from the body

Q

quackery marketing of unreliable and ineffective services, products, or information under the guise of curing disease or improving health

R

range of motion distance through which a joint can be moved; measured in degrees

rape an act of violence against another person wherein that person is forced to engage in sexual activities

recovery stage stage of an infectious disease at which the body's immune system has overcome the infectious agent and recovery is under way; convalescence stage

reflexology massage applied to specific areas of the feet to treat illness and disease in other areas of the body

refractory errors incorrect patterns of light wave transmission through the structures of the eye

refractory phase that portion of the male's resolution stage during which sexual arousal cannot occur

regulatory genes genes within the cell that control cellular replication and specialization

relaxation response physiological state of opposition to the fight-or-flight response of the general adaptation syndrome

resolution stage fourth stage of the sexual response pattern; the return of the body to a preexcitement state

retinal hemorrhage uncontrolled bleeding from arteries within the eye's retina

rheumatic heart disease chronic damage to the heart (especially heart valves) resulting from a streptococcal infection within the heart; a complication associated with rheumatic fever

rheumatoid arthritis the result of autoimmune deterioration of the joints

rigor mortis rigidity of the body that occurs after death

role of health mission of health within a person's life cycle

rubella German (or 3-day) measles

rubeola red or common measles

S

sadism sexual excitement achieved while inflicting injury or humiliation on another person

sadomasochism combination of sadism and masochism into one sexual activity

salt sensitive descriptive of people whose bodies overreact to the presence of sodium by retaining fluid and thus increasing blood pressure

satiety state in which there is no longer a desire to eat; fullness

saturated fats dietary fats that influence the formation of cholesterol

sclerotic changes thickening or hardening of tissues

screenings relatively superficial evaluations designed to identify deviations from normal

secondary bacterial infection bacterial infection that develops as a consequence of a primary infection

selective estrogen receptor modulators (SERMs) the first drugs able to prevent the development of breast cancer in some women at high risk

self-actualization highest level of personality development; self-actualized people recognize their roles in life and use personal strengths to reach their fullest potential

self-antigen cells that the immune system identifies as "foreign," (not self), thus triggering an immune response

self-care movement trend toward individuals taking increased responsibility for prevention or management of certain health conditions

self-esteem the quality of feeling good about yourself and your abilities

self-limiting capable of not progressing beyond a specific point; self-correcting

semen secretion containing sperm and nutrients discharged from the male urethra at ejaculation

serum lipid analysis analysis of fat substances in the bloodstream; includes cholesterol and triglyceride measurements

set point a genetically programmed range of body weight beyond which a person finds it difficult to gain or lose additional weight

sex flush reddish skin response that results from increasing sexual arousal

sex reassignment operation surgical procedure designed to remove the external genitalia and replace them with genitalia appropriate to the opposite gender

sexual fantasies fantasies with sexual themes; sexual daydreams or imaginary events

sexual harassment unwanted attention of a sexual nature that creates embarrassment or stress

sexuality the quality of being sexual; can be viewed from many biological and psychosocial perspectives

sexually transmitted diseases (STDs) infectious diseases that are spread primarily through intimate sexual contact

sexual victimization sexual abuse of children, family members, or subordinates by a person in a position of power

shaft body of the penis

shingles viral infection affecting the nerve endings of the skin

shock profound collapse of many vital body functions; evident during acute alcohol intoxication and other serious health emergencies

sidestream smoke the smoke that comes from the burning end of a cigarette, pipe, or cigar

singlehood the state of not being married

six dimensions of health important areas of health in which specific strengths or limitations will be found: physical, emotional, social, intellectual, spiritual, and occupational

skinfold measurement measurement to determine the thickness of the fat layer that lies immediately beneath the skin

sliding scale method of payment by which patient fees are scaled according to income levels

smegma cellular discharge that can accumulate beneath the clitoral hood and the foreskin of an uncircumcised penis

smokeless tobacco tobacco products (chewing tobacco and snuff) that are chewed or sucked rather than smoked

snuff finely shredded smokeless tobacco; used for dipping

social anxiety the clinical label for chronic shyness that inhibits social interaction

spermatogenesis process of sperm production

spermicides chemicals capable of killing sperm

stalking a crime involving an assailant's planned efforts to pursue an intended victim

starch complex carbohydrate; a polysaccharide; a compound of long-chain glucose units

static stretching the slow lengthening of a muscle group to an extended level of stretch followed by holding the extended position for a recommended time period

sterilization generally permanent birth control techniques that surgically disrupt the normal passage of ova or sperm

stillborn baby that is dead at the time of birth

stimulants psychoactive drugs that stimulate the function of the central nervous system

stress the physiological and psychological state of disruption caused by the presence of an unanticipated, disruptive, or stimulating event

stressors factors or events, real or imagined, that elicit a state of stress

stress test examination and analysis of heart-lung function while the body is undergoing physical exercise; generally accomplished when the client walks or runs on a treadmill while being monitored by a cardiograph

subcutaneous fat fat layer immediately beneath the skin

sudden cardiac death immediate death resulting from a sudden change in the rhythm of the heart

surrogate parenting one of several arrangements in which a woman becomes pregnant and gives birth for an infertile couple

sympto-thermal method method of periodic abstinence that combines the basal body temperature method and the cervical mucus method

synapse location at which an electrical impulse from one neuron is transmitted to an adjacent neuron

synergistic drug effect heightened, exaggerated effect produced by the concurrent use of two or more drugs

synesthesia perceptual process in which a stimulus produces a response from a different sensory modality

systolic pressure blood pressure against blood vessel walls when the heart contracts

T

tar particulate phase of tobacco smoke with nicotine and water removed

target heart rate (THR) number of times per minute that the heart must contract to produce a training effect

technical nurses registered nurses (RNs) who hold diplomas or associate degrees from schools of nursing or university nursing programs

telomerase an enzyme produced by cancer cells; it short circuits the biological clocks of normal cells, thus giving the cancer cells an infinite life expectancy

testes male reproductive structures that produce sperm and the gonadal hormone testosterone

testosterone male sex hormone that stimulates tissue development

therapeutic humor humor incorporated into a patient's treatment for illness or injury

thorax the chest; portion of the torso above the diaphragm and within the rib cage

titration determining a particular level of a drug within the body

tolerance an acquired reaction to a drug; continued intake of the same dose has diminished results

total person holistic view of the person, incorporating the dynamic interplay of physical, emotional, social, intellectual, spiritual, and occupational factors

toxic shock syndrome (TSS) potentially fatal condition resulting from the proliferation of certain bacteria in the vagina, whose toxins enter the blood circulation

trace elements minerals whose presence in the body occurs in very small amounts; micronutrient elements

training effect significant positive effect that exercise has on the heart, lungs, and blood vessels

transcenders self-actualized people who have achieved a quality of being ordinarily associated with higher levels of spiritual growth

transcervical balloon tuboplasty the use of inflatable balloon catheters to open blocked fallopian tubes; a procedure used for some women with fertility problems

transient ischemic attack (TIA) temporary spasm of a cerebral artery that produces symptoms similar to those of a minor stroke; often a forewarning of a true cerebrovascular accident

transition the third and last phase of the first stage of labor; full dilation of the cervix

transsexualism the profound rejection of the gender to which the individual has been born

transvestism recurrent, persistent crossdressing as a source of sexual excitement

trimester three-month period of time; human pregnancies encompass three trimesters

tropical oils oils extracted from coconut, palm, and palm kernel that contain much higher levels of saturated fat than other vegetable oils

tubal ligation sterilization procedure in which the fallopian tubes are cut and the ends tied back or cauterized

tumescence state of being swollen or enlarged

tumor mass of cells; may be cancerous (malignant) or noncancerous (benign)

type I alcoholism inherited predisposition supported by environmental factors favoring alcoholism

type II alcoholism male-limited alcoholism; an inherited form of alcoholism passed from father to son

U

unbalanced diet diet lacking adequate representation from each of the five food groups

underweight condition in which body weight is below desirable weight

unintentional injuries injuries that occur without anyone's intending that harm be done

unsubstantiated claim a claim that cannot be supported by valid scientific evidence

urethra passageway through which urine leaves the urinary bladder

urethritis infection of the urethra

V

vacuum aspiration abortion procedure in which the cervix is dilated and vacuum pressure is used to remove the uterine contents

vaginal contraceptive film (VCF) spermicide-containing film that clings to the cervical opening

variant different from the statistical average

vascular system body's blood vessels; arteries, arterioles, capillaries, venules, and veins

vas deferens (pl. vasa deferentia) passageway through which sperm move from the epididymis to the ejaculatory duct

vasectomy surgical procedure in which the vasa deferentia are cut to prevent the passage of sperm from the testicles; the most common form of male sterilization

vasocongestion retention of blood within a particular tissue

vegan vegetarian diet vegetarian diet that excludes the use of all animal products, including eggs and dairy products

very-low-density lipoprotein (VLDL) the type of lipoprotein that transports cholesterol and other lipid material from the liver into the bloodstream

vicariously formed stimuli erotic stimuli that originate in one's imagination

virulent capable of causing disease

vitamins organic compounds that facilitate the action of enzymes

voyeurism watching others undressing or engaging in sexual activities

vulval tissues tissues surrounding the vaginal opening

W

warm-up physical and mental preparation for exercise

wellness a broadly based process used to achieve a highly developed level of health

will legal document that describes how a person wishes his or her estate to be disposed of after death

withdrawal illness uncomfortable, perhaps toxic response of the body as it attempts to maintain homeostasis in the absence of a drug; also called *abstinence syndrome*

work movement of mass over distance

Y

yeast single-cell plant responsible for the fermentation of plant products

young adult years segment of the life cycle from ages 18 to 22; a transitional period between adolescence and adulthood

yo-yo syndrome The repeated weight loss, followed by weight gain, experienced by many dieters

Z

zero tolerance laws laws that severely restrict the right to drive for underage drinkers who have been convicted of driving under the influence of *any* alcohol

zoophilia sexual contact with animals as a preferred source of sexual excitement; bestiality

Exam Prep

chapter 1

Shaping Your Health

MULTIPLE CHOICE

1. What health strategy involves following specific eating plans or exercise programs?
   A. Health screenings
   B. Education activities
   C. Behavior changes
   D. Regimentation
2. Why is it necessary to formulate an initial adult identity?
   A. So you can answer the question, "Who am I?"
   B. To have a productive and satisfying life
   C. It will help you move through other stages of development
   D. All of the above
3. Which developmental task involves using your own resources to follow a particular path?
   A. Forming an initial adult identity
   B. Assuming responsibility
   C. Establishing independence
   D. Developing social skills
4. Which of the following statements is *false?*
   A. The deeper the emotional relationships a person has, the better.
   B. Maintaining and improving your health is an important responsibility.
   C. The need to interact socially will at times negatively influence your health.
   D. Development of social skills can enhance your independence from your family.
5. Which of the following is *not* a dimension of health?
   A. Transitional dimension of health
   B. Emotional dimension of health
   C. Holistic dimension of health
   D. Both A and C
6. Which dimension of health do some professionals believe to be the "core of wellness"?
   A. Emotional
   B. Spiritual
   C. Social
   D. Intellectual
7. Why is the occupational dimension of health important?
   A. Because you won't be happy unless you make a lot of money after graduation.
   B. Because both external and internal rewards from work affect your happiness.
   C. Because when people feel good about their work, they are more likely to live a healthier lifestyle.
   D. Both B and C
8. Which of the following is a strategy for changing your behavior?
   A. Make a personal contract to accomplish your goals.
   B. "Go it alone!" It is better not to involve family or friends.
   C. Don't reward yourself until you get to the final outcome.
   D. Don't let any obstacles occur or you will fail.

CRITICAL THINKING

1. What is health?

2. What is meant by the term *wellness?*

3. How does *empowerment* affect overall health and well-being?

4. Which dimensions of your health would you like to improve, and why?

5. How do you plan to successfully complete your developmental tasks?

chapter **2**

Achieving Psychological Wellness

MULTIPLE CHOICE

1. Emotionally well people:
   A. Experience the full range of human emotions, but are not overcome by them.
   B. Are only concerned with their own well-being.
   C. Set goals that are far and above what they can realistically accomplish.
   D. Trust only those who have proven their worth.

2. What factors shape self-esteem?
   A. Warm and supportive physical contact
   B. Religious indoctrination leading to guilt
   C. Failure to be successful in early undertakings
   D. All of the above

3. What three traits show a person's *hardiness?*
   A. Success, direction, and ability
   B. Commitment, control, and challenge
   C. Commitment, self-control, and self-esteem
   D. None of the above

4. What type of depression may occur after the death of a spouse or some other period of difficulty?
   A. Primary depression
   B. Reactive depression
   C. Chemically induced depression
   D. None of the above

5. Which is the most mature form of conflict resolution?
   A. Dialogue
   B. Submission
   C. Persuasion
   D. Aggression

6. What is the first step toward taking a proactive approach to life?
   A. Undertaking new experiences
   B. Taking risks
   C. Accepting mental pictures
   D. None of the above

7. Which of the following are motivational needs defined by Maslow?
   A. Physiological needs
   B. Economic needs
   C. Sexual needs
   D. Material needs

8. Which of the following statements describes creative individuals?
   A. They are intuitive and open to new experiences.
   B. They are less interested in detail than in meaning and implications.
   C. They are flexible.
   D. All of the above

CRITICAL THINKING

1. What is meant by a "normal range of emotions"?

2. What are some ways to overcome feelings of loneliness and shyness?

3. What are the warning signs of suicide, and how should they be treated?

4. What is the four-step process that allows one to control the outcomes of experiences and learn about one's emotional resources?

5. How do faith and spirituality affect emotional well-being?

chapter **3**

Managing Stress

MULTIPLE CHOICE

1. An event that produces stress is called a:
   A. Response
   B. Stressor
   C. Type B
   D. None of the above

2. Positive stress is called:
   A. Eustress
   B. Distress
   C. Type R stress
   D. None of the above

3. Which of the following is *not* a stage in Selye's general adaptation syndrome model?
   A. Alarm reaction stage
   B. Relaxation stage
   C. Resistance stage
   D. Exhaustion stage

4. Which part of the body is responsible for the interconnection between the nervous system and the endocrine system?
   A. Hypothalamus
   B. Pituitary gland
   C. Adrenal gland
   D. None of the above

5. When the body perceives stress, a number of responses are brought about by the epinephrine (adrenaline) and corticoids released. Which of the following is an expected response?
   A. Decreased cardiac and pulmonary function
   B. Increased digestive activity
   C. Decreased fat use
   D. Altered immune system response

6. PMR, or progressive muscular relaxation, is:
   A. A procedure of alternately contracting and relaxing muscle groups.
   B. A correct way of breathing, by relaxing the diaphragm.
   C. An Eastern relaxation technique that employs the use of a mantra.
   D. A form of self-hypnosis that costs between $250 to $400 to learn.

7. Which of the following diseases have some origin in unresolved stress?
   A. Irritable bowel syndrome
   B. Allergies
   C. Asthma
   D. All of the above

8. Which of the following personality traits fosters high levels of stress?
   A. Self-confidence and practicality
   B. Anger and cynicism
   C. Both A and B
   D. Neither A nor B

9. Stress is best described as:
   A. Something completely beyond your control.
   B. The leading cause of cynicism.
   C. A physical and emotional response to change.
   D. A realistic and positive outlook on life.

10. What two areas of the body prepare the body to respond to stressors?
    A. Circulatory system and lymphatic system
    B. Nervous system and endocrine system
    C. Muscular tissue and nervous system
    D. Heart and lungs

CRITICAL THINKING

1. What is stress? Give an example of a stressful situation and how the person might feel.

2. Can stress be positive? Give an example.

3. What physiological reactions occur in the body because of stress?

4. How can repeated stress, if not dealt with properly, affect long-term health?

5. What are some healthy ways to deal with stress? Which would you choose to adopt, and why?

chapter **4**

Becoming Physically Fit

MULTIPLE CHOICE

1. Which of the following is *not* a benefit of physical fitness?
   A. The person can engage in various tasks and leisure activities.
   B. Body systems function efficiently to resist disease.
   C. Body systems are healthy enough to respond to emergency (threatening) situations.
   D. All of the above are benefits.

2. Which of the following areas of physical fitness do exercise physiologists say is most important?
   A. Muscular strength
   B. Muscular endurance
   C. Cardiorespiratory endurance
   D. Flexibility

3. Anaerobic, or oxygen-deprived, energy production:
   A. Is the result of low-intensity activity.
   B. Is the result of short-duration activities that quickly cause muscle fatigue.
   C. Is the result of activities such as walking, distance jogging, and bicycle touring.
   D. None of the above

4. Which of the following types of training exercises are based on the *overload principle?*
   A. Isometric exercises
   B. Progressive resistance exercises
   C. Isokinetic exercises
   D. All of the above

5. Of the following statements, which accurately describes flexibility?
   A. It is relatively the same throughout your body.
   B. Not every joint in your body is equally flexible.
   C. Nothing alters the flexibility of a particular joint.
   D. Gender and age do not affect flexibility.

6. The ability of a muscle group to continue to contract is a definition of which physical fitness component?
   A. Muscular strength
   B. Muscular endurance
   C. Agility
   D. Flexibility

7. The American College of Sports Medicine recommends six significant areas to consider for achievement of cardiorespiratory fitness. Which of these is *not* one of the areas?
   A. Mode of activity
   B. Frequency of training
   C. Intensity of training
   D. Popularity of activity

8. What is target heart rate (THR)?
   A. An intensity level of between 65% and 90% of maximum heart rate
   B. An intensity level of between 70% and 100% of maximum heart rate
   C. The maximum number of times your heart should contract each minute to give your respiratory system a work overload
   D. The rate at which you become so fatigued that you must stop exercising

9. What are the three basic parts of a good training session?
   A. Running, weightlifting, stretching
   B. Warm-up, workout, cooldown
   C. Warm-up, stretching, cooldown
   D. Mental warm-up, socialize, workout

10. Which of these is an abnormal sign to be aware of, during or after exercise?
    A. A delay of over 1 hour in your body's return to a fully relaxed, comfortable state after exercise
    B. Difficulty sleeping
    C. Noticeable breathing difficulties or chest pains
    D. All of the above

CRITICAL THINKING

1. What are the differences between osteoporosis and osteoarthritis?

2. How serious is low back pain, and what should a person do to alleviate or prevent it?

3. Explain what steps you would take to develop a cardiorespiratory fitness program, taking into account all six areas recommended by the American College of Sports Medicine.

4. What are the three major components of the Female Athlete Triad?

5. Why is steroid use dangerous?

chapter **5**

Understanding Nutrition and Your Diet

MULTIPLE CHOICE

1. What three nutrients provide the body with calories?
   A. Sugar, amino acids, and supplements
   B. Carbohydrates, fats, and proteins
   C. Tropical oils, food additives, and carbohydrates
   D. None of the above
2. Which of the following statements accurately describes carbohydrates?
   A. They occur in two forms only, depending on the number of proteins that make up the molecule.
   B. About 20% of our calories comes from carbohydrates.
   C. Carbohydrates are combinations of sugar units, or saccharides.
   D. Each gram of carbohydrate contains 400 calories.
3. Which of the following statements is *false?*
   A. Fats are important nutrients in our diets.
   B. Fats make it impossible for our bodies to absorb vitamins A, D, E, and K.
   C. Fat insulates our bodies, helping us retain heat.
   D. Most of the fat we eat is "hidden" in food.
4. What are vitamins?
   A. Inorganic materials necessary for tissue repair and disease prevention
   B. Pills that can be taken each morning to give the body energy all day
   C. Organic compounds that are required in small amounts for normal growth, reproduction, and maintenance of health
   D. Nutrients that provide more than half our body weight
5. Which of the following nutrients could the body not live without for over a week?
   A. Minerals
   B. Fiber
   C. Vitamins
   D. Water
6. Which of the following is a recommendation based on the USDA Food Guide Pyramid?
   A. Adults should eat two to four servings from the fruit group each day.
   B. Three to five servings from the vegetable group each day are recommended for an adult.
   C. Adults should consume two to three servings from the milk, yogurt, and cheese group each day.
   D. All of the above
7. What are phytochemicals?
   A. Physiologically active components that function as antioxidants and may deactivate carcinogens
   B. The additives used in foods that preserve freshness or enhance flavor, color, or texture
   C. The chemicals used to enrich breads and cereals
   D. None of the above
8. What kind of vegetarian eats milk products but not eggs?
   A. Ovolactovegetarian
   B. Macrobiotic vegetarian
   C. Lactovegetarian
   D. Vegan vegetarian

9. What factors may influence nutritional changes as a person ages?
   A. Changes to the structure and function of the body resulting from age
   B. The progressive lowering of the body's basal metabolism
   C. Both A and B
   D. Neither A nor B

10. Which of the following is a suggested step toward increasing the availability of food?
    A. Increase the yield of land under cultivation.
    B. Increase the amount of land under cultivation.
    C. Use water more efficiently for the production of food.
    D. All of the above

CRITICAL THINKING

1. Based on your personal assessment of your current diet, are you getting all the nutrients you need? In which areas do you need to improve?

2. What role does cholesterol play in the diet?

3. Explain the difference between *water-soluble* and *fat-soluble* vitamins and the characteristics of each.

4. Would you consider becoming a vegetarian? Why or why not?

5. What is *nutrient density?* Why is it important to consider this concept when making food choices?

chapter 6

Maintaining a Healthy Weight

MULTIPLE CHOICE

1. Which weight measurement technique precisely measures relative amounts of fat and lean body mass by comparing underwater weight with out-of-water weight?
   A. Skinfold measurements
   B. Body mass index (BMI)
   C. Electrical impedance
   D. Hydrostatic weighing
2. Which may be the simplest method of determining a person's amount of body fat?
   A. Appearance
   B. Height-weight tables
   C. Body mass index (BMI)
   D. Waist-to-hip ratio
3. What influences obesity?
   A. Environment
   B. Genetics
   C. Both environment and genetics
   D. None of the above
4. Which area(s) within the hypothalamus tell the body when it should begin and end food consumption?
   A. Feeding and satiety centers
   B. Central nervous system (CNS)
   C. Thyroid and pituitary glands
   D. None of the above
5. Which of the following statements describes "brown fat"?
   A. It is located in small amounts in the upper back between the shoulder blades.
   B. There is a renewed interest in the study of it.
   C. It burns calories as heat without generating energy units that are stored in fat cells.
   D. All of the above
6. Which of Sheldon's three body types is characterized by a tall, slender build?
   A. Ectomorph
   B. Mesomorph
   C. Endomorph
   D. None of the above
7. What is hypercellular obesity?
   A. The increase of fat cells later in life as a result of being overfed in infancy or substantially gaining weight in childhood or adolescence
   B. When fat cells increase in size as a result of long-term positive caloric balance in adulthood
   C. Excessive fat around the waist, which can contribute to the onset of diabetes mellitus
   D. None of the above
8. What would most experts cite as the most important reason for the widespread problem of obesity?
   A. Family dietary practices
   B. Endocrine influence
   C. Infant feeding patterns
   D. None of the above
9. What is basal metabolic rate (BMR)?
   A. The rate of caloric intake to caloric output
   B. The minimum amount of energy the body requires to carry on all vital functions
   C. The rate of a food's thermic output
   D. None of the above
10. Which weight management technique involves the use of pharmaceuticals?
    A. Balanced diets supported by portion control
    B. Fad diets
    C. Hunger/satiety-influencing products
    D. Self-help weight reduction programs

CRITICAL THINKING

1. What factors influence your body image and self-concept?

2. What steps might you take to successfully control your weight throughout your lifetime?

3. Why is dieting alone not a good technique for achieving and maintaining weight loss?

4. What are reasons someone might develop anorexia nervosa or bulimia? How should a person be treated for these disorders?

5. What does it mean to exercise or eat compulsively?

chapter **7**

Making Decisions About Drug Use

MULTIPLE CHOICE

1. Which of these is an aspect of addictive behavior?
   A. Exposure
   B. Compulsion
   C. Loss of control
   D. All of the above

2. What kind of drugs alter the user's feelings, behaviors, or moods?
   A. Medicines
   B. Over-the-counter drugs
   C. Psychoactive drugs
   D. Steroids

3. Which type of dependence creates *full* withdrawal symptoms when the drug use is stopped?
   A. Psychological
   B. Physical
   C. Cross-tolerant
   D. None of the above

4. What are neurotransmitters?
   A. Chemical messengers that transmit electrical impulses
   B. Organic messengers that transmit the chemicals in drugs directly to the brain
   C. Hallucinogenic drugs that are currently popular with college students
   D. None of the above

5. How do drugs "work"?
   A. By blocking the production of a neurotransmitter
   B. By forcing the continued release of a neurotransmitter
   C. Either A or B
   D. Neither A nor B

6. Which type of psychoactive drug *excites* the activity of the central nervous system (CNS)?
   A. Inhalants
   B. Hallucinogens
   C. Narcotics
   D. None of the above

7. What is "crack"?
   A. Powdered cocaine that is alkalized in benzene or ether and smoked through a waterpipe
   B. A small, rocklike crystalline material made from cocaine hydrochloride and baking soda
   C. A white powder that is snorted in "lines" through a rolled dollar bill or tube
   D. A pure form of methamphetamine that looks like rock candy

8. Which type of psychoactive drug *slows down* the function of the central nervous system (CNS)?
   A. Inhalants
   B. Hallucinogens
   C. Cannabis
   D. Depressants

9. What is THC?
   A. A hallucinogen derived from the peyote cactus plant
   B. A drug popular in the 1960s
   C. The active ingredient in marijuana
   D. A new "designer" drug

10. Which drugs are among the most dependence-producing?
    A. Inhalants
    B. Hallucinogens
    C. Depressants
    D. Narcotics

CRITICAL THINKING

1. What is the difference between drug *misuse* and drug *abuse?*

2. What are the dangers posed by the drugs Rohypnol, GHB, and Ketamine?

3. What are possible long-term effects of marijuana use?

4. What is a synergistic effect, and why is it dangerous?

5. What do you think about the legalization of drugs and about drug testing?

chapter **8**

Taking Control of Alcohol Use

MULTIPLE CHOICE

1. What is *binge drinking?*
   A. The practice of drinking and then purging
   B. A harmless activity popular among college students
   C. The practice of consuming five drinks in a row, at least once during the previous 2-week period
   D. The practice of consuming two drinks in a row, at least once a day

2. What is the alcohol content of a bottle of 140-proof gin?
   A. 140% of the fluid in the bottle
   B. 70% of the fluid in the bottle
   C. 14% of the fluid in the bottle
   D. 1.4% of the fluid in the bottle

3. What type of drug is alcohol?
   A. Stimulant
   B. Hallucinogen
   C. Depressant
   D. Narcotic

4. What should be done with people who become unconscious resulting from alcohol consumption?
   A. They should be given a cold shower to wake them up.
   B. They should be made to drink coffee.
   C. They should be taken to bed and left undisturbed for several hours.
   D. They should be put on their side and monitored frequently.

5. Which of the following leading causes of accidental death has connections to alcohol use?
   A. Motor vehicle collisions
   B. Falls
   C. Drownings
   D. All of the above

6. Which of the following is a good guideline to follow for responsibly hosting a party?
   A. Make alcohol the primary entertainment, especially with a keg or other popular way to serve alcohol.
   B. Ridicule those who are too afraid to drink.
   C. If friends say they are just fine to drive home even though they have been drinking, let them go.
   D. None of the above

7. Which alcohol awareness group promotes responsible party hosting among university students?
   A. AA
   B. MADD
   C. BACCHUS
   D. SADD

8. What is the main difference between problem drinking and alcoholism?
   A. Problem drinkers stay away from hard liquor.
   B. Alcoholics usually don't engage in binge drinking.
   C. Alcoholism involves a physical addiction to alcohol.
   D. Problem drinking is easier to detect.

9. Which support group appeals to the children of alcoholics?
   A. Al-Anon
   B. AA
   C. Alateen
   D. MADD

10. Which of the following drugs, approved by the FDA, is being used to treat alcoholism?
    A. Naltrexone
    B. Zocor
    C. Heroin
    D. Maltodextrine

CRITICAL THINKING

1. Why do people drink alcohol?

2. What physiological differences in women make them more susceptible to the effects of alcohol?

3. What are the possible effects of drinking alcohol while pregnant?

4. What role does alcohol use play in violent crime, family violence, and suicide?

5. Explain *denial, enabling,* and *codependence* as they occur with alcoholism.

chapter 9

Rejecting Tobacco Use

MULTIPLE CHOICE

1. Which factor most affects a person's decision to smoke?
   A. Gender
   B. Age
   C. Education
   D. Race

2. What are psychosocial factors of tobacco dependence?
   A. Manipulation
   B. Advertising
   C. Modeling
   D. Both A and C

3. What consumer group is the FDA focusing its education efforts on to discourage increased tobacco use?
   A. Women
   B. African-American men who attend predominately black universities
   C. Teens
   D. Older adults who began smoking before health risks were known

4. Which phase of tobacco use includes nicotine, water, and a variety of powerful chemical compounds known collectively as *tar?*
   A. Active phase
   B. Particulate phase
   C. Gaseous phase
   D. Nicotine phase

5. What signals the beginning of lung cancer?
   A. Changes in the basal cell layer resulting from constant irritation by accumulating tar in the airways
   B. An inability to breathe normally
   C. A "smoker's cough"
   D. Mucus swept up to the throat by cilia, where it is swallowed and removed through the digestive system

6. What is COLD?
   A. Chronic obstructive lung disease
   B. A chronic disease in which air flow in and out of the lungs becomes progressively limited
   C. A disease state made up of chronic bronchitis and pulmonary emphysema
   D. All of the above

7. Which of the following statements is *false?*
   A. It is strongly recommended that women who smoke not use oral contraceptives.
   B. Chewing tobacco and snuff generate blood levels of nicotine in amounts equivalent to those seen in cigarette smokers.
   C. Contrary to some claims, secondhand smoke is not a serious health threat.
   D. Children of parents who smoke are twice as likely to develop bronchitis or pneumonia during the first year of life.

8. Which of the following statements is *true?*
   A. Chewing tobacco is a safe alternative to smoking.
   B. Sidestream smoke makes up only 15% of our exposure to involuntary smoking.
   C. Spouses of smokers may have a 30% greater risk of lung cancer.
   D. The only effective way to quit smoking is to go "cold turkey."

9. Which is more effective as a means of quitting smoking?
   A. Nicotine-containing chewing gum
   B. Transdermal patch
   C. Neither A nor B work
   D. Both A and B are equally effective

10. What is the main debate concerning smoking today?
    A. The validity of health warnings
    B. The rights of the nonsmoker vs. the rights of the smoker
    C. The rights of young adults to buy cigarettes
    D. None of the above

CRITICAL THINKING

1. What advertising tactics do tobacco companies use to offset the potential decline in sales from reports of health risks?

2. In what ways is tobacco addictive?

3. How does smoking adversely affect health?

4. Why should a pregnant or breastfeeding woman refrain from smoking?

5. Do you think smoking should continue to be banned from public places? Why or why not?

chapter **10**

Reducing Your Risk of Cardiovascular Disease

MULTIPLE CHOICE

1. Why has the rate of death caused by cardiovascular disease declined?
   A. Changing American lifestyles
   B. Medical advances in diagnosis and treatment
   C. A breakthrough new drug
   D. Both A and B

2. What is the nation's number one "killer"?
   A. AIDS
   B. Lung disease
   C. Cancer
   D. Cardiovascular disease

3. Which of the following is a function of the blood?
   A. Regulation of water content of body cells and fluids
   B. Transportation of nutrients, oxygen, wastes, and hormones
   C. Buffering to help maintain appropriate pH balance
   D. All of the above

4. What are three cardiovascular risk factors that cannot be changed?
   A. Age, gender, body composition
   B. Heredity, weight, glandular production
   C. Age, heredity, and metabolism
   D. None of the above

5. What is a risk factor that can be changed?
   A. Tobacco smoke
   B. Physical inactivity
   C. High blood pressure
   D. All of the above

6. Which disease predisposes people to developing heart disease?
   A. Cancer
   B. Epilepsy
   C. Diabetes
   D. Multiple sclerosis

7. Which form of cardiovascular disease involves damage to the vessels that supply blood to the heart muscle?
   A. Hypertension
   B. Stroke
   C. Coronary heart disease
   D. Congenital heart disease

8. What is cholesterol?
   A. The oil used to fry food
   B. A soft, fatlike material manufactured by the body
   C. A material necessary for reproduction of blood
   D. None of the above

9. What is hypertension?
   A. A consistently elevated blood pressure
   B. Stress on arterial walls resulting from plaque build-up
   C. The tendency for blood to clot
   D. Abnormally low blood pressure

10. What is the name of the cardiovascular disease that begins as a streptococcal infection of the throat?
    A. Peripheral artery disease
    B. Rheumatic heart disease
    C. Phlebitis
    D. Congestive heart failure

CRITICAL THINKING

1. What components make up the cardiovascular system? How does the system work?

2. Do you exhibit any risk factors for cardiovascular disease? What steps can you take to change them, if they can be changed?

3. What is the difference between HDLs and LDLs?

4. How can hypertension be prevented?

5. What are the different causes of stroke?

chapter **11**

Living with Cancer and Chronic Conditions

MULTIPLE CHOICE

1. What changes characterize cancer cells?
   A. Their normal behavior ceases.
   B. They become severely dysfunctional.
   C. Neither A nor B
   D. Both A and B
2. What are protooncogenes?
   A. Genes that repair damaged cells
   B. Genes that suppress the immune system
   C. Genes that have the potential to become cancerous
   D. Abnormal genes
3. What is the Human Genome Project?
   A. The testing of new cancer-fighting drugs
   B. A scientific study of genes
   C. A secret military project that exposed World War II troops to carcinogens
   D. The study of cancer-producing viruses
4. Which type of cancer is found in cells of the blood and blood-forming tissues?
   A. Lymphoma
   B. Neuroblastoma
   C. Carcinoma
   D. Leukemia
5. Which is the most common site of the body to develop cancer in women?
   A. Breast
   B. Uterus
   C. Lung
   D. Skin
6. Which test greatly improves the chances of preventing cervical cancer?
   A. Mammography
   B. MRI
   C. Pap test
   D. Biopsy
7. Which type of cancer is referred to as the "silent" cancer because of its vague symptoms?
   A. Ovarian
   B. Prostate
   C. Vaginal
   D. Lung
8. Which traditional method of cancer treatment has had many successful advances in recent years?
   A. Surgery
   B. Chiropractic manipulation
   C. Chemotherapy
   D. Radiation
9. Which chronic disease most often appears in early adulthood and continues intermittently for the next 20 to 25 years?
   A. Diabetes mellitus
   B. Sickle cell trait
   C. Multiple sclerosis
   D. Asthma

CRITICAL THINKING

1. What social and environmental factors contribute to the onset of cancer?

2. What steps can women take to prevent cancer or to detect the early stages of cancer?

3. What steps can men take to prevent cancer or to detect the early stages of cancer?

4. What are the seven warning signs of cancer?

5. What are the differences and similarities between type 1 and type 2 diabetes?

chapter **12**

Preventing Infectious Diseases

MULTIPLE CHOICE

1. What is a pathogen?
   A. A disease-causing agent
   B. A virus, bacterium, or fungus
   C. Neither A nor B
   D. Both A and B

2. What is the function of a reservoir in the chain of infection?
   A. To cause disease
   B. To offer a favorable environment in which an infectious agent can thrive
   C. To act as a portal of exit
   D. To transmit the agent from person to person

3. Which term describes insects, animals, or birds that carry diseases from human to human?
   A. Vectors
   B. Pathogens
   C. Reservoirs
   D. Agents

4. During which of the following stages of infection is the infected person *most* contagious?
   A. Prodromal stage
   B. Clinical stage
   C. Decline stage
   D. Incubation stage

5. Which type of immunity is the result of vaccination or immunization?
   A. Naturally acquired immunity
   B. Artificially acquired immunity
   C. Passively acquired immunity
   D. None of the above

6. Which viral infection has mental fatigue and depression as side effects?
   A. Influenza
   B. Common cold
   C. Mononucleosis
   D. Pneumonia

7. What is chronic fatigue syndrome (CFS)?
   A. A mononucleosis-like condition most commonly seen in women in their thirties and forties
   B. A condition that may be linked to neurally mediated hypotension
   C. A condition that may be a psychological disorder
   D. All of the above

8. How is Lyme disease transmitted?
   A. Through droplet spread
   B. Through fecal-oral spread
   C. Through the deer tick nymph
   D. Through inhalation

9. Which sexually transmitted disease occurs as blister-like lesions on the genitals or lips?
   A. Herpes simplex
   B. Gonorrhea
   C. Syphilis
   D. Human papillomavirus

10. Of the following STDs, which has no cure?
    A. Vaginal infections
    B. Cystitis and urethritis
    C. Herpes simplex
    D. Gonorrhea

CRITICAL THINKING

1. What are the two main components to the body's protective defense? How do they work?

2. Why do the elderly and people with additional health complications need to take extra precaution to avoid contracting influenza?

3. Why should people pay close attention to their immunization history, especially college-aged students?

4. What precautions should women take when using tampons to avoid toxic shock syndrome?

5. How is AIDS transmitted, and what precautions can be taken to avoid contracting it?

chapter **13**

Understanding Sexuality

MULTIPLE CHOICE

1. Which basis for biological sexuality refers to the growing embryo's development of gonads?
   A. Genetic
   B. Gonadal
   C. Structural
   D. None of the above

2. At which age are typical children able to correctly identify their gender?
   A. 4 years
   B. 2 years
   C. 18 months
   D. 6 months

3. What part of the testis produces sperm?
   A. Seminiferous tubules
   B. Scrotum
   C. Epididymis
   D. Interstitial cells

4. Which is the most sensitive part of the female body?
   A. Mons pubis
   B. Vagina
   C. Clitoris
   D. Prepuce

5. During which phase of the menstrual cycle does ovulation occur?
   A. Menstrual
   B. Proliferative
   C. Secretory
   D. None of the above

6. Which phase of the sexual response pattern prevents men from having multiple orgasms?
   A. Excitement
   B. Plateau
   C. Orgasmic
   D. Refractory

7. Which of the following statements is *not* true about celibacy?
   A. Celibate people may have intimate relationships without sex.
   B. It is defined as the self-imposed avoidance of sexual contact.
   C. Psychological complications often result from a celibate lifestyle.
   D. All are true.

8. Which type of oral-genital stimulation involves kissing and licking the vulva of the female?
   A. Foreplay
   B. Fellatio
   C. Cunnilingus
   D. None of the above

9. Which type of love is enduring and capable of sustaining long-term mutual growth?
   A. Infatuation
   B. Passionate love
   C. Companionate love
   D. Devotional love

10. Which of the following statements is *not* true of cohabitation?
    A. It is an alternative to marriage.
    B. It can sometimes exist between people sharing a platonic relationship.
    C. In the U.S., the number of unmarried couples that live together is rising.
    D. In the U.S., older adults rarely live in cohabitation.

CRITICAL THINKING

1. How do biological and psychosocial factors contribute to the complex expression of our sexuality?

2. How has a blending of feminine and masculine qualities benefitted society?

3. What differences and similarities exist between the male sexual response pattern and the female sexual response pattern?

4. What changes, both physiological and psychological, might menopause create in a woman's life?

5. What effect does the aging process have on the sexual response pattern?

chapter **14**

Managing Your Fertility

MULTIPLE CHOICE

1. Which form of birth control *does not* prevent STDs?
   A. Withdrawal
   B. Calendar method
   C. IUD
   D. All of the above

2. Which two forms of birth control, when used together, provide a high degree of contraceptive protection *and* disease control?
   A. IUD and spermicides
   B. Spermicides and condoms
   C. Calendar method and spermicides
   D. Oral contraceptive and spermicides

3. Which of the following statements is *not* true of oral contraceptives?
   A. The use of antibiotics lowers their contraceptive effectiveness.
   B. They regulate a woman's menstrual cycle.
   C. The user may experience more frequent vaginal infections, weight gain, mild headaches, and mild depression.
   D. They are useful in the prevention of STDs.

4. What are "minipills"?
   A. Smaller versions of the regular oral contraceptive that can be swallowed more easily
   B. The placebo pills taken between cycles
   C. Oral contraceptives that contain no estrogen—only low-dose progesterone
   D. Less expensive versions of the pill that are slightly less effective

5. What are Depo-Provera and Lunelle?
   A. Injectable contraceptives
   B. Subdermal implant contraceptives
   C. Types of diaphragms
   D. Brands of oral contraceptives

6. Which type of abortion is performed in the earliest stages of the first trimester?
   A. Menstrual extraction
   B. Dilation and curettage
   C. Dilation and evacuation
   D. Hypertonic saline procedure

7. What is mifepristone?
   A. The "morning after" pill
   B. The process of using prostaglandin to influence muscle contractions that expel uterine contents
   C. A hypertonic saline solution
   D. A drug whose use produces a medical abortion

8. The most common method of female sterilization is:
   A. Vasectomy
   B. Tubal ligation
   C. Colpotomy
   D. Hysterectomy

9. Which of the following is an obstacle to pregnancy?
   A. 200 to 500 million sperm cells are deposited in each ejaculation.
   B. Sperm cells are capable of moving quickly.
   C. The acidic level of the vagina is destructive to sperm.
   D. Once inside the fallopian tubes, sperm can live for days.

10. Which type of artificial fertilization involves transferring fertilized ova from a laboratory dish into the fallopian tubes?
    A. In vitro fertilization and embryo transfer (IVF-ET)
    B. Gamete intrafallopian transfer (GIFT)
    C. Zygote intrafallopian transfer (ZIFT)
    D. Surrogate parenting

CRITICAL THINKING

1. What factors should you consider when choosing a method of birth control?

2. Which of the available methods of birth control would you be most likely to use, if you needed to?

3. What are your feelings about the use of emergency contraception? Do they differ from your feelings about using drugs to produce a medical abortion?

4. What serious questions need to be considered before deciding to have children?

5. Describe the birth process from beginning to end.

chapter **15**

Becoming an Informed Health-Care Consumer

MULTIPLE CHOICE

1. Which of the following statements is *false?*
   A. The accuracy of health information from friends and family members may be questionable.
   B. The mass media routinely supply public service messages that give valuable health-related information.
   C. Never trust the labels and directions on prescription medication; it is usually misleading and intended to make you buy more of the product.
   D. Folk wisdom is on occasion supported by scientific evidence.
2. Which health resource has the most effective way of distributing information to the public by mail?
   A. On-line computer services
   B. Voluntary health agencies
   C. Government agencies
   D. Qualified health educators
3. What is the difference between allopathy and osteopathy?
   A. Osteopaths engage in quackery.
   B. Allopathic physicians are board-certified; osteopaths are not.
   C. Osteopaths perceive themselves as being more holistic.
   D. Only osteopaths function as primary care physicians.
4. Which type of health-care professional provides services relating to understanding behavior patterns or perceptions but does not dispense drugs?
   A. Dentist
   B. Psychiatrist
   C. Podiatrist
   D. Psychologist
5. What does an optician do?
   A. Specializes in vision problems due to refractory errors
   B. Provides prescriptions for eyewear products
   C. Grinds lenses according to a precise prescription
   D. Specializes in vision care with a base in general medicine
6. What type of nursing position is helping to provide communities with additional primary care providers?
   A. Nurse practitioner
   B. Registered nurse
   C. Licensed practical nurse
   D. Technical nurse
7. The established amount that the insuree must pay before the insurer reimburses for services is:
   A. Fixed indemnity
   B. Coinsurance
   C. Deductible
   D. Exclusion
8. Which of the following is a sign of quackery?
   A. Makes promises of quick, dramatic, painless, or drugless treatment
   B. Claims a product provides treatment for multiple illnesses
   C. States that the treatment is secret or not yet available in this country
   D. All of the above

CRITICAL THINKING

1. What are some pros and cons of obtaining health information from mass media?

2. What are some sources of health information available to you?

3. What are some alternative health-care practices? Would you be willing to try them?

4. How can self-care benefit both individuals and the health-care industry as a whole?

5. In terms of FDA regulations, how do food supplements differ from prescription and OTC medications?

chapter **16**

Protecting Your Safety

MULTIPLE CHOICE

1. The annual homicide rate in the United States has ____________ over the past decade.
   A. Increased
   B. Stayed the same
   C. Declined
   D. None of the above

2. Who is most often a victim of intimate abuse?
   A. Prostitutes
   B. Teenage girls
   C. Spouses or former spouses of the assailant
   D. Men

3. Which form of child abuse occurs most frequently?
   A. Neglect
   B. Physical
   C. Psychological
   D. Sexual

4. Crimes directed at individuals or groups because of racial, ethnic, religious, or other differences are called:
   A. Hate crimes
   B. Assault crimes
   C. Global crimes
   D. Difference crimes

5. Aside from the physical harm of rape, what other effects may occur?
   A. Posttraumatic stress syndrome
   B. Guilt
   C. Emotional damage resulting from "broken trust"
   D. All of the above

6. Which of the following constitutes sexual harassment?
   A. Excessive pressure for dates
   B. Sexually explicit humor
   C. Unwanted physical contact
   D. All of the above

7. Which of the following can help increase safety around your home?
   A. Make sure your name is spelled correctly in the phone book.
   B. Try to live in apartments on the first floor.
   C. Require repair people to show valid identification.
   D. Leave windows unlocked in case you need to escape in a hurry.

8. Over half of all murders result from:
   A. Random crime
   B. Domestic abuse
   C. Arguments between acquaintances or relatives
   D. None of the above

9. Which of the following persons is a highly probable candidate for death by motor vehicle accident?
   A. Male, 55–65 years of age, driving in rainy conditions on a weekend afternoon
   B. Female, 35–45 years of age, driving on a freeway with the noise of children playing in the back seat
   C. Female, 65–75 years of age, driving in rush-hour traffic
   D. Male, 15–25 years of age, driving on a two-lane rural road on a Saturday night

10. Which of the following resources will help improve your safety on campus?
    A. University-approved escorts
    B. Campus security departments
    C. Campus counseling center
    D. All of the above

CRITICAL THINKING

1. What factors may have contributed to a drop in U.S. homicide rates?

2. How should suspected child abuse be properly handled?

3. What is rape? What is acquaintance rape? What is date rape?

4. How can you increase your personal safety?

5. What steps can you take to protect children and the elderly?

chapter **17**

Accepting Dying and Death

MULTIPLE CHOICE

1. Which of the following is a criterion by which death may be determined?
   A. Lack of heartbeat and breathing
   B. Lack of central nervous system function
   C. Presence of rigor mortis
   D. All of the above

2. Which type of euthanasia is generally illegal in the United States?
   A. Direct euthanasia
   B. Indirect euthanasia
   C. Both A and B
   D. Neither A nor B

3. What does the physician's order "DNR" stand for?
   A. Death not recorded
   B. Do not resuscitate
   C. Do not release
   D. Do not recognize

4. Which psychological stage for dying people serves as the earliest temporary defense mechanism?
   A. Denial
   B. Anger
   C. Bargaining
   D. None of the above

5. Which of the following describes the appropriate way to act toward someone who is dying?
   A. Refrain from crying so as not to upset them
   B. Remain optimistic even when there is no hope for recovery
   C. Try to be genuine and honest
   D. Try to distract the person from talking about death

6. Adults coping with the death of a child should:
   A. Have another child and name that child after the deceased.
   B. Move to a different home for a change of environment.
   C. Give themselves time and space to grieve.
   D. All of the above

7. Which of the following is *not* a normal, healthy expression of grief over the loss of a loved one?
   A. Physical discomfort
   B. Sense of numbness
   C. Guilt
   D. Extreme hostility

8. How long do periods of grief usually last?
   A. A few weeks
   B. 2 to 5 years
   C. A few months to a year
   D. 10 years or more

9. What is a wake?
   A. An established time for friends and family to share emotions and experiences about the deceased
   B. A formaldehyde-based fluid used to replace blood components during embalming
   C. A container for ashes from cremation
   D. None of the above

10. Which of the following is the word for a notice of death printed in a newspaper?
    A. Eulogy
    B. Epitaph
    C. Obituary notice
    D. None of the above

CRITICAL THINKING

1. What are living wills and medical power of attorney documents? Why would it be prudent to have these documents?

2. How do the emotional stages of dying described by Elisabeth Kübler-Ross affect those close to the dying person?

3. Describe what might occur during an out-of-body experience.

4. How does a hospice differ from a traditional hospital with respect to care of the terminally ill?

5. In what ways do death rituals aid people in dealing with death?

answers

CHAPTER 1

1. C; 2. D; 3. C; 4. A; 5. D; 6. B; 7. D;
8. A

CHAPTER 2

1. A; 2. D; 3. B; 4. B; 5. A; 6. D; 7. A;
8. D

CHAPTER 3

1. B; 2. A; 3. B; 4. A; 5. D; 6. A; 7. D;
8. B; 9. C; 10. B

CHAPTER 4

1. D; 2. C; 3. B; 4. D; 5. B; 6. B; 7. D;
8. A; 9. B; 10. D

CHAPTER 5

1. B; 2. C; 3. B; 4. C; 5. D; 6. D; 7. A;
8. C; 9. C; 10. D

CHAPTER 6

1. D; 2. A; 3. C; 4. A; 5. D; 6. A; 7. A;
8. D; 9. B; 10. C

CHAPTER 7

1. D; 2. C; 3. B; 4. A; 5. C; 6. D; 7. B;
8. D; 9. C; 10. D

CHAPTER 8

1. C; 2. B; 3. C; 4. D; 5. D; 6. D; 7. C;
8. C; 9. C; 10. A

CHAPTER 9

1. C; 2. D; 3. C; 4. B; 5. A; 6. D; 7. C;
8. C; 9. A; 10. B

CHAPTER 10

1. D; 2. D; 3. D; 4. D; 5. D; 6. C; 7. C;
8. B; 9. A; 10. B

CHAPTER 11

1. D; 2. C; 3. B; 4. D; 5. A; 6. C; 7. A;
8. C; 9. C

CHAPTER 12

1. A; 2. B; 3. A; 4. B; 5. B; 6. C; 7. D;
8. C; 9. A; 10. C

CHAPTER 13

1. B; 2. C; 3. A; 4. C; 5. B; 6. D; 7. C;
8. C; 9. C; 10. D

CHAPTER 14

1. D; 2. B; 3. D; 4. C; 5. A; 6. A; 7. D;
8. B; 9. C; 10. C

CHAPTER 15

1. C; 2. C; 3. C; 4. D; 5. C; 6. A; 7. C;
8. D

CHAPTER 16

1. C; 2. C; 3. A; 4. A; 5. D; 6. D; 7. C;
8. C; 9. D; 10. D

CHAPTER 17

1. D; 2. A; 3. B; 4. A; 5. C; 6. C; 7. D;
8. C; 9. A; 10. C

Credits

Chapter 1: p. 2 (Figure 1-1), Men's Health Magazine/CNN; **p. 5 (Star Box),** Source: Guyton R, et al: College students and national health objectives for the year 2000: a summary report, *Journal of American College Health,* July 1989, 38:9-14; **p. 5 (Table 1-1),** Data from Kochanek KD, Smith BL, Anderson RN: Deaths: preliminary data for 1999. *National Vital Statistics Reports,* 49:3, 1–49, 2001; **p. 6 (Star Box),** Data from *Healthy People 2000: Midcourse Review and 1995 Revisions,* Department of Health and Human Services, Washington, DC, 1996, and *Developing objectives for healthy people 2010,* Washington, DC, 1997, U.S. Department of Health and Human Services, Office of Disease Prevention and Health Promotion.

Chapter 2: p. 21 (Star Box), From Depression is a sign of illness, not a sign of weakness, *Ball State University Campus Update,* Dec 12, 1988, p. 1; **p. 29 (Figure 2-2),** "Hierarchy of Needs" from Motivation and Personality, 3rd ed., by Abraham H. Maslow. Revised by Robert Frager, James Fadiman, Cynthia McReynolds, and Ruth Cox. Copyright 1954, © 1987, Harper and Row, Publishers, Inc. Copyright © 1970 by Abraham H. Maslow. Reprinted by permission of HarperCollins Publishers Inc.; **p. 33 (Personal Assessment),** From Study Guide and Personal Explorations for *Psychology applied to modern life; adjustment in the 80s,* by Wayne Weiten. Copyright © 1983 by Wadsworth, Inc. Reprinted by permission of Brooks/Cole Publishing, Pacific Grove, CA 93950; **p. 35 (Figure),** Yankelovich Partners for Lutheran Brotherhood.

Chapter 3: p. 40 (Figure 3-1), Data from US Department of Labor; **p. 42 (Figure 3-2),** Data from The Wirthlin Report; **p. 53 (Personal Assessment),** Modified from Holmes TH, Rahe RH: The social adjustment rating scale, *Journal of Psychosomatic Research* 11:213-218, 1967; **p. 55 (Personal Assessment),** Source: Self-Development Center, A service of the Counseling and Students Development Center, George Mason University: *Time Management Tips.*

Chapter 4: p. 63 (Figure 4-1), Data from The Wirthlin Report; **pp. 66, 71 (Star Boxes),** From Prentice WE: *Fitness for college and life,* ed 4, St. Louis, 1994, Mosby; **pp. 74-75 (Star Box),** Copyright 1986, *USA Today,* excerpted with permission, art by Donald O'Connor; **p. 78 (Figure 4-2),** Copyright 1984, *USA Today,* excerpted with permission, art by Donald O'Connor; **p. 79 (Table 4-1),** From Prentice WE: *Fitness for college and life,* ed 5, St. Louis, 1997, McGraw-Hill; **pp. 83-84 (Personal Assessment),** Data from the National Fitness Foundation.

Chapter 5: p. 96 (Figure 5-1), US Department of Agriculture/US Department of Health and Human Services, August, 1992; **p. 97 (Figure 5-2),** US Department of Agriculture; **p. 98 (Table 5-1),** From Wardlaw G, Insel P: *Perspectives in nutrition,* ed 3, St. Louis, 1996, Mosby; **p. 99 (Table 5-2),** Modified from Food and Nutrition Board, National Research Council: *Recommended dietary allowances,* ed 10, Washington, DC, 11989, National Academy of Sciences; **pp. 100-101 (Table 5-3),** Modified from Hegarty V: *Decisions in nutrition,* St. Louis, 1988, Mosby, 132-133; **p. 104 (Figure 5-3),** Source: Food and Drug Administration, and Wardlaw G, Insel P: *Perspectives in nutrition,* ed 3, St. Louis, 1996, Mosby; **p. 106 (Table 5-4),** US Department of Health and Human Services, Public Health Service: *The Surgeon General's report on nutrition and health,* Washington, DC, 1988, US Government Printing Office; **p. 106 (Star Box),** From *Nutrition and your health: dietary guidelines for Americans,* ed 4, 1995, USDA, Home & Garden Bulletin no. 232; **p. 107 (Figure 5-4),** National Dairy Council, Rosemont, IL; **p. 108 (Figure 5-5),** National Dairy Council, Rosemont, IL; **pp. 113-114 (Personal Assessment),** From *Nutrition for a healthy life,* courtesy of March Leeds.

Chapter 6: p. 121 (Star Box), Data from C. Everett Koop Foundation, American Diabetes Association; **p. 121 (Table 6-1),** Reprinted with permission of Metropolitan Life Insurance Company; **p. 123 (Figure 6-1),** Modified from George A. Bray; **p. 129 (Table 6-3),** Based on data from Bannister EW, Brown SR: The relative energy requirements of physical activity. In HB Falls, editor: *Exercise physiology,* New York, 1968, Academic Press Inc.; Howley ET, Glover ME: The caloric costs of running and walking a mile for men and women, *Medicine and Science in Sports* 6:235, 1984; and Passmore R, Durnin JVGA: Human energy expenditure, *Physiological Reviews* 35:801, 1955; **p. 132 (Figure 6-4),** Opinion Research Corporation for *Simply Lite Foods;* **pp. 133-134 (Table 6-4),** Modified from Guthrie H: *Introductory nutrition,* ed 7, St. Louis, 1989, Mosby, pp. 226-227; **p. 143 (Personal Assessment),** Data from Wardlaw GM, Kessel M: *Perspectives in nutrition,* ed 5, New York, 2002, McGraw-Hill, p. 540; **p. 145 (Personal Assessment),** Modified from Foreyt J, Goodrick GK: *Living without dieting,* Houston: Harrison Publishing.

Chapter 7: p. 159 (Table 7-1), Modified from Muncie Star © 1987. Reprinted with permission; **p. 161 (Figure 7-2),** Source: American Management Association Survey; **p. 169 (Personal Assessment),** US Department of Education, *A Parents' Guide to Prevention.*

Chapter 8: p. 178 (Figure 8-1), Data from Core Institute: *2000 Statistics on alcohol and other drug use on American campuses,* Center for Alcohol and Other Drug Studies, Student Health Programs, Southern Illinois University at Carbondale, 2000; **p. 178 (Table 8-1),** US Department of Health and Human Services: Alcohol and health: fourth special report to the US Congress, Washington, DC, 1981, DHS Pub No ADM 81-1080; **p. 181 (Figure 8-2),** Data from Core Institute: *2000 Statistics on alcohol and other drug use on American campuses,* Center for Alcohol and Other Drug Studies, Student Health Programs, Southern Illinois University at Carbondale, 2000; **p. 181 (Table 8-2),** US Department of Transportation, National Highway Safety Administration: Modified from *Alcohol and the impaired driver* (AMA); **p. 185 (Figure 8-3),** From Wardlaw G, Insel P: *Perspectives in nutrition,* ed 3, St. Louis, 1996, Mosby; **p. 192 (Changing for the Better),** Modified from brochure of the Indiana Alcohol Countermeasure Program; **p. 194 (Star Box),** Modified from Woititz JG: *Adult children of alcoholics,* Pompano Beach, FL, 1983, Health Communications, Inc. In Pinger R, Payne W, Hahn D, Hahn E: *Drugs: issues for today,* St. Louis, 1991, Mosby; **p. 199 (Personal Assessment),** From *Are You Troubled by Someone's Drinking?,* 1980, by Al-Anon Family Group Headquarters, Inc. Reprinted by permission of Al-Anon Family Group Headquarters, Inc.

Chapter 9: p. 204 (Figure 9-1), Centers for Disease Control and Prevention.

Chapter 10: p. 230 (Figure 10-1 and Table 10-1), Data from American Heart Association: 2001 *Heart and stroke statistical update,* 2000, The Association; **p. 236 (Figure 10-3),** Reproduced with permission, © 1988, American Heart Association: Heart Facts; **p. 238 (Table 10-2),** Report of the Expert Panel on Detection, Evaluation and Treatment of High Blood Cholesterol in Adults, US Department of Health and Human Services (DHS: NIH Pub No 89-2925), 1989, Washington, DC, US Government Printing Office; **p. 239 (Figure 10-4),** 1990 Heart Facts, art by Donald O'Connor; **p. 244 (Star Box),** Data from American Heart Association; **pp. 247-248 (Personal Assessment),** From Howard E: *Health Risks,* Tucson, 1985, Body Press.

Chapter 11: p. 254 (Figure 11-1), Data from National Cancer Institute: *Horizons of cancer research,* NIH Pub No 89-3011, © 1989; **p. 255 (Figure 11-2),** Reprinted with permission of the American Cancer Society; **pp. 256, 258, 261 (Changing for the Better)** and **p. 263 (Star Box),** Reprinted with permission of the American Cancer Society; **p. 262 (Changing for the Better),** Courtesy of the American Academy of Dermatology; **pp. 275-276 (Personal Assessment),** Reprinted with permission of the American Cancer Society.

Chapter 12: p. 282 (Table 12-1), Data from Centers for Disease Control and Prevention and American Academy of Pediatrics; **p. 289 (Table 12-2),** Courtesy of the National Institute of Allergy and Infectious Diseases; **p. 298 (Figure 12-4),** Report on the Global HIV/AIDS Epidemic: Global summary of the HIV/AIDS epidemic, end 1999, UNAIDS, 2000; **p. 298 (Figure 12-5),** Source: Michael RT, Gagnon JH, Laumann EO, Kolata G: *Sex in America: A Definitive Study;* **p. 307 (Personal Assessment),** Centers for Disease Control and Prevention.

Chapter 13: p. 333 (Changing for the Better), Adapted from Haas K, Haas A: *Understanding sexuality,* ed 3, St. Louis, 1993, Mosby; **p. 341 (Personal Assessment),** Modified from *USA Today.*

Chapter 14: p. 349 (Table 14-1), Modified from Lisken L, et al: Youth in the 1980s: social and health concerns, Population Reports, Series M, No. 9, Population Information Program, Johns Hopkins University, November-December 1985; **p. 363 (Figure 14-8),** *Abortion Laws,* Allen Guttmacher Institute (website [www.usa.org] accessed Sept. 18, 2001); **p. 373 (Personal Assessment),** From Haas K, Haas A: *Understanding sexuality,* ed 3, St. Louis, 1993, Mosby.

Chapter 15: p. 381 (Figure 15-1), Cyber Dialogue/ Find SVP; **p. 386 (Changing for the Better),** Source: Pell AR: *Making the Most of Medicare,* DCI Publishing, 1990, in *in-synch,* Erie, PA, Spring, 1994, Erie Insurance.

Chapter 16: p. 408 (Figure 16-1), Courtesy of the National Committee to Prevent Child Abuse, Chicago, IL; **p. 415 (Changing for the Better),** From the American College Health Association; **p. 418 (Figure 16-2),** Data from National Highway Traffic Safety Administration: *Traffic Safety Facts 1999,* December 2000 (DOT-HS-B09-100), p. 98; **p. 419 (Changing for the Better),** Adapted from Pynoos J, Cohen E: *Creative ideas for a safe and livable home,* Washington, DC, American Association of Retired Persons, 1992; and Van Tassel D: *Home, safe home,* St. Louis, 1996, GenCare Health Systems.

Chapter 17: p. 432 (Star Box), Courtesy of Partnership for Caring, Inc.; **p. 441 (Figure 17-2),** The National Kidney Foundation Uniform Donor Card is reprinted with permission from the National Kidney Foundation, Inc. Copyright 2000, New York, NY.

PHOTO CREDITS

Photos by FPG International unless otherwise noted.

Chapter 4: pp. 75, 83-84, 85, Stewart Halperin.

Chapter 8: p. 186 (Figure 8-4), George Steinmetz; **p. 186 (lower),** Mothers Against Drunk Driving.

Chapter 9: pp. 212 (lower)-213, Custom Medical.

Chapter 11: p. 263, From Thibodeau G, Patton K: *Anatomy & physiology,* ed 3, St. Louis, 1996, Mosby.

Chapter 13: p. 344, Stewart Halperin.

Chapter 14: p. 352, Courtesy of Ortho Pharmaceutical Corp.; **p. 353 (left),** Courtesy of Apothocus, Inc.; **p. 353 (right),** Stewart Halperin; **p. 354,** Linsley Photographics; **pp. 355, 356,** Laura J. Edwards; **p. 357 (left),** Stewart Halperin; **p. 357 (right),** Courtesy of the Alza Corporation; **p. 359,** Courtesy of Wyeth-Ayerst Laboratories; **p. 364,** Photo Researchers; **p. 365,** Science Photo Library/Photo Researchers.

Chapter 16: p. 405, Associated Press.

Chapter 17: p. 430, The Gamma Liaison Network; **p. 438,** Associated Press.

Index

Q

R

S